Methods in Pharmacology and Toxicology

Series Editor
Y. James Kang

For further volumes:
http://www.springer.com/series/7653

The Handbook of Metabolomics

Edited by

Teresa Whei-Mei Fan and Richard M. Higashi

Department of Chemistry, Center for Regulatory and Environmental Analytical Metabolomics (CREAM), and James Graham Brown Cancer Center, University of Louisville, Louisville, KY, USA

Andrew N. Lane

Departments of Medicine and Chemistry, Center for Regulatory and Environmental Analytical Metabolomics (CREAM), and James Graham Brown Cancer Center, University of Louisville, Louisville, KY, USA

Humana Press

Editors
Teresa Whei-Mei Fan
Department of Chemistry
Center for Regulatory and Environmental
Analytical Metabolomics (CREAM),
and James Graham Brown Cancer Center
University of Louisville
Louisville, KY, USA

Andrew N. Lane
Departments of Medicine and Chemistry
Center for Regulatory and Environmental
Analytical Metabolomics (CREAM),
and James Graham Brown Cancer Center
University of Louisville
Louisville, KY, USA

Richard M. Higashi
Department of Chemistry
Center for Regulatory and Environmental
Analytical Metabolomics (CREAM),
and James Graham Brown Cancer Center
University of Louisville
Louisville, KY, USA

ISSN 1557-2153 ISSN 1940-6053 (electronic)
ISBN 978-1-4939-6043-9 ISBN 978-1-61779-618-0 (eBook)
DOI 10.1007/978-1-61779-618-0
Springer New York Heidelberg Dordrecht London

Printed on acid-free paper

Humana Press is a brand of Springer
Springer is part of Springer Science+Business Media (www.springer.com)

Preface

Metabolomics is a rapidly expanding field that provides a link between functional biology (phenotypes) and the inner workings of cells in tissues or whole organisms. The technologies of metabolomics are being taken up by academic researchers, increasingly in the medical field, and especially by the biotech and pharmaceutical companies.

The goal of the handbook is to provide readers with the current state of metabolomic development and the integration of metabolomics with transcriptomics and proteomics. These aspects are illustrated by research efforts related to toxicology and pharmacology.

The 14 contributions deal with a critical discussion of topics ranging from sample preparation and considerations (both laboratory and clinical), analytical methodologies for metabolite and isotopomer profiling, to metabolic flux modeling, database construction, and integration of "omics" for systems biochemical understanding. The handbook includes extensive bibliographies and resources.

Louisville, KY, USA

Teresa Whei-Mei Fan
Andrew N. Lane
Richard M. Higashi

Contents

Contributors

MICHAEL BOUSAMRA II • *Department of Surgery, University of Louisville, Louisville, KY, USA*
MARTA CASCANTE • *Department of Biochemistry and Molecular Biology, Associated Unit to CSIC, Institute of Biomedicine of University of Barcelona (IBUB) and IDIBAPS (Institut d'Investigacions Biomèdiques August Pi i Sunyer), Barcelona, Spain*
TERESA CASSEL • *Center for Regulatory and Environmental Analytical Metabolomics (CREAM), University of Louisville, Louisville, KY, USA*
JAMIE DAY • *James Graham Brown Cancer Center, University of Louisville, Louisville, KY, USA*
BRIAN J. DEWAR • *Department of Pharmacology, University of North Carolina School of Medicine, Chapel Hill, NC, USA*
TIMOTHY C. ELSTON • *Department of Pharmacology, University of North Carolina School of Medicine, Chapel Hill, NC, USA*
TERESA WHEI-MEI FAN • *Department of Chemistry, Center for Regulatory and Environmental Analytical Metabolomics (CREAM), and James Graham Brown Cancer Center, University of Louisville, Louisville, KY, USA*
OLEG FAVOROV • *Department of Biomedical Engineering, University of North Carolina School of Medicine, Chapel Hill, NC, USA*
LEE M. GRAVES • *Department of Pharmacology, University of North Carolina School of Medicine, Chapel Hill, NC, USA*
ADRIAN D. HEGEMAN • *Department of Horticultural Science, University of Minnesota, St. Paul, MN, USA*
ROB HENRY • *Thermo Fisher Scientific, Bremen, Germany*
RICHARD M. HIGASHI • *Department of Chemistry, Center for Regulatory and Environmental Analytical Metabolomics (CREAM), and James Graham Brown Cancer Center, University of Louisville, Louisville, KY, USA*
EKHSON HOLMUHAMEDOV • *Department of Cell and Molecular Biology, University of North Carolina School of Medicine, Chapel Hill, NC, USA*
REX E. JEFFRIES • *Department of Biomedical Engineering, University of North Carolina School of Medicine, Chapel Hill, NC, USA*
MALIACKAL POULO JOY • *Department of Pharmacology, University of North Carolina School of Medicine, Chapel Hill, NC, USA*
GOETZ KLOECKER • *Department of Medicine and James Graham Brown Cancer Center, University of Louisville, Louisville, KY, USA*
JOHN KURHANEWICZ • *Departments of Radiology and Pharmaceutical Chemistry, University of California at San Francisco, San Francisco, CA, USA*
ANDREW N. LANE • *Departments of Medicine and Chemistry, Center for Regulatory and Environmental Analytical Metabolomics (CREAM), and James Graham Brown Cancer Center, University of Louisville, Louisville, KY, USA*

IAN A. LEWIS • *Department of Biochemistry, University of Wisconsin-Madison, Madison, WI, USA*
JEFFREY M. MACDONALD • *Department of Biomedical Engineering, University of North Carolina School of Medicine, Chapel Hill, NC, USA*
JOHN L. MARKLEY • *Department of Biochemistry, University of Wisconsin-Madison, Madison, WI, USA*
DONALD M. MILLER • *Department of Medicine, Center for Regulatory and Environmental Analytical Metabolomics (CREAM), and James Graham Brown Cancer Center, University of Louisville, Louisville, KY, USA*
PETER PEDIATITAKIS • *Department of Biomedical Engineering, University of North Carolina School of Medicine, Chapel Hill, NC, USA*
KAYVAN RAHIMI-KESHARI • *Department of Biomedical Engineering, University of North Carolina School of Medicine, Chapel Hill, NC, USA*
ANTONIO RAMOS-MONTOYA • *Department of Biochemistry and Molecular Biology, Associated Unit to CSIC, Institute of Biomedicine of University of Barcelona (IBUB) and IDIBAPS (Institut d'Investigacions Biomèdiques August Pi i Sunyer), Barcelona, Spain*
PEDRO ROMERO • *School of Informatics, Indiana University-Purdue University, Indianapolis, IN, USA; Center for Computational Biology and Bioinformatics, Indiana University School of Medicine, Indianapolis, IN, USA*
VITALY SELIVANOV • *Department of Biochemistry and Molecular Biology, Associated Unit to CSIC, Institute of Biomedicine of University of Barcelona (IBUB) and IDIBAPS (Institut d'Investigacions Biomèdiques August Pi i Sunyer), Barcelona, Spain*
MICHAEL R. SHORTREED • *Department of Chemistry, University of Wisconsin-Madison, Madison, WI, USA*
ABIGAIL TODD • *Department of Pharmacology, University of North Carolina School of Medicine, Chapel Hill, NC, USA*
DANIEL VIGNERON • *Departments of Radiology and Pharmaceutical Chemistry, University of California at San Francisco, San Francisco, CA, USA*
JASON H. WINNIKE • *Department of Biomedical Engineering, University of North Carolina School of Medicine, Chapel Hill, NC, USA*
JUSTYNA WOLAK • *Department of Biomedical Engineering, University of North Carolina School of Medicine, Chapel Hill, NC, USA*
TAE HOON YANG • *Genomatica, Inc., San Diego, CA, USA*
M. CECILIA YAPPERT • *Department of Chemistry, University of Louisville, Louisville, KY, USA*

Chapter 1

Introduction to Metabolomics

Teresa Whei-Mei Fan, Andrew N. Lane, and Richard M. Higashi

Abstract

We provide an overview of metabolomics in its current practices, including sample processing, major techniques, example applications, and useful resources to the readership, as described in detail in the various chapters of the handbook. In our view, metabolomics can be defined as "a systematic interrogation of the metabolome in terms of metabolite concentration, structure, and transformation pathways." We emphasize the use of stable isotope tracing methodologies both in vitro and in vivo. We further provide a brief introduction to some concepts of flux analyses at steady state and nonsteady state.

Key words: Stable isotope editing, Metabolic pathways, Flux analysis

1. Overview

In this handbook, we aim to provide an overview of metabolomics in its current practices, including sample processing, major techniques, example applications, and useful resources to the readership. In our view, metabolomics can be defined as "a systematic interrogation of the metabolome in terms of metabolite concentration, structure, and transformation pathways." We have emphasized the use of stable isotope tracing methodologies both in vitro and in vivo. This is complementary to the metabonomics approaches that employ largely statistical analysis of very large numbers of biofluid samples, which have been extensively reviewed elsewhere (1–5). We also illustrate how stable isotope-resolved metabolomics (SIRM) can be integrated with transcriptomic and proteomic interrogations to achieve systems' biochemical level of understanding.

As the majority of the metabolomic studies deal with biofluids or tissue extracts, considerations of sample handling and extraction techniques are extremely important. T. W-M. Fan provided an overview and comparison of common approaches in Chap. 2. For experimentation with human subjects, specific protocols that are required by

Teresa Whei-Mei Fan et al. (eds.), *The Handbook of Metabolomics*, Methods in Pharmacology and Toxicology,
DOI 10.1007/978-1-61779-618-0_1,

Internal Review Board, HIPAA regulations, and ethical standards are described in Chap. 3 by M. Bousamra et al. This is followed by Chaps. 4–6 on the basics of organic mass spectrometry (MS) (R.M. Higashi), elemental and organometallic MS (R. Henry and T. Cassel), and NMR (A.N. Lane) for metabolomic analyses. In Chap. 7, Lewis et al. described the effort on NMR database for metabolites, approaches to automated NMR assignment, and some novel NMR and MS approaches to metabolomic studies. Although there are certainly many other techniques that are useful for probing specific questions in metabolic studies, the extremely information-rich NMR and MS technologies are central to metabolomic investigations due to their enormous metabolite coverage. Equally valuable is the ability of the two techniques to provide detailed stable isotopic-labeled patterns of metabolites (isotopomers and isotopologues, see Chaps. 4 and 6) that cannot be readily acquired with any other techniques.

This knowledge, together with the quantitative information obtainable by NMR and MS, is essential to metabolic network modeling, as described in Chaps. 8–10 of two different approaches, i.e., steady-state and nonsteady-state flux analysis. For the steady-state approach, T.H. Yang (Chap. 8) described the principles of metabolic flux analysis, and M.P. Joy et al. (Chap. 9) gave a brief introduction to the metabolic control analysis (MCA). The latter was utilized by M. Cascante et al. in a nonsteady state approach to metabolic flux modeling (Chap. 10). These chapters also discussed the needs for stable isotope tracing for flux modeling, which can be performed in vitro in defined cell cultures or in vivo in live organisms, including human subjects.

Chapter 11 by Wolak et al. described noninvasive NMR approaches to fluxomics, with a section on the emerging technology of dynamic nuclear polarization (DNP) that gives a much-needed boost to in vivo NMR sensitivity. Although MS is not suited for in vivo applications, emerging research on utilizing MS for in situ imaging of phospholipids is described by M. C. Yappert in Chap. 12, along with combining MS and ^{31}P NMR techniques for phospholipid analysis.

To reconstruct metabolic networks based on the limited data typically acquired from metabolomic analysis, it is essential to have robust and comprehensive metabolic databases. In Chap. 13, P. Romero described the establishment of an in silico human metabolic database based on annotated human genomic sequence information. Finally, T. W-M. Fan in Chap. 14 illustrates how metabolomic data can be synergistically integrated with transcriptomic data (e.g., metabolomics-edited transcriptomic analysis or META) and target protein analysis for discerning perturbations in molecular regulation in response to stress.

Although not explicitly discussed in all chapters, it is imperative to recognize the importance of "precision" and "accuracy" of metabolomic analysis. The large number of metabolites and their enriched isotopomers and isotopologues in metabolomic studies present a difficult challenge for precise quantification and accurate determination of biological trend. Precision of analysis can be calculated from replication of individual samples (also called technical replicates) (see Chap. 7) while biological accuracy and variability can be assessed from sufficient replications of biological experiments.

In view of the complexity of living organisms and the plethora of environmental factors that they interact with, the technologies and approaches introduced in this handbook should greatly accelerate our ability to decipher the many "black boxes" common to life sciences. Although a useful stand-alone, the metabolomic approach maximizes its value by serving as the functional link in the "omics" world to achieve a systems biochemical level of understanding. Such utility is generally applicable in any biological system, including human subjects, which has been demonstrated recently in both animals (6, 7) and human lung cancer patient studies (8–10).

If metabolomics is defined as the technologies for describing the metabolic state of a cell, organ, or organism and how the metabolic state evolves in time owing to some external perturbation, then it is necessary to be able to measure accurately and reliably the time dependence of concentrations of a large number of metabolites. However, intracellular metabolic concentrations generally do not vary much (an example of homeostasis). Therefore, in order to understand how individual interacting pathways within a network are affected by external perturbation, it is essential to be able to measure the flow of individual atoms from a source molecule, such as labeled glucose, through the metabolic network, and preferably obtain actual flux information. This is a challenging problem, and can be achieved only by using tracer technologies. As described above, there are different solutions to tracer technologies, depending on whether the tracer approaches a steady state or whether the full time dependence is taken into account, as described in the Chaps. 8–10 and as outlined below.

2. Fluxes: Steady-State and Nonsteady-State Kinetics

Consider a simple reaction A⇔B

The rate in the forward direction $db/dt = k_1 a$, and in the reverse direction $da/dt = k_{-1} b$

The net rate or flux is $J = db/dt - da/dt = k_1 a - k_{-1} b$

This can be rewritten as $J = k_1 a(1 - k_{-1} b / k_1 a)$

As k_{-1}/k_1 is $1/K$, and b/a is the activity ratio, Γ, the flux is simply

$$J = k_1 a(1 - \Gamma / K)$$

Thus, if $\Gamma/K < 1$, the reaction proceeds toward B, whereas if it is >1 the flux is negative and the reaction goes from B to A. The flux in this case will be time dependent because the ratio of b to a will change until it reaches the equilibrium value at which point the flux is zero.

At equilibrium, the concentrations do not change on average (all considerations refer to bulk ensemble-averaged events; at very low amounts of materials, fluctuations become statistically relevant, and can be detected by appropriate techniques). Furthermore, the flux is zero. Thus, equilibrium is a special case of a more general condition, the steady state, in which concentrations are constant, but the flux is nonzero. A nonequilibrium steady state is at a higher energy, and is less stable to perturbation than an equilibrium steady state.

Consider a simple pathway:

$$\overset{k_1}{\underset{k_{-1}}{S \Leftrightarrow}} \overset{k_2}{X \Leftrightarrow} P$$

S represents a source molecule, which for simplicity is assumed to be held constant, and P the pathway product that is removed constantly (rendering this segment effectively irreversible). X is an intermediate.

The flux, J, through the pathway is:

$$J = k_2 x$$

Lower case denotes concentration of the species in upper case

$$dx/dt = k_1 s - (k_{-1} + k_2)x \quad (1)$$

The exact solutions to (1) are given by:

$$x(t) = x(0) + k_1 s[1 - \exp(-k_{-1} + k_2)t]/(k_{-1} + k_2) \quad (2)$$

$$p(t) = p(0) + k_1 k_2 s[t - (1 - \exp(-k_{-1} + k_2)t)/(k_{-1} + k_2)]/(k_{-1} + k_2) \quad (3)$$

After an initial period determined by $k_{-1} + k_2$, the concentration of x reaches a steady state, i.e., its concentration becomes constant, and $dx/dt = 0$.

Once this condition is reached, the steady state concentration of x is simply

$$x_{ss} = k_1 s/(k_{-1} + k_2)$$

Hence,

$$J = k_1 k_2 s/(k_{-1} + k_2) \quad (4)$$

Under these circumstances, there are three unknowns, and only two experimentally accessible parameters, namely, x_{ss} and $p(t)$. The ratio of J to x_{ss} gives k_2, but k_1 and k_{-2} are undetermined.

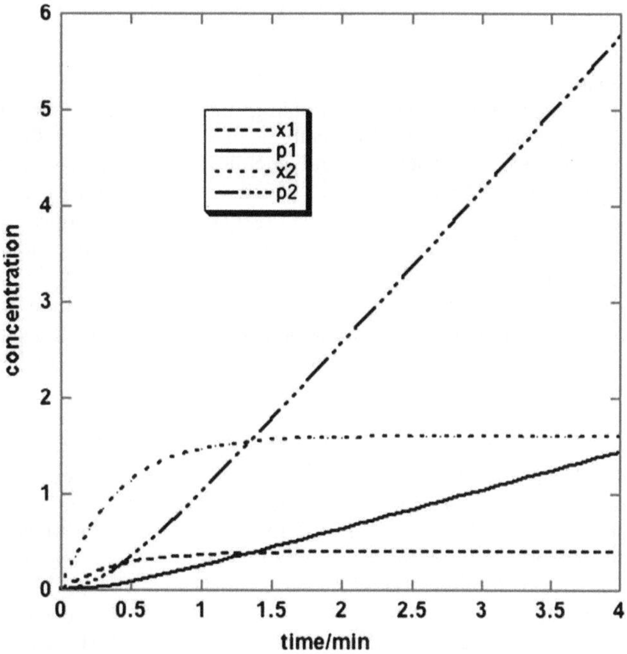

Fig. 1. Approach to steady state for tracers: $k_1 = 1$ mM^{-1} min^{-1}; $k_{-1} = 0.5$ mM^{-1}; and $k_2 = 2$ min^{-1}. $S = 1$ and 4 mM. The lag time is defined as the time at which the linear portion extrapolates back to $p = 0$. This time is equal to $1/(k_{-1} + k_2)$ in this model.

Under nonsteady state conditions, the sum $k_{-1} + k_2$ can also be determined either from the approach of x to the steady state or from the lag period in the production of P, as shown in Fig. 1. The point is that under steady state conditions the information content is lower than under nonsteady state conditions. If a bolus of a tracer is added to a system in a biochemical steady state, the label can be followed as a function of time from a low initial value and thus from the time course, permitting extraction of rate parameters that are otherwise inaccessible. The cost is that considerably greater sophistication is needed for the modeling and data analysis.

There are many statistical approaches to analyzing metabolomics (11, 12) data, where steady states are assumed and tracers are not used. These typically involve variants on cluster analyses analogous to the techniques widely used in gene array data sets and PCA or partial least squares approaches. These technologies are not covered here, but there are several general reviews of these techniques as applied to metabolomics data (13, 14).

Standardization for data acquisition and databasing is a significant issue in the metabolomics field and others. Several initiatives for standards of data reporting have appeared (15–18), and general resources can be found at http://msi-workgroups.sourceforge.net/.

References

1. Harrigan GG, Brackett DJ, Boros LG (2005) Medicinal chemistry, metabolic profiling and drug target discovery: a role for metabolic profiling in reverse pharmacology and chemical genetics. Mini Rev Med Chem 5(1):13–20
2. Whitfield PD, German AJ, Noble PJM (2004) Metabolomics: an emerging post-genomic tool for nutrition. Br J Nutr 92(4):549–55
3. Kaddurah-Daouk R, Kristal BS, Weinshilboum RM (2008) Metabolomics: a global biochemical approach to drug response and disease. Annu Rev Pharmacol Toxicol 48:653–683
4. Nicholson J (2005) Metabonomics and global systems biology approaches to molecular diagnostics. Drug Metab Rev 37:10–10
5. Bollard ME, Stanley EG, Lindon JC, Nicholson JK, Holmes E (2005) NMR-based metabonomic approaches for evaluating physiological influences on biofluid composition. NMR Biomed 18(3):143–62
6. Fan TW-M, Lane AN, Higashi RM, Yan J (2011) Stable isotope resolved metabolomics of lung cancer in a SCID mouse model. Metabolomics 7:257–69
7. Beger RD, Hansen DK, Schnackenberg LK, Cross BM, Fatollahi JJ, Lagunero FT, Sarnyai Z, Boros LG (2009) Single valproic acid treatment inhibits glycogen and RNA ribose turnover while disrupting glucose-derived cholesterol synthesis in liver as revealed by the [U-^{13}C6]-D-glucose tracer in mice. Metabolomics 5:336–45
8. Fan TW-M, Lane AN, Higashi RM, Bousamra M, Kloecker G, Miller DM (2009) Erlotinib-sensitive and resistant lung tumors show radically different metabolic profiles. Exp Mol Pathol 87:83–6
9. Fan TW, Lane AN, Higashi RM, Farag MA, Gao H, Bousamra M, Miller DM (2009) Altered regulation of metabolic pathways in human lung cancer discerned by ^{13}C stable isotope-resolved metabolomics (SIRM). Mol Cancer 8:41
10. Lane AN, Fan TW-M, Bousamra M II, Higashi RM, Yan J, Miller DM (2011) Clinical applications of stable isotope-resolved metabolomics (SIRM) in non-small cell lung cancer. Omics 15:173–82
11. Dieterle F, Ross A, Schlotterbeck G, Senn H (2006) Metabolite projection analysis for fast identification of metabolites in metabonomics. Application in an amiodarone study. Anal Chem 78(11):3551–61
12. Kettaneh N, Berglund A, Wold S (2005) PCA and PLS with very large data sets. Comput Stat Data Anal 48(1):69–85
13. Trygg J, Holmes E, Lundstedt T (2007) Chemometrics in metabonomics. J Proteome Res 6 (2):469–79
14. Vaidyanathan S, Harrigan GG, Goodacre R (2005) Metabolome analyses: strategies for systems biology. Springer, Boston
15. Sumner LW, Amberg A, Barrett D, Beger R, Beale MH, Daykin C, Fan TW-M, Fiehn O, Goodacre R, Griffin JL, Hardy N, Higashi RM, Kopka J, Lindon JC, Lane AN, Marriott P, Nicholls AW, Reily MD, Viant M (2007) Proposed minimum reporting standards for chemical analysis. Metabolomics 3:211–21
16. Castle AL, Fiehn O, Kaddurah-Daouk R, Lindon JC (2006) Metabolomics Standards Workshop and the development of international standards for reporting metabolomics experimental results. Brief Bioinform 7(2):159–65
17. Sansone SA, Fan T, Goodacre R, Griffin JL, Hardy NW, Kaddurah-Daouk R, Kristal BS, Lindon J, Mendes P, Morrison N, Nikolau B, Robertson D, Sumner LW, Taylor C, van der Werf M, van Ommen B, Fiehn O (2007) The metabolomics standards initiative. Nat Biotechnol 25(8):844–8
18. Goodacre R, Broadhurst D, Smilde AK, Kristal BS, Baker JD, Beger R, Bessant C, Connor S, Calmani G, Craig A, Ebbels T, Kell DB, Manetti C, Newton J, Paternostro G, Somorjai R, Sjostrom M, Trygg J, Wulfert F (2007) Proposed minimum reporting standards for data analysis in metabolomics. Metabolomics 3(3):231–41

Chapter 2

Considerations of Sample Preparation for Metabolomics Investigation

Teresa Whei-Mei Fan

Abstract

Sample preparation is the gateway to metabolomic analysis, the importance of which cannot be overemphasized. There are general rules of thumb for sample preparation that help maximize sample integrity and metabolite recovery. The wide range of variations in metabolite functional groups, polarity, sizes, and stability precludes the use of a single extraction method in metabolomic studies. Common extraction methods for polar metabolites that utilize trichloroacetic acid or aqueous acetonitrile are suitable for both nuclear magnetic resonance (NMR) and mass spectrometry (MS) analysis while others that use chloroform/methanol/water partition or boiling water may not. Control of extract pH is crucial for consistent NMR assignments and chemical derivatization-linked MS analysis. Sequential polar and lipid extractions reduce sample size requirement and provide a better coverage for direct-infusion MS analysis of lipids, possibly by removing interfering salts. Cleanup of sample extracts, such as removal of fine particles or interfering cations, is often necessary but should be limited to reduce loss of metabolites.

Key words: NMR, GC-MS, FT-ICR-MS, Trichloroacetic acid, Perchloric acid, Chloroform/ methanol/water, Acetonitrile, Boiling water, Mouse liver, Human lung

1. Introduction

Sample preparation is a crucial factor in metabolomic research, although this aspect is generally not sufficiently discussed in many metabolomic publications. The quality of the analytical output and subsequent data analysis are critically dependent on the sample history and preparation methods in the first place. The nature of metabolomic analyses demands the maintenance of the integrity of a large number of metabolites ranging widely in concentrations and chemical properties. This is not a trivial task and may have considerations specific to the sample types and sizes, range of analytes, instrument platforms, etc. However, there are general

Teresa Whei-Mei Fan et al. (eds.), *The Handbook of Metabolomics*, Methods in Pharmacology and Toxicology, DOI 10.1007/978-1-61779-618-0_2, © Springer Science+Business Media New York 2012

guidelines on good practices of sample preparation. These include, but are not limited to, the following:

1. Maximize sample integrity during handling, storage, and processing
2. Optimize sample sharing for different applications
3. Optimize metabolite recovery both in terms of number and concentrations of metabolites as well as reproducibility
4. Versatility for analysis by different instrument platforms

In this chapter, the general practices are presented along with examples of specific considerations.

2. Sample Integrity

Immediately following the biological experimentation, sample integrity should be maintained to prevent unwanted metabolic changes. This is commonly achieved by flash freezing in liquid N_2 (−196°C) (1–3) or in acetone/dry ice bath (−78°C, http://en.wikipedia.org/wiki/Freezing_mixture) when liquid N_2 is not available. However, samples may need to be manipulated, e.g., washing or centrifugation to remove extraneous metabolites, before flash freezing. In such cases, samples should be kept cold (e.g., 4°C) and processed as soon as possible to minimize metabolic changes. Appendices 1 and 2, respectively, provide protocols for preparing mammalian cell cultures and blood plasma, which are routinely employed in our laboratory. For harvesting adherent mammalian cells, cells can be detached by treatment with trypsin, followed by centrifugation and PBS wash to remove medium components before flash freezing in liquid N_2. Both wet and dry weights of the cell mass can be readily measured for normalizing metabolite content. However, this method could introduce metabolic artifacts due to the trypsinization procedure.

To minimize this problem, cell metabolism can be quenched rapidly with cold methanol (e.g., (4)) or acetonitrile (Fan, published data), which can also be integrated with subsequent metabolite extraction using the water–chloroform partition method (cf. Appendix 1). Dilute acids (e.g., ice-cold 6% perchloric acid (PCA)) (5) have also been reported for quenching cellular metabolism, although acid-labile metabolites are lost with such method. An example comparison of the metabolite profiles of human adenocarcinoma A549 cell extracts obtained from the trypsinization and methanol quench methods is shown in Fig. 1. The ^{1}H nuclear magnetic resonance (NMR) profiles of the two cell extracts differed quantitatively for some of the resonances. Most notably, the peak ratio of phosphocholine (P-choline) resonance at 3.22 ppm to the

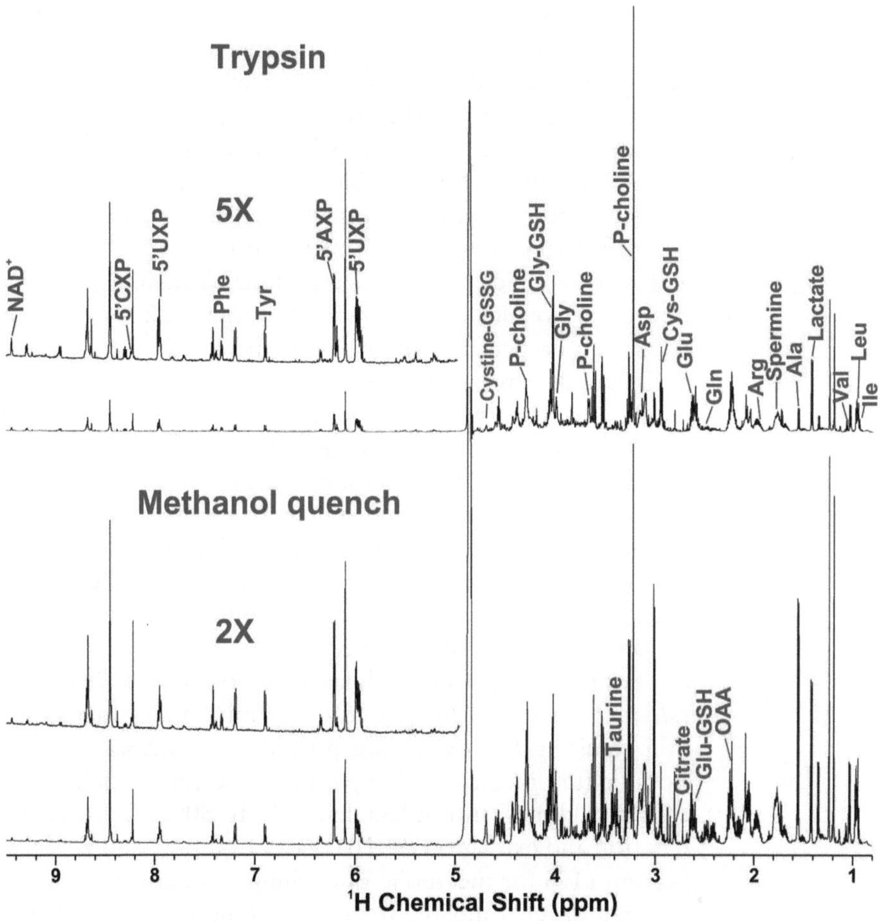

Fig. 1. Comparison of 1-D ^{1}H NMR profiles of human lung adenocarcinoma A549 cell extracts obtained from two cell harvest methods. The trypsinization and methanol quench methods were performed on the same batch of cells as described in Appendix 1. The ^{1}H NMR spectra of the two extracts were acquired at 14.1 T on a Varian Inova spectrometer system using an HCN triple-resonance cold probe. The spectral assignment was made as described in 16. The two spectral insets were overscaled relative to the largest resonance, i.e., the methyl resonance of phosphocholine (P-choline) at 3.22 ppm. *GSH* reduced glutathione; *OAA* oxaloacetate; *GSSG* oxidized glutathione; *UXP* uracil nucleotides; *AXP* adenine nucleotides; *CXP* cytosine nucleotides; *NAD* nicotine adenine dinucleotide.

rest of the resonances was much higher for the trypsinization than the methanol quench method. Marked differences in peak ratios were also evident for Ala, lactate, oxaloacetate (OAA), Gln, taurine, and NAD^{+}. These distinctions could reflect some metabolic alterations caused by the trypsin treatment. On the other hand, it is nontrivial to normalize metabolite content for the direct methanol quench method, as cell weights or counts are not practical to obtain, as for the trypsinization method. Without normalization, it would be difficult to compare metabolite content of cells harvested from individual culture vessels. This is because cell mass of each vessel varies significantly, even grown under the same condition. This problem is even more pronounced in the case of time course analysis, where cell mass is expected to change several folds over a 48-h period, depending on the cell doubling time. Thus, reliable normalization method for metabolite content needs to be carefully explored for the solvent quench method. These could include total protein or glycerol lipid analysis.

For biofluids other than blood (e.g., urine and bronchioalveolar fluids), they can be flash frozen and stored untreated at −20 to −80 °C before further processing (6, 7). Sodium azide (e.g., 0.1% w/v) can be added to biofluids to minimize bacterial contamination (7). When necessary, biofluids can be filtered through 0.22- or 0.45-μm filters to remove particulate matter before analysis. It is also important to avoid repeated freeze–thaw cycles of biofluids by flash freezing multiple aliquots. For tissues, small samples (e.g., ≤5 mm diameter) can be preserved by flash freezing in liquid N_2 directly after blotting excess blood or other biofluids. To ensure fast and even freezing, it is advisable to freeze large pieces of tissue samples by freeze clamping in liquid N_2 (cf. Appendix 3). We have observed a significant buildup of lactate by leaving resected human lung tissues on ice for 15 min as opposed to freeze clamping tissues from the same source without delay (T. W-M. Fan and A.N. Lane, unpublished result).

For microorganisms with fast metabolic rates such as *Escherichia coli*, metabolic quenching is crucial to minimizing metabolic distortion resulting from sampling procedures, such as separating cells from culture media (8). A typical method for quenching is placing cells in cold methanol at less than −20 to 50°C, followed by centrifugation and extraction (9, 10). Fast filtration (<30 s) (11) and fast heating (12) for metabolic quenching have also been introduced. A recent paper compared the extent of metabolite loss between the cold methanol quenching and fast filtration method, and concluded that the latter method coupled with a wash solution isotonic (e.g., 2.6% NaCl) with the culture medium was suitable for recovering intracellular metabolites from different bacteria (8). However, metabolite recovery for the popular methanol quenching method can be improved by including glycerol in the quenching solution (e.g., 60% (v/v) methanol/glycerol (13) or glycerol/NaCl at 13.5 g/L (v/v) 3/2 (14)). Regardless of the quenching method employed, leakage of intracellular metabolites into the culture medium may be inevitable (15, 16), which should be taken into account in subsequent data analysis and interpretation.

3. Sample Processing

3.1. Sample Homogenization

In order to maximize and reproduce extraction efficiency, it is imperative that tissue or cell masses are homogenized into fine particles (e.g., <10-μm size) while maintaining their biochemical integrity. Pulverization in liquid N_2 before metabolite extraction is a method of choice. This can be achieved by manual grinding with a mortar

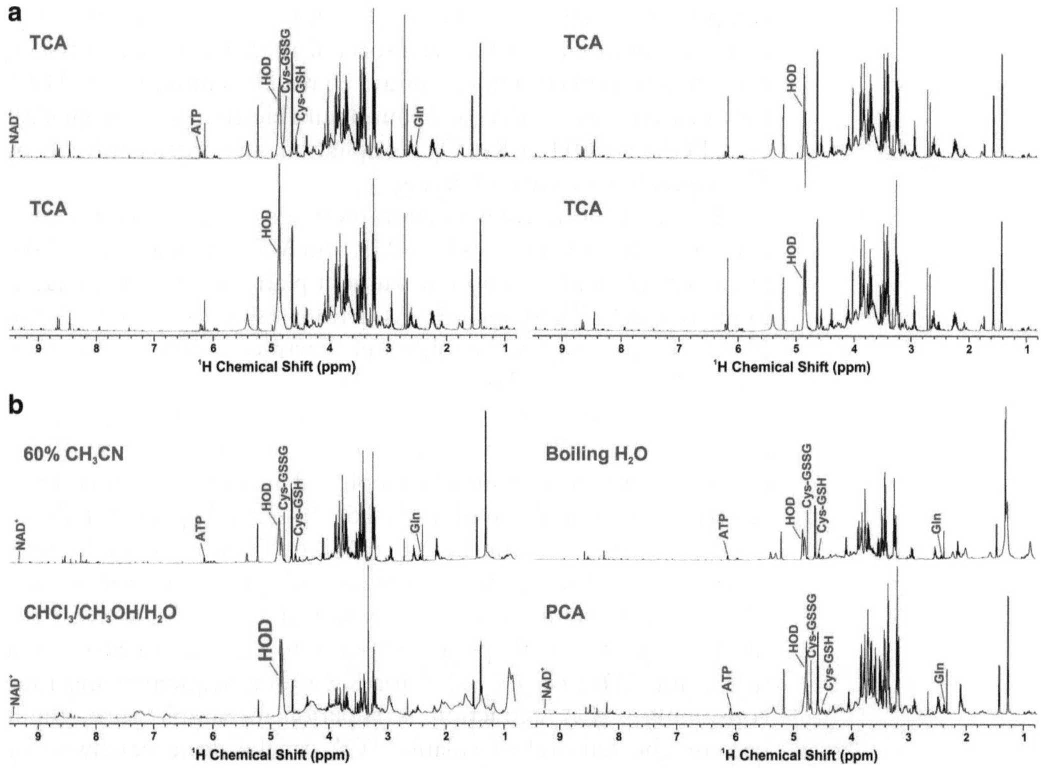

Fig. 2. 1-D ^{1}H NMR analysis of extracts of pulverized mouse liver using five different extraction methods. (**a**) illustrates four separate TCA extractions while (**b**) displays four other types of extractions (performed in duplicates) from the same batch of the liver sample (3.1–4.8 mg dry weight each). Reproducible NMR spectra were obtained from duplicate extraction for all five methods. The ^{1}H NMR spectra were acquired on a Varian Inova 600 MHz instrument (Varian, Inc., Palo Alto) using a PRESAT pulse sequence, where the HOD signal was saturated. Cys-GSH and Cys-GSSG are the cysteine residue of reduced (GSH) and oxidized (GSSG) glutathione.

and pestle equilibrated in liquid N_2 or by liquid N_2-compatible mechanical homogenizers (cf. Appendix 8). We have obtained consistent ^{1}H NMR profiles of mouse liver extracts by pulverizing tissues in a liquid N_2-based freezer mill (Retsch, Inc, Newtown, PA) (cf. Fig. 2). Tissue homogenization into frozen powder also allows the same sample to be shared for different analytical purposes, including analysis of metabolites, proteins, polysaccharides, and nucleic acids. Cell pellets can be homogenized with glass beads using a micro ball mill (e.g., MM200, Retsch, Inc.) directly in buffers or solvents that denature and precipitate proteins and other macromolecules which interfere with metabolite profiling by NMR (nuclear magnetic resonance) or MS (mass spectrometry) (see Sect. 2).

3.2. Sample Extraction

3.2.1. NMR Analysis

Extraction of Polar Metabolites

For extracting polar metabolites, various methods have been employed in the metabolomic literature (3, 8, 16–23). These methods invariably adopt acids, solvents, ultrafiltration, or heating to quench enzyme activities while minimizing the extraction of lipids and macromolecular components, such as proteins, nucleic acids, and complex carbohydrates. In addition, to avoid major spectral interferences or excess salts, extraction solvents or buffers should be readily removed, e.g., H_2O, trichloroacetic acid (TCA), and ammonium bicarbonate by lyophilization, PCA by KOH or K_2CO_3 precipitation, and organic solvents by N_2 evaporation or vacuum drying.

In this section, five extraction methods are discussed for their compatibility with analyses by NMR and MS, which are two of the most versatile and common instrument platforms used in metabolomic research. These include extractions using ice-cold TCA and PCA, chloroform/methanol/water partition, 60% acetonitrile, and boiling water (3, 16, 17, 24–30).

The TCA (e.g., 10% w/v, minimum extraction ratio v/w 40:1) and PCA (e.g., 5% w/v, minimum extraction ratio v/w 40/1) methods have been routinely employed in our laboratory for a variety of biological samples (3, 16, 25–29). Appendix 4 lists a detailed protocol for the TCA extraction. TCA or PCA efficiently denatures and precipitates proteins and other macromolecules while the extractant itself can be removed as stated above. As the titration of PCA with potassium salts to the equivalence point (pH 7 for KOH or pH 3–3.5 for K_2CO_3) is sequential and time consuming, TCA extraction is superior in sample throughput because the removal of volatile TCA can be done batchwise by lyophilization. However, some metabolites, such as glutamine, are more prone to degradation with this method due to a more acidic end point (pH 2–2.5) of lyophilized TCA extracts. Example ^{1}H NMR analysis of TCA and PCA extracts of pulverized mammalian tissues is shown in Fig. 2a, b, respectively. Also illustrated in Fig. 2a is the reproducibility of the TCA extraction when the same batch of pulverized sample was extracted four times by two different operators. These strong acid agents are well suited for NMR analysis as relatively flat spectral baselines are routinely obtained, and the spectra are free of all but the smallest peptides, which are themselves of interest to metabolomic studies (e.g., glutathione).

Although efficient in removing macromolecules and lipids, acid-based extraction methods are unsuitable for extracting acid-labile metabolites, such as fructose-2,6-bisphosphate, UDP-*N*-acetylglucosamine, NAD(P)H, or dGTP. Aqueous solvent mixtures (e.g., 60% acetonitrile or 50% methanol) can be used instead. When necessary, a volatile neutral buffer (e.g., ammonium bicarbonate) can be added to buffer the pH during extraction and subsequently removed by lyophilization. Example extraction protocols using 60% acetonitrile or chloroform/methanol/water partition are described in Appendices 5 and 6, respectively. As indicated in the previous section, the solvent extraction method can be integrated with the solvent quenching method and an example protocol is given in Appendix 1.

Figure 2 illustrates the 1-D ^{1}H NMR analysis of the solvent-based extracts of mouse liver (Fig. 2b) in comparison with those using TCA, PCA, or boiling water. Unlike the extraction for mammalian cells (cf. Fig. 1), the aqueous solvent extraction is not as efficient in removing macromolecular interference as the acid-based extraction. This is evidenced by the presence of broad ^{1}H resonances in the aliphatic and aromatic regions (e.g., 0.8–1 and 7–8 ppm of Fig. 2). Such interference is most pronounced for the chloroform/methanol/water method (cf. Fig. 2b), which may be reduced by ultrafiltration (e.g., through 3.5–5 kDa MWCO membranes). As ultrafiltration membranes are typically conditioned with glycerol, the added filtration step will require an extensive water rinse of the filter in order to minimize glycerol contamination. It should also be noted that different extraction methods yield somewhat different ^{1}H NMR profiles, except for the TCA and PCA methods, which give comparable results. This generally precludes comparison of metabolite profiles obtained from different extraction methods.

Although commonly used for GC-MS analysis, the chloroform/methanol/water method (the solvent ratio used often varies in the literature) (17, 31) gives a distorted ^{1}H NMR spectrum of mouse liver extract, particularly in terms of the resonances of ATP, NAD^+, and reduced/oxidized glutathione (GSH/GSSG), compared with those obtained from the other four extraction methods (Fig. 2). A similar problem is also evident with the $CHCl_3$/methanol/water extraction of human lung tissues (32). The broad resonances present in the spectrum further interfere with the 2D total correlation spectroscopy (TOCSY) analysis (Fig. 3 and see Chap. 6 for more information about this analysis). Compared with the TOCSY spectrum of the TCA extract (Fig. 3d), the TOCSY spectrum of the $CHCl_3$/methanol/water extract (Fig. 3b) exhibits a number of broad cross-peaks, which obscure many of the sharper cross-peaks arising from metabolites, such as Leu, Ile, spermine, Pro, and Arg. These interferences interfere with many of the metabolite assignments by TOCSY while jeopardizing the use of TOCSY for isotopomer determination (see Chaps. 2 and 6 (21, 33, 34)).

Broad interfering resonances and spectral distortion also occur in the boiling water extract, as shown in Fig. 2b. In addition to a reduced intensity of GSH/GSSG, Gln, and ATP resonances, those of NAD^+ are absent in the ^{1}H NMR spectrum of the boiling water extract. As high heat is destructive to a number of important but heat-labile metabolites, this method is not advisable for general use in metabolomic investigations.

pH Control

The solution pH is a very important parameter for sample preparation and subsequent analysis. As discussed above, modulating the pH of the extraction buffer is important for metabolite extraction. Appropriate pH is also required for derivatization in preparation for GC-MS analysis as discussed below, and in Chap. 4 by Higashi.

For NMR analysis, controlling the pH is critical because the spectral appearance of many metabolites, including amino acids, organic acids, and phosphorylated compounds, is very sensitive to pH so that their chemical shifts and/or spin coupling can vary greatly for relatively small changes in pH. Variable pH makes spectral assignment more difficult. Many NMR databases of metabolites are acquired with standards at a specific pH, such as pH 7.0, 7.4, or acidic pH, where most metabolites are in the fully protonated forms (see Chaps. 6 and 7 for further discussion of this point). It is, therefore, critical to adjust all samples to a pH value similar to that of the standard (less than ±0.05 pH, if the pH is near the pK value) prior to NMR analysis.

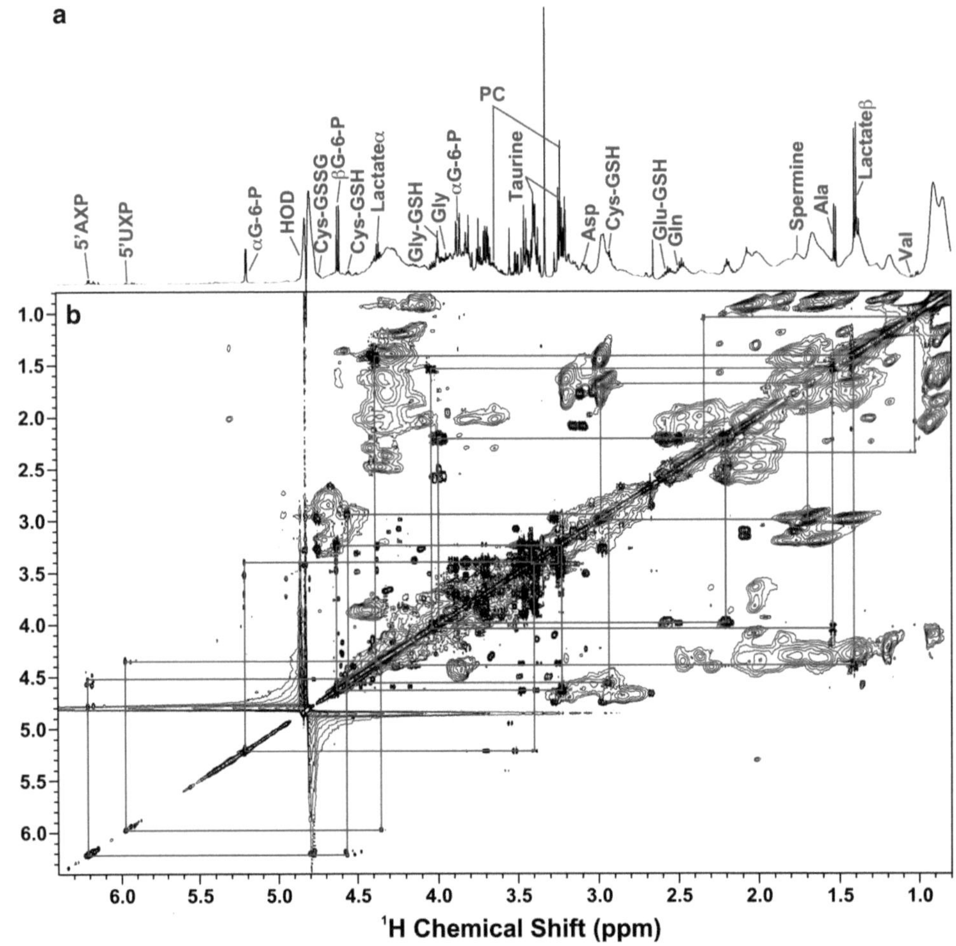

Fig. 3. 2D ^{1}H TOCSY analysis of TCA and chloroform/methanol/water extracts of mice liver. The extracts from Fig. 2 were analyzed on the same instrument using a standard 2D TOCSY pulse sequence. **b** and **d** are the 2D contour maps of the TCA and chloroform/methanol/water extracts, respectively, while **a** and **c** are the corresponding high-resolution 1-D ^{1}H NMR spectra.

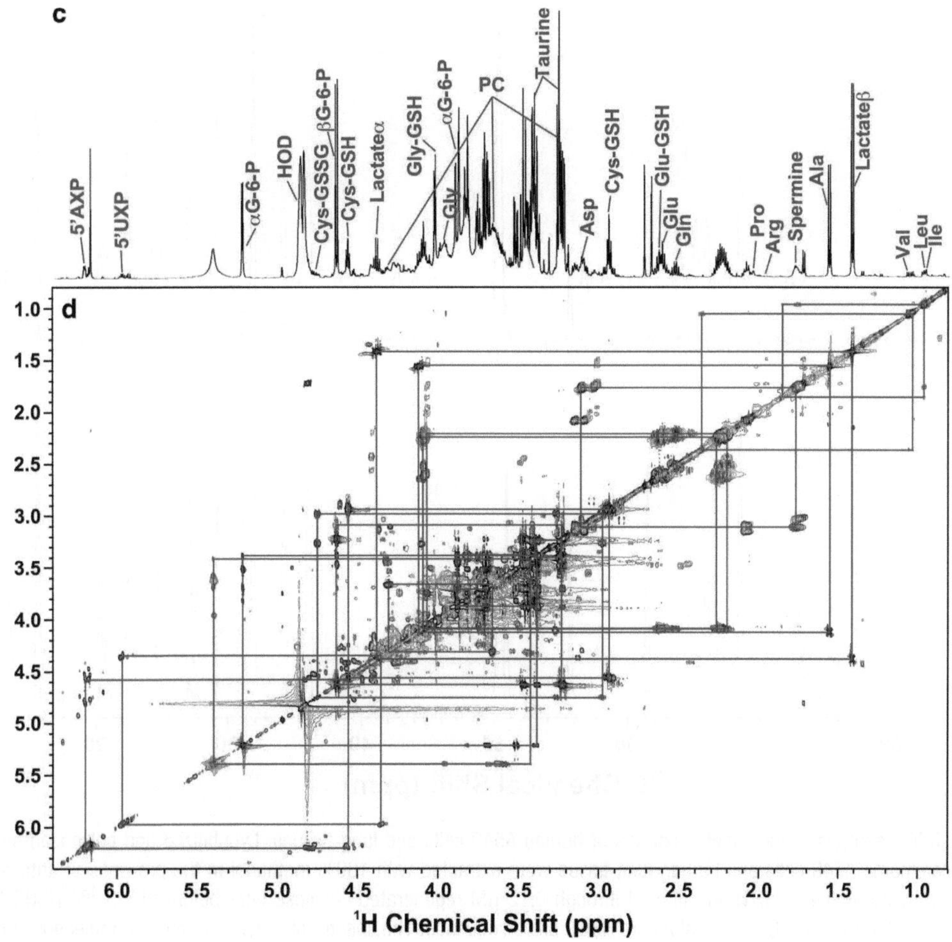

Fig. 3. (continued)

Extraction of Low-Polarity Metabolites

For extracting low-polarity metabolites, such as glycerolipids, sphingolipids, and cholesterol, methanol or chloroform/methanol (e.g., 2:1, v/v) mixtures are suitable. Methanolic extraction favors phospholipids (PLs) and sphingolipids, whereas chloroform/methanol mixtures better extract neutral lipids (35, 36). A protocol for methanol extraction is described in Appendix 6. Figure 4 illustrates the lipid profiles of methanolic extracts of human lung cancer cells and tissues, as analyzed by 2D ^{1}H-^{13}C heteronuclear single quantum coherence spectroscopy (HSQC). The spectra shown are the 1-D projection along the ^{13}C dimension of the 2D data. The antioxidant butylated hydroxytoluene (BHT) was included during the extraction to protect polyunsaturated lipids from oxidation. The large peak near 56 ppm is assigned to the *N*-methyl group of the phosphocholine (P-choline) head group, which indicates the abundance of phosphatidylcholine and/or sphingolipids. Also present in the extracts are cholesterol and phosphatidylethanolamine

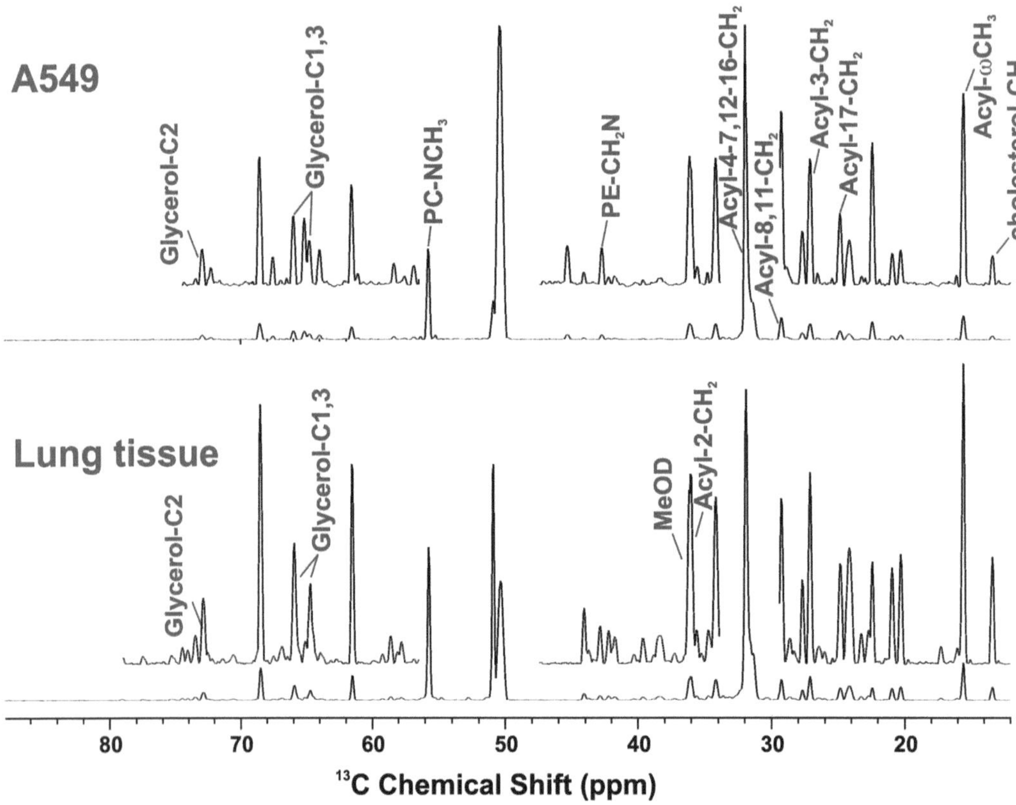

Fig. 4. HSQC analysis of methanolic extracts of human A549 cells and lung tissues. Lyophilized and pulverized human adenocarcinoma A549 cells and human lung tissue were extracted with 100% methanol in the presence of antioxidant butylated hydroxytoluene (BHT) and filtered through 0.22-μM regenerated cellulose filter before 2D ^{1}H-^{13}C HSQC NMR analysis at 14.1 T and 20°C using a standard HSQC pulse sequence. The spectra displayed are the 1-D projection spectra along the ^{13}C dimension. The inset spectra are four times magnified over the corresponding full spectra. ^{13}C chemical shift was referenced to methanol-d$_6$ (MeOD) at 36.07 ppm and peak assignments are made according to Fan and Lane (21).

lipids. The lipid profiles of lung cells and tissues show both similarity and differences. However, detailed lipid composition is not practical to determine with the HSQC analysis of such mixtures (see FT-ICR-MS analysis below for lipid speciation).

3.2.2. MS Analysis

The five polar extracts from Fig. 2 were also analyzed by GC-MS after derivatization with the silylation agent *N*-methyl-*N*-(*tert*-butyldimethylsilyl)trifluoroacetamide (MTBSTFA) (see Chap. 4 for discussion of MS-based methods). A comparison of the absolute content of various metabolites in these extracts as quantified by GC-MS is shown in Table 1. It is clear that the TCA extraction method performed the best overall while the CMW method was the worst in terms of the recovery of acid-resistant polar metabolites. In many cases, the recovery of the CMW method was several fold to more than an order of magnitude less than that of the TCA method for mouse liver tissues. The boiling water method was also less

Table 1
Comparison of GC-MS-analyzed metabolite profiles in extracts obtained using five different extraction methods[a]

Average[b]	PCA	TCA	ACN[c]	Water	CMW[c]	*Error*	PCA	TCA	ACN[c]	Water	CMW[c]
Lactate	32.92	12.69	36.17	50.72	2.10	Lactate	3.38	0.03	1.82	3.06	0.11
Ala	41.07	46.37	33.67	26.52	3.18	Ala	6.33	1.83	9.80	2.85	0.26
Gly	2.05	3.13	3.96	1.60	0.59	Gly	0.24	0.19	0.46	0.06	0.07
Val	0.38	0.51	0.37	0.31	0.11	Val	0.04	0.02	0.01	0.01	0.01
Leu	0.36	0.84	0.45	0.36	0.10	Leu	0.04	0.06	0.02	0.02	0.00
Ile	0.18	0.45	0.20	0.19	0.05	Ile	0.00	0.03	0.02	0.01	0.01
Succinate	3.03	4.89	2.20	1.86	0.55	Succinate	0.55	0.09	0.47	0.12	0.03
Fumarate	0.08	0.54	0.68	0.25	0.01	Fumarate	0.01	0.04	0.17	0.02	0.01
Pro	0.29	0.42	0.35	0.25	0.09	Pro	0.02	0.01	0.04	0.04	0.02
Ser	0.17	0.52	0.28	0.20	0.07	Ser	0.03	0.00	0.05	0.01	0.01
Thr	0.48	0.89	0.59	0.43	0.23	Thr	0.06	0.03	0.11	0.03	0.02
Phe	0.18	0.31	0.24	0.16	0.05	Phe	0.01	0.00	0.04	0.01	0.01
Malate	0.45	0.77	0.10	0.19	0.09	Malate	0.07	0.02	0.02	0.01	0.02
Asp	0.57	1.00	0.53	0.07	0.21	Asp	0.06	0.06	0.05	0.02	0.01
Asn	0.19	0.66	0.46	0.25	0.08	Asn	0.01	0.04	0.04	0.03	0.01
Lys	0.03	0.29	0.42	0.09	0.05	Lys	0.00	0.03	0.06	0.01	0.05
Gln	9.56	12.34	14.61	6.00	2.94	Gln	0.65	0.10	2.11	0.39	0.46
a-G3P[c]	1.08	2.91	1.85	1.10	0.31	a-G3P[c]	0.01	0.05	0.32	0.03	0.02
Citrate	0.07	0.02	0.04	0.01	0.00	Citrate	0.02	0.00	0.00	0.00	0.00
Tyr	0.11	0.23	0.21	0.15	0.02	Tyr	0.02	0.00	0.02	0.02	0.01
Ascorbate	0.00	1.75	0.12	0.00	0.03	Ascorbate	0.00	0.19	0.04	0.00	0.00

[a] The same set of extracts from Fig. 1
[b] Average of duplicate samples in μmole/g tissue dry wt
[c] *ACN* 60% acetonitrile method; *CMW* chloroform/methanol/water partition method; *a-G3P* α-glycerol-3-phosphate

desirable than the TCA or 60% acetonitrile methods, particularly in terms of Gly, fumarate, Asp, Asn, Lys, Gln, citrate, and ascorbate. The poor yield of the antioxidant metabolites ascorbate (Table 1) and GSH (Fig. 2) in the boiled water extracts is presumably due to their sensitivity to high temperatures, which makes the boiling water method unsuitable for antioxidant determination. PCA extraction also performed poorly on selected metabolites, e.g., fumarate, Asn, Lys, and ascorbate.

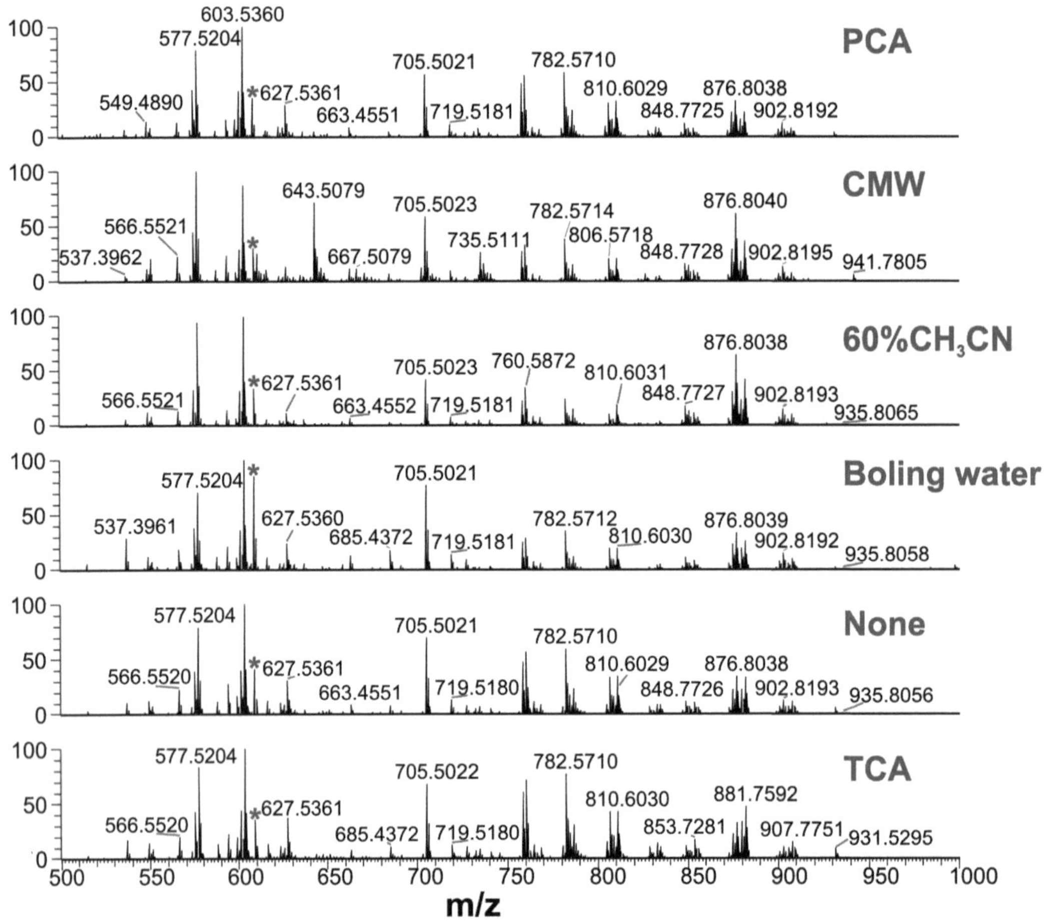

Fig. 5. FT-ICR-MS analysis of methanolic extracts of pulverized mice liver tissues. Except for the chloroform/methanol/water (CMW) extraction, the tissue residues from the other four polar extraction protocols in Fig. 2 were extracted with 100% methanol plus 1 mM BHT to recover lipid components. The PCA- and TCA-extracted residues were washed in nanopure water to remove acids and lyophilized before the methanol extraction. The CMW method simultaneously extracted lipid components in the chloroform partition. Duplicate liver samples with no prior extraction (none) were also extracted with methanol plus BHT for comparison. All lipid extracts in 500 μL methanol were diluted 100-fold in the spray solvent mixture CH_3Cl–methanol–2-propanol (1:2:4, v/v) plus 7.5 mM ammonium acetate (all in HPLC grade) and internal calibration standard reserpine at 1 ng/μL (37). The diluted lipid mixtures were introduced into an LTQ-FT-ICR-MS (ThermoFinnigan) using a NanoMate device (Advion). The exact mass analysis was performed in the positive mode with a mass resolution of 200,000. The *asterisk* marks the mass ion arising from reserpine (*m/z* 609.28213).

Subsequent to the polar extraction, the tissue or cell residues can be extracted for low-polarity components using methanol or other lipophilic solvents. Such sequential extraction is highly desired when samples are limited in amounts, such as human biopsy samples. The polar extraction can also serve as a cleanup step for the liphophilic extractions. Thus, it is useful to evaluate the recovery of low-polarity components from the sequential polar-lipophilic extraction protocols described above. Figure 5 shows the ultra-high-resolution and accurate mass FT-ICR-MS profiles of the

Table 2
Summary of FT-ICR-MS analysis of PLs extracted from mouse liver tissues pre-extracted with different polar solvents

Sample	# PLs	# Assigned peaks	# False compounds	# False peaks
Blank + reserpine	4	7	0	0
PCA	39	68	1	2
CMW	35	64	1	3
60% CH_3CN	35	63	1	4
Boiling water	33	55	2	3
None	40	70	1	3
TCA	42	75	1	2

methanolic extracts subsequent to PCA, TCA, 60% acetonitrile, and boiling water extractions, for comparison with those obtained from the chloroform partition of the CMW extraction and from direct methanol extraction of lyophilized liver powder. All extraction procedures give an overall qualitatively similar FT-ICR-MS profile with some minor differences. For example, the CMW method yielded an additional cluster of ions in the neighborhood of *m/z* 643.5079 while the TCA method gave a more significant ion cluster at 931.5295. In contrary to the poor recovery of polar metabolites, the CMW method gave a better response for low-polarity metabolites (when normalized to the standard reserpine as noted by asterisk) than the other four extraction methods. Quantitatively, the boiling water method had the lowest response for all mass ions, when normalized to reserpine.

The ultrahigh mass resolution and accuracy of the FT-ICR-MS analysis allow the exact mass of hundreds to thousands of observable ions to be determined, which in turn provides the molecular formulae information. The exact mass data is also valuable for high-throughput automated assignment by matching with the theoretical mass calculated from known molecular formulae (see Chap. 4 for details). This has been developed in our laboratory and applied to the assignment of mammalian phospholipids (PLs) based on the FT-ICR-MS data of crude mammalian extracts. The algorithm used for this purpose is called PRecalculated Exact Mass Isotopomer Search Engine (PREMISE, Higashi, Fan et al., in preparation). PREMISE search was performed for the six methanolic extracts in Fig. 5 and a summary of the output is shown in Table 2. The TCA pretreatment gave the highest number of assignable mass ion peaks, which corresponded to the highest number of identified PLs, while the boiling water pretreatment yielded the lowest number of identified PLs and assigned mass ion peaks. There were only a few falsely assigned peaks and compounds using the PREMISE algorithm. Example lipid species identified in the spectra acquired using the positive mode of FT-ICR-MS include phosphatidylcholines (e.g., C16:0/C22:4; C18:1/C20:5; C16:0/C24:0), phosphatidylethanolamines (e.g., C18:0/C20:4; C18:1/C20:5; C22:0/C20:4), sphingolipids (e.g., C18:1/C22:0; C18:1/C24:1; C18:1/C24:0), and phosphatidic acids (C20:0/C20:5; C18:0/C18:3; C18:0/C20:5).

In addition to PL assignment, PREMISE also identifies the isotopomer(s) of a given lipid species. Isotopomers are molecules with identical chemical structures but differing in isotopic composition at individual atoms (see Chap. 1 for details). For example, ^{13}C-1-alanine is an isotopomer of ^{13}C-2-alanine. Such automated assignment of isotopomers is excellently suited for FT-ICR-MS data, which routinely yield mass resolution of a neutron or electron. When coupled with ^{13}C tracer (e.g., uniformly ^{13}C-labeled glucose) study, the ability to profile ^{13}C isotopomers of various PLs is unprecedented and extremely valuable for tracing the metabolic pathways of specific lipids, which has not been possible using conventional approaches.

3.3. Sample Cleanup

For NMR analysis, extract sample cleanup mainly involves removing particulate matters and paramagnetic ions, such as Fe^{3+}, Cu^{2+}, and Mn^{2+}, that can lead to resonance line broadening or distortion. Centrifugation at a high speed (e.g., $\geq$18,000 g) for 20–30 min helps remove insoluble materials while passage through a cation exchange resin, such as Chelex-100, is effective in removing interfering cations but time consuming (cf. TCA extract in Fig. 2). A quicker alternative is to add chelating agents, such as EDTA, to the extract to bind interfering cations. However, excess EDTA produces a large singlet at ca 3.65 ppm in the ^{1}H spectrum, which obscures peaks around that region. Thus, it is important to optimize the amount of added EDTA or use the commercially available perdeuterated form which is typically 98 atom% ^{2}H.

For GC-MS analysis, extracts are normally derivatized using silylating or alkylating agents. For example, MTBSTFA is commonly used as a derivatizing agent for polar extracts and its efficiency is best at acidic conditions in aprotic solvents. Therefore, extracts should be acidified to pH 2–3, lyophilized to remove water before reaction with MTBSTFA in acetonitrile (28). It is common to have insoluble salts in the derivatization mixture, which should be removed by centrifugation. For direct-infusion nanospray MS or LC-MS, it is common practice to filter extracts through a 0.45- or 0.22-μm membrane filter to remove fine particles. If excess salts are present, it is important to reduce the salt content by passing through a hydrophobic column cartridge (e.g., C-18 cartridge), provided that the metabolites of interest are retained by the column material. It should be kept in mind that extensive sample cleanup can lead to distortion of metabolite profiles, which could defeat the purpose of metabolomic analysis.

In conclusion, sample preparation is the gateway to metabolomic analysis, the importance of which must be underscored. Sample preparation schemes may vary with sample nature or types of metabolites to be recovered but a given protocol should maximize sample integrity and metabolite recovery. It is also advantageous to implement sequential extraction methods that are applicable to different analytical purposes to minimize sample requirement and cleanup.

Acknowledgments

This work was supported in part by the National Cancer Institute grants # 1R01 CA101199-01 and 1R01CA118434-01A2, NIH Grant Number RR018733 from the National Center for Research Resources, National Science Foundation EPSCoR grant # EPS-0447479, Kentucky Challenge for Excellence, and the Brown Foundation. Dr. Zhengzhi Xie and Ms. Vennila Arumugum are acknowledged for respective assistance in sample processing and FT-ICR-MS analysis.

Glossary

BHT	Butylated hydroxytoluene
CMW	Chloroform/methanol/water partition
FT-ICR-MS	Fourier transform-ion cyclotron resonance mass spectrometry
GC-MS	Gas chromatography-mass spectrometry
GSH	Reduced glutathione
GSSG	Oxidized glutathione
HSQC	Heteronuclear single quantum coherence spectroscopy
Isotopomer	Compounds of identical chemical structure but differing in isotopic composition at individual atoms
LC-MS	Liquid chromatography-mass spectrometry
MTBSTFA	*N*-methyl-*N*-(*tert*-butyldimethylsilyl)trifluoroacetamide
PCA	Perchloric acid
TCA	Trichloroacetic acid
TOCSY	Total correlation spectroscopy

Appendices

Protocol for Preparing Adherent Mammalian Cells for Metabolite Extraction

Trypsinization Method

1. When feasible, keep cells ice cold during all processing steps prior to freezing.
2. Harvest cells by trypsinization and centrifugation at 280 × *g* for 5 min at 4°C.
3. Wash cell pellet by resuspension in excess ice-cold phosphate-buffered saline (PBS) (e.g., 10–15 mL per 10^7 cells), followed by centrifugation at 280 × *g* for 5 min at 4°C.
4. Resuspend cell pellet in ice-cold PBS (e.g., 1 mL per 10^7 cells) and transfer cell suspension to a pre-tared microfuge tube.
5. Centrifuge cell suspension at 1,700 × *g* (or at maximal g force without disrupting cell integrity) for 5 min at 4°C so that as much PBS as possible can be removed by pipetting with a fine-tip transfer pipette.

   Note: PBS contributes salts to the sample, which can be problematic for both MS and NMR analyses.
6. Obtain wet weight of cell pellet before flash freezing in liquid N_2.
7. Store frozen cell pellet at −80°C or lyophilize and obtain dry weight before storage.

Solvent-Quenching Method

1. Place cell culture plate on ice, remove culture medium by vacuum suction, and wash cells three times with ice-cold PBS by vacuum suction.
2. In the last wash, slant plate to drain PBS and remove as much PBS as possible by vacuum suction. Keep plate on ice for all subsequent procedures.

   Note: This is important to minimize salt contribution.
3. Add cold methanol (kept at −80°C) or acetonitrile (kept at −20°C) to drained plate to quench cell metabolism. Adjust solvent volume so that the plate surface is covered fully with solvent, e.g., 1 mL for 10-cm-diameter plate or 2.5 mL for 15-cm-diameter plate.
4. Scrape plate with a cell scraper to collect cell mass and transfer cell mass to a 15-ml conical polypropylene (PP) centrifuge tube.
5. Add another equal volume of cold methanol or acetonitrile to plate; scrap and collect cells as in step 4.
6. Add nanopure water to plate in a ratio of water:methanol (1:1) or water:acetonitrile (1.5:2); scrap and collect cells as in step 4.

7. Add chloroform to the cell homogenate in a ratio of $CHCl_3$:water:methanol (1:2:2) or $CHCl_3$:water:CH_3CN (1:1.5:2).

   Note: All solvents used should be of optima or HPLC grade.

8. Mix aqueous and $CHCl_3$ layers rigorously in the 15-mL tube before centrifugation at 3,000xg for 20 min at 4°C to separate the layers.

9. Transfer the upper aqueous and lower chloroform layers to 1.5-mL PP microfuge tube and 1.5-mL screw-cap glass vials, respectively, using a fine-tip transfer pipet for aqueous layer and PP gel-loading tip for chloroform layer.

   Note: Avoid pipetting the protein/cell debris in between the aqueous and chloroform layers.

10. Dry aqueous and chloroform extracts in a vacuum centrifuge.

Protocol for Preparing Blood Plasma for Metabolite Extraction

1. Collect blood into purple-top vacutainer containing K_3-EDTA as anticoagulant. Care should be taken to avoid lysis of the blood.

   Note: EDTA is compatible with both MS and NMR analyses; for NMR, it helps remove the influence of interfering cations, such as paramagnetic Fe^{3+} and Cu^{2+}.

2. Immediately keep blood sample on ice during transport.
3. Centrifuge blood (within 30 min–1 h of collection) at 3,939 × g for 15 min at 4°C.
4. Aliquot plasma into separate microfuge tubes and flash freeze in liquid N_2.
5. Store plasma samples at −80°C until analysis.

Protocol for Freeze Clamping

1. Immerse an aluminum clamping device (cf. Fig. 6) in liquid N2 bath to preequilibrate.
2. Place tissue(s) in the middle of the frozen clamp and quickly close the handles to flatten the sample(s), immediately followed by immersing in liquid N_2 to freeze.

Protocol for TCA Extraction

1. All extraction steps are carried out at 0–4°C (e.g., on ice).
2. Extract frozen or lyophilized powders (e.g., 30–40 mg) in microfuge tubes with 4–6:1 or 40–60:1 (v/w) volumes of 10% (w/v) ice-cold TCA, respectively. Vortex the mixture rigorously into a homogenous suspension. If homogenization is difficult by vortexing, it can be aided by a pellet pestle for microfuge tubes (cf. Fig. 7). If frozen powder is extracted, make sure that the homogenate is completely thawed before centrifugation.
3. Centrifuge the homogenate in a refrigerated centrifuge (set at 4°C) at ≥15,000 rpm in a microfuge rotor for 20–30 min.
4. Recover the supernatant with a fine-tip transfer pipette and store on ice. It is important to avoid pipetting tissue powder into the supernatant.

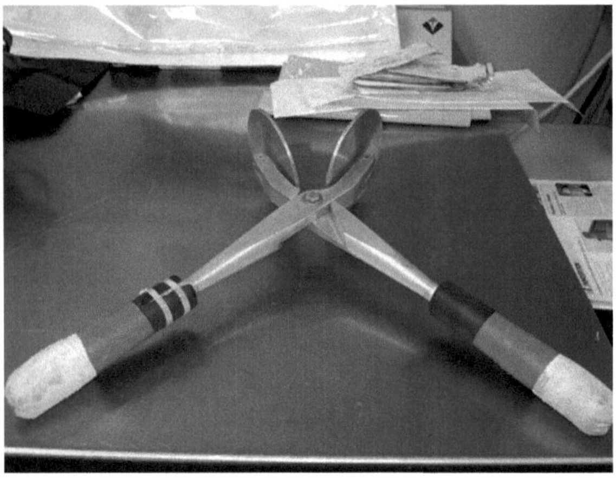

Fig. 6. Freeze clamp.

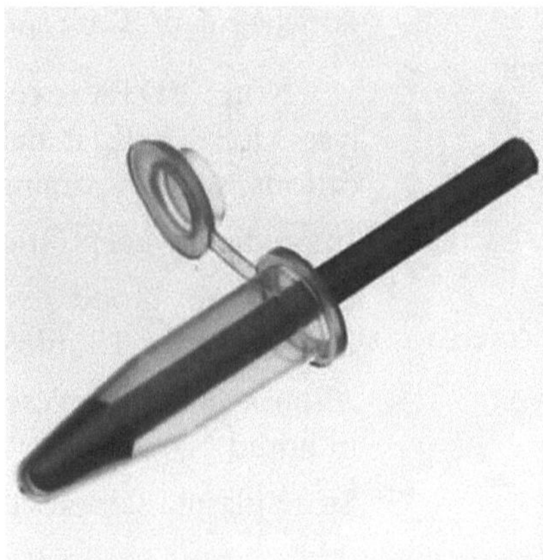

Fig. 7. Pellet pestle for microfuge tubes.

5. Extract the residue again according to Step 2 and centrifuge according to Step 3.
6. Pool supernatants from the two extractions and lyophilize using a liquid N_2 pretrap to prevent TCA vapor from reaching the vacuum pump.
7. Store lyophilized extract at −80°C until further analysis.

Protocol for 60% Acetonitrile Extraction

1. Homogenize 5 mg of lyophilized tissue powder or cell mass in ≥0.4 mL (1:80 w/v) 60% acetonitrile (HPLC or higher solvent grade). Homogenization is achieved by rigorous vortexing or by mechanical shaking in glass beads using a micro ball mill (e.g., MM200, Retsch, Inc.).
2. Incubate the homogenate for 30 min at −80°C to facilitate precipitation of macromolecules.

3. Centrifuge the thawed sample at ≥15,000 *g* for 20–30 min at 4°C.
4. Recover supernatant using a fine-tip transfer pipette into a 2-mL polypropylene microfuge tube or a 7-mL scintillation vial.
5. Repeat steps 1–3 (the −80°C step can be omitted) and pool supernatants.
6. Lyophilize extract using a liquid N_2 pretrap to prevent acetonitrile vapor from reaching the vacuum pump.
7. Store lyophilized extract at −80 C until analysis.

Protocol for Chloroform/Methanol/Water Extraction

1. Homogenize 5 mg of lyophilized tissue powder or cell mass in 0.4 mL methanol in a 2-mL microfuge tube by rigorous vortexing or by mechanical shaking in glass beads for 1 min at 30 Hz using a micro ball mill (e.g., MM200, Retsch, Inc.). *Alternatively, tissue or cell residue after polar metabolite extraction can be sequentially extracted with methanol for lipid components. For PCA- or TCA-extracted residues, remove acids with two to three times wash in nanopure water. All residues are lyophilized before lipid extraction.*
2. Incubate the homogenate for 20 min at 60 C.
3. Cool and centrifuge sample at ≥15,000 *g* for 30 min at 4 C.
4. Recover supernatant using a fine-tip transfer pipette into a screw-cap glass vial.
5. Add 0.4 mL nanopure water and 0.2 mL chloroform and shake rigorously for 2 min.
6. Centrifuge the biphasic solvent mixture at ≥14,000 *g* for 10 min at 4°C to separate the two phases.
7. Recover the top aqueous layer using a fine-tip transfer pipette into a 2-mL microfuge tube or a 7-mL scintillation vial. *Avoid transferring the protein pellet at the interface of the aqueous and chloroform layers.*

   Note: The bottom chloroform layer can also be recovered for nonpolar metabolites.
8. Lyophilize extract using a liquid N_2 pretrap to prevent solvent vapor from reaching the vacuum pump.
9. Store lyophilized extract at −80°C until analysis.

Protocol for Methanol Extraction of Lipids

1. Homogenize medium-free lyophilized cell mass or tissue powder (e.g., 1–5 mg) in 100% methanol (HPLC or MS grade) using a ratio of dry weight:methanol volume ≥100:1 plus 1 mM butylated hydroxytoluene (BHT, as antioxidant).

Homogenization can be done by mechanically beating the pellet with glass beads in a micro ball mill (e.g., MM200, Retsch, Inc.) for 1 min at 30 Hz *or by a pellet pestle in microfuge tubes.*

2. Let the homogenate stand at room temperature in the dark for 30 min.
3. Centrifuge at ≥18,000 × g for 10–20 min at 4°C.
4. Repeat step 1 with another aliquot of 100% methanol and centrifuge as in step 2.
5. Pool both supernatants and dry under vacuum in a Speedvac or lyophilizer with a liquid N_2 pretrap.
6. Dissolve lipid residue in methanol or other appropriate solvents and store in Teflon-faced septum screw-cap glass vials at −80°C until analysis.

   Note: Lipid extract should be filtered through 0.45-μM solvent-compatible filters (e.g., regenerated cellulose, Alltech Assoc.) prior to NMR or MS analysis.

References

1. De Vos RC, Moco S, Lommen A, Keurentjes JJ, Bino RJ, Hall RD. Untargeted large-scale plant metabolomics using liquid chromatography coupled to mass spectrometry. Nat Protoc. 2007;2:778–91.
2. Lu X, Xu G. LC-MS metabonomics methodology in biomarker discovery. In: Wang F, editor. Biomarker methods in drug discovery and development. Totowa, NJ: Humana press; 2008. p. 291–315.
3. Fan TWM, Colmer TD, Lane AN, Higashi RM. Determination of metabolites by proton NMR and GC analysis for organic osmolytes in crude tissue extracts. Anal Biochem. 1993;214:260–71.
4. Sellick CA, Hansen R, Maqsood AR, et al. Effective quenching processes for physiologically valid metabolite profiling of suspension cultured mammalian cells. Anal Chem. 2009;81:174–83.
5. Troy H, Chung Y-L, Mayr M, et al. Metabolic profiling of hypoxia-inducible factor-1beta-deficient and wild type Hepa-1 cells: effects of hypoxia measured by 1H magnetic resonance spectroscopy. Metabolomics. 2005;1:293–303.
6. Lutz U, Lutz RW, Lutz WK. Metabolic profiling of glucuronides in human urine by LC-MS/MS and partial least-squares discriminant analysis for classification and prediction of gender. Anal Chem. 2006;78:4564–71.
7. Azmi J, Connelly J, Holmes E, Nicholson JK, Shore RF, Griffin JL. Characterization of the biochemical effects of 1-nitronaphthalene in rats using global metabolic profiling by NMR spectroscopy and pattern recognition. Biomarkers. 2005;10:401–16.
8. Bolten CJ, Kiefer P, Letisse F, Portais JC, Wittmann C. Sampling for metabolome analysis of microorganisms. Anal Chem. 2007; 79:3843–9.
9. de Koning W, van Dam K. A method for the determination of changes of glycolytic metabolites in yeast on a subsecond time scale using extraction at neutral pH. Anal Biochem. 1992;204:118–23.
10. Buchholz A, Hurlebaus J, Wandrey C, Takors R. Metabolomics: quantification of intracellular metabolite dynamics. Biomol Eng. 2002;19:5–15.
11. Wittmann C, Kromer JO, Kiefer P, Binz T, Heinzle E. Impact of the cold shock phenomenon on quantification of intracellular metabolites in bacteria. Anal Biochem. 2004; 327:135–9.
12. Schaub J, Schiesling C, Reuss M, Dauner M. Integrated sampling procedure for metabolome analysis. Biotechnol Prog. 2006;22:1434–42.
13. Link H, Anselment B, Weuster-Botz D. Leakage of adenylates during cold methanol/glycerol quenching of *Escherichia coli*. Metabolomics. 2008;4:240–7.

14. Villas-Buas SG, Bruheim P. Cold glycerol-saline: the promising quenching solution for accurate intracellular metabolite analysis of microbial cells. Anal Biochem. 2007;370:87–97.
15. Winder CL, Dunn WB, Schuler S, et al. Global metabolic profiling of *Escherichia coli* cultures: an evaluation of methods for quenching and extraction of intracellular metabolites. Anal Chem. 2008;80:2939–48.
16. Fan TWM, Bandura L, Higashi RM, Lane AN. Metabolomics-edited transcriptomics analysis of Se anticancer action in human lung cancer cells. Metabolomics. 2005;1:325–39.
17. Villas-Boas SG, Hojer-Pedersen J, Akesson M, Smedsgaard J, Nielsen J. Global metabolite analysis of yeast: evaluation of sample preparation methods. Yeast. 2005;22:1155–69.
18. Liang YS, Kim HK, Lefeber AW, Erkelens C, Choi YH, Verpoorte R. Identification of phenylpropanoids in methyl jasmonate treated Brassica rapa leaves using two-dimensional nuclear magnetic resonance spectroscopy. J Chromatogr. 2006;1112:148–55.
19. Barsch A, Patschkowski T, Niehaus K. Comprehensive metabolite profiling of Sinorhizobium meliloti using gas chromatography–mass spectrometry. Funct Integr Genomics. 2004; 4:219–30.
20. Bolling C, Fiehn O. Metabolite profiling of Chlamydomonas reinhardtii under nutrient deprivation. Plant Physiol. 2005;139:1995–2005.
21. Fan TW-M, Lane AN. Structure-based profiling of metabolites and isotopomers by NMR. Prog NMR Spectr. 2008;52:69–117.
22. Lane AN, Fan TWM, Higashi RM. Isotopomer-based metabolomic analysis by NMR and mass spectrometry. Methods Cell Biol. 2008; 84:541–88.
23. Fan TWM, Kucia M, Jankowski K, et al. Rhabdomyosarcoma cells show an energy producing anabolic metabolic phenotype compared with primary myocytes. Mol Cancer. 2008;7:79.
24. Fiehn O, Kopka J, Dormann P, Altmann T, Trethewey RN, Willmitzer L. Metabolite profiling for plant functional genomics. Nat Biotechnol. 2000;18:1157–61.
25. Gradwell MJ, Fan TWM, Lane AN. Analysis of phosphorylated metabolites in crayfish extracts by two-dimensional 1H-31P NMR heteronuclear total correlation spectroscopy (hetero TOCSY). Anal Biochem. 1998;263:139–49.
26. Fan TWM, Lane AN, Higashi RM. Selenium biotransformations by a euryhaline microalga isolated from a saline evaporation pond. Environ Sci Technol. 1997;31:569–76.
27. Fan TWM, Higashi RM, Macdonald JM. Emergence and recovery response of phosphate metabolites and intracellular pH in intact Mytilus edulis as examined in situ by in vivo phosphorus-31 NMR. Biochim Biophys Acta. 1991;1092:39–48.
28. Fan TWM, Higashi RM, Lane AN, Jardetzky O. Combined use of proton NMR and gas chromatography-mass spectra for metabolite monitoring and in vivo proton NMR assignments. Biochim Biophys Acta. 1986;882:154–67.
29. Fan TWM, Lane AN, Shenker M, Bartley JP, Crowley D, Higashi RM. Comprehensive chemical profiling of gramineous plant root exudates using high-resolution NMR and MS. Phytochemistry (Oxford). 2001;57:209–21.
30. Lewis IA, Schommer SC, Hodis B, Robb KA, Tonelli M, Westler WM, Suissman MR, Markley JL. Method for determining molar concentrations of metabolites in complex solutions from two-dimensional H-1-C-13 NMR spectra. Anal Chem. 2007;79:9385–90.
31. Fiehn O, Kopka J, Trethewey RN, Willmitzer L. Identification of uncommon plant metabolites based on calculation of elemental compositions using gas chromatography and quadrupole mass spectrometry. Anal Chem. 2000;72:3573–80.
32. Fan TW-M, Lane AN. Structure-based profiling of metabolites and isotopomers by NMR. Prog NMR Spectrosc. 2008;52:69–117.
33. Lane AN, Fan TW-M, Higashi RM. Isotopomer-based metabolomic analysis by NMR and mass spectrometry. Methods Cell Biol. 2008;84:541–88.
34. Lane AN, Fan TW-M. Quantification and identification of isotopomer distributions of metabolites in crude cell extracts using 1H TOCSY. Metabolomics. 2007;3:79–86.
35. Rujoi M, Jin J, Borchman D, Tang D, Yappert MC. Isolation and lipid characterization of cholesterol-enriched fractions in cortical and nuclear human lens fibers. Invest Ophthalmol Vis Sci. 2003;44:1634–42.
36. Yappert MC, Rujoi M, Borchman D, Vorobyov I, Estrada R. Glycero- versus sphingo-phospholipids: correlations with human and non-human mammalian lens growth. Exp Eye Res. 2003;76:725–34.
37. Schwudke D, Oegema J, Burton L, et al. Lipid profiling by multiple precursor and neutral loss scanning driven by the data-dependent acquisition. Anal Chem. 2006;78:585–95.

Chapter 3

Clinical Aspects of Metabolomics

Michael Bousamra II, Jamie Day, Teresa Whei-Mei Fan, Goetz Kloecker, Andrew N. Lane, and Donald M. Miller

Abstract

Clinical metabolomics using stable isotope tracing represents an important new approach to obtaining metabolic parameters in human subjects in situ. In this chapter, the considerations for such clinical metabolomics are outlined and discussed. Descriptions include the essentials of patient accrual, permission, and institutional review approvals as well as specifics of treatments, tissue and biofluid collection, and curation. Although procedures vary among Institutes, the basic features for clinical research are common. Here, we illustrate the process from concept to analysis with an example from a recent study on non-small cell lung cancer metabolomics. This powerful new approach has already provided important new insights into metabolic adaptations in lung cancer cells.

1. Introduction

Metabolomics has been defined and described in Chap. 1 of this volume and elsewhere (1) to be the application of appropriate technologies to defining metabolic profile and responses of an organism, tissue, or cells under defined conditions. In other chapters (e.g., Chaps. 10 and 11) specific applications of metabolomics to analysis of drug effects are treated for cells in culture.

There is a hierarchy of complexity from the laboratory-based studies with cells in culture which can be manipulated at will, through organ studies, animal models, to the clinical setting with human subjects. For a variety of reasons, both ethicolegal and logistical, studies with human subjects cannot be as well controlled as animal models or laboratory-based experiments. To understand the etiology of a disease state in humans (and other vertebrates for that matter) and their response to treatments requires information from all of these levels of complexity (1–3). Ultimately, however, the physician wants to know how accurate is the diagnosis, how well the treatment is working, and what is the best prognosis.

Teresa Whei-Mei Fan et al. (eds.), *The Handbook of Metabolomics*, Methods in Pharmacology and Toxicology,
DOI 10.1007/978-1-61779-618-0_3, © Springer Science+Business Media New York 2012

Compared with the laboratory-based biomedical research, working with human subjects requires an additional set of considerations, both legal and ethical, and these have profound implications for experimental design. In this chapter, we present an overview of the processes that are needed to start a clinical investigation, and then considerations for tissue collection and storage. Although these considerations are identical for any clinical investigation study, for illustrative purposes here we use our own experience obtained from an ongoing lung cancer metabolomics study.

2. Experimental Design and Protocols

By their very nature, clinical investigations necessarily deal with a very heterogeneous population of subjects that certainly in early stages is likely to involve small numbers of subjects. Therefore, the initial experimental design must consider not only the logistics of sample and data collection (see next section) but also the expected outcomes of the study prior to beginning the work. Institutional Review Boards (IRB) review not only the scientific content (see below) but also the expected outcome, which requires a detailed discussion of the statistical techniques and estimates of the power that may be achieved given the proposed sample size.

The experimental design should also take into account the costs of such a study and the institutional rules that govern sample handling and biorepositories, some of which are not compatible with an ideal design.

An investigational metabolomics study in humans generally requires the assembly of a large team of professionals from very different backgrounds. This will include the originators of the study idea, the laboratory-based scientists, physicians, surgeons, biostatisticians, support staff (technicians, nursing staff, phlebotomists, etc.). Furthermore, there needs to be effective liaison with the clinical trials office, pathologists, pharmacy staff, and considerable clerical help for overseeing IRB proposals and amendments (see below), ensuring study orders are made up on time, responsibility for records being maintained under HIPAA rules. There is usually a research staff member that acts as the overall coordinator for the necessary extensive bureaucratic component, who may be associated with the clinical trials office or equivalent.

All personnel who are involved in samples or data collection at any stage must be HIPAA certified, and if institutionally required, CITI certified. Furthermore, the personnel who directly handle tissue or biofluids must have all the appropriate training (e.g., blood borne pathogen training). The details of how these certifications and requirements are organized are institution dependent.

It also cannot be overemphasized how important standardization of protocols, compliance, and accurate up-to-date record keeping is. All metadata pertaining to sample collection and handling should be recorded immediately, and preferably electronically. The records of course must be stored under HIPAA-compliant conditions (i.e., in a locked room, and electronic records accessible only by authorized personnel and with password protection).

The laboratory and storage space for tissue handling and workup for analysis must be designated as such, and be appropriate for the proposed work. Human tissue should be handled in a category II laboratory, and appropriate measures for disposal are available, as covered by Institutional Biosafety Committee certifications (IBC).

2.1. In Vivo vs. In Vitro Studies

For a metabolomics study, the monitoring may require taking samples of urine, hair, fingernails, etc. for analysis from subjects grouped according to diet, age, body mass index, etc. to determine response to dietary supplements (4); obtaining tissue samples from a biorepository; collecting tissue samples specifically for the study, e.g., in response to an experimental therapeutic approach; continuous monitoring of a subject over a period of time in response to an intervention using spectroscopy/imaging such as NMR (MRI/MRS) or PET imaging as described for animals by Wolak et al. (Chap. 11) and for human subjects by the Yale group (5).

A clinical metabolomics investigation can involve analysis of collected biofluids such as urine from two or more cohorts to determine whether there is a significant difference in metabolic profile between the normal and disease groups. This may be purely investigational, or combined with a therapy such as an investigational drug or device. The requirements for these modes are quite different. Considerably more invasive are procedures that involve needle biopsies or actual surgery to obtain tissue, which may or may not be combined with an investigational therapy for example.

The most invasive study would involve continuous monitoring of patient during an investigational procedure, such as infusion of ^{13}C-labeled glucose (dextrose) (NMR) or ^{18}F-2DG (PET) during the imaging or spectroscopy. However, where appropriate, this approach can produce extremely detailed information about metabolic processes in situ (5, 6) (Chap. 11).

2.2. Oral vs. IV Agent Introduction

If a drug or a labeled tracer such as ^{13}C-glucose is to be administered, there are choices about route. Injection into the blood stream is in many ways preferred as the agent distributes systemically very quickly, and this is straightforward with a surgical subject who has a central line (see below). Injection may also be appropriate for localized accessible lesions such as skin, though salves may also be possible for this purpose (e.g., in melanoma). For drugs, these must be GMP grade. Injectable agents also must undergo extensive pyrogen and sterility testing, and be certified. Although purely synthetic agents are unlikely to contain bacteria-derived pyrogens, they must be certified as being endotoxin-free. There are services that can provide such certification (cf. Resources) for a moderate fee. Injectables must also be certified sterile, which includes also the delivery vehicle, and be maintained under the control of the pharmacy. According to FDA regulations, 20% of the material must be tested for sterility and certified though less may be used in practice. The sterility testing typically takes of the order a week or more from submission to results. As the certification is valid for only 6 months, it is important to consider the costs of repeated certification, time, and the need for excess material for each certification commensurate with patient accrual rates.

The alternatives are mainly via the GI tract. The oral route has some practical advantages in that there are lesser requirements for sterility and pyrogen testing, and is less stressful to the subject (for a preoperative subject with a central line, this is a minor consideration). Drinking 50 mL of a sterile 20% solution of glucose solution (total 10 g) is a minor undertaking. The oral route however means that the absorption is slower, even on an empty stomach, so that the delivery lies somewhere between a pulse (bolus) and continuous infusion, the two ideal approaches. Continuous infusion will eventually reach isotopic steady state, which can make analysis more straightforward (cf Chap. 8), but requires a large total input of reagent. Pulse and pulse chase experiments also have analytical advantages for kinetic analyses, but necessarily result in isotopic dilution with time, and consequent analytical accuracy. In studies with brain chemistry, it has been shown that oral intake produces comparable results to continuous infusion but with lower precision (5).

2.3. Stable Isotopes

Stable isotopes have several major advantages for metabolic labeling compared with radioisotopes. First is that they are not radioactive, so there are no radiochemical concerns with infusion, nor with disposal. Second, they can be detected by two independent and complementary platforms, namely NMR, which responds to the magnetic moment of the isotope (cf. Chap. 6), and mass spectrometry, which measure the difference in mass between isotopes (cf. Chap. 4). Third, the commonly used stable isotopes (^{15}N, ^{13}C) are normally present in metabolites, albeit to a low extent. For example, the natural abundance of ^{13}C is 1.1%. However, the (bio)chemistry of the heavier isotope is essentially identical to that of the more abundant lighter isotope, such that there is no discernible effect on cellular biochemistry. This is especially so with ^{13}C substituting for ^{12}C or ^{15}N substituting for ^{14}N. The only potential concern may be with kinetic isotope effects on biochemical reactions. For this to be significant, there must be a rate-limiting bond cleavage in a metabolic pathway that involves the labeled compound. Furthermore, the difference in the light and heavy compounds must be large which effectively means substitution of deuterium for hydrogen. The maximum kinetic isotope effect is normally up to sevenfold for $^2H/^1H$. However, in practice, a bond-breaking step in a pathway is unlikely to be fully rate limiting (cf. Chap. 9). Indeed, deuteriated water slows the growth of cells, but only at high concentrations (>10% or so). Substitution of ^{13}C for ^{12}C has a very much smaller kinetic isotope effect than deuteration, and is not detectable on the flux through glycolysis in cultured cells (7). Thus, stable isotopes of common element such as carbon and nitrogen have no discernible physiological effects at the doses used for metabolomics. We have observed no adverse effects from administration of 10 g glucose iv.

Many metabolic studies are carried out using ^{13}C isotopomers of glucose, which is present in preprandial blood at a concentration of about 5 mM, rising to 10–15 mM after a sugar-rich meal. Indeed, glucose tolerance tests require drinking a large amount of glucose (up to 75 g), and the time taken for the glucose to clear from the blood is monitored. In nondiabetic humans, this is of the order 1 h or so whereas in diabetics, the blood glucose may remain above 10 mM for 2 h after ingestion (8). Ingested ^{13}C glucose is taken up by tissue from the blood, and metabolized to, for example, lactate and other compounds in the same way as the ^{12}C isoform.

^{13}C glucose isotopomers (and other labeled precursors) are readily available. At the time of writing, the list prices of [U-^{13}C]-glucose or [^{13}C-1]-glucose are about $160–180/g. However, the cost per gram is generally much lower when purchased in bulk, e.g., at the 100 g level. Thus, assuming 5–10 g per patient, the cost of isotopes becomes a relatively small fraction of the total study cost per subject.

2.4. Patient Accrual

The manner in which subjects are accrued depends on the kind of study. In cases where only readily obtainable biofluids are needed, such as urine or blood, it is possible to advertise within a university for example, or recruit relatives of subjects who will undergo treatment. For metabolomic studies, valuable information can be obtained from such biofluids (9–11). However, where more invasive procedures are indicated, such as surgery, chemo or radiotherapy, accrual is generally done in the physician's office. In all cases, potential research subjects must be carefully informed of any risks involved with participation in the study, its aims and potential benefits, prior to obtaining a signed informed consent form (see below).

In some cases, payment in the form of gift vouchers or for meals may be appropriate, within ethical guidelines (NIH and HIPAA) that in effect cover costs of attending a clinic to draw blood, etc. Again, depending on the study, once a subject has agreed, it is usual to obtain information that is relevant to the study, for the purposes ultimately of accounting for confounding factors such as age, gender, medical history, and so forth.

All such material must be collected and stored under HIPAA rules by trained personnel.

In the following, we give an outline of the procedures used in a lung cancer study at the University of Louisville under an IRB-approved protocol for studying metabolomics in non-small cell lung cancer patients.

2.4.1. Accrual to a Lung Cancer Metabolomics Study

Patients visiting the Thoracic Oncology Clinic for their lung cancer and that are evaluated for resectability of their lung cancer are offered participation in this trial. Those patients found to have resectable lung cancer and that agreed to participate were accrued.

Patients must have had a pathological diagnosis of lung cancer, all subtypes were permitted. Resectability and ability to sign informed consent were the primary eligibility criteria. In this particular study, special consideration was given to patients who had impaired glucose tolerance, but diabetics were specifically excluded. The majority of patients invited to participate agreed to do so. There was no advertisement for the trial and patients did not receive any reward for participating.

The recording of medical history is normal at presentation. It can be useful also to record additional data that are especially relevant to the study, for example smoking history (for lung cancer), general medical health, diet. For other kinds of studies, a detailed questionnaire may be prepared, which requires considerable expertise, and for which guidelines are published by NIH (e.g., http://dceg.cancer.gov/QMOD/).

2.4.2. Clinician's Office

The Thoracic Multimodality Clinic at the JG Brown Cancer Center is held one day a week. Thoracic Surgery, Radiation Oncology, Interventional Pulmonary and Medical Oncology staffs are seeing patients together with ancillary services (e.g., clinical coordinator, oncology nurse, social worker, phlebotomist). A meeting is held and all new cases are discussed as well any follow-up provided to patients already in treatment. Most patients in the Thoracic Multimodality Clinic are new patients. Follow-up for actively treated patients or for those under surveillance is scheduled on other clinic days according to the appropriate specialty.

2.4.3. Criteria for Inclusion/Exclusion

The criteria for inclusion or exclusion in a study must be included in the IRB, and adhered to. These criteria will vary considerably depending on the nature of the study. For example, in a pilot study where only a small number of subjects will be accrued, it may be useful to choose one gender and rough age matching to increase the statistical power (see below). In a larger or follow on study, careful study design may allow for extracting any gender specific or ethnicity effects with sufficient numbers. There are numerous confounding variables which need to be considered, but in the context of the study itself. For example we excluded diabetics because of (brief) hyperglycemia from the glucose bolus. Where biomarkers are sought from biofluids, then other medical history components such as prior cancer may be a reason for exclusion. In a revised version of our IRB, where urine in addition to blood was collected, subjects with a history of prior cancer were excluded. In practice, for lung cancer the majority of patients who present with a resectable tumor are older, and rough age matching occurs naturally (e.g., all >55 years of age).

2.4.4. Payments/Gift Cards

Payment for donating tissue is complex and raises ethical issues. It is not unusual to offer limited recompense, especially for out of pocket expenses if a special visit is required to donate biofluids for example. This can be done in the form of a cash payment, a gift card, etc. For surgery, where the visit to the clinic and the hospital is part of the treatment, and where blood will be drawn as a matter of course for clinical workup, such payments are less appropriate. In the lung cancer study, no financial inducements were made. Blood for the study was drawn at the time of surgery and during surgery, as described below.

2.4.5. Considerations Within Study Design

The study design, which is detailed in the specific IRB (see below) must consider the logistics of patient recruitment within the allotted time frame, which may be determined by funding. This needs careful consideration of the rate of uptake of the offer to participate in a study with respect to the total number of potential subjects passing through the clinic for example. In our pilot lung cancer study, we were able to accrue 24 patients suitable for surgical resection of NSCLC in less than 2 years. Since the Thoracic Multimodality Clinic sees 250 new patients per year, 50 patients with potentially resectable lung cancers were screened for the trial. This suggest that a larger study over a 5 year period could accrue of the order 250 subjects from this one site, which with the particulars of the study design would give considerable statistical power for determining the difference between normal and NSCLC of different grades and types (e.g., squamous cell carcinoma vs. adenocarcinoma) (and see Sect. 4).

The costs of such studies are high. In addition to the ^{13}C-labeled glucose, and the costs of sterile testing all other consumables and services must be borne by the study. This includes additional pathological workups, the costs of laboratory analytical services, blood draws, and associated supplies.

In our pilot study, all research related expenses were paid by the study funds. There were no additional expenses to the patient or the insurance. There were no additional office visits. For a follow-up study, with a larger patient cohort, further funds are necessary.

2.4.6. Compliance Issues

For investigational drug studies, there are significant issues of compliance, such as were the drugs taken, in the correct number and at the right times. In the lung cancer study, the main issue of compliance was related to the needs for fasting prior to surgery.

This is also necessary for control subjects who do not undergo surgery, but who donate blood and urine for analysis. The requirement for a 12 h fast effectively means providing blood or urine before taking breakfast. As this can be burdensome, it is not unreasonable to supply a voucher for a meal after donation.

There was no problem with fasting or compliance with the study. Patients had to follow standard procedures for surgery (e.g., NPO after midnight) and the [U-^{13}C]-glucose infusion was given right before surgery in the preoperative area. The surgical personnel helped with the infusion of the [U-^{13}C]-glucose. Actual compliance can often be ascertained from analysis of blood, which is rather sensitive to recent food intake.

2.5. Study Orders

Once the funding and IRB procedures have been approved, and patient accrual is underway, the detailed study can commence. For investigational drugs, detailed study orders must be available that provide instructions to ancillary staff involved in the project. This would include the nursing staff, phlebotomist, and contact with the pharmacy. It is usual also to have clear discussion with the pathology department, as the rules for tissue handling vary from institution to institution. Appendix 1 shows an example study order.

Nursing staff is very busy. It is often valuable that a senior member of the study is present at the preoperative area, both to ascertain that the study orders are being followed to the letter, to answer questions (e.g., about blood draw and the kind of receptacle needed; if necessary the study can provide the required vacutainers), and even discuss with the patient and family members the purpose of the study and its importance. Involving the staff and subjects in this way is not only a courtesy, but also can have a beneficial influence on the study procedure.

2.6. Tissue Collection

For example, collection of tissue of any kind must be standardized so at least to obtain reproducibility in the handling (and see Chap. 2). Unfortunately, metabolism is generally rather rapid compared with, for example, cell division, so to capture a snapshot of the metabolism at a given time as it was in situ requires very fast quenching techniques. Regrettably this is not always compatible with standards of care in an operating theater, or even with local rules. For this reason, many metabolic studies are conducted with readily collected biofluids such as blood, urine, sputum or BALF, breath, CSF, nipple aspirate, saliva, etc. (9, 12). The choice of biofluid to collect clearly depends on the goals and scope of the study, as well as for other more mundane reasons of expediency of cost, analytical capability, patient accrual and so forth. These may in some instances have greater selectivity as they are more proximal to the organ of interest, for example BALF reports on lung epithelial activity, and CSF on central nervous system functions. Many of these studies are directed toward the search for metabolic disease biomarkers (1, 13–18).

2.6.1. Blood

Blood draws can be taken by trained personnel in the clinic, preoperatively and during surgery. It is imperative that the drawn blood be chilled immediately and taken for processing as soon as possible. To prevent coagulating of the blood and hemolysis, the fresh blood should be placed in a chilled vacutainer containing the anticoagulant. Of the three main anticoagulation agents used, we have found that for metabolomics studies, the best is K_3-EDTA, which is very effective in preventing hemolysis (assuming careful handling of the blood), and does not interfere with subsequent analysis (unlike citrate or heparin). K_3-EDTA vacutainers have purple or lavender tops (cf. Becton, Dickinson & Co. http://www.bdbiosciences.com/index.shtml) and differ in that one is a liquid, the other is spray dried on the walls of the tube. EDTA has the additional benefit of chelating paramagnetic cations, and therefore improving subsequent NMR spectral analysis. We typically use 5-mL vacutainers (smaller volume, gives more rapid cooling) and can be centrifuged at 3,500 × *g*. Centrifugation of whole blood at low speed (3,500 × *g*, swingout rotor, 15 min 4°C) separates into three fraction: the packed red cells at the bottom of the tube, the yellowish plasma at the top, and the creamy "buffy" coat at the interface of these two major phases. Great care should be taken to avoid hemolysis, as this can seriously interfere with subsequent metabolic and protein analyses of the plasma. The fractions are separated by aliquotting the plasma phase. A detailed protocol is provided in Chap. 2 by Fan. It is also important to keep accurate notes of the timings of collection (draw), temporary storage on ice or in the refrigerator, and use a standardized protocol for phase separations.

Manual aspiration is relatively slow, albeit carried out on ice and aliquotting into ice-cold (plastic) receptacles. An alternative once the sample has been centrifuged is to flash-freeze the whole tube. The frozen phases can then be separated physically by sawing off the end of the (plastic) collection tube, and expelling the solid pellets sequentially, all under frozen conditions (e.g., on a liquid nitrogen cooled stage in a designated class II microbiology hood—the sawing may aerosolize the blood to some extent).

The buffy coat can be further purified by ficoll (cf. Histopaque, Sigma-Aldrich) gradient centrifugation if desired, such as to separate different cell types (http://www.stemcell.com/technical/RosetteSep_Buffy_Coat_Procedure.pdf).

Even storage at 4°C causes morphological changes in the platelets, related to membrane lipid phase transition and actin reorganization analogous to activation (19, 20).

The minimal amount of sample handling compatible with downstreamanalysis is needed to minimize time during which metabolites can change. As individuals have different metabolic activity, longer preparation times increase variance across the samples.

2.6.2. Urine

Even urine requires care in sampling and storage, as bacterial contamination can change the metabolic profile (21, 22), and there appear to be both biogenic and nonbiogenic reactions occurring in urine that is left to stand for even short periods (23). For surgical subjects, urine can be taken from the catheterized bladder and chilled on ice for temporary storage.

3. Ethical and Legal Considerations

In order to protect individuals from inappropriate use of their medical records, the need for all subjects who participate in clinical research, and to ensure that any experiments are ethically conducted, a number of ethical and legal regulations have been established.

3.1. HIPAA Regulations

HIPAA (Health Insurance Portability and Accountability Act (1996)) regulations were established to protect the subject from abuse, or in the case of genetic analysis, from discrimination in the workplace or for insurance purposes. The HIPAA regulations are relatively stringent, and have been criticized for being overly strict to the possible detriment of patients for future treatments (24). Nevertheless, in practical terms, all human-based studies must comply with these regulations, which requires considerable patience and planning by the study personnel. All personnel involved in the study, and with any aspect of handling samples or have access to data must be HIPAA certified. This requires an initial extensive examination, followed by regular recertification.

All aspects of primary data (medical records) fall under the HIPAA regulations. In practice, this means that data must be stored in a secure facility, with access to authorized personnel only. Electronic data stored on computers must be password protected. Our primary data are stored on designated computers in a secured Clinical Trials Office.

Similar considerations apply also to tissues stored in Biorepositories. Access to tissue samples for research purposes is determined in large measure by how the repository was established. All subsequent use nevertheless requires IRB approval consistent with HIPAA regulations. In this regard, the language of the protocol, the informed consent and the HIPAA documents should be consistent.

This is generally more straightforward for deidentified samples or records, which must be devoid of any of 18 category identifiers of the source.

The HIPAA regulations are both prescriptive and proscriptive but unfortunately, the implementation of the rules is left to individual institutions. Here we can only outline the general procedures at UofL, that are relevant to metabolomics studies.

3.2. Institutional Review Board (IRB)

The IRB is a committee that certifies that a study is ethical and adheres to the highest standards. The IRB document is generally submitted after vetting by other committees who comment on the value of the study (e.g., potential benefit), budget and statistical considerations. The full IRB document briefly describes the background and purpose of the study, and then sets out the conditions under which the study will be conducted. For an investigational study, the details of any drug that is to be used must be supplied including its status as IND, approved uses, etc. The criteria for inclusion or exclusion of subjects in the study must be provided, and with reasons. The details of the treatment plan are provided, e.g., route of administration, dose, method of administration as well as the toxicities that may occur, and procedures for reporting any adverse reactions. Particular attention must be paid to potential risks to study participants. Any nonstandard procedures must be included for drug administration or any departure from best standards of care practices. Details of the tissue and biofluid collection are included, and all appropriate ethical and legal information about participation. An example IRB application is shown in Appendix 2.

The IRB certification has a fixed term, which may be renewed if necessary subject to progress reports.

3.3. Amendments

During a study, it may become apparent that changes to procedures would improve the tissue collection, storage or data analysis. Such changes can only be made with an amendment to the original IRB. Depending on the extent of the amendment, the revised IRB may require convening the whole committee for approval, or can be approved by the committee chair if the changes meet the appropriate criteria. An example of a minor amendment would be a change in the rate or timing of the ^{13}C glucose. A major amendment would include substantial changes in the experimental design of the study such as altering the patient population or adding invasive procedures.

Only in rare instances are exceptions permitted, as documented in the extensive HIPAA documentation.

3.4. Informed Consent

A fundamental ethical concern that has been in place for decades is the principle of informed consent. This means that any subject recruited to a research study must be made fully aware of the risks involved as well as the purpose of the study. This may also have implications for inclusion or exclusion criteria, such as age of consent, the ability to comprehend, and for questionnaire-based studies fluency in the language of the study (e.g., English in the USA). It is essential that any subject entering into a research study signs an informed consent form, which must detail not only what the procedures are, but also any future uses of tissue or information that is obtained. Samples may be used only for those purposes specified in the IRB and agreed by the subject. Thus, careful wording of the IRB becomes critical (see above), such as specifying all research purposes. Such language must also be included in the consent forms (and see above). The preparation of consent forms must follow specific guidelines, including federally mandated as well as local rules. Appendix 3 gives a checklist of such requirements.

4. Statistics

The level of statistical analysis depends on the scope and phase of the study. In a pilot study, where there are no prior relevant data available, and a small number of subjects will be accrued, then there is a lesser requirement for detailed statistics, as the point is to demonstrate feasibility. In these cases, descriptive statistics can be used, also with simple measures of mean and standard error and similar descriptors of the data. In a large-scale study following on from initial or other studies, much more detailed statistics are required, both in the design phase (power analysis for sample size determination) as well as in the final reckoning. The considerations can be very complex with real populations, and may require professional assistance from biostatisticians. The nature of the analytical data from metabolomics studies also requires specialized techniques for dealing with very large, multivariate data sets.

4.1. Paired Samples or Unpaired Samples?

For simple studies of prechosen biomarkers, ANOVA and *t*-tests are adequate. For metabolite profiling, multivariate procedures must be used (variants on PCA, OPLS, etc.) (25–27). The standard *t*-test has to be applied with care because of the uncertainty about the number of corrections to make for multiple comparisons between linked (i.e., metabolites) objects.

4.2. Power Analysis

Power analysis is often expected as part of a study design. For a simple comparison of a few variables, if the variance of the control and treatment groups is known or can be reasonably estimated (sic), then it is possible to calculate the power of a study to detect a particular difference between the groups at a given significance (p value, often arbitrarily chosen to be 0.05 (28)). Thus in a prospective power analysis, it is possible to estimate the number of subjects needed to detect a particular difference between the groups at that power level, often chosen to be 80% or better at a significance level of 0.05, and thus inform on the size of the study to be undertaken. With a pilot study where there is no reasonable estimate of the sample variance, such a power analysis cannot be sensibly conducted. However, a *retrospective* power analysis can, and should, be done, in preparation for larger study.

As one might expect, the power of a study using matched pairs is much greater than one in which the groups are not matched.

The analytical platforms used in our lung cancer study were NMR and MS (see Chaps. 3 and 5). NMR peaks were identified according to in-house databases (7, 29, 30). Peak areas were normalized to that of the internal concentration standard DSS at known concentration to determine the concentration in the NMR tube (7, 31). The analytical accuracy associated with this procedure is better than 5%.

The concentrations of tissue metabolites determined by MS and NMR are normalized to tissue dry weight (i.e., biomass). For initial visualization, these are displayed as fold changes and heat maps, which gives a rapid readout of the major differences between treatment and control.

4.3. Statistical Significance

Paired t-tests were used for ^{13}C enrichment in glucose and glucose-6-phosphate, lactate, alanine and glutamate, aspartate and nucleotide riboses. The paired t-tests for ^{13}C enriched metabolites from 7 samples showed a statistical power ranging from 50% (lactate) to 92% (alanine) at $p = 0.05$ (32). Differences in the enrichment of such metabolites for as few as ten subjects then give statistically significant differences ($p < 0.05$) in ^{13}C-containing metabolites with a power of >80% (28). The steady state concentrations of many intracellular metabolites differed considerably between cancerous and normal lung tissue. Based on the experimental variances, a power of >90% can be expected at $p < 0.05$ for ten or more subjects, and in many instances, considerably better statistics. We have subsequently analyzed 40 paired subjects, and for pyruvate carboxylase expression in human lung tumors, the p value in the paired t-test was 0.0001 (ratio of the means was 8) (unpublished data).

5. Example: Metabolomics Lung Cancer Study

Here we give an outline of a metabolomics study of NSCLC to determine the metabolic differences between cancerous and non-cancerous lung tissue, using ^{13}C isotope tracing (9, 32–34). This study involved collaboration and organization of a large number of personnel. In addition to the surgeon and his team, the study required the oncologist, research coordinator, laboratory PIs and their teams, phlebotomist, pharmacy and nursing staff. Tissue collection was done by groups of trained personnel for initial blood draws (preoperatively) and to oversee the administration of the glucose. In the operating theater, two or three personnel were required. They carried out rapid freezing of tissue, recorded the surgical procedures and timing of tumor removal, and prepared samples for pathology (slides of specimens) (35).

5.1. Study Design

The experimental design was to analyze paired samples of lung tissue from the same patient who were scheduled for surgery for NSCLC. In this case, the lung cancer and a piece of nontumorous tissue from the same lung were analyzed approximately 3 h after infusion of a bolus of [U-^{13}C]-glucose. Tissue and blood samples were to be analyzed by NMR and mass spectrometry for metabolite profiles and incorporation of ^{13}C from the source glucose. Specific mRNAs and proteins associated with the metabolic differences observed between the noncancerous lung tissue and the tumor were probed by gene array, qRTPCR, Western blots and enzyme activity as desired. As described above, the statistical power under this design allowed for small numbers of subjects.

All procedures were carried out according to the authorization under IRB approval for this study. The IRB allowed for any research use of the excised tissue.

Subjects were accrued to the study as described in Sect. 2. There were two phases to the study, first to ascertain appropriate times for infusion ^{13}C glucose prior to resection, and second to determine the metabolic profiles of lung tumor and noncancerous lung tissue after the time of glucose infusion. In the first phase, 10 g ^{13}C glucose were administered iv approximately 12 h prior to surgery. Blood samples were taken immediately prior to glucose infusion, immediately after infusion, and then at intervals up to the time of surgery. Blood ^{13}C glucose and ^{13}C lactate were measured using ^{1}H NMR of the separated plasma to establish the rate of glucose utilization and the rate of metabolism by tissue into secreted lactate (^{13}C lactate derives exclusively from the ^{13}C glucose supplied). It was discovered that for metabolic purposes, glucose infusion about 3 h prior to resection gave a significant amount of label in tissue metabolites as determined NMR and mass spectrometry. Tissues were also analyzed by pathology (for staging), and paraffin embedded H&E slides were prepared for the research arm of the study. H&E (hematoxylin and eosin) are commonly used dual stains that respectively show acidic structures such as the nucleus as blue, and the cytoplasm pink. Frozen tissue was also used for mRNA analysis of targeted metabolites by qRTPCR.

5.2. Stratification

There was no attempt to stratify by gender in this initial study of fifty five subjects including controls. Only nondiabetic patients were allowed. Although not specified, the age range was 44–80 years (median 62 years), which reflects the usual range for tobacco induced NSCLC (36). Less than five percent of subjects were nonsmokers. Fifty-four percent of the subjects were male. About 2/5 of the cancers were squamous cell carcinoma, the remainder being adenocarcinoma, large cell or (rarely) the bronchioalveolar carcinoma (BAC) subtype. Two thirds of the tumors were stage I (no involvement of lymph nodes) and the rest were stage II or rarely III/IV. The statistics are given in Table 1.

Table 1
Statistics of surgical NSCLC subjects at Louisville

Factor	Statistic ($n = 55$)
Ethnicity	70% Caucasian, 25% African American, 5% other
Gender	54% Male, 46% female
Median, mean age (year); range	62, 61.8 ± 9; 44–80
Stage	67% I, 19% II, 14% III + IV
Subtype	29% Adenocarcinoma 42% Squamous cell carcinoma 4% BAC 25% Large cell + adenosquamous

5.3. Equipment Needed for Tissue Collection

Liquid nitrogen Dewar (4 L) (flash freezing at −196°C)

Additional working container for lN_2 (actual freezing)

Ice bucket + ice

Ice bucket for lN_2 freezing of tissue samples

Freeze clamp

Precut heavy-duty aluminum foil

Forceps

Very sharp scissors

Weigh boats or thick Al foil

Deionized (pure) water in 50-mL Falcon or equivalent (for washing and wetting implements)

4× 10% buffered formalin (histology grade) in labeled screw-cap containers (ca. 20 mL formalin)

6× Empty 15-mL Falcon tubes with screw caps in a rack

Stopwatch

Notebook, marker pens

Digital camera for documenting in situ tumor and tissue after excision

5.4. Preoperative Procedures

5.4.1. ^{13}C Glucose Infusion

[U-^{13}C]-glucose was purchased from Isotec as a pyrogen-free powder at 99 atom% ^{13}C. The powder was dissolved in sterile water, and aliquotted, and sent for endotoxin and sterility testing. The certified glucose was kept frozen in the pharmacy until required. The solutions were prewarmed and sent to the preoperative facility on demand.

The glucose was infused iv under gravity feed as a 50 mL solution, followed by an equal volume flush of normal saline, which takes about 5 min. Blood was drawn in the presence of study personnel immediately prior to and post infusion, and placed on ice. The blood was separated into plasma and cells by centrifugation at 4°C within 30 min of drawing, flash-frozen in lN_2, then stored at −85°C until needed for analysis (see below and cf. Chap. 2).

5.5. Operating Theater

5.5.1. Methods

All relevant times were recorded, e.g., infusion with ^{13}C glucose, time of anesthesia, time of chest opening, time to tie vein and artery, time of tissue excision, time of tissue into lN_2 and in formalin. The times at which the blood (and urine) samples were actually collected were recorded. Such metadata are essential for subsequent data analysis (37, 38).

Additional critical data recorded were the time of incision into the thoracic cavity, and the amount of time the lungs were inflated. The latter is critical to monitor the duration of hypoxia during surgery The surgeon described the state of the lung, location of the lesion, and visual characteristics, as well as the kind of resection (e.g., wedge resection, lobectomy, pneumonectomy, etc.). To minimize hypoxia, the lungs are kept inflated as long as possible. Furthermore, whenever indicated, localized tumors are wedge resected which is very fast, and the tissues can be snap-frozen within 5 min of excision.

Following resection samples of tissue were chosen by the surgeon and placed on weigh boats on ice (separate boat for each tissue sample, e.g., tumor vs. normal tissue). The surgeon's experience was vital for tumor identification and finding the margins of viable tumors. In these studies, the surface located, well-differentiated NSCL tumors could be found accurately using a combination of palpation and visual scrutiny, as the masses have a distinct feel. The generally poorer vascularization makes them visually distinctive (paler tissue) (cf Fig. 1). Some larger tumors were necrotic, which was easily observed once the tissue was sliced. All such information was recorded, and necrotic tissue was separated from nonnecrotic tissue at the site, and frozen separately. Photographs including a ruler were taken for estimating tissue and tumor size as well as providing a permanent record of appearance of the fresh tissue.

Separate samples of tissue were sent to the pathology laboratory for microscopic evaluation, along with any lymph nodes to determine metastatic spread. The final detailed pathology report included tumor stage, histology and various microscopic features. These data were incorporated into the record for subsequent comparative analysis and interpretation of the metabolomics results.

The excised tissue samples were placed on the bottom plate of the freeze clamp precooled in lN_2, and immediately clamped to form a thin cake (Fig. 1b). The freezing was held for a least 30 s, and then the tissue cake was carefully (!) dropped onto a prelabeled

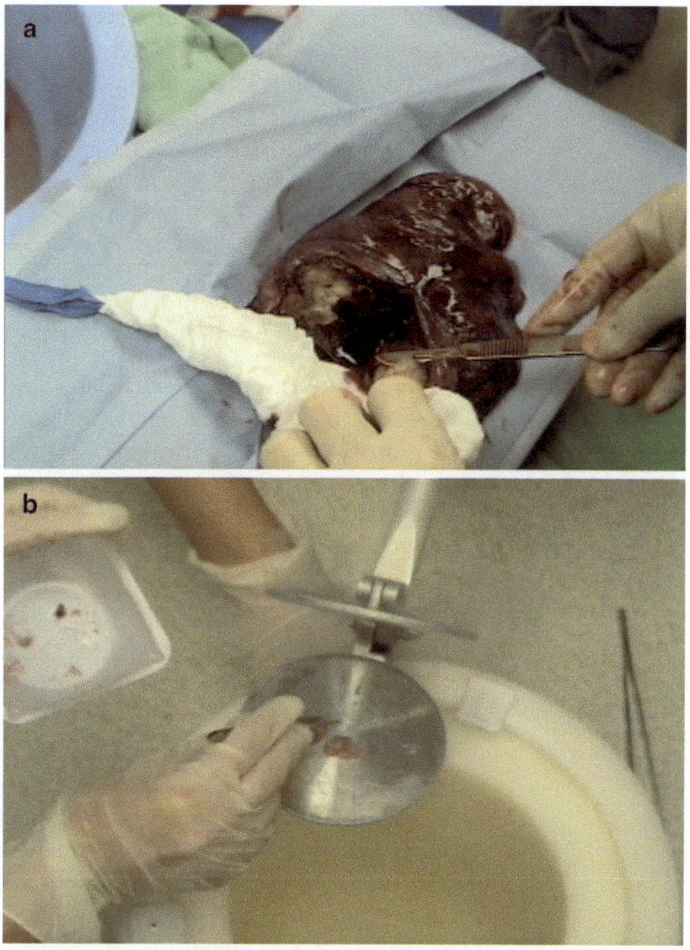

Fig. 1. Resected lobe of a lung cancer patient. The lobe was resected 3 h after infusion of 10 g [U-^{13}C]-glucose. (**a**) The lung was sliced in half on a table in the sterile area adjacent to the operating table, and slices of tumor (light, poorly vascularized lesion) and nonadjacent nontumorous lung tissue (*dark*) were immediately placed between the aluminum plates of a freeze clamp device (**b**) precooled in liquid nitrogen.

Al foil floating on lN_2. This was then folded and kept in the lN_2. A small piece of each tissue sample was separately dropped into 10% buffered formalin (source) for histological analysis. This process typically took less than 5 min.

A blood sample (ca. 10 mL) was drawn into 2× 5-mL purple-top vacutainers and immediately placed on ice. All samples were transported cold (lN_2 for tissue or ice for blood) to the laboratory for immediate processing.

Blood samples: whole blood aliquots 1 × 1 mL + 4 × 100 μL were placed in screw-cap microfuge tubes under sterile conditions and flash-frozen in lN_2. Remaining blood is centrifuged at 4°C for 15 min at 3,500 × *g* using a swing-out rotor. Plasma aliquots

(100 μL) were pipetted into screw-cap microfuge tubes on ice and flash-frozen in lN_2 (1 mL each per tube and any remaining plasma frozen separately). The plasma is then pipetted into a cold container, and separately frozen (lN_2) from the packed red cells. These samples were stored at −85°C prior to workup for metabolomic, proteomic and/or RNA analysis.

6. Conclusions

For a variety of ethical, legal, and logistical reasons, studies with human subjects cannot be as well controlled as animal models or laboratory-based experiments. However, clinical metabolomics provides a powerful opportunity to generate detailed metabolic data in humans who are either normal (control) subjects or patients with a specific disease. In the laboratory it is possible to manipulate the conditions essentially at will, and work with genetically well-defined systems, and ultimately with pure cell lines in culture. This makes it possible to define the range of possible responses to external conditions or to drug treatment for example. Which of these behaviors accessible to the cells actually occurs in vivo remains the province of clinical experimentation. Ultimately, the physician wants to know how accurate is the diagnosis, how well the treatment is working, and what factors will improve survival.

Clinical metabolomics is highly desirable so that the information obtained in laboratory studies can be translated into the clinical setting either in biomarker discovery, for diagnosis or for prognosis. Concentrations of specific metabolites or groups of metabolites present in serum or other accessible biofluids may vary according to disease state, thus providing a set of biomarkers that correlate with clinical outcomes.

Generally, the metabolomics approach does not lead to mechanistic understanding of the disease progression, and therefore does not necessarily help with the development of new treatments or early detection methods. However, stable isotope tracing provides an additional dimension, in that specific pathways in the tissue can be delineated, and how they differ from the same pathways present in the normal tissue (39, 40). Such information is extremely valuable for understanding the biochemistry of cancer. Such knowledge may then lead to novel avenues of cancer therapy. Although invasive, such studies can be extended to less invasive procedures such as tissue biopsy. Needle biopsies are common interventions for several cancers, including breast and prostate. Furthermore, with modern ultrasensitive technologies such as FT-ICR-MS (see Chap. 4), the amount of tissue available is sufficient for a study of this kind. The use of stable isotope tracing would greatly increase the specific information content from tumor biopsies.

In contrast, in biofluid analysis, the origin of the molecule is unclear. An additional advantage of stable isotope tracing is that if a product metabolite contains the stable isotope, then there is a connection to the original source provided (e.g., glucose), which shows that it originated from metabolic processes within the subject, and not as some adventitious contaminant from the local environment.

Such studies in vivo clinical are inherently more involved than pure laboratory-based metabolomics, with a very strong emphasis on teamwork. Nevertheless, the clinically relevant information content is sufficiently high as to make such approaches with stable isotope tracing more prevalent in the future.

Resources

HIPAA information from NIH: http://www.hhs.gov/ocr/hipaa/
http://www.hipaa.org/
http://www.accessdata.fda.gov/scripts/cdrh/cfdocs/cfcfr/CFRSearch.cfm?fr=610.12
IRB: http://en.wikipedia.org/wiki/Institutional_Review_Board
Pyrogen testing: http://www.fda.gov/ora/inspect_ref/itg/itg32.html
Associates of Cape Cod, Inc. http://www.acciusa.com/cts/
USP Sterility testing: http://www.usp797.org/index.html
http://www.mobio.com/services/services_view.php?id=8 http://www.clongen.com/endotoxin_testing.php?PHPSESSID=add6af185852e68a9909b8726a0eaea8

Sources of Isotopes
Spectra Stable gases: http://www.spectrastableisotopes.com/
Cambridge Isotopes: http://www.isotope.com/cil/index.html
Isotec(Sigma): http://www.sigmaaldrich.com/Area_of_Interest/Chemistry/Stable_Isotopes_ISOTEC_.html

Sample Size Calculators
For the difference between two proportions: http://newton.stat.ubc.ca/~rollin/stats/ssize/b2.html
For the difference between two means: http://newton.stat.ubc.ca/~rollin/stats/ssize/n2.html
For the ratio of two hazard rates: http://hedwig.mgh.harvard.edu/sample_size/time_to_event/para_time.html

Glossary

Buffy coat — It is the fraction of an anticoagulated blood sample after centrifugation that contains most of the white

	blood cells and platelets. It comprises the interstitial layer between the red cells and the plasma, and accounts for <1% of the total volume of the blood sample, and contains most of the white blood cells and platelets. It this contains the DNA component of (mammalian) blood.
CITI	Collaborative Institutional Training Initiative is an organization that provides a (subscription) service in ethics for researchers, and includes modules in patient privacy and biomedical research. Participating organizations require annual training and certification.
HIPAA	Health Insurance Portability and Accountability Act (1996).
IND	Investigational new drug. FDA approval for use of an agent in a manner different from its original designation, such as a New indication; Change in the approved route of administration or dosage level; Change in the approved patient population (e.g., pediatric) or a population at greater or increase of risk.
IBC	Institutional Biosafety Committee. All biological tissues and recombinant material must be approved by a biological safety committee that determines the level of risk from exposure. Human tissues require strict regulations for handling owing to the potential for disseminating disease, viruses, etc. Only authorized personnel may handle such specimens, and they must be provided with appropriate safety clothing, containment facilities and adequate sterilization procedures. This usually also requires undertaking additional biological safety training and blood borne pathogen training.
IRB	Institutional Review Boards. Ethical oversight committees for all biomedical experimentation. Ethical issues, statistical and basic science are all assessed for quality and legal requirements, and the committee can approve or deny any specific research project. This is designed to protect the subject as well as the institution and the researchers from ethicolegal breaches.
MRI/MRS	Magnetic resonance imaging/magnetic resonance spectroscopy. These are clinical manifestations of the NMR experiment (cf. Chap. 6). The former uses pulsed field gradients to obtain spatial resolution of an intense signal intrinsic to the object (usually tissue water), and produces high-resolution anatomical images especially of soft tissue. Some biochemical information can be obtained using

	chemical shift imaging. MRS is explicitly a spectroscopic approach that can be combined with imaging (image guided spectroscopy) and provides direct information about spatial distribution and concentrations of certain abundant metabolites. Variants of the approach can be used to obtain very detailed metabolic information in situ in an alert subject.
NSCLC	Non small cell lung cancer is a class of lung carcinoma that involves a variety of cell types that are distinguishable from the small cell type. Small cell carcinoma is usually not treatable by surgery, and generally chemotherapeutic regimens differ from the NSCLC. NSCL cancers comprise squamous cell carcinoma, adenocarcinoma (the two most common varieties), bronchioalveolar carcinoma (BAC) which is a subset of adenocarcinoma, and large cell carcinomas ("other") (36).
PET	Positron emission tomography is an imaging modality that detects the gamma photons emitted when a positron annihilates an electron. The positron is emitted from an unstable nuclide such as ^{18}F (half-life ca. 110 min) that is incorporated into a marker metabolite for injection. A common compound is ^{18}F-2-deoxyglucose, which is taken up by cells by the usual glucose transported, and phosphorylated by hexokinase. The resulting 6-phosphate is not further metabolized, so the radionuclide accumulates in cells that have active glucose transport, such as cancer cells (which also often have downregulated G6P phosphatase, thereby maintaining a high concentration of the labeled sugar).
PHI	Public health information covered under HIPAA rules regarding any health information of individuals.
Stable isotope	Isotopes are variants of an element that differ in the number of neutrons, but have the same number of protons (or atomic number). A stable isotope is one that does not decay into another elements or isotope. For example, there are three isotopes of hydrogen, containing 1 proton and 0 (protium, ^{1}H 99.99%), 1 (deuterium, ^{2}H 0.01%) or 2 (tritium, ^{3}H) neutrons. Protium and deuterium are stable, whereas tritium is radioactive, and emits a low energy electron (beta particle) to decay to a form of ^{3}He with a half-life of 12.32 years.
USP	US Pharmacopeia produces standards for drug safety that are effectively ratified by the FDA.

Appendices

Appendix 1: Example Study Order

Study Title: Metabolomic Analysis of Tissue: A Translational Clinical Trial

IRB# xxx

Patient # __________

1. Enroll patient ______________________ in IRB# xx, Hospital study number yyy "Metabolomic Analysis of tissue: A Translational Clinical Trial"

2. Dr. X or designee to begin infusion of study drug: 10 grams of ^{13}C-glucose in 50 ml sterile water for injection, I.V. piggy back, 100 cc hr, 2-6 hours prior to scheduled surgery time. Allow to run by gravity, no pump necessary.

   -Study drug will be supplied by pharmacy.

3. Follow study drug infusion with 50 cc normal saline to "flush" tubing. Heplock i.v. site after study med and normal saline flush.

<u>CAUTION</u> - DO NOT ADMINISTER ANY OTHER GLUCOSE-CONTAINING SOLUTIONS (MAINTENANCE IV FLUIDS ETC.) FROM TIME OF ADMISSION UNTIL AFTER SURGERY

4. NPO until after surgery once glucose bolus initiated

5. Serum Glucose check five minutes after glucose infusion begins

6. Draw purple top tube for study analysis x 2 – 15 minutes prior to infusion, 5 minutes after infusion completion. Study personnel will come to pick up the blood at the scheduled draw times.

6. Vital signs routine

For questions contact:

AB , RN (study nurse): mmm pgr.

CD (pharmacy): nnn pgr.

Appendix 2: Example IRB

Metabolomic Analysis of Lung Cancer: A Translational Clinical Trial of the Brown Cancer Center

Participants
Donald M. Miller, MD, PhD
Andrew Lane, PhD
Teresa Fan, PhD
Michael Bousamra, MD
Goetz Kloecker, MD
Agents: [U-^{13}C]-glucose

Objectives

Although it has been known for almost 80 years that cancer cells have marked changes in energy metabolism, the exact extent of these abnormalities in humans is completely unknown. The development of structural biology technologies which use NMR and mass spectroscopy has allowed scientists to analyze the metabolic characteristics of tumors at the *atomic* level. The development of metabolomics provides the ability to gather metabolic information which will drive the development of more effective and less toxic targeted therapies. The Cancer Center has a unique combination of infrastructure and expertise to perform *the first in situ metabolomic study of human cancer.* This protocol will use the infusion of uniformly ^{13}C labeled-glucose ([U-^{13}C]-Glc) 3 h prior to surgery to analyze the metabolic characteristics of these tumors.

The objectives of this protocol are:

1. To characterize the metabolism of glucose by the tumors of patients undergoing surgical resection of non-small cell lung cancer.
2. To characterize glycolytic metabolism in patients as demonstrated in serum metabolite analysis after C^{13}-glucose administration.

Background

Anaerobic glucose metabolism involving glycolysis evolved to produce energy for ancient anaerobic life forms before the existence of atmospheric oxygen. The glycolytic pathway and its enzymes, which convert glucose to pyruvate using the oxidative potential of NAD$^+$, are among the most ancient molecular metabolic networks. In the absence of oxygen, NAD$^+$ is regenerated from reduced NADH by the conversion of pyruvate to lactate. Glycolysis has been highly conserved among species, even after the emergence of atmospheric oxygen, which provided a means to further oxidize pyruvate by oxidative phosphorylation, resulting in a high yield of energy. Although ambient expression of glycolytic enzymes is necessary for steady-state glucose metabolism, the coordinated increased expression of genes encoding glycolytic enzymes is particularly important for adaptation to hypoxia.

Although the first observation that most tumor cells have a marked increase in glycolysis was made at least 100 years ago, the relationship between the abnormal proliferation of tumor cells and these metabolic changes has been unclear. However, it is apparent that increased activity of the glycolytic pathway results in the decreased pH which is characteristic of most human tumors. There is considerable evidence that the altered metabolism of cancer cells plays a role in the growth advantage, which these cells enjoy.

The development of metabolomics provides the opportunity to investigate changes in cellular metabolism in human tumors and patients with cancer. It is likely that these changes will be quite different from those seen in cancer cells in culture. These studies have not been done.

This section can be as long or short a needed for the particular study, and could include preliminary data and a generalized description of the analytical techniques for example.

Drug Information

[U-^{13}C]-glucose (dextrose).

Eligibility Criteria

Each of the criteria in the following section must be met in order for a patient to be considered eligible for registration. Use the spaces provided to confirm a patient's eligibility. For each patient, this section must be photocopied, completed and submitted to the Clinical Research Office.

1. Only patients with resectable lung cancer will be eligible to participate in this nontherapeutic study. Patients with non-small cell lung cancer will be eligible.
2. All patients must have general medical conditions to allow them to undergo surgical resection of their primary tumor.
3. Patients must be informed of the investigational nature of this study and sign and give written informed consent in accordance with institutional and federal guidelines.

Stratification Factors

All patients will have resectable lung cancer. Patients will be stratified into adeno and squamous cell non-small cell lung cancer for purposes of data analysis.

Treatment Plan

Each patient will receive 10 g of ^{13}C-glucose orally 3–12 h prior to scheduled resection of primary lung cancer. ^{13}C-glucose is nonradioactive and has no known toxicity. In fact, ^{13}C-glucose is present as approximately 1% of glucose in nature. Blood samples will be taken at 0, 3 and 12 h after oral administration of ^{13}C-glucose.

Criteria for Removal from Protocol Treatment

The patient may withdraw from the study at any time up to surgical resection for any reason.

Toxicities to be Monitored

The only potential toxicity with this treatment will be the possibility of hyperglycemia. Plasma glucose levels will be monitored at 0, 3 and 12 h after initiation of the glucose infusion. General medical conditions (vital signs) will be monitored at hourly intervals during the glucose infusion.

Statistical Considerations

1. The primary objective of this study is to determine the metabolic characteristics of primary lung tumors. The data will be analyzed for each patient individually. Patient response or life expectancy will not be taken into account.

Descriptive statistics will be computed for all subjects. Adverse events and toxicities will be summarized as well. Results will be reported for the patient group as a whole and for non-small cell tumor types as well. Where relevant, paired *t*-tests will be used for ^{13}C-labeled metabolites

Discipline Review

Pathology

(a) The goals of this pathology review are to verify the diagnosis of appropriate stage malignant melanoma, in order to validate patient eligibility; and to record detailed information about morphologic and histological features of the lesions, which will then be available for analyses of prognosis.
(b) Failure to submit the materials necessary for review will render the patient ineligible.
(c) The materials to be submitted are as follows: 5 H&E stained section from the primary lesion and nearby noncancerous lung tissue.

Registration Guidelines

1. Patients must be registered prior to initiation of treatment (no more than 5 working days prior to planned start of treatment).

To register a patient the following must be done (in order):

- Notification of the Clinical Trials Office at the Cancer Center
- Documentation of eligibility
- Execution of an informed consent
- Initiation of protocol treatment

Data Submission Schedule

1. Data must be submitted according to the protocol requirement; for *ALL* patients registered, whether or not assigned treatment is administered, including patients deemed to be ineligible.
2. Master forms are included in Sect. 18.
3. Once off treatment submit every 6 months until 5 years after registration then annually thereafter until 10 years after registration or death (whichever comes first).

Sample Collection

Peripheral blood will be obtained prior to administration of C^{13}-glucose (after registration) and at 3 and 12 h (after administration). Blood will be collected in a single purple top tube at each time point. Plasma will be prepared by centrifugation. White blood cells will be purified by Ficoll-Hypaque centrifugation.

Ethical and Regulatory Considerations

The following must be observed to comply with Food and Drug Administration regulations for the conduct and monitoring of clinical investigations; they also represent sound research practice:

Informed Consent

The principles of informed consent are described by Federal Regulatory Guidelines (Federal Register Vol. 46, No. 17, January 27, 1981, part 50) and the Office for Protection from Research Risks Reports: Protection of Human Subjects (Code of Federal Regulations 45 CFR 46). They must be followed to comply with FDA regulations for the conduct and monitoring of clinical investigations.

Institutional Review

This study must be approved by an appropriate institutional review committee as defined by Federal Regulatory Guidelines (Ref. Federal Register Vol. 46, No. 17, January 27, 1981, part 56) and the Office for Protection from Research Risks Reports: Protection of Human Subjects (Code of Federal Regulations 45 CFR 46).

Adverse Experiences

All adverse experiences must also be reported to the Institutional Review Board within 10 days and documentation of this report sent to the Clinical Trials Office.

All adverse experiences must also be recorded in the appropriate section of the case report form. The report should include, whenever possible, the investigator's written medical judgment as to relationship of the adverse experience to study medication(s) (i.e., "probable," "possible" or "unrelated").

Monitoring: This trial will be monitored by the Clinical Trials Office on a quarterly basis.

Adverse Reactions: Although we do not anticipate any adverse reactions from the administration of ^{13}C-glucose all patients will be carefully monitored for any evidence of hyperglycemia. Any complications attributable to administration of ^{13}C-glucose will be reported immediately to the Clinical Studies Unit of the Cancer Center.

Inclusion of Women and Minorities

The gender and race distribution in lung cancer studies reflects the unique risk factors for this disease. In Kentucky, 33% of all lung cancer patients are female and 25% are minority. We anticipate that these percentages will also apply to individuals entered on this study.

Appendix 3: Example Consent Form

This checklist is from the University of Louisville IRB committee and contains both federal and local requirements for generating specific consent forms.

Reference this checklist to your prepared informed consent. List the location of each of the requested checklist items by completing the Page number, paragraph number and line number information listed on the left side of the checklist.

*An asterisk following the item number indicates that the information is to be included in the informed consent if it is relevant to the study in question.

Page	Para	Line	Item #	Statement Descriptions	Source of Requirement
			1.	**INTRODUCTION AND BACKGROUND INFORMATION** State that the subject is invited (not asked) to participate.	Local IRB
			2.	Indicate it is a research study.	Federal, basic
			3.	Name the sponsor. Identify the University department, as well as any sponsoring agencies.	Local IRB
			4.*	Indicate the approximate number of local subjects in the study.	Federal, when appropriate
			5.*	Indicate the place where the study will be conducted, e.g., campus, school, office or home.	Local IRB
			6.	**PURPOSE** State the scientific purpose of the study in non-technical language. Give the background of the study including the reason for the study and rationale for conducting the study.	Federal, basic
			7.	**PROCEDURES** Describe the procedures to be performed in the study, acknowledging those that are experimental by using the word "experimental". Use language a middle school student could understand.	Federal, basic, Local IRB
			8.*	**If the study involves randomization, state this and explain the term; e.g., a process 'like flipping a coin'.**	Local IRB, interpretation of federal
			9.	Indicate the expected duration of the subject's participation in the study (days or hours).	Federal, basic
			10.*	If the study involves multiple sessions with the subject, estimate the amount of time for each session.	Local IRB, interpretation of federal
			11.	**POTENTIAL RISKS** Describe any reasonably foreseeable physical risks and/or discomforts to subjects. If questions are to be asked that may be sensitive and produce discomfort (e.g., recollections of past stressful situations), state this. If some of the questions to be answered are incriminating, state that there is a risk of prosecution. If there are no reasonably foreseeable risks, so state. There may also be risks with associated procedures performed as part of the research study. Include the risks associated with the clinical procedures that are part of the study. Other risks that should be included are: psychological risks, social risks, economic risks, and/or legal risks.	

(continued)

Page	Para	Line	Item #	Statement Descriptions	Source of Requirement
			12.*	State that there may be unforeseeable risks to the subject.	Federal, when appropriate
			13.	**BENEFITS** Describe any benefits to subjects or to others that may be reasonably expected from the research. If none, then so state. State: Although the information collected may not benefit the subject directly, the informed may be helpful to others.	Federal, basic
			14.*	**COMPENSATION** If applicable, state whether there is payment for participation and the amount to be paid. Do not state that subjects will be paid for their participation. State, rather, that they will be compensated for their time, inconvenience, and expenses.	Local IRB
			15.*	State that payment for participation will be prorated in the event the subject withdraws before completion of the study.	Local IRB
			16.*	**RESEARCH RELATED INJURY – Review and use the template language on who pays for injury.** State whether medical treatment is available.	Federal, basic
			17.*	State who will pay for the treatment. If industry sponsored, pick the option that best matches the proposed contract language.	Federal, basic; Local IRB interpretation
			18.*	State who to contact about the research related injury.	Federal, basic
			19.*	State whether there is any additional financial compensation to cover items such as lost wages, inconvenience, discomfort, etc.	Federal, basic
			20.	**CONFIDENTIALITY** Acknowledge that total confidentiality cannot be guaranteed. ***Note:** Not needed if the subject will be identified. If so, state this in the consent form.	Federal, basic; Local IRB interpretation
			21.	State that in all other respects the data will be held in confidence to the extent permitted by law.	Federal, basic; Local IRB interpretation
			22.	State that, should the data be published, the subject's identity will not be revealed.	Federal, basic; Local IRB interpretation
			23.	Indicate who may look at the subject's medical and research records. Use the following recommended list. This information should also be included in Section 3 of the Research Authorization. • The sponsor and others hired by the sponsor to oversee the research (include only is the study is sponsored) • The University of Louisville Institutional Review Board, Human Subjects Protection Program Office, Privacy Office, and others involved with research administration (include Privacy Office only if HIPAA is involved) • People who are responsible for research and HIPAA oversight at the institutions where the study is conducted (include only is study conducted in a covered entity) • Government agencies, such as: (List all that apply) o Office for Human Research Protections (OHRP),	Federal, basic; Local IRB interpretation

Page	Para	Line	Item #	Statement Descriptions	Source of Requirement
				o Office of Civil Rights (include if HIPAA is required) o Other (please specify) • People who make sure that billing is submitted correctly.	
			24.*	State how the data collected will be kept private and secure. The description should include how the subjects data will be protected from disclosure and physically secured.	Federal, basic; Local IRB interpretation
			25.	**CONFLICT OF INTEREST – Include if this is a sponsored study.** This study involves a conflict of interest because (***Select one of the following three options. Delete the remaining options and instructions prior to submission.*** (1) the institution, (2) the investigator or (3) the institution and investigator) will be compensated for your participation in it. Ask the investigator how ***Select one of the following three options. Delete the remaining options and instructions prior to submission.*** (1) the institution, (2) the investigator or (3) the institution and investigator) will benefit by your participation in the study.	Local IRB
			26.*	**HIPAA Research Authorization – This section should only be included if the PI will access PHI. Use the statement shown below exactly.** **The Health Insurance Portability and Accountability Act of 1996 (HIPAA) provides federal safeguards for protected health information (PHI). Examples of PHI are your name, address, and birth date. PHI may also include your medical history, results of health exams and lab tests, drugs taken and results of this research study. Your PHI cannot be used or shared without your agreement, unless it meets one of the HIPAA exceptions. You will be asked to sign a "Research Authorization" form. This allows the use and sharing of your PHI by those listed in the "Research Authorization."**	Federal, when appropriate
			27.	**VOLUNTARY PARTICIPATION** Indicate that participation is voluntary.	Federal, basic
			28.	State that the subject may refuse to participate without incurring any penalty or losing any benefits to which he/she is otherwise entitled.	Federal, basic
			29.	State that the subject may discontinue participation at any time without incurring any penalty or losing any benefits to which he/she is otherwise entitled.	Federal, basic
			30.*	State that any new findings that could affect willingness to participate will be shared with the subject.	Federal, when appropriate
			31.	**RESEARCH SUBJECT'S RIGHTS, QUESTIONS, CONCERNS, COMPLAINTS** State: "If you have any concerns or complaints about the study or the study staff, you have three options. You may contact the principal investigator at XXX-XXXX. If you have any questions about your rights as a study subject, questions, concerns or complaints, you may call the Human Subjects Protection Program Office (HSPPO)	Federal, basic; Local IRB interpretation

(continued)

Page	Para	Line	Item #	Statement Descriptions	Source of Requirement
				at (502) 852-5188. You may discuss any questions about your rights as a subject, in secret, with a member of the Institutional Review Board (IRB) or the HSPPO staff. The IRB is an independent committee composed of members of the University community, staff of the institutions, as well as lay members of the community not connected with these institutions. The IRB has reviewed this study. ***(Do not state approved. This section is mandatory for all studies.)*** If you want to speak to a person outside the University, you may call 1-877-852-1167. You will be given a chance to talk about any questions, concerns, or complaints in secret. This is a 24 hour hot line answered by people who do not work at the University of Louisville.	
			32.	State: This paper tells you what will happen during the study if you choose to take part. Your signature means that this study has been discussed with you, that your questions have been answered, and that you will take part in the study. This informed consent document is not a contract. You are not giving up any legal rights by signing this informed consent document. You will be given a signed copy of this paper to keep for your records.	Federal, basic; Local IRB interpretation
			33.	Provide a line and caption for the "Printed name of the subject/legal representative."	Local IRB
			34.*	Provide lines for the signatures of the parties involved (subject/legal representative, and investigator). Include a separate "date signed" line for each signature line. In studies involving minors aged seven or above, the minor involved will sign an assent form to indicate awareness of his/her role in the study.	Federal, basic
			35.*	Provide a line for "Person Explaining Consent if other than the Investigator". Include a "date signed" line.	Local IRB

References

1. Kaddurah-Daouk R, Kristal BS, Weinshilboum RM. Metabolomics: a global biochemical approach to drug response and disease. Annu Rev Pharmacol Toxicol. 2008;48: 23.21–32.31.
2. Fan TW-M, Lane AN, Higashi RM. The promise of metabolomics in cancer molecular therapeutics. Curr Opin Mol Ther. 2004;6:584–92.
3. Serkova NJ, Spratlin JL, Eckhardt SG. NMR-based metabolomics: translational application and treatment of cancer. Curr Opin Mol Ther. 2007;9:572–85.
4. Di Buono M, Jones PJH, Beaumier L, Wykes LJ. Comparison of deuterium incorporation and mass isotopomer distribution analysis for measurement of human cholesterol biosynthesis. J Lipid Res. 2000;41:1516–23.
5. Mason GF, Petersen KF, de Graaf RA, Kanamatsu T, Otsuki T, Rothman DL. A comparison of C-13 NMR measurements of the rates of glutamine synthesis and the tricarboxylic acid cycle during oral and intravenous administration of 1-C-13 glucose. Brain Res Protoc. 2002;10:181–90.
6. Patel AB, de Graaf RA, Mason GF, Rothman DL, Shulman RG, Behar KL. The contribution of GABA to glutamate/glutamine cycling

and energy metabolism in the rat cortex in vivo. Proc Natl Acad Sci USA. 2005;102:5588–93.
7. Fan TW, Lane AN. Structure-based profiling of metabolites and isotopomers by NMR. Prog NMR Spectrosc. 2008;52:69–117.
8. Mayes PD, Bender DA. In: Murray RK, Granner DK, Mayes PA, Rodwell VW, editors. Harper's illustrated biochemistry. 26th ed. McGraw-Hill: New York; 2003.
9. Lane AN, Fan TW-M, Higashi RM. Stable isotope assisted metabolomics in cancer research. IUBMB Life. 2008;60:124–9.
10. Lindon JC, Holmes E, Nicholson JK. Toxicological applications of magnetic resonance. Prog Nucl Magn Reson Spectrosc. 2004; 45:109–43.
11. Bollard ME, Stanley EG, Lindon JC, Nicholson JK, Holmes E. NMR-based metabonomic approaches for evaluating physiological influences on biofluid composition. NMR Biomed. 2005;18:143–62.
12. Lindon JC, Nicholson JK, Everett JR. Annual reports on NMR spectroscopy, vol. 38. San Diego: Academic Press; 1999. p. 1–88.
13. Fan TWM, Lane AN, Higashi RM. The promise of metabolomics in cancer molecular therapeutics. Curr Opin Mol Ther. 2004;6:584–92.
14. Griffin JL, Kauppinen RA. Tumour metabolomics in animal models of human cancer. J Proteome Res. 2007;6:498–505.
15. Ippolito JE, Xu J, Jain SJ, Moulder K, Mennerick S, Crowley JR, Townsend RR, Gordon JI. An integrated functional genomics and metabolomics approach for defining poor prognosis in human neuroendocrine cancers. Proc Natl Acad Sci U S A. 2005;102:9901–6.
16. Zimmermann D, Hartmann M, Moyer MP, Nolte J, Baumbach JI. Determination of volatile products of human colon cell line metabolism by GC/MS analysis. Metabolomics. 2007;3:13–7.
17. Kind T, Tolstikov V, Fiehn O, Weiss RH. A comprehensive urinary metabolomic approach for identifying kidney cancer. Anal Biochem. 2007;363:185–95.
18. Beger RD, Schnackenberg LK, Holland RD, Li DH, Dragan Y. Metabonomic models of human pancreatic cancer using 1D proton NMR spectra of lipids in plasma. Metabolomics. 2006;2:125–34.
19. Hoffmeister KN, Falet H, Toker A, Barkalow KL, StosselDagger TP, Hartwig JH. Mechanisms of cold-induced platelet actin assembly. J Biol Chem. 2001;276:24751–9.
20. Tablin F, Oliver AE, Walker NJ, Crowe LM, Crowe JH. Membrane phase transition of intact human platelets: correlation with cold-induced activation. J Cell Physiol. 1996;168:305–13.
21. Saude EJ, Sykes BD. Urine stability for metabolomic studies: effects of preparation and storage. Metabolomics. 2007;3:19–27.
22. Saude EJ, Adamko D, Rowe BH, Marrie T, Sykes BD. Variation of metabolites in normal human urine. Metabolomics. 2007;3:439–51.
23. Viant MR, Ludwig C, Rhodes S, Günther UL, Allaway D. Validation of a urine metabolome fingerprint in dog for phenotypic classification. Metabolomics. 2007;3:453–63.
24. Wilson JF. Health Insurance Portability and Accountability Act Privacy Rule causes ongoing concerns among clinicians and researchers. Ann Intern Med. 2006;145:313–6.
25. Harrigan GG, Goodacre R, editors. Metabolic profiling: its role in biomarker discovery and gene function analysis. New York: Springer; 2003.
26. Trygg J, Holmes E, Lundstedt T. Chemometrics in metabonomics. J Proteome Res. 2007;6:469–79.
27. Kettaneh N, Berglund A, Wold S. PCA and PLS with very large data sets. Comput Stat Data Anal. 2005;48:69–85.
28. Rossner B. Fundamentals of biostatistics. 6th ed. Belmont: Thomson; 2006.
29. Fan TWM. Recent advances in profiling plant metabolites by multinuclear and multidimensional NMR. In: Shachar-Hill Y, Pfeffer PE, editors. Nuclear magnetic resonance in plant biology, Vol 16. American Society of Plant Physiologists, Rockville; 1996. p. 181–254.
30. Fan TWM. Metabolite profiling by one- and two-dimensional NMR analysis of complex mixtures. Prog Nucl Magn Reson Spectrosc. 1996;28:161–219.
31. Lane AN, Fan TW. Quantification and identification of isotopomer distributions of metabolites in crude cell extracts using ^{1}H TOCSY. Metabolomics. 2007;3:79–86.
32. Fan TW, Lane AN, Higashi RM, Farag MA, Gao H, Bousamra M, Miller DM. Altered regulation of metabolic pathways in human lung cancer discerned by ^{13}C stable isotope-resolved metabolomics (SIRM). Mol Cancer. 2009;8:41.
33. Lane AN, Fan TW, Higashi RM, Tan J, Bousamra M, Miller DM. Prospects for clinical cancer metabolomics using stable isotope tracers. J Exp Mol Pathol. 2009;86:165–73.
34. Fan TW-M, Lane AN, Higashi M, Bousamra M, Kloecker G, Miller DM. Erlotinib-sensitive and resistant lung tumors show radically different metabolic profiles. Exp Mol Pathol. 2009;87:83–6.

35. Lane AN, Fan TW-M, Bousamra II M, Higashi RM, Yan J, Miller DM. Clinical applications of stable isotope-resolved metabolomics (SIRM) in non-small cell lung cancer. Omics. 2011;15:173–182.
36. Edelman RJ, Gandara DR. Lung Cancer. In: Casciato DA, editor. Manual of clinical oncology. 5th ed. Philadelphia: Lippincott Williams & Wilkins; 2004.
37. Griffin JL, Nicholls AW, Daykin CA, Heald S, Keun HC, Schuppe-Koistinen I, Griffiths JR, Cheng LL, Rocca-Serra P, Rubtsov DV, et al. Standard reporting requirements for biological samples in metabolomics experiments: mammalian/in vivo experiments. Metabolomics. 2007;3:179–88.
38. Goodacre R, Broadhurst D, Smilde AK, Kristal BS, Baker JD, Beger R, Bessant C, Connor S, Calmani G, Craig A, et al. Proposed minimum reporting standards for data analysis in metabolomics. Metabolomics. 2007;3:231–41.
39. Boros LG. Metabolic targeted therapy of cancer: current tracer technologies and future drug design strategies in the old metabolic network. Metabolomics. 2005;1:11–5.
40. Harrigan GG, Brackett DJ, Boros LG. Medicinal chemistry, metabolic profiling and drug target discovery: a role for metabolic profiling in reverse pharmacology and chemical genetics. Mini Rev Med Chem. 2005;5:13–20.

Chapter 4

Structural Mass Spectrometry for Metabolomics

Richard M. Higashi

Abstract

Structural mass spectrometry (MS) is a chemical structure-revealing analytical technique that measures mass/charge ratio of ions. Biochemical analyses in the context of metabolomics—which seeks chemical descriptions of cellular, organismal, and even community biology—pose challenges distinct from past applications of MS. The scientific need for both far greater depth and breadth of metabolic analytes is manifested analytically in two general approaches: the "Biomarker" approach and the "Pathway" approach. In this chapter, the basic principles of mass spectrometry relevant to these two approaches to metabolomics are reviewed. The emphasis is on practical aspects of how experimental design interacts with instrument designs and capabilities. Both simulated theoretical and real-life analyses are used to illustrate the key concepts and their ramifications.

Key words: High resolution MS, Stable isotope resolved metabolomics, Isotopologue analysis, Metabolic pathways

Abbreviations

ddMSn	Data-dependent MSn
FT-ICR	Fourier transform ion cyclotron resonance
GC	Gas chromatography
HIT	High information throughput
ICP-MS	Inductively coupled plasma MS
IR	Infrared
LC	Liquid chromatography
MDLs	Minimum detectable limits
MQLs	Minimum quantifiable limits
MRM	Multiple reaction monitoring
MS	Mass spectrometry
MS2	MS to the 2nd or tandem MS
MSn	MS to the nth
NA	Natural abundance
NMR	Nuclear magnetic resonance spectroscopy
PC	Phosphatidylcholine

Teresa Whei-Mei Fan et al. (eds.), *The Handbook of Metabolomics*, Methods in Pharmacology and Toxicology, DOI 10.1007/978-1-61779-618-0_4, © Springer Science+Business Media New York 2012

RF Radio frequency
SIRM Stable isotope-resolved metabolomics
ToF Time of flight
UV Ultraviolet visible

1. Introduction to MS

1.1. What is MS? The MS Experiment

Structural mass spectrometry (MS) is a chemical structure-revealing analytical technique that measures mass/charge ratio of ions. If the ion is singly charged, then it measures the putative molecular mass. Often, the ions decompose in the MS, leading to fragmentation that is rich in chemical structure information (see Fig. 1), sometimes revealing even the subatomic composition. All of these properties are extremely useful in metabolomics, as will be seen. The use of mass spectrometers for nonstructural analyses, such as ICP-MS and isotope-ratio MS, is beyond the scope of this chapter; ICP-MS is treated in Chap. 5.

Most structure-revealing analytical measurements are spectroscopies that use ranges of the electromagnetic spectrum; for example, NMR is in the radio frequency (RF) range, and ESR is in the microwave region. In fact, the names of the techniques are often descriptive of their frequency range (IR, near IR, visible, UV, X-ray, etc.).

In contrast, MS is found nowhere in the electromagnetic spectrum. As illustrated in Fig. 1, it is a technique that is based on physical–chemical reactions and ionic separations, and therefore is an "experiment" in the same sense of the NMR experiment. One does not just "take a spectrum" or "analyze by MS," but rather has to plan the MS experiment to conduct. MS is also distinguished by

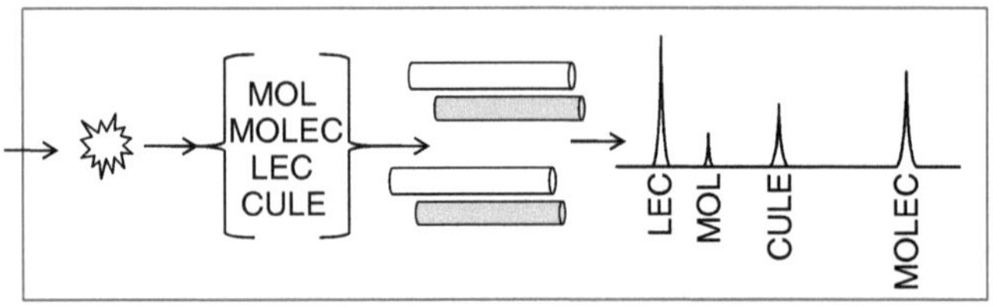

Fig. 1. Schematic illustration of the mass spectrometry (MS) "experiment." Ionized molecules are fragmented, and the fragment ions of a single mass/charge ratio (*m/z*) are passed by a "quadrupole" MS instrument; this acts as a filter and all other ions are rejected during that period. By rapidly changing the *m/z* that is to be passed, a spectrum of intensity vs. time is generated. The time abscissa is then calibrated to *m/z* to produce a mass spectrum. Here, the molecule MOLECULE is fragmented into a pattern that is representative of the original structure. Unlike most forms of spectroscopy, MS entails degradative physical–chemical reactions; experimental control over these reactions produces the desired type of data.

the fact that it necessarily destroys the sample. This in part accounts for the use of the term "spectrometry" to describe the technique, and is usually distinct from other forms of "spectroscopy."

1.2. Why MS for Metabolomics? Perspective from Modern MS

It is vital to note that this chapter covers MS usage for "metabolomics." Although the century-long history of MS can provide valuable lessons and insights, the marriage of MS with metabolomics is a comparatively recent event. Thus, the historical perspective is evoked only when deemed necessary. For an appreciation of historic MS development, the reader is referred to older books (1). For over half a century, MS has been a tool of choice for the study of the "metabolism" of drugs, pesticides, nutrients, pollutants, and other xenobiotics; for those perspectives, the reader is referred to the many excellent books and reviews on these topics.

Biochemical analyses in the context of metabolomics—which seeks chemical descriptions of cellular, organismal, and even community biology—pose challenges distinct from past applications of MS. First, the problem in metabolomics is to distinguish small differences in metabolite patterns in the presence of an overwhelmingly greater background of the same metabolites. Second, this feat must be accomplished on literally many orders of magnitude more analytes than in past applications of MS. Third, the concentration ranges needed to solve metabolomic problems can span 12 orders of magnitude. These analytical problems are far greater than any single analysis can address.

This scientific need for both far greater depth and breadth of metabolic analytes is manifested analytically in two general approaches: the "Biomarker" approach and the "Pathway" approach. In the former, MS is utilized for its capability of high sensitivity and selectivity, with acceptable precision. This helps to *statistically* distinguish concentration profiles of mixtures of analytes, which is the chemical signature that is sought. In the Pathway approach, MS is used to distinguish among isotopologues (sometimes also called "mass isotopomers") of metabolites with high sensitivity, which yields the biochemical signatures. In both cases, the information generated by MS is highly complementary to NMR, and in effect is the only practical analytical partner to NMR for the Pathway approach. Generally, these two are the only analytical techniques that can distinguish and quantify the necessarily large number of metabolites together with their isotopomers, across the necessary span of concentrations.

The current state of MS instrument development enables interfacing to most separation techniques (see below), with high sensitivity down to the sub-pM range, structural information from pmole amounts of analyte, and rapid generation of spectral data. Moreover, the technology is experiencing extremely active developments on all fronts, generally leading to greater performance at lower costs or extended performance at the high end of MS instrumentation, and improved ease of use and reliability.

2. Information Encoded by the Mass Spectrum

2.1. The Mass Spectrum

In order to understand the uses of MS in metabolomics, it is crucial to first understand the types of information provided by MS. It is instructive to start with the traditional graphical conveyance of MS information: the mass spectrum.

Shown in Fig. 2 is a mass spectrum of the reduced form of nicotinamide adenine dinucleotide reduced form (NADH) along with the historically more prevalent representation, the mass histogram. The histogram is summary of the actual spectrum via a process called "centroiding." As will become clear later, this distinction is important. The abscissa in Fig. 2 reflects the second central concept

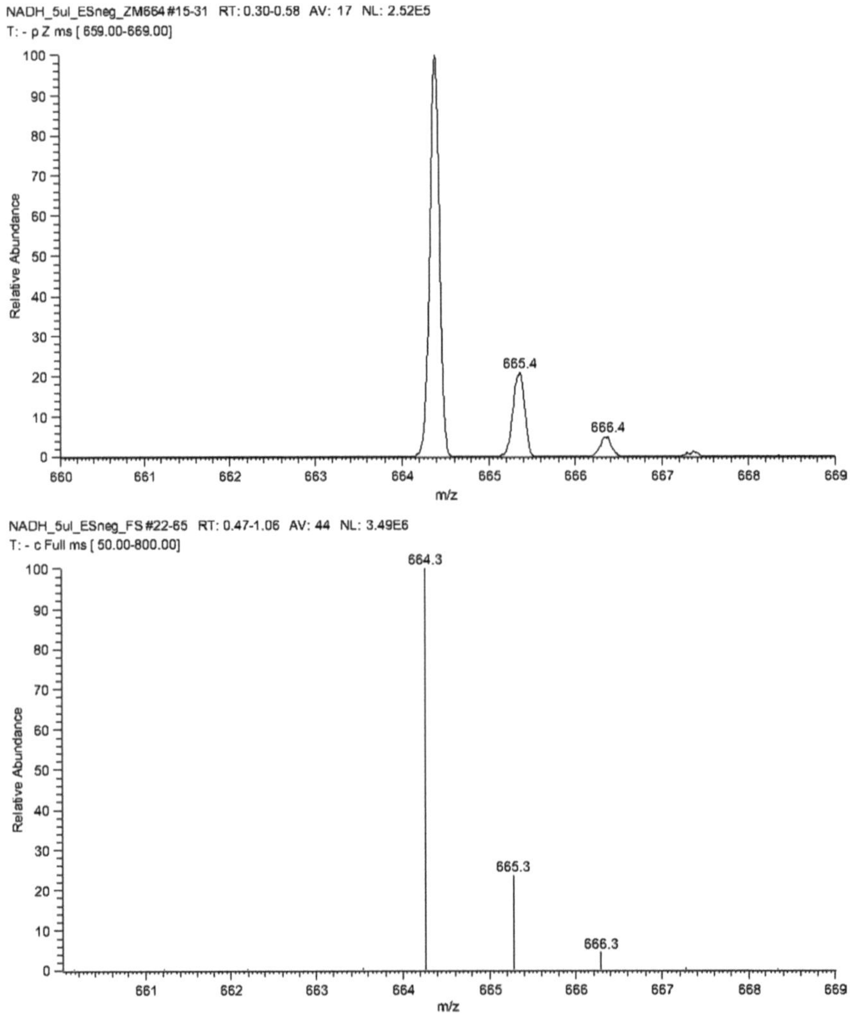

Fig. 2. *Top panel*: Mass spectrum of nicotinamide adenine dinucleotide reduced form (NADH). *Bottom panel*: Mass histogram of NADH. Both are unpublished data by the author.

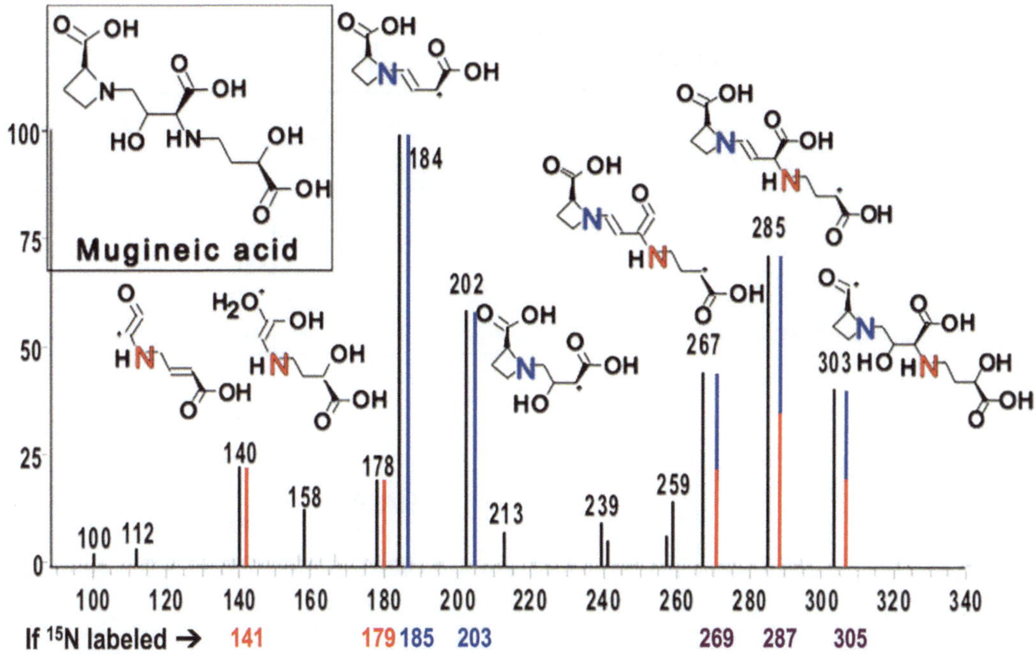

Fig. 3. Fragmentation of mugineic acid illustrating how fragmentation (Fig. 1) conveys structural information, including isotopic composition. The black-line portion of the figure represents the mass histogram of unlabeled mugineic acid, with the corresponding fragment structures assigned above each bar. Such mass histograms are often not interpreted for fragment structures at all, but instead the pattern is used for confirming identity by comparison with authentic standards. The red- and blue-colored lines represent the mass histogram if both nitrogens were labeled with ^{15}N, with the resulting *m/z* of the fragment ions listed below the abscissa. Note that some of the ions shift 1 *m/z* (*red* or *blue*) while others shift 2 *m/z* (*red* + *blue* lines denoted by purple values) because they contain one or two ^{15}N, respectively. In this fashion, it is possible to determine if a metabolite had zero, one, or two ^{15}N, and the relative amount of label in each position. Redrawn from 10.

that an MS instrument measures mass-to-charge ratios (m/z), not mass. A third central concept is that only charged ions are measured; neutral molecules are not measured by MS instruments.

Figure 3 illustrates several aspects of a fourth concept: fragmentation. The mass histogram consists of many ions of different m/z from a single molecule, described in Fig. 3 and its legend. Fragmentation of the molecular ion conveys structural information, the pattern of which is used for identification by comparison with fragmentation patterns of authentic chemical standards or for interpretation of structure. The use of fragment information varies enormously by discipline. For example, in drug analysis, fragment patterns are the most important information for identification, since the structures are known and authentic standards are available; thus, interpretation of fragment patterns is rarely performed. In contrast, MS-based proteomics uses fragment patterns almost exclusively for sequence structure interpretation, and comparison with authentic standards is generally not done because it is often extremely impractical.

In Biomarker and Pathway metabolomics approaches, both uses of fragment patterns are practiced for confirming identities of

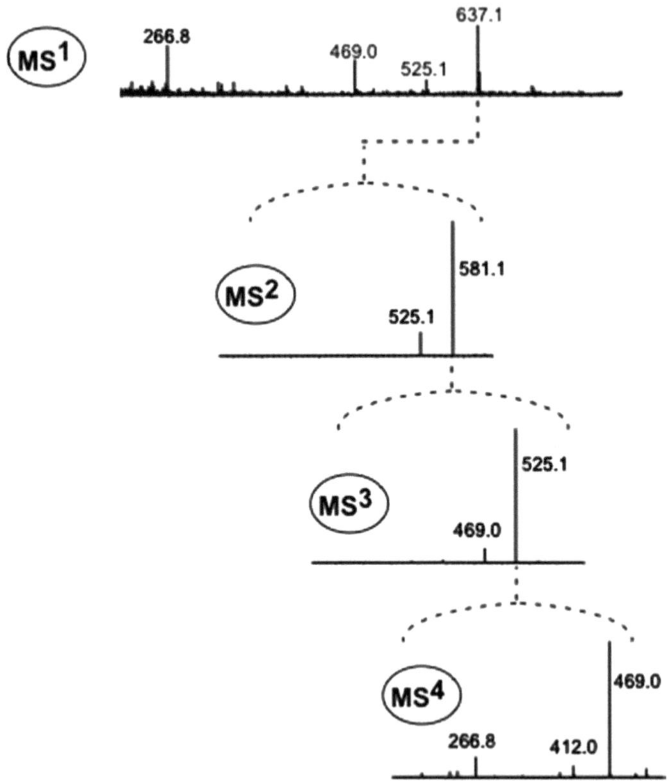

Fig. 4. Illustration of tandem MSn. These spectra were obtained directly from a crude extract of wheat plant under continuous nanoelectrospray ion trap MS, total acquisition time was <30 s, and the precursor ion of 637.1 *m/z* is an unknown metabolite. MSn attains sequential control of fragmentation, thus establishing the provenance of the *m/z* ions labeled in the MS1 spectrum. Figure redrawn from 10.

known metabolites, as well as attempting to identify unknown or unexpected metabolites. In addition, there is a third use of fragment patterns for only the Pathway approach: submolecular localization of isotopic incorporation. Figure 3 illustrates how the locations and number of ^{15}N atoms incorporated can be discerned, which are direct pathway clues. This has been used, for example, to follow the fate of N from nitrate by rice coleoptiles (2).

The overarching importance of fragmentation led to the development of “tandem” MS or, more generally, “MS to the nth” (MSn). Figure 4 and its legend illustrate this fifth concept, whereby a series of related MS spectra are generated, roughly analogous to 1D vs 2D-NMR. The practice of MSn attains sequential control over fragmentation, allowing unambiguous assignment of fragment ions to their source molecule. For example, two phosphatidylcholine (PC) metabolites with acyl chains of C16:O and C18:3 (PC1) or C16:1 and C18:2 (PC2) have the identical molecular ion exact-mass of 756.554321 m/z (M + H), thus unresolvable in a single-spectrum MS. However, the two PC lipids have different

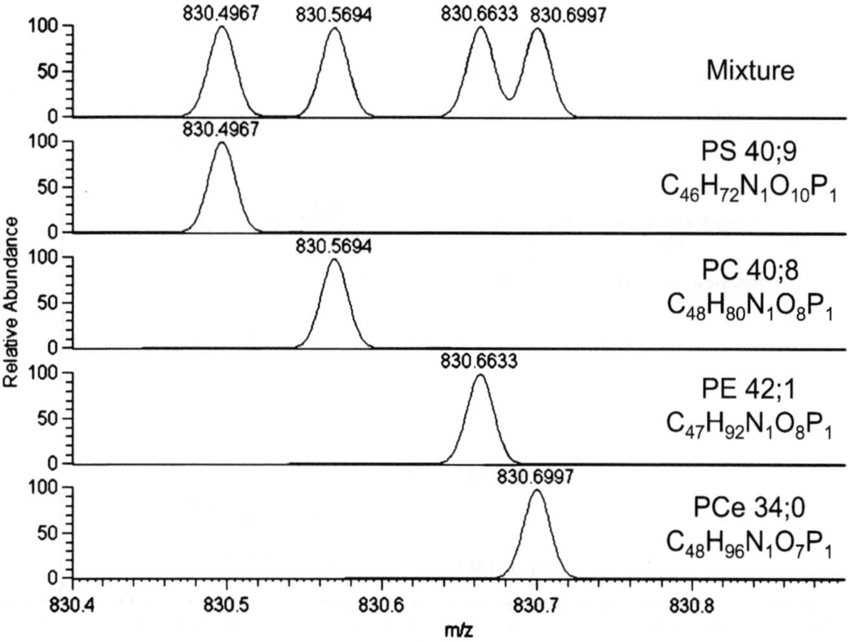

Fig. 5. Spectral simulations of protonated adducts of four diacyl glycerophospholipids (gPLs) illustrating an important use of accurate mass. In this case, accurate mass is used to distinguish, in a mixture, among these four different classes of lipids that have very similar *m/z* near 830.6. They differ in molecular formulae, and thus differ also in their accurate mass. The spectral range shown is 0.5 Da, and sufficient resolution was simulated to distinguish the four lipid species. The naming conventions are *PS* phosphatidyl serine; *PC* phosphatidylcholine; *PE* phosphatidyl ethanolamine; *PCe* phosphatidylcholine plasmalogen (ether linkage). The numerals denote the total [# C]; [# unsaturations] across the two acyl chains.

tandem MS fragments from, e.g., loss of different acyl chains. Namely, the ions of 501.321916 *m/z* (loss of C16:0) and 479.337566 *m/z* (loss of C18:3) are indicative of PC lipid with C16:0 and C18:3 acyl chains while the mass of 503.337566 *m/z* (loss of C16:1) and 477.321916 *m/z* (loss of C18:2) can be assigned to PC lipid with C16:1 and C18:2 acyl chains. Thus, tandem MS can distinguish different structures with the same molecular ion (identical molecular formulae).

A sixth concept is that of "exact" mass, also called accurate mass, illustrated in Fig. 5. The major utility of accurate mass is the determination of molecular formulae. In metabolomics, a given molecular formula usually corresponds to just a handful of known metabolites given the biological source; hence, an array of accurate mass information alone can enable assignment (tentative identities) to many hundreds, sometimes thousands, of peaks in a single spectrum. However, the attainment of sufficiently accurate mass data is technically demanding and not achieved by most MS instruments on the market today. One interesting fact shown in Fig. 5 is that very close (<1 *m/z*) peaks are *not* closely related structures; rather, they are substantially different in molecular formula.

A seventh concept conveyed by the mass spectrum is that of resolving power or resolution. The resolution of an MS instrument

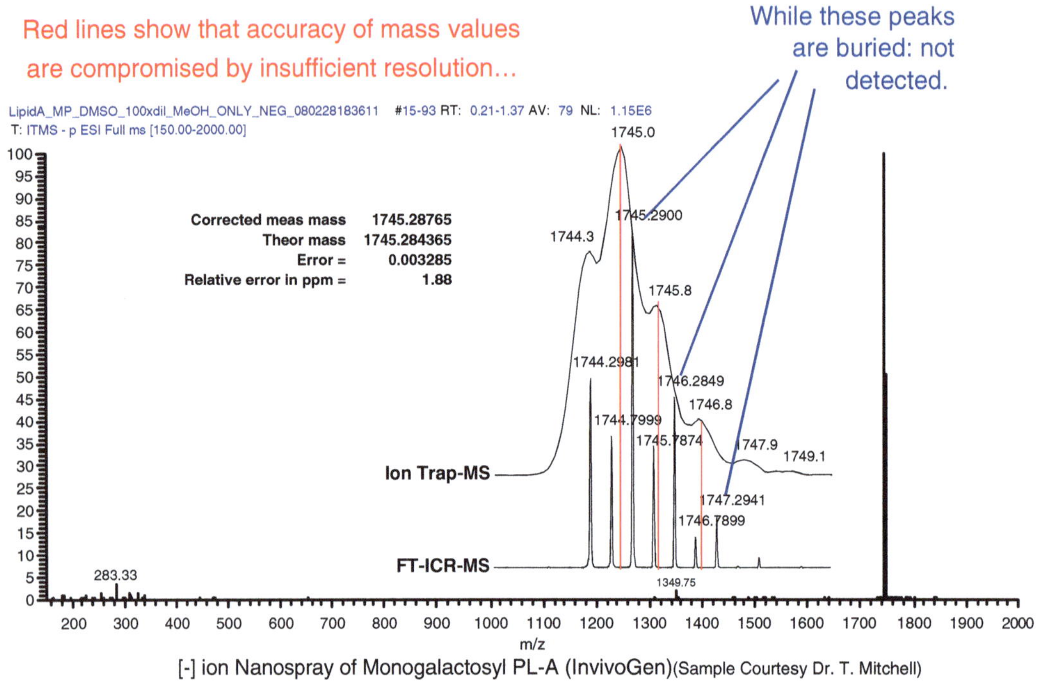

Fig. 6. Negative ion mass spectra of monogalactosyl PL-A (InvivoGen) illustrating the influence of resolution on mass accuracy. Spectra were obtained using a Thermo LTQ-FT MS hybrid ion trap/FT-ICR-MS instrument. Under continuous spray, spectral acquisition was alternated between low resolution (ion trap MS) and high resolution (FT-ICR-MS) repeatedly so that the spectra shown are a true average over a 5-min acquisition span. Note that low resolution returns average values that are nonexistent *m/z* peaks (false positive), as shown by the red lines; here, as in other cases, the reader is reminded that averages are values that do not actually exist. At the same time, low resolution fails to reveal the presence of some peaks that actually do exist (false negative), as shown by the *blue lines*. Unpublished data by the author.

is generally defined as $m1/(m1 - m2)$, where $m1$ and $m2$ are two peaks of equal intensity with 10% overlap. A common practice is to set $m1 = 400\ m/z$ because the actual resolving power varies across the spectrum depending on the design of the instrument. By selecting a single m/z, specifications can be compared. Thus, *resolving power* $= R(400\ m/z, 10\%) = 4{,}000$ means that the MS instrument is able to discriminate unambiguously (with only 10% overlap) between two equally sized peaks at 400.0 and 400.1 m/z. It is important to note that such a specification is dependent on the m/z; thus, if $R(400\ m/z, 10\%) = 4{,}000$ but the analyte of interest is $m1 = 800\ m/z$, then that same resolution specification is theoretically reduced to 2,000 for the analyte of interest. It is also important to note that a mass histogram contains no information regarding resolving power.

It turns out that "sufficient" resolution must be achieved in order to obtain useful accurate mass, as previously shown in Fig. 5 (where $R = 40{,}000$ was used) and further shown in Fig. 6 and its legend. In this illustration, the accuracy of the m/z (intensity-weighted center of an m/z peak) is affected by the "purity" of

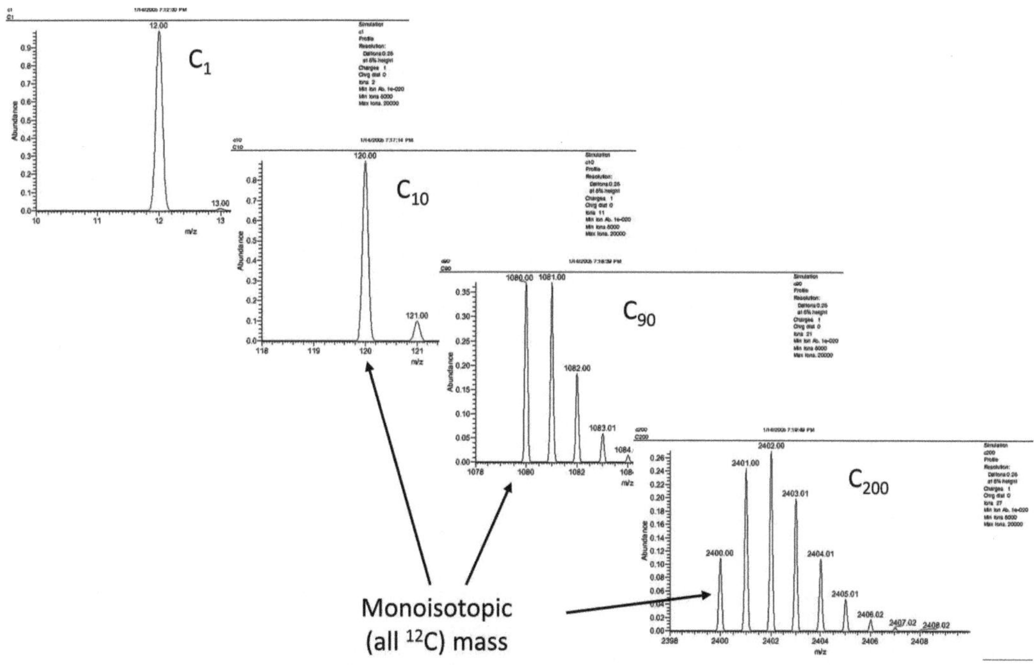

Fig. 7. Illustration of isotopic abundance dependence on number of carbons. The series of simulated spectra are of pure carbon compounds of the designated number of carbons. In the C_1 spectrum, the $^{13}C_1$ peak ($m + 1$ isotopologue) has the expected natural abundance (intensity) of approximately 1.1%. For the C_{10} spectrum, the $m + 1$ isotopologue has ten possible locations to populate, increasing by 10× the probability of the molecule harboring a single ^{13}C isotope. Thus, the $^{12}C_9{}^{13}C_1$ peak is $1.1\% \times 10 = 11\%$ the abundance. At C_{90}, the $m + 1$ isotopologue is approximately the same abundance as the monoisotopic. Furthermore, the $^{12}C_{89}{}^{13}C_1$ peak itself has a natural abundance peak of one more ^{13}C ($m + 2$, or $^{12}C_{88}{}^{13}C_2$) and so forth, forming a cluster of molecular ions. Note that at C_{200} the molecular ion cluster is dominated by the various ^{13}C isotopologues.

each *m/z* peak, which in turn is a function of the resolution. Note that insufficient resolution in this case led to both false positives and false negatives with regards to the mass spectral peaks, even in this simplest case of a pure standard. A further consequence of insufficient resolution is also seen in Fig. 6, namely, that intensities are nonrepresentative of the individual peaks, hampering quantification if these peaks had originated from different metabolites.

Thus, MS instruments sporting excellent accurate mass specifications cannot realize this advantage on real-life complex samples (or even the pure standard in Fig. 6) without sufficiently good resolving power. As is the case with accurate mass, the attainment of very high resolution is technically demanding and not achieved by most MS instruments. In fact, the need to achieve simultaneous accurate mass with high resolution only compounds the difficulty.

An eighth key concept is isotopic abundances. In Fig. 7, the theoretical natural-abundance (NA) ^{13}C isotope peaks are shown as simulated mass spectra for increasing number of carbons per molecule. As is evident from Fig. 7, the ^{13}C isotopic mass isomers

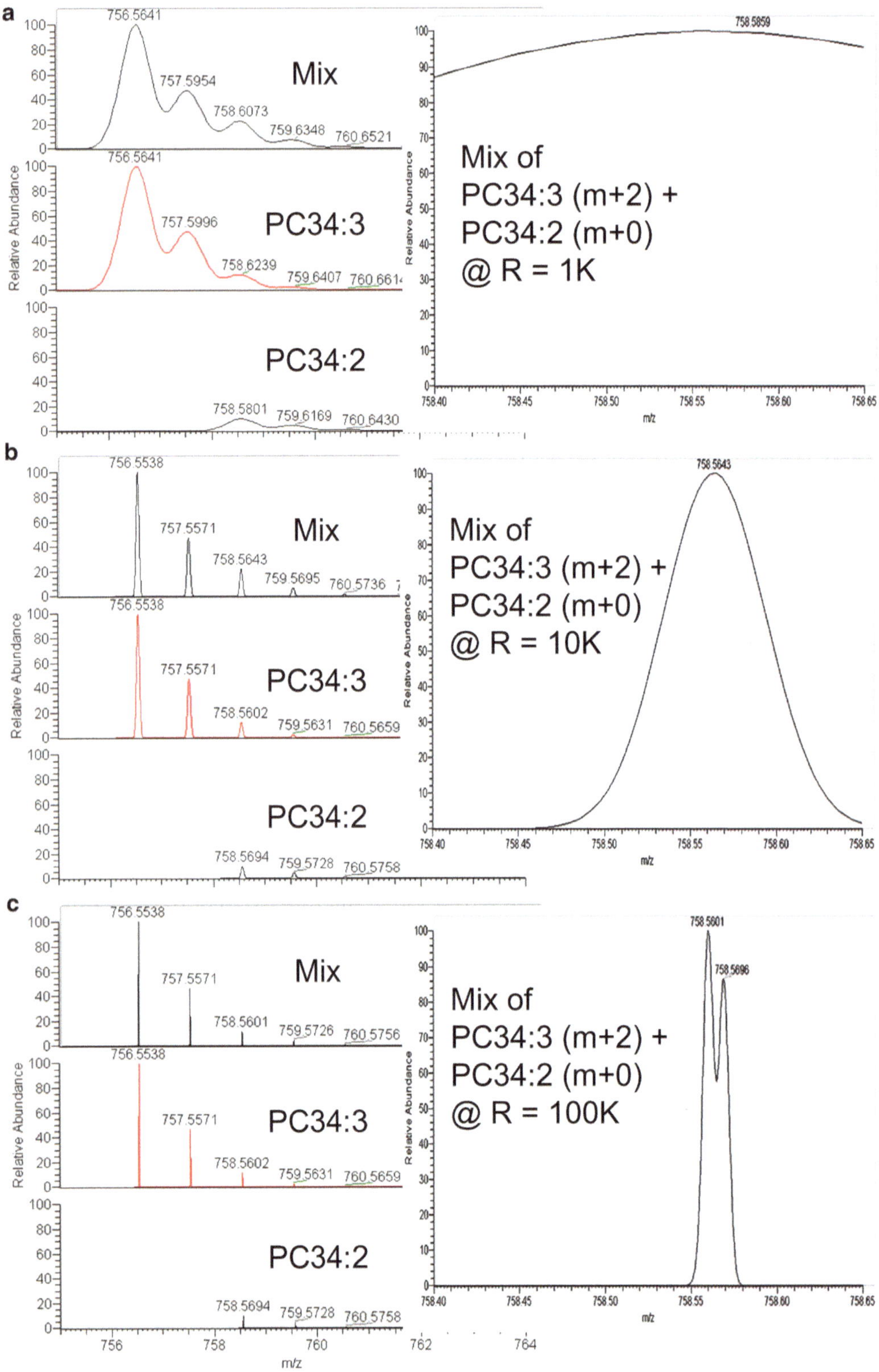
a
Mix
PC34:3
PC34:2
Mix of
PC34:3 (m+2) +
PC34:2 (m+0)
@ R = 1K
b
Mix
PC34:3
PC34:2
Mix of
PC34:3 (m+2) +
PC34:2 (m+0)
@ R = 10K
c
Mix
PC34:3
PC34:2
Mix of
PC34:3 (m+2) +
PC34:2 (m+0)
@ R = 100K
Relative Abundance
m/z

(isotopologues) increase with the carbon-skeleton size of the molecule, which has two main advantages in metabolomics: (a) for the Biomarker approach, the relative intensities of the natural-abundance ^{13}C isotopomer peaks can be used for structure confirmation; (b) for the Pathway approach, the isotopomer intensities that are in excess of natural abundance are useful in that they encode metabolic pathway information (3, 4).

Figure 6 illustrates "sufficient" resolution on a pure standard—so how much resolution is sufficient for real samples? Of course, this depends on the goal and particular sample, but the Pathway approach will be far more demanding than the Biomarker approach. For the latter, it is feasible to calculate the natural-abundance isotopologues for each known analyte, and subtract all the NA isotopologues using a "deisotoping" algorithm based on the known metabolite identity (5). However, deisotoping obviously cannot be done for unknowns, and also cannot be done in the Pathway approach, because the isotopic variation is the very experimental variable that is sought. Figure 8 and its legend illustrate the *minimum* resolution that is needed for assignments of molecular ions for the *simplest* case—that is, the Biomarker approach assuming NA isotopologues—for an idealized mixture of two lipid metabolites. Figure 9 and its legend illustrate the greater resolving power needed for the same two metabolites, by simply having a larger abundance of an ($m + 2$) isotopologue, a common occurrence in an actual experimental sample. Here, it is seen that the $m + 2$ isotopologue peak of one lipid overlaps considerably with the monoisotopic peak of another lipid species such that $R = 200{,}000$ must be used to distinguish the peaks. Figure 9 also shows the application to a real sample of the apparently "sufficient" resolution with accurate mass.

The lessons from Figs. 8 and 9 point to at least three important ramifications of insufficient resolution: (a) in a ^{13}C isotope-based study (Pathway approach), the MS would fail to distinguish among the ^{13}C isotopologues of numerous compounds; (b) if metabolite X were known to be unlabeled (i.e., Biomarker approach) but at far higher in concentration than metabolite Y, the natural-abundance isotopologues of *X* will be sufficiently large to

Fig. 8. Illustration of "sufficient resolution" for the simplest case of two metabolites with natural-abundance isotopic distributions. Spectra were simulated at different resolutions of a mixture of PC34:3 and PC34:2, the former at tenfold the concentration of the latter. (**a–c**) each show mixture spectra at the top, PC34:3 alone, and PC34:2 alone, respectively, at R (400 m/z, 10%) = 1 K, 10 K, and 100 K. The insets to the right zoom in on the 0.15-Da spectral region corresponding to an overlap of PC34:3 ($m + 2$) isotopologue and PC34:2 monoisotopic peaks. Note that at least $R = 100$ K is required to begin to distinguish these two molecular species. In principle, for the Biomarker approach, it is possible to calculate the natural abundance contribution of the PC34:3 ($m + 2$) to "deisotope" the peak, if these two species were the only compounds in the mixture. However, in practice, it is common to have isotopologues of many molecular species crowded into even such a narrow region, making "deisotope" data analyses techniques extremely difficult.

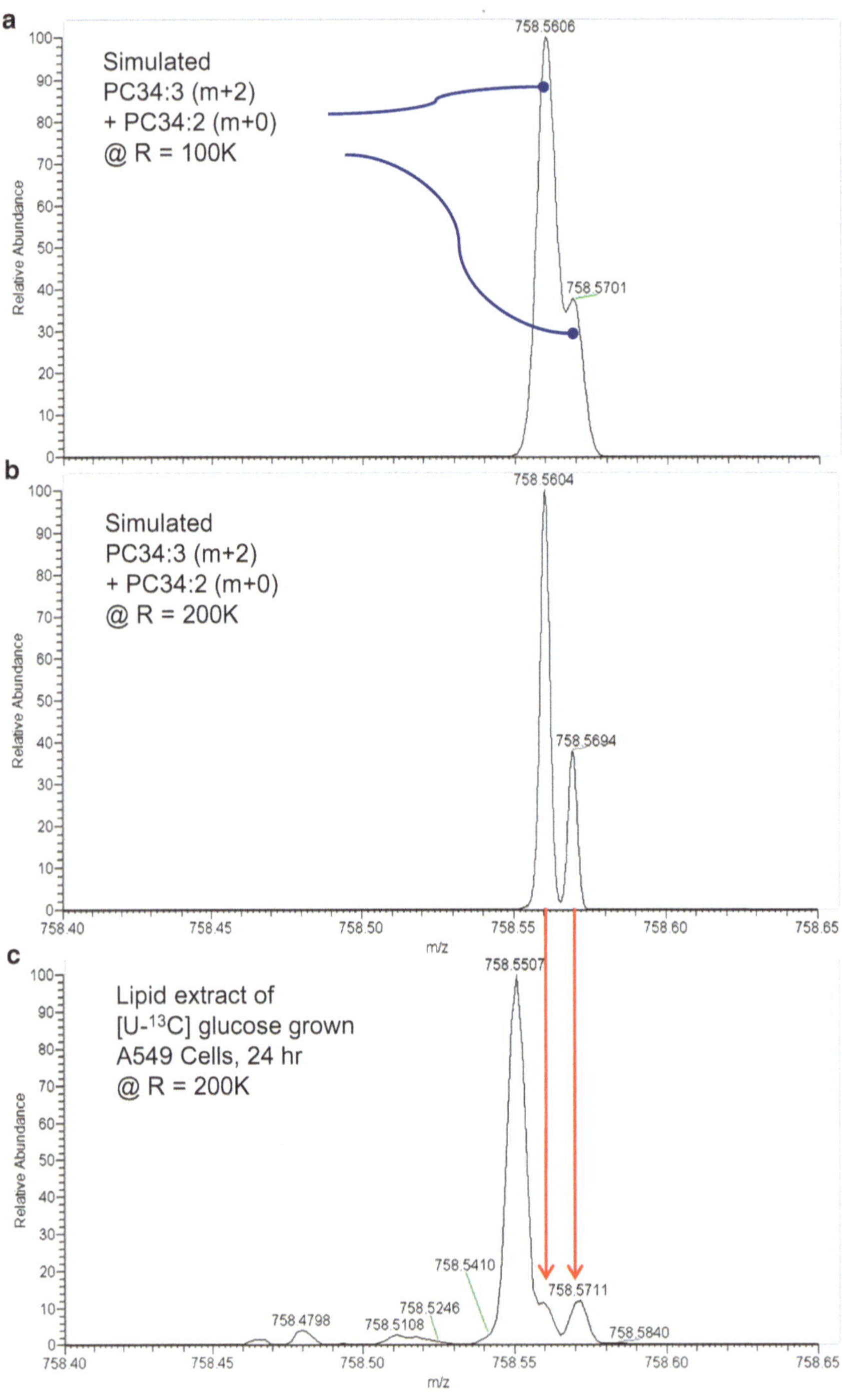

Fig. 9. Illustration of the greater demand for "sufficient resolution" in a ^{13}C-labeled Pathway approach, 0.15-Da *m/z* window. The simulated spectral mixture from Fig. 8c is now tenfold enriched in [$^{13}C_2$] PC34:3 such that there is much more PC34:3 ($m + 2$) than PC34:2 ($m + 0$). As shown in (**a**), this simple change in only one of the isotopologues renders insufficient the $R = 100$ K spectrum that previously appeared to be adequate (Fig. 8c). (**b**) Illustrates that $R = 200$ K is now needed to cleanly resolve the PC34:3 ($m + 2$) isotopologue ion from the PC34:2 ($m + 0$) ion. (**c**) A spectrum from a methanolic extract of [U-^{13}C] glucose-grown human lung adenocarcinoma (A549) cell culture illustrates that even the $R = 200$ K is barely adequate for real samples due to the presence of other metabolites, such as the much more abundant one at 758.5507 *m/z*. The concentrations of the gPLs were in the low picomolar range, analyzed using a continuous nanoelectrospray Fourier-transform ion-cyclotron resonance mass spectrometry (FT-ICR-MS) instrument. The assignments of corresponding peaks for PC34:3 ($m + 2$) and PC34:2 ($m + 0$) are shown by the arrows in (**c**) (the accurate mass is in slight error which is readily corrected by an internal mass accuracy standard). (**c**) Is unpublished data by the author.

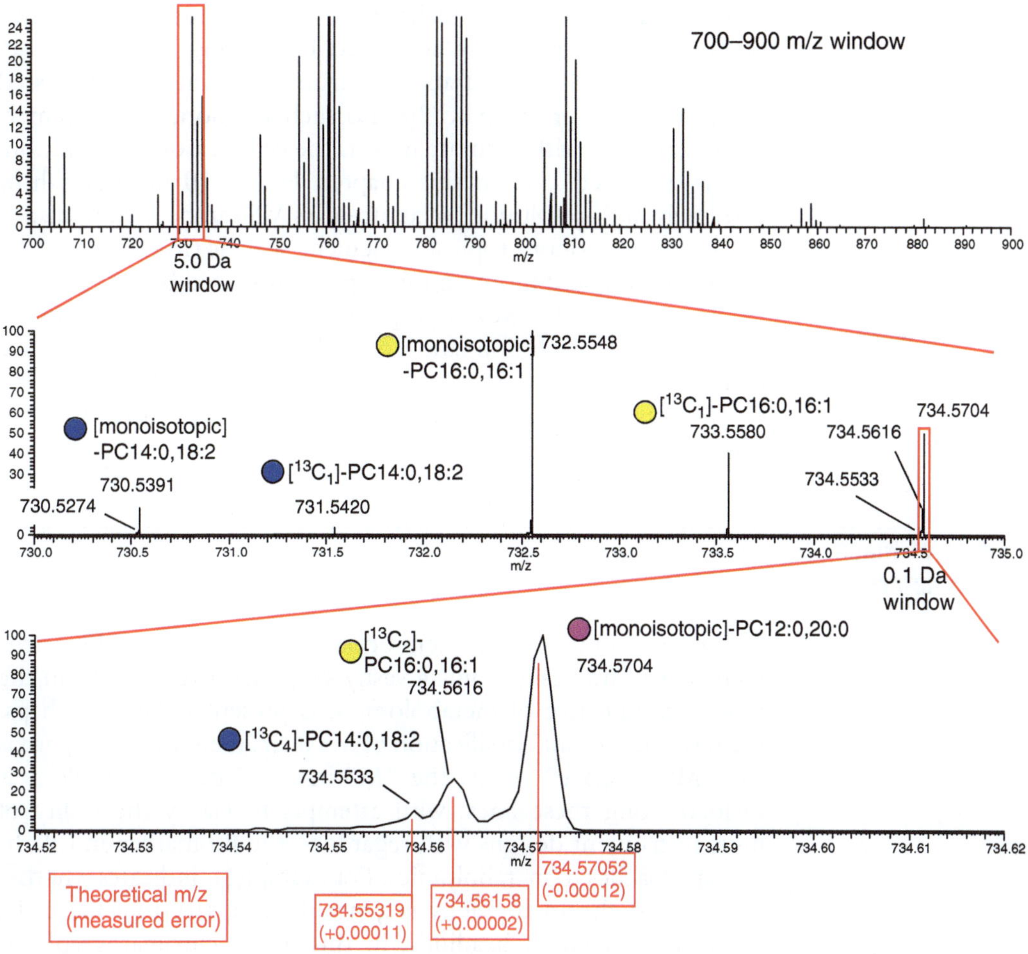

Fig. 10. Continuous nanoelectrospray FT-ICR-MS spectrum, obtained at an R(400 *m/z*, 10%) = 200,000, of a methanolic extract of human lung adenocarcinoma (A549) cell culture grown in [U-^{13}C]-glucose. The *top panel* shows the region of 700–900 *m/z* which is dominated by gPLs, consisting of >1,500 distinct ion peaks, many of which is not visible at this graphical scale. The 5.0-Da window denoted by the rectangle is expanded into the *middle panel*, where gPLs of identical structures are indicated by the colored dots; they are isotopologues of each other. Due to the extremely high resolution, the peaks are widely separated; however, there is a tight clustering at the right. This 0.1-Da-wide region is expanded into the *bottom panel* that shows gPLs of three different structures that are nearly isobaric (same molecular mass). As illustrated by Fig. 9 and its legend, these would not have been distinguished at lower resolutions. The boxes below the *bottom panel* show the comparison of theoretical and measured *m/z*; recall from Fig. 6 that such small errors in mass accuracy require simultaneous extremely high resolution. These *m/z* errors are small enough to readily distinguish incremental addition of protons (+1.00782 *m/z* each) which denote different gPL structures, from among isotopologues achieved through incremental additions of neutrons in ^{13}C (+1.00336 *m/z* each), deuterium (+1.00618 *m/z* each), ^{15}N (+0.99703 *m/z* each), ^{18}O (+1.99668 *m/z* each), ^{34}S (+1.99580 *m/z* each), etc. Thus, the *blue* and *yellow dot* peaks in the *bottom panel* can be confidently assigned as ^{13}C isotopologues (and not of other elements) of the same dot color in the *middle panel*, and clearly distinct from another, third monoisotopic gPL (*purple dot*). Unpublished data by the author.

skew the quantification of the Y monoisotopic peak and its isotopologues (Fig. 9); (c) insufficient resolution would preclude the use of the extremely powerful multielement labeling approaches for Pathway metabolomics, an approach that is readily accommodated by NMR techniques. It turns out that problems (a) and (b) can be partly addressed by turning to tandem MS or coupling MS to separation instruments, which is discussed later. However, problem (c) has no such solution, and extremely high resolution with accurate mass is the only reasonable solution; this is discussed later in this chapter. Figure 10 illustrates how extremely high-resolution, accurate-mass MS can be used to distinguish among monoisotopic and element-specific (in this case, ^{13}C) isotopologues, and more on this topic is discussed below.

In summary, the key concepts six through eight, respectively, accurate mass, resolution, and isotopologues, interplay to produce confounding interferences or rich information, or both, depending on the perspective and instrument capabilities. The latter aspect is now considered.

3. Types of Mass Spectrometers

As there are numerous excellent books on the subject of MS instrument types and design, only a vastly simplified overview, from the unique perspective of metabolomics, is presented here. Perhaps, the most significant classification of MS instruments in this regard is the "MS-in-space" versus the "MS-in-time" designs. Table 1 is divided along these lines, with attempts to clarify the utility of most instrument designs with regards to the Biomarker and Pathway approaches to metabolomics. For example, it indicates whether coupling to chromatography is generally necessary to achieve the tasks in the column headings; in this sense, chromatography is called upon to solve inadequate MS capability. The first six columns are the various modes of measurement supported by the instrument type, which are very useful to the Biomarker approach. The last three columns state additional requirements by the Pathway approach, indicating whether the instrument type supports sufficient resolution simultaneously with sufficient mass accuracy in order to distinguish isotopologues from nearly isobaric monoisotopic peaks, and whether isotopologues of multiple-element-labeled metabolites can be distinguished. The resolution required to achieve unambiguous distinction among combinations of ^{13}C isotopologues in natural abundance (Biomarker) and enriched (Pathway) was illustrated earlier in Figs. 8–10.

3.1. MS-in-Space Designs

The top part of Table 1 lists the metabolomics capabilities of the MS-in-space designs. The MS-in-space designs comprise most of the instruments historically, and modern ones are at the state of the art in speed and sensitivity. They are characterized principally by reliance on spatial transport of ions to achieve fragmentation experiments and additional resolution of m/z;

Table 1
Metabolomics[a] capabilities[b] of MS instrument types

	Basic need	Modes for advanced confirmation or structural assignment[c]					Pathway metabolomics demands[e]: suf ficient R&A for metabolites <1,000 Da		
Design[d]	Confirmation using standards	MS2	MS ($n > 2$)	Collision-induced dissociation	Other dissociation modes	Fixed (F) or multiple (M) ion sources	Nat. abund.	Single-element isotopomer	Multielement isotopomer
MS-in-space types									
Single quadrupole	1					F	1	1	n/a
Triple quad	0	0		0		M	1	1	n/a
ToF	1				PSD	F	1	1	n/a
ToF-ToF	0	0		0	PSD	F	1	1	n/a
Hybrid quadrupole-ToF	0	0		0		M	1	1	n/a
Dual-sector magnetic + electrostatic	0	0		0		M	0	1	n/a
MS-in-time types									
IT/LIT	1	0	0	0	ETD	M	1	1	n/a
Hybrid quadrupole-LIT	0	0	0	0		M	1	1	n/a
Hybrid LIT-Markarov trap (Orbitrap®)	0	0	0	0	ETD	M	0	0	1
Hybrid quadrupole/LIT-ICR	0	0	0	0	ETD,IRMPD	M	0	0	0
Dual-setor magnetic + electrostatic-IT	0	0	0	0		M	0	1	n/a

0 = Yes, or standalone use possible, 1 = usually requires coupling with separations techniques, n/a = not applicable

[a]"Metabolomics" implies extremely complex organic and orgonometallic mixtures, with minimal sample cleanup to enable discovery of unexpected and unknown metabolites

[b]The capabilities implied here, of course, depend on a number of analytical factors, including but not limited to experimental design, sample preparation, specifics of instrument design, practicality of sample throughput for a biochemical study (as opposed to the ability to perform on only very few samples before maintenance is required), and chemo/bioinformatics

[c]"Assignment" in this context means temporary structural assignment, with identification or confirmation to follow, if necessary

[d]These are instrument designs the reader is most likely to encounter. The list is not intended to be exhaustive

[e]See text for further explanation

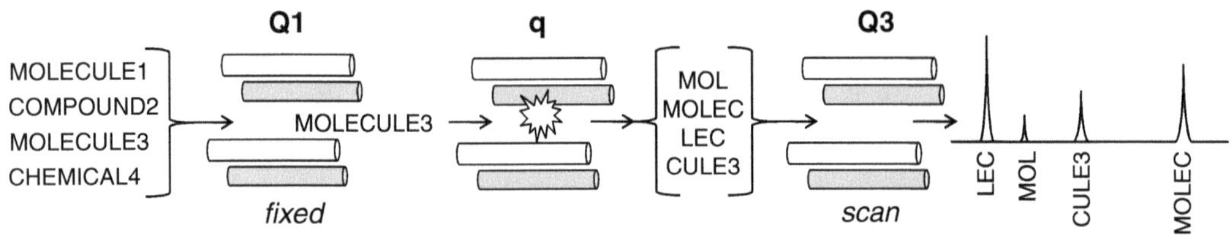

Fig. 11. Illustration of the basic mode of tandem MS for an MS-in-space instrument. The original design, schematized here, consisted of three physical quadrupole MS instrument sections, hence the traditional name of "triple quad." See Table 1 for a listing of design variations. In comparison with Fig. 1, note that Q3 is the basic MS instrument, and the added front sections Q1 and *q* attain the reaction control for the tandem MS experiment. In this experiment, Q1 is set to pass a desired *m*/*z*, which is collided in *q* to generate fragments, which are sorted and detected in Q3. Since the operations for MSn occur in different physical sections of the MS instrument, this is called MS in space.

a considerable practical consequence of the MS-in-space designs is that additional physical sections are required in order to achieve MSn (illustrated in Fig. 4). They range from the historically common quadrupole MS instruments to high-end "hybrid" instruments combining quadrupole with time-of-flight (ToF) and other designs.

Many MS instruments in use are MS-in-space designs, such as those dedicated to GC, rapid very-high-sample throughput nucleotide sequencing, portable field instruments, etc. Often, the more affordable instruments are also of this category, which is a very important advantage, although there is considerable overlap of prices with MS-in-time designs. At the high end, the MS-in-space designs include some of the highest sensitivity "tandem" MS (MS/MS) instruments available for preselected analytes or structural classes, such as for drug analysis, their toxicodynamics, and abuse testing.

Tandem MS, or MSn, is an extremely powerful technique that greatly enhances the detection of target analytes. It is instructive to describe how the MSn concept (Fig. 4) is translated into hardware operation, which is illustrated by Fig. 11 and its legend. In the most basic use, *Q1* is set to pass the target molecular ion (*m*/*z* corresponding to MOLECULE3 in the example) that is then fragmented by collision with Ar gas in the "*q*" section, from which the mass spectrum of the fragments is obtained by scanning *Q3* (the operation is, thus, $Q1_{\text{fixed}}/q/Q3_{\text{scan}}$). An LC-triple-quad MS instrument will, thus, continuously acquire full spectra on only molecules that pass selection in *Q1*. This results in very good detection due to the specificity of *Q1* while *Q3* provides structural confirmation fragments. Figure 12 shows an operational mode for further s/n improvement, whereby *Q1* and *Q3* can both cycle through a list of preselected pairs of *m*/*z* (for each pair, $Q1_{\text{fixed}}/q/Q3_{\text{fixed}}$), which would continuously detect MS/MS products of multiple analytes in a technique called mutiple reaction monitoring (MRM). This second operational mode eschews confirmation spectra in order to

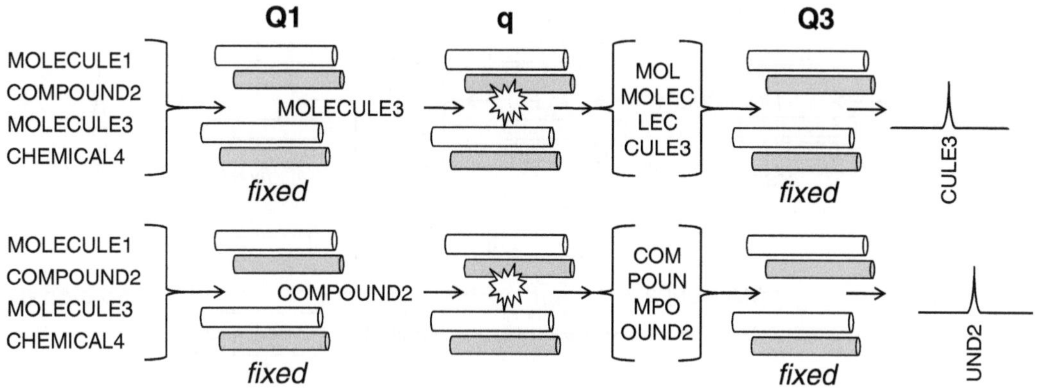

Fig. 12. Illustration of a second mode of operation for tandem MS on the "tripleOquad" MS-in-space instrument. Q1 and Q3 can be programmed to pass many such fixed pairs of *m/z*, which is called MRM as described in the text. Two such fixed pairs are shown here. Since all of the *m/z* values are fixed, there is no mass spectrum acquired in this mode of operation.

gain the advantage of improved detection by higher throughput of only the target ion(s), since the instrument does not waste time collecting unwanted "noise" portions that can constitute the major portion of mass spectra.

An interesting use of the high-end tandem MS-in-space instruments for metabolomics is substructure monitoring. The most common use of this capability is shown in Fig. 13, a simulation of an LC-"triple-quad" MS instrument. In this third mode of operation, which flips the operation from that shown in Fig. 11, *Q1* is set to obtain full-scan spectra while *Q3* is fixed on a given *m/z* (hence, $Q1_{scan}/q/Q3_{fixed}$). Operated in this manner, the LC-triple-quad MS will continuously detect a given fragment from any compound as it elutes from the LC, resulting in a chromatogram consisting of all compounds that contain that fragment (and thus presumably the desired substructure). In the example shown, if the interest was only in metabolites that contain MOLEC moieties, both known and unknown, then *Q1* can be set to full scan while *Q3* can be fixed on a particular fragment, in this case the *m/z* corresponding to the MOLEC substructure.

Table 1 also alludes to some of the *metabolomic* considerations of MS-in-space instruments. Note that most of the instrument configurations have a "0" designation, meaning that for extremely complex metabolomic samples it is possible to perform unassisted MS (e.g., without prior chromatographic separation). However, note that for the Pathway approach, which entails analysis of isotopologues, the designations mostly have a "1," which means that some assistance such as prior chromatographic separation is needed in order to reduce overlaps in the spectra (see Fig. 9). Also note that none of these instruments are generally capable of multielement isotopologue analysis due to lack of sufficient resolution and mass accuracy.

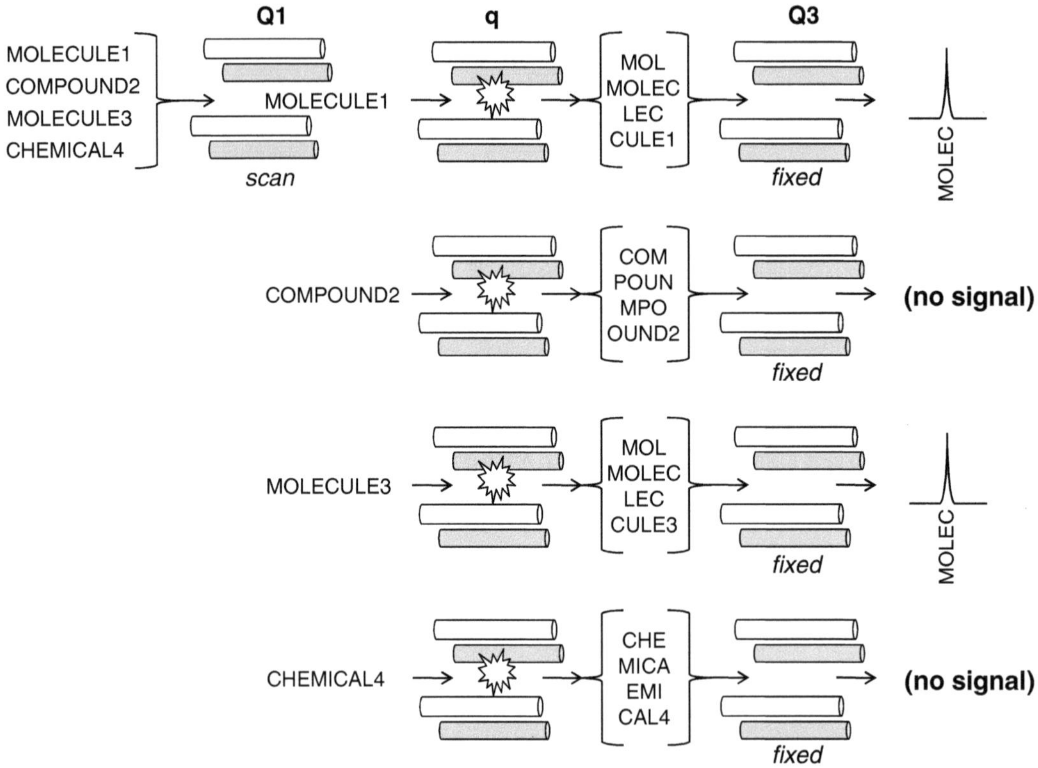

Fig. 13. Illustration of a third mode of operation for tandem MS on the "triple-quad" MS-in-space instrument. In this mode, the MS instrument is used to detect any substructure of interest. Here, Q1 scans allow one *m/z* metabolite at a time, which undergoes the fragmentation process in q as usual; however, Q3 is set to pass *m/z* ions corresponding only to MOLEC. Thus, any metabolite—including unknowns—with *m/z* corresponding to MOLEC is detected while all others are rejected. In a sense, this is an "any-and-all" MRM mode that does not have a predefined molecular *m/z* list, which is useful for unknown or unexpected metabolites.

3.2. MS-in-Time Designs

The bottom part of Table 1 lists some of the most common MS-in-time designs. MS-in-time instruments—at least ones available for purchase—appeared historically later than the MS-in-space instruments. This instrument strategy is based on first trapping ions in a confined space, and then mass spectrometry by manipulations (usually radio-frequency pulses) in the same physical device over time, rather than spatially across discrete devices. Thus, one of the reasons for the later historic appearance is a much greater need for integrated computer control, the technology for which greatly accelerated in the 1980s. An important practical consequence of the MS-in-time designs is that MSn is achieved in the same physical device, unlike MS-in-space designs. The MS-in-time instruments range from the early retail-available "ion trap" MS to high-end hybrid instruments combining ion traps or quadrupoles on the front end with ICR or even another ion trap and other MS designs at the back. In short, hybrid instruments can, in principle, utilize any combination MS-in-space and MS-in-time devices. The basic operation of an ion trap MS instrument is illustrated in Fig. 14.

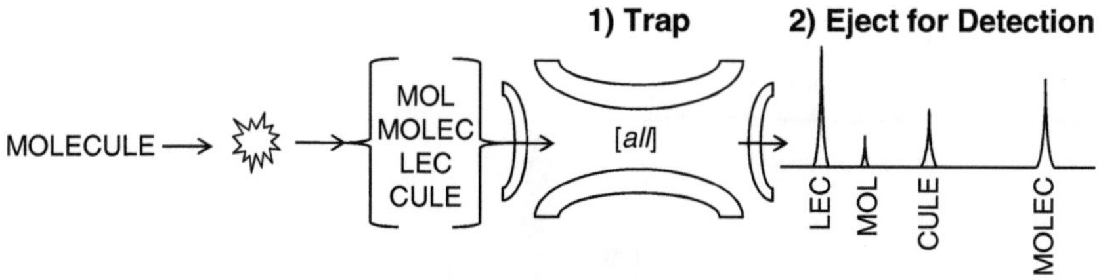

Fig. 14. Illustration of the basic mode of operation for "ion trap" MS-in-time instrument. Most MS-in-time instruments are ion traps of some sort. A major type of ion trap design features a two-dimensional cross section of four curved surfaces facing each other, schematized here as curved plates. Other types of ion traps can differ considerably in both hardware and principle of operation; see Table 1 for a listing of some of the designs. Compare to Fig. 1: ion traps first collect all of the ions with the assistance of He gas to "cool" (*slow*) down the ions, and then eject them by *m/z* over time. The time abscissa is calibrated to *m/z* to produce a mass spectrum.

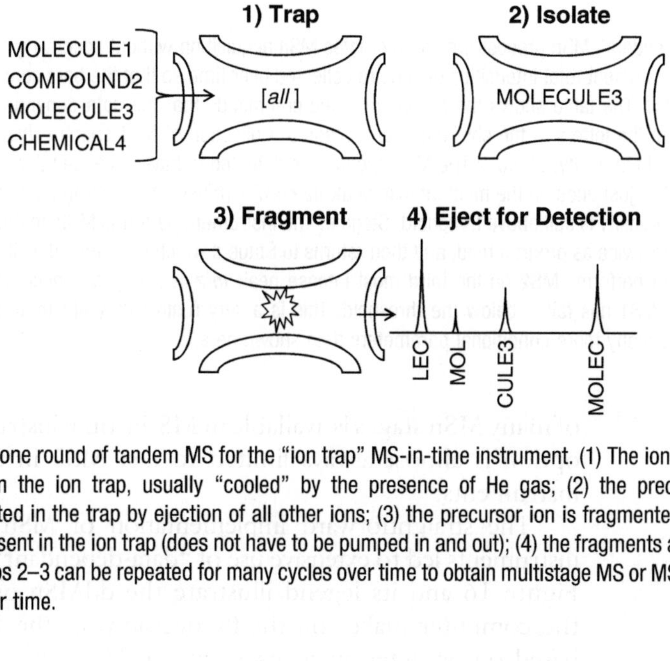

Fig. 15. Illustration of one round of tandem MS for the "ion trap" MS-in-time instrument. (1) The ions comprising the MS1 spectrum is stored in the ion trap, usually "cooled" by the presence of He gas; (2) the precursor ion of interest (MOLECULE3) is isolated in the trap by ejection of all other ions; (3) the precursor ion is fragmented by collision with He gas that is always present in the ion trap (does not have to be pumped in and out); (4) the fragments are scanned out of the trap as in Fig. 14. Steps 2–3 can be repeated for many cycles over time to obtain multistage MS or MSn. Hence, this type of MSn is called MS over time.

Tandem MS, or MSn, is achieved in MS-in-time instruments in the manner shown in Fig. 15; compare this with MS2 on the MS-in-space instruments (Figs. 11–13). Achievement of multiple MS stages is, thus, a matter of repeating steps 2 and 3, for which the isolation and fragmentation steps over time (as explained in Fig. 15 legend) are readily controlled by the computer. A practical limitation of requesting many steps in MSn is that the population of available ions decreases dramatically at each MSn step; thus, analytical utilization of MS10, for example, is very rare while up to MS5 is not unusual. Another practical limitation is that many stages in MSn take considerable time, usually many milliseconds per step, thus limiting MSn stages in applications where the analytes are available to the MS instrument for only a short time, such as in LC-MS. This argument is often countered by pointing out that at least the option

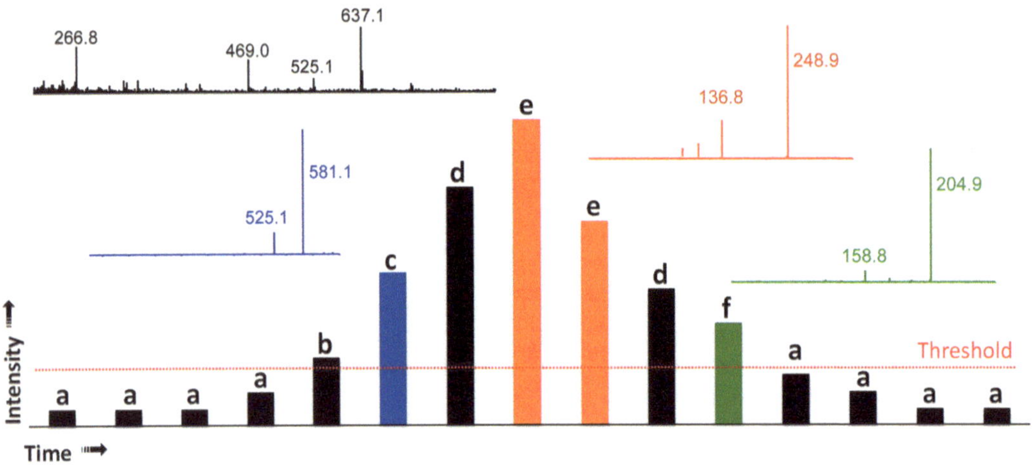

Fig. 16. The "data-dependent" MSn process which automates MSn acquisition without specifying a predetermined list of analyte *m/z*. The bars represent total intensities of spectra collected over time so that the bars comprise a chromatogram peak eluting from an LC. The table shows the preprogrammed commands that the data-dependent MSn uses, and the stages corresponding to the letters in the chromatogram. Stage a: Collection of MS1 spectra (*black*) remaining below a preprogrammed threshold intensity. Stage b: The MS1 spectra are detected to have exceeded the threshold. Stage c: The instrument performs MS2 just once on the most intense peak *m/z* 637.1 (*blue*), as programmed. Stage d: Returns to MS1 which shows that the intensity is still above threshold. Stage e: The instrument performs MS2 on the second most intense peak *m/z* 266.8 (*orange*) twice as programmed, and then returns to Stage d which finds the intensity still above threshold. Stage f: The instrument performs MS2 on the third most intense peak *m/z* 469.0 (*green*) once. Stage g: This is never executed because the MS1 has fallen below the threshold. This is a very rudimentary illustration and data-dependent acquisition can include many more conditional parameters than shown here.

of many MSn stages is available in MS-in-time instruments while the option is almost always limited to just MS2 in the MS-in-space instruments.

The straightforward implementation of MSn on MS-in-time instruments led to extensive use of "data-dependant" MSn (ddMSn). Figure 16 and its legend illustrate the ddMSn process, in which the computer makes on-the-fly decisions of the MSn acquisition based on predetermined user criteria. Note that ddMSn requires switching between different operational modes of an MS instrument, which can introduce significant time-consuming steps; in fact, a consequence of this time limitation is illustrated in Fig. 16, where the command stage "g" is never executed because the LC peak is no longer present. Generally, ddMS2 is performed less commonly in MS-in-space instruments. To see why, using a triple- quad MS as an example, a $Q1_{scan}$ first finds the target *m/zs*, followed by $Q1_{fixed}/q/Q3_{scan}$, and then cycling back to the $Q1_{scan}$. This takes considerable time because the fragmentation is achieved in the collision cell by the physical presence of the collision gas, which must be introduced and stabilized between the two steps and then pumped out again, all of which take many seconds. Thus, a typical LC peak elution of 20 s duration misses much of data while the triple-quad MS is switching modes. In contrast, in, e.g., an ion trap, the collision

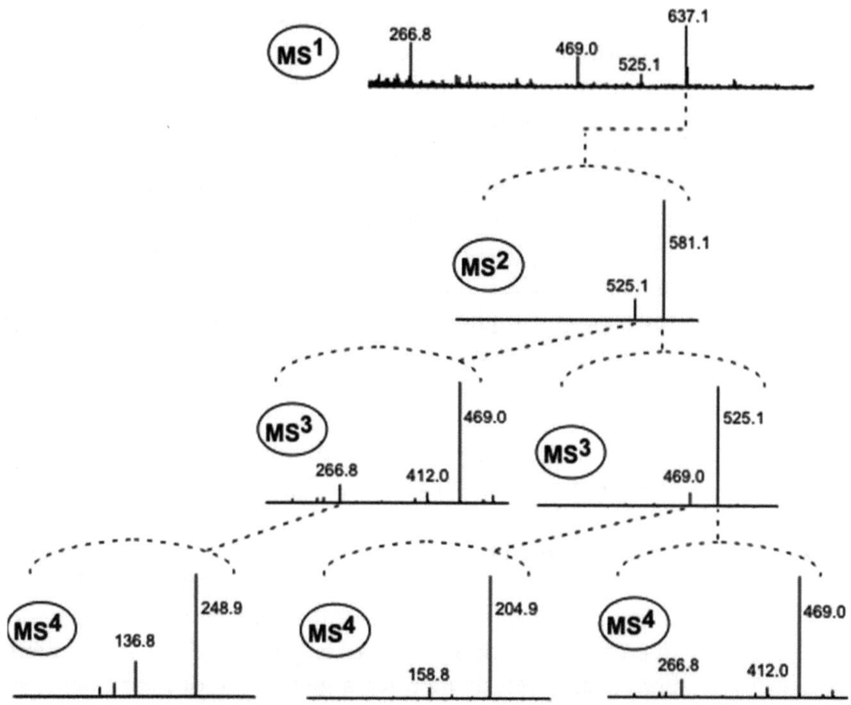

Fig. 17. The "data-dependent" MSn process as applied to ion trees. These spectra were obtained directly from a crude extract of wheat plant under continuous electrospray into an ion trap MSn instrument, total acquisition time was <30 s, and the precursor ion of 637.1 *m/z* is an unknown metabolite. The MS instrument was programmed to automatically obtain up to MS4 spectra for each of the two most intense ions in a spectrum, thus yielding an extremely detailed, sequentially controlled fragmentation for interpretation without prior knowledge of the structure or expected ions. Figure redrawn from 10 using unpublished data by the author.

gas is always present and fragmentation is induced by excitation of ions using an RF pulse. Although such switching modes by RF pulses is far faster, even the ion trap needs time to switch operational modes because ions still have a physical settling time after fragmentation, isolation, ejection, etc., all of which take many milliseconds. In summary, the advantages and disadvantages between MS-in-space and MS-in-time instruments for ddMS2 depend on the specific features of each model and how they are implemented. However, for ddMSn where $n > 2$, the MS-in-time instruments are usually the only choice because the MS-in-space instruments simply lack the required hardware sections.

An example of intensive ddMSn by MS-in-time instruments is the generation of an "ion tree." Figure 17, which is effectively a multiple version of Fig. 4, illustrates how ddMSn can be used to automatically investigate multiple parallel fragmentation pathways of a substance. If the ion tree is generated at accurate mass (recall that this also requires sufficiently high resolution), the ion tree can reveal details regarding the substructures of a given molecular ion, even in the highly complex sample illustrated here. Ion tree generation can take many seconds to minutes, making it practical only for direct infusion that provides a continuous source of molecular ions, as in the case of Fig. 17.

The bottom part of Table 1 lists the *metabolomic* considerations of MS-in-time instrument types. Note that all of these are capable of MSn of $n > 2$, which as discussed previously is an intrinsic advantage of the MS-in-time design strategy. Because MSn implies advanced applications of MS, many instruments are generally richer in features (i.e., noncollision dissociation modes, variety of ion sources, and higher accuracy and resolution), at of course correspondingly greater cost. However, for metabolomics, the advantages of such capabilities can be considerable. Lastly, note that this category represents the only instruments that have sufficient resolution and mass accuracy to perform multielement isotopologue analysis for advanced Pathway approaches, discussed below.

3.3. Sensitivity

Sensitivity is a general term that can have many meanings to different users, but in MS analysis the main concept is that of signal to noise ratio (s/n). Most chemists are familiar with concepts and determination of s/n for data generated by instruments, which are usually well defined for a given type of instrument, and is also sample specific. One common determination of the analytical s/n of a mass spectrometer is the signal strength (i.e., in ion counts) of series of known constituent mass spectra that is acquired over time on an actual sample, in comparison to a blank sample. Thus, if the total spectral ion count for NADH from Fig. 2 averaged 12,000 and the blank under identical conditions averaged 200 counts, then $s/n = 60$. However, the total spectral ion count includes spectral noise in between fragment m/z peaks, so if only the actual fragment m/z peaks of NADH were used the s/n would very likely be far better. This, in turn, means that dozens to hundreds of combinations of m/z peaks can be custom specified to optimize the s/n of each metabolite such that the s/n is often determined post acquisition at the time of data processing, and can be a different specification for each sample. Such myriad s/n complications have led to much simpler, single-numerical value standards, such as minimum detectable limits (MDLs) or minimum quantifiable limits (MQLs), as the most widely used metrics for sensitivity in MS analysis.

However, for metabolomics, since structure-revealing *spectral* data are critical to the extremely complex sample analyses, MDL and MQL are *not* useful metrics of s/n because they are specified for a very limited set of analytes, and not readily applied to submolecular parts (fragments) which are sometimes the key metabolomic data sought. Furthermore, MDL and MQL cannot be specified for unknown analytes or cases, whereby authentic standards are not available, both of which are extremely important for metabolomics.

Thus, for metabolomics, such simplified mass spectrometry conventions need to be disregarded.

The analytical *s*/*n* of MS is intrinsically the best among structure-revealing analytical techniques, but it depends heavily on the instrument design, operational mode, and analytical intention, such as having a preset list of analytes versus profiling of unknowns. In case of the latter, *s*/*n* is effectively impossible to determine since it is not known which *m*/*z* peaks "belong" to the unknown. Thus, a discussion of MS spectral *s*/*n* in metabolomic applications threatens to span several chapters of discussion, at the end of which no general conclusions can be drawn. Ultimately, the *adequacy* of *s*/*n*—and not *s*/*n* as some citable numerical standard—is what should be addressed. Adequate s/n must be couched in terms of supporting the findings of an experimental study, and is not a consideration of the analytical platform alone. For example, a very basic and common question such as "Will the MS have enough sensitivity to analyze NADH at picomolar levels in my samples?" may need much discussion and testing to answer because it depends on the intended interpretation of such data. For discovery or hypothesis-generating studies, the intended interpretation is not known prior to analysis.

From a hardware perspective, the discussion of *s*/*n* is simplified because in most cases the MS sensitivity is limited by the ion source, and not the design of the MS itself. The classical ion source is electron ionization, which is variously estimated to have <1% ionization efficiency (1). This is in contrast with the electrospray source, which for a species with permanent charge, such as quaternary ammonium compounds (e.g., cholines, betaines), has a theoretical ionization efficiency of 100%. Actual efficiency is less than 100% and depends on the particular design and operation of both the ion source and MS, as well as the general nature of the sample (e.g., 1, 5).

The foregoing discussion touched upon just a few of the numerous considerations of *s*/*n* in MS analysis, and a comprehensive coverage is far beyond the scope of this chapter. The important practical parameter for sensitivity in metabolomics is how much material is needed to obtain a spectrum of experimentally adequate s/n across numerous analytes in a given analysis time. Modern electrospray MS instruments can routinely obtain experimentally adequate spectra from subpicomoles of each substance in an extremely complex metabolomic extract (e.g., 6). In contrast, NMR requires much larger amounts of each analyte in a complex mixture, on the order of nanomoles of each metabolite. It must be kept in mind that the metabolomic information from these two techniques is highly complementary so that this large difference in sensitivity alone is *not* a useful criterion in choosing one technique over the other.

4. Chromatography-MS

Although it is well beyond the scope of this chapter to cover metabolomic uses of chromatography—a vast field by itself—some perspectives with specific regards to MS in metabolomics are warranted. As stated earlier, chromatography interfaced to MS is a result of inadequate MS capability. For example, there are many metabolites that are isobaric compounds (identical molecular formulae), principally structural isomers, which can give essentially the same fragmentation pattern, and thus are indistinguishable even by MSn; simple examples of this are leucine vs. isoleucine, Z vs. E fatty acids, and so on. The most difficult is distinguishing stereoisomers, which is usually best left to NMR, although there are chiral chromatography columns that are useful for resolving enantiomers and diastereomers, if the samples are of relatively simple composition. However, it should be kept in mind that, as stated at the onset of this chapter, the analytical needs of metabolomics usually entail highly complex samples driven by the need for very rich data sets.

A major contribution of interfacing chromatography to MS instruments is to reduce the complexity of the sample presented to the MS instrument at any given time, thus reducing spectral ambiguity and improving s/n (however, that is defined). For example, the significant spectral overlap problems illustrated by Fig. 8 could possibly be addressed by chromatography which can separate the PC34:3 from PC34:2. This would allow the use of low- resolution MS instruments, which is a considerable cost and possible ease-of-use advantage. Among the most affordable MS instruments is GC-MS. Figure 18 and its legend illustrate the use of GC-MS to analyze silyl-derivatized amino and organic acids for their isotopologues. It should be noted that, due to the nonvolatile nature of almost all of the metabolome, and even with derivatization, the limitations on molecular mass imposed by the requirement of volatility, GC-based techniques are intrinsically poorly suited for metabolomics. Their broad and decades-long usage—including by this author—is principally due to the low cost and practical robustness of the technique. Such factors should be weighed against the paucity of metabolomic coverage by GC-MS, which imposes severe limits on research progress or diagnostic potential. Thus, it is expected that GC-MS usage will be phased out from metabolomics as other MS techniques develop.

Chromatography can help, but not necessarily solve, the problems faced by many Pathway approach samples. Figure 9 presents a very elementary example to revisit in this regard. As there are potentially scores of isotopologues for each gPL, they overlap the entire *m/z* range of gPLs. Thus, there is no assurance that any

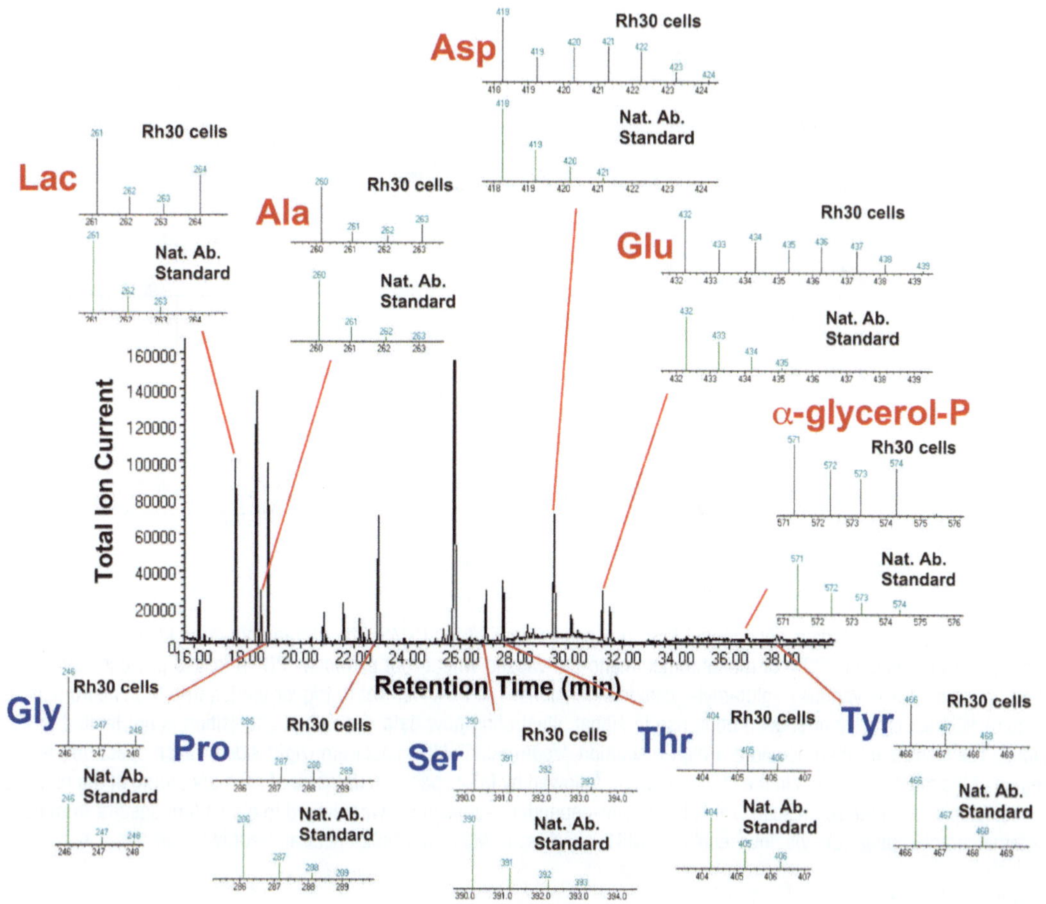

Fig. 18. GC-MS analysis of silyl-derivatized organic and amino acids, revealing isotopologue patterns from crude extracts of rhabdomyosarcoma cells grown in the presence of [U-^{13}C]-glucose. For each metabolite, the corresponding molecular ion region of the tert-butyldimethylsilyl derivative is shown for analyses of both natural isotopic abundance chemical standard and cellular extract ("Rh 30 cells"). The total ion chromatogram is shown for the Rh 30 sample while the chromatogram for the standards is not shown. By comparison of the spectra, it is immediately apparent that some metabolites are heavily and multiply labeled (*red lettering*) while others are not (*blue lettering*), rapidly providing a glimpse into the glucose-utilization networks by these cancer cell lines. This would not have been apparent using unlabeled cell cultures, which would instead require extensive experimentation, tedious quantification of concentrations, and modeling of pathways to interpret the concentrations, just to obtain a similar glimpse. Redrawn from 10, 11.

of the peaks detected by insufficient-resolution MS are free of interference from isotopologues of other lipid species; this point was illustrated in Figs. 9 and 10. There is currently no practical chromatographic solution that can separate all of the thousands of possible gPLs. Additionally, chromatography cannot ensure adequate separation of metabolites that are unknown, unexpected, or unavailable as authentic standards; all of these categories are of key importance to metabolomics.

An example of combining chromatography with data-dependent acquisition is shown in Fig. 19 and its legend. Note that data-dependent acquisition is not limited to MS instruments;

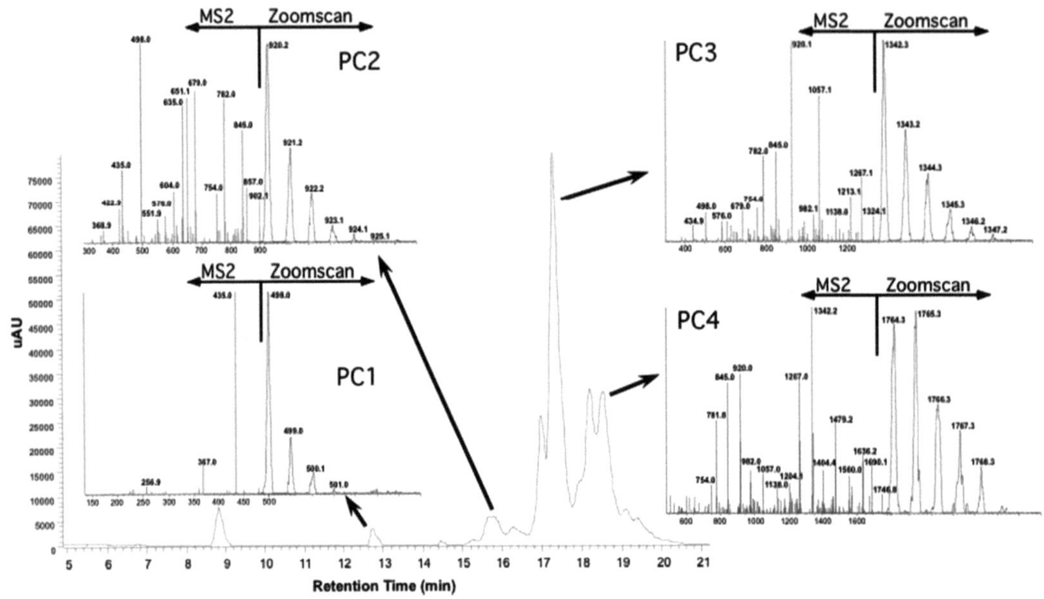

Fig. 19. Example of the "data-dependent" MSn process as applied to LC-MS. The chromatogram is LC-photodiodearray total spectrum detection (PDA) of monobromobimane-derivatized wheat root extracts. "PC" refers to phytochelatins and the numerals refer to various γ-glutamyl-cysteine extensions. The PDA was set to trigger the ion trap MSn instrument to acquire MS1 spectrum (not shown) upon rise in signal, illustrating how data-dependent acquisition is not limited to MS alone. The instrument then acquired a high-resolution "zoom-scan" MS1 spectrum (*right side* of each spectrum) in the region of the most intense ion in the MS1 spectrum, followed by MS2 spectrum (*left side* of each spectrum) of the putative monoisotopic ion in the zoom scan. Thus, three data-dependent acquisitions were linked to obtain four spectra from each chromatographic peak (UV–vis, low-resolution MS1, zoom-scan MS1, and MS2 spectra). Redrawn from ref. 19.

in this case, a UV-visible detector was used to ensure acquisition of mass spectra only when there was sufficient material eluting from the LC. It is important to keep in mind that, as discussed for Fig. 16, chromatography can also severely limit the utility of ddMSn due to the short time the analyte is present at the MS interface as well as the constantly changing concentration of analytes in the ion source.

5. Biomarkers vs. Pathway Approaches for MS

5.1. Biochemical Information Content

Ultimately, the *information* generated from MS analysis—not the data per se—is the objective of any analysis. Thus, the analysis must go well beyone the past exercise of merely obtaining metabolite concentration data, to providing key information on metabolic response differences (e.g. control vs. treatment) of hundreds or even thousands of metabolites, and doing so in the presence of a large background of the very same metabolites, including unknown or unexpected metabolites. This is an unprecedented challenge, as these requirements are completely beyond all other current applications of MS, such as clinical diagnostics, drug analysis, biotechnology, security, and environmental pollution, to name just a few.

The brief discussion above regarding *s/n* in MS focused mainly on spectral data. But determining the *s/n* for *information* is even less straightforward. Assuming that the data *s/n* is adequate—which is the initial step—we quickly find that the really important task is to determine *s/n* of information content. To assess this, we must necessarily include metadata, such as the experimental or diagnostic purpose and biochemical interpretation, other MS data, as well as data from other types of measurements. For the Biomarker approach, adequate information *s/n* would mean that the data can be used to statistically detect differences between biological treatment and control; thus, in this case, *information s/n* is a direct function of data *s/n*. For the Pathway approach, the detection must be (at the least) for differences between *biochemical pathways* of treatment and control samples; thus, data s/n alone is insufficient to judge the adequacy of MS analysis for a given study.

Figure 18 can be revisited as a simple example to compare the potential *information* s/n for both Biomarker and Pathway approaches. For the purposes of this discussion, the data s/n is assumed to be very good and thus have no influence on this discussion. For the Biomarker approach, which uses no stable-isotope labeling, this GC-MS run would consist of only of spectra identical to the natural abundance standards (only the bottom spectra for each metabolite in Fig. 18). This figure would convey almost no *information* s/n for the Biomarker approach; that is, there is no statistical significance that can be gleaned from runs of one chemical standard versus one sample.

For the Pathway approach, the data set from the same two GC-MS runs would include the isotopologue data (top spectra for each metabolite in Fig. 18), from which we can readily obtain hints of glucose metabolism pathways. Of course, there is almost no *scientific* information in Fig. 18 alone (to obtain that, the corresponding control samples must be run), but there is clear evidence for the analytical approach to be able to distinguish biochemical pathways, which clearly conveys the potential to gain scientific information from continued experimentation and analysis. In summary, from two GC-MS runs—one standard and only one sample—the Biomarker approach would gain next to no information (conceptually, information $s/n \leq 1$) while the Pathway approach already yields some useful information (conceptually, information $s/n > 1$).

Once it is established that the information $s/n > 1$ for a given analytical approach, then the next focus of MS analysis for metabolomics should be high information throughput (HIT), not per se high sample or data throughput. The reasoning behind HIT is simple: obviously, high data or sample throughput that yields data with information $s/n < 1$ is in essence useless. HIT is not a function of the analytical technique alone. HIT requires the interaction of MS considerations with experimental design, quality of its execution, sampling, sample preparation, other non-MS considerations, such as other analytical instruments, most notably NMR, and data reduction.

Although HIT might at first sound like huge sample numbers or large data sets, that is not necessarily true. For an illustration of this, we turn once again to Fig. 18 and its legend, where arguably the most powerful "analytical" tool is the ^{13}C labeling of the experiment, and otherwise utilized the least-expensive and least-sophisticated MS instrument type. Compared with nonlabeled experimentation of the Biomarker approach, the Pathway approach of Fig. 18 illustrates far greater potential for HIT because of its much greater information s/n, without the need to improve the data s/n, analysis speed, cost, sophistication, sample preparation, or any other aspect of the instrumental analysis. The greater HIT from labeling experiments, in turn, provides a major basis for far less experimentation as compared to nonlabeled experiments, which in turn accelerates scientific discovery and hypothesis testing. In this way, pursuit of HIT can lead to experimental designs with far less samples than would be needed otherwise. The approach has been used for a number of publications in stable isotope-resolved metabolomics (SIRM) which involved this author (2–4, 7–13).

However, modern MS instruments can readily provide HIT for the Biomarker approach as well. An example of this is shown in Fig. 20 and its legend. This is a case, where the number of samples is necessarily limited (resected tissue from human subjects) which makes HIT approaches indispensable. The information content of lipid analysis by FT-ICR-MS is a very high data throughput technique, with several thousand lipid metabolites analyzed in 10 min (6); more explanation of such use of FT-ICR-MS follows below. This makes it a true HIT for the Biomarker approach. The very high data content combined with rapid sample preparation and comprehensiveness of gPL analysis supplies extremely detailed, very high coverage data for comparative statistical analyses. The key point conveyed by Fig. 20 is that such surgically obtained human samples will rarely reach large sample numbers for optimal statistical needs. Therefore, alternative high sample throughput techniques that sacrifice HIT (e.g., fast MSn analysis of only 50 gPLs) would not be desired in such cases.

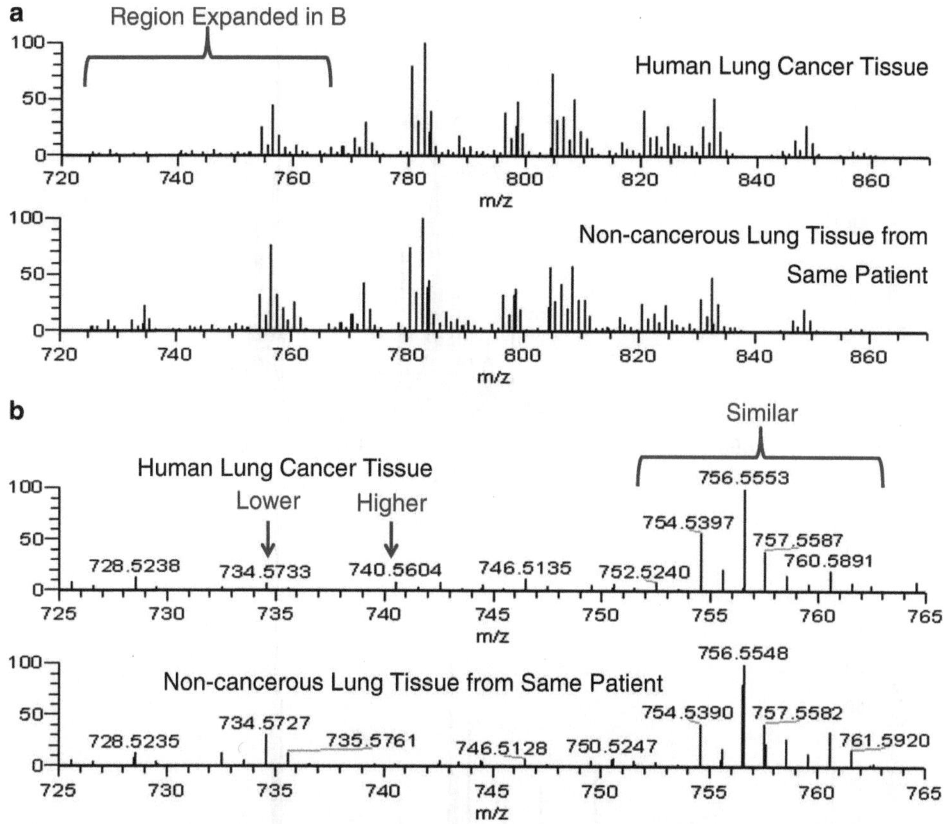

Fig. 20. Comparison of glycerophospholipid (gPL) profiles from cancerous and noncancerous lung tissues from the same human subject using the method similar to Fig. 10. (**a**) Shows FT-ICR-MS analyses of gPL extracts. Note that overall the spectra look similar to each other, which is expected since the most abundant gPL serves functional roles, such as membrane structure. (**b**) Shows the expansion of the region indicated in (**a**), illustrating the three general categories of results for the thousands of *m/z* ions obtained from each such 10-min sample run. As indicated, the most abundant lipids tend to be similar in profile while many of the less abundant lipids decrease or increase in lung cancer relative to the noncancerous lung tissue from the same human subject. In this particular example, there are >1,000% differences in the indicated lipids, which are only two out of many dozens of differences in this concentration range that are present. This is a high-information throughput (HIT) technique for the Biomarker approach; high sample throughput techniques at the expense of HIT are not needed, nor desired, nor even feasible in such a limited-subject study. Figure redrawn from 8.

Figure 21 illustrates HIT in the Pathway approach. Considerable information exists even in these spectra from just two extracts of A549 cancer cells grown on [U-^{13}C]-glucose. As explained in more detail in the legend, ^{13}C incorporation into fatty acids was inhibited without affecting whole gPL synthesis; thus, one possible explanation is inhibition of the fatty acid synthase system (FAS) that would utilize glucose-metabolism sources of carbon. Such information can already be discerned from analyzing just two samples! In fact, many more clues lie in the detailed pattern of labeling (not shown) of Fig. 21 and other spectra from related experiments so that it is possible that there are hundreds of pieces of biochemical information embedded in these spectra.

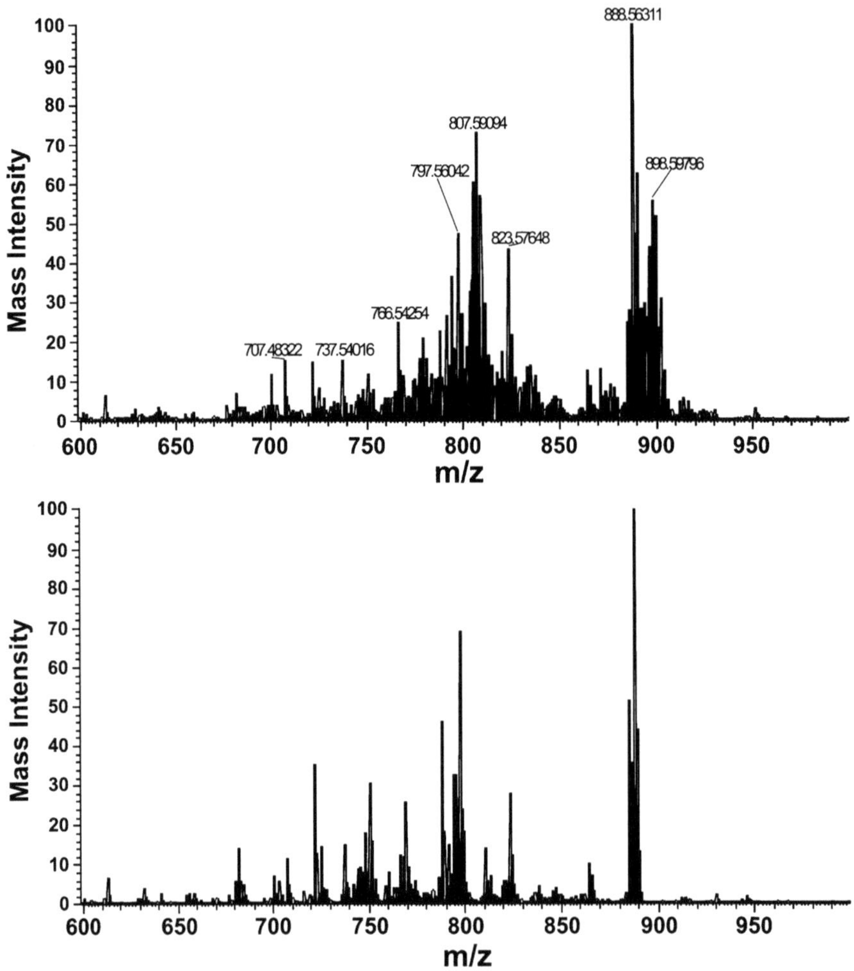

Fig. 21. Continuous nanoelectrospray FT-ICR-MS analysis of methanolic extracts of human lung adenocarcinoma (A549) cells using the method similar to Fig. 10. The A549 cells were grown in [U-^{13}C]-glucose in the absence (control, *top panel*) or presence of selenite (*bottom panel*). The accurate mass data (numerals on peaks) usually provides sufficient information for assignment of all gPLs to the head group and total acyl chain level of detail, including all of the corresponding isotopologues (6). Extensive incorporation of ^{13}C from [U-^{13}C]-glucose into the acyl chains of gPLs is evident from detailed data analysis of neutron mass incorporation (see Fig. 10 for explanation). The detailed data analysis (not shown) also revealed that the very substantial difference in the appearance of the two spectra was due to the lack of ^{13}C labeling in the fatty acyl chains of gPLs in the selenite treatment. Since the gPL head groups were ^{13}C labeled in similar fashion in the two treatments, whole gPLs were being synthesized at similar rates; yet the fatty acyl chain portions of the gPLs were not. Therefore, one plausible explanation is inhibition of fatty acid synthesis by selenite; since much of that occurs by the fatty acid synthase multienzyme complex (FAS) that utilizes glucose-metabolism sources of carbon (e.g., via acetyl-CoA), that could be one of the targets of selenite effects. Unpublished data from T. Fan, A.N. Lane, and the author.

5.2. The Natural Abundance Problem in Enrichment Quantification

Several of the key fundamental concepts above come into play when labeling patterns are complex, which as mentioned earlier can be rich in information but confounding if it cannot be dealt with. First and foremost, each isotopologue itself has contributions from natural-abundance isotopologues, which in turn means that each

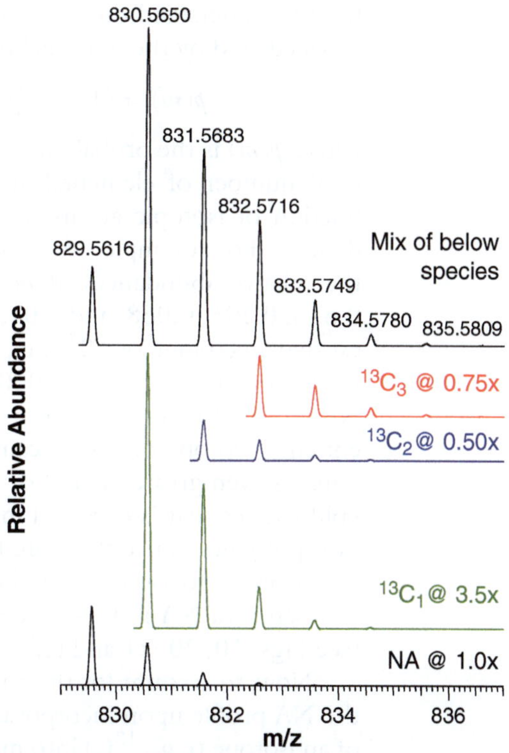

Fig. 22. Illustration of the complexity and problems regarding multiply ^{13}C-enriched isotopologues of a single compound. Simulated spectra represent, from bottom, respectively, several isotopologues of PC 34:3 with their relative levels of enrichment: *black* = natural abundance 1.0×; *green* = $^{13}C_1$ 3.5×; *blue* = $^{13}C_2$ 0.5×; *red* = $^{13}C_3$ 0.75×. The spectrum at the top is the mixture of these four isotopologues, as would be acquired from an actual sample. The problem is, except for the monoisotopic *m/z* 829.5616, each of the exact masses in the top spectrum harbors multiple ^{13}C isotopologues of the same metabolite. Moreover, neither the number of isotopologues present nor their intensities are known; in fact, this is precisely the experimental data that is desired from the analysis. Most frustratingly, because natural-abundance and enriched isotopologues are physically–chemically identical in every way, there will be no MS measurement solution to this problem; there will be no chromatographic, no mass spectrometric technique forthcoming, ever, that can distinguish between sources of these chemically identical isotopologues. However, there is an informatics solution to this as described in the text.

isotopologue must itself consist of a mixture of enriched and natural-abundance isotopes; the latter commensurate with the structure. Because the amount of enrichment is unknown, the amounts of the corresponding NA isotopologues are also unknown.

These statements are better understood by the example in Fig. 22 and its legend. A key concept from the figure is that these isotopologue mixtures are not resolvable by chromatography or mass spectrometry; thus, there is no measurement solution to this problem. In order to deal with this complexity, we first have to understand distributions at natural abundance, which can be calculated by the binomial theorem (1):

$$p(m) = (1 - f)^n f^m n!\,(1)/[m!(n - m)!], \tag{1}$$

where $p(m)$ is the probability of finding m isotopic atoms, n is the total number of elemental atoms in the molecule, and f is the fraction of isotopic atoms (e.g., $^{13}C = 1.108\%$ at natural abundance). For example, for carbon in PC 34:1, $n = 42$, and the relative abundances of $m + 0$, $m + 1$, $m + 2$, and $m + 3$ are 0.626, 0.295, 0.068, and 0.01, respectively. Thus, for even a modest dynamic range of 10^3 (i.e., the largest and smallest peaks have intensity differences of 1,000-fold), in this case at least four NA isotopologues must be taken into account for each of the enriched isotopologues. Because in real applications the dynamic range is even greater at 10^4 or more, this means that even a single lipid species that is enriched in ^{13}C can have many dozens of NA isotopologues. Since there are hundreds of lipid species in a single spectrum, it follows that a single spectrum can easily consist of thousands of NA isotopologues. This is, in fact, what is observed (see Figs. 10, 20, 21 and refs. 3, 4, 6, 7).

Now, to account for the enrichment—effectively the change in the NA profile upon incorporation of multiple unknown numbers of an isotope (e.g., ^{13}C) into molecules—an exact solution was not available until recently, when an iterative NA isotope stripping approach was developed for pathway metabolomics (6, 14). This is based on eventually decaying binomial terms (2) that describe the multiple possible combinations of ^{13}C incorporation for a particular molecule,

$$B(n,k) = \binom{C_{\text{Max}} - n}{k - n} \text{NA}_{13_\text{C}}^{k-n} (1 - \text{NA}_{13_\text{C}})^{C_{\text{Max}} - k},$$

$$B\ \text{Sum}(n) \sum_{k=n+1}^{C_{\text{Max}}} B(n,k), \tag{2}$$

where C_{Max} is the number of carbon atoms in the molecule and NA (0.01108) is the fractional natural abundance for ^{13}C. In the presence of ^{13}C enrichment, the effects of the natural abundance can be calculated using a series of decaying binomial terms as described by (3) representing the contributions from ^{13}C natural abundance for each mass isotopologue.

$$I_{M+i} = \frac{I_{M+i,\text{NA}} - \sum_{X=0}^{X<i} I_{M+x} B(x,i)}{1 - B\ \text{sum}(i)} \tag{3}$$

starting with $i = 0$. I is the intensity of the ith species, with $B(x, i)$ defined in (2).

In essence, then, the complex isotopologue pattern acquired in the MS (e.g., top spectrum of Fig. 22) contains sufficient information to strip the NA contributions and, thus, reveals the biologically enriched contributions of each isotopologue. This is an illustration of the crucial importance of *chemical informatics* as an integral part of MS for metabolomics.

5.3. A Model Approach for Metabolomic MS Analysis

Thus far, this chapter has addressed separately the various analytical concepts for the use of MS in metabolomics. So how does it all come together? One analytical approach is to exploit the simultaneous accurate mass, extremely high resolution capability of the FT-ICR-MS (Table 1) to perform a broad-coverage, isotopologue-resolving, metabolite-identifiable, rapid, and sensitive analysis of a crude biological extract (5, 6). Figures 10 and 21 illustrate just such analyses, each consisting of >1,500 analytes including isotopologues, at picomole amounts, acquired in just 10 min of FT-ICR-MS time from biological samples using a simple and rapid extraction. In other words, a true HIT analysis: note that the Fig. 21 legend is able to discuss possible biological interpretations from the general appearance of just two spectra.

Beyond general spectral appearance, it is completely feasible to obtain extremely detailed metabolite information by this approach. A hint of this data richness was presented in Figs. 10 and 20, showing specific lipid isotopologue assignments and specific lipid differences, respectively. From any of these spectra, a long list of the m/z values can be exported, assigned, and sorted, as illustrated by Fig. 23 and its legend. In this way, the thousands of metabolites from a single spectrum can be tentatively assigned by relatively simple matching of m/z values. Once assigned, the NA isotopic contributions can be stripped from each lipid as described in the preceding section to yield the isotopic enrichment of *each* of the thousands of gPL isotopologues present in the spectrum.

Because this method uses one-dimensional MS, it is at once sensitive, rapid, and of high coverage that includes unknown or unexpected metabolites, with the caveat of tentative assignments. It fully supports secondary analyses by MSn for confirmatory and more detailed structural studies of selected metabolites. Thus, the method is amenable to both Biomarker (Fig. 20) and Pathway (Fig. 21) approaches, but places an ever-greater burden on chemical informatics.

Figure 24 and its legend describe how advanced experimental design can be supported by FT-ICR-MS analysis. This spectrum clearly shows ATP pools that have *eight* different metabolic "histories," seven of them unambiguously involving exogenous glutamine. The remainder of this spectrum (not shown) contains similar detail of information regarding hundreds of other metabolites so that it becomes apparent that far more than pathway information is encoded in the MS spectrum with this approach. The experimental design in combination with the FT-ICR-MS yields information on the kinetics of multiple pathways interacting in the metabolic network of the cells. The data processing of such complex MS spectra that is required to extract the metabolic network information,

Accurate Mass Peak List from ICR-MS

of ^{13}C (blank= Monoisotopic)

Metabolite Identity Descriptors

Difference from Theoretical Mass

Abundance

Color-coding helps to visualize identical molecular formulae isotopologues

Intensity	Input m/z	C13 Info.	Head Group	R1	R2	Adduct	Delta
7614	718.5392		PE	18;0	16;1	[+H]	0.00053
10533	720.5549		PE	12;0	22;0	[+H]	0.00058
114220	725.5579		SM	18;1	16;0	[+Na]	0.00056
12117	726.5051		PC	12;0	18;1	[+Na]	0.00014
23696	726.5610	1C13	SM	18;1	16;0	[+Na]	0.00025
7180	728.5122	2C13	PC	12;0	18;1	[+Na]	0.00039
171713	728.5210		PC	12;0	18;0	[+Na]	0.00039
42327	729.5243	1C13	PC	12;0	18;0	[+Na]	0.00005
21034	730.5274	2C13	PC	12;0	18;0	[+Na]	0.00031
77177	730.5391		PC	14;0	18;2	[+H]	0.00043
6105	731.5420	1C13	PC	14;0	18;2	[+H]	0.00045
588032	732.5548		PC	16;0	16;1	[+H]	0.00048
242923	733.5580	1C13	PC	16;0	16;1	[+H]	0.00015
5602	734.5533	4C13	PC	14;0	18;2	[+H]	0.00078
73200	734.5616	2C13	PC	16;0	16;1	[+H]	0.00009
296498	734.5704		PC	12;0	20;0	[+H]	0.00043
13183	735.5649	3C13	PC	16;0	16;1	[+H]	0.00004
119581	735.5737	1C13	PC	12;0	20;0	[+H]	0.00005
5458	736.5689	4C13	PC	16;0	16;1	[+H]	0.00068
35466	736.5771	2C13	PC	12;0	20;0	[+H]	0.00001
27978	740.5209		PE	18;0	16;1	[+Na]	0.00029
10570	742.5366		PE	12;0	22;0	[+Na]	0.00034

Fig. 23. Illustration of data output from precalculated mass isotopologue search engine (PREMISE). The first two columns consist of a small portion of text output from the FT-ICR-MS (spectrum shown in Fig. 10), in this case a Thermo LTQ-FT using Xcalibur software. Then, PREMISE compared this accurate mass list with a simple spreadsheet containing theoretical *m/z* of every possible mammalian gPL (including those never before observed, but theoretically possible): all known head groups (PC, SM, PE, PS, PI, etc.) were combined with every possible pair of known saturated and unsaturated fatty acid chains, utilizing both ester and ether linkages. This results in a tentative assignment of the gPL adducts (columns 4–7) and their isotopologue identity (column 3) of the thousands of peaks in column 2. The last column shows the extremely small deviation from the theoretical *m/z* of each peak, giving some measure of the confidence of the assignment. A second analysis using FT-ICR tandem MS can confirm the assignments of a select number of these gPLs.

but the current state of the technology is well suited to fully harness parallel advances in SIRM bioinformatics (15–18).

6. Concluding Remarks

Mass spectrometry continues its breakneck pace of instrument development, for which metabolomics is a major beneficiary. For metabolomics, because of the extreme complexity of samples and need for very high metabolite coverage, there is a critical need to consider the difference between structural data content and biochemical information content in MS spectra. Figure 25 is a conceptual diagram that describes the relationship between spectral resolution and its analytical content for a ~400 *m/z* metabolite.

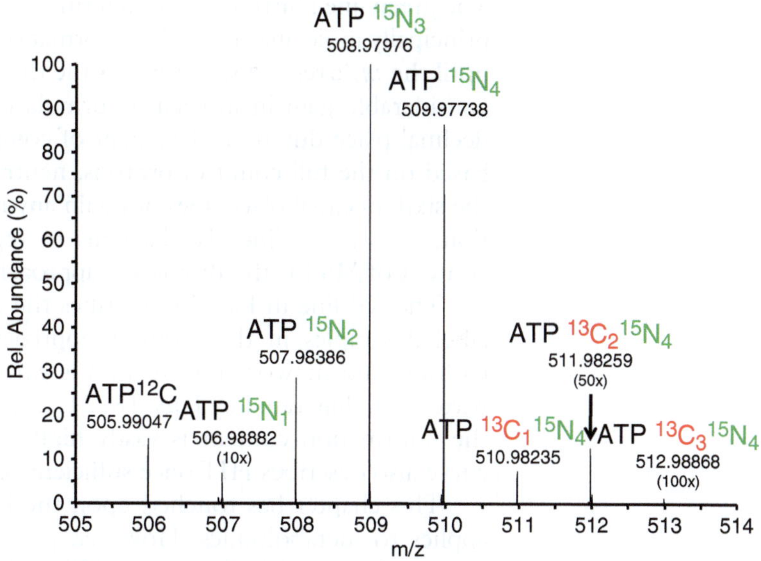

Fig. 24. Negative ion nanoelectrospray FT-ICR-MS spectrum, acquired at $R = 200{,}000$ in less than 10 min, showing the region of the ATP molecular ion cluster, analysis of an extract of A549 cancer cells grown with [U-^{13}C][U-^{15}N] glutamine in the vehicle. Note that the last two labeled peaks are expanded on the ordinate to make them visible. The spectral quality is sufficient to detect that, for example, the $m + 5$ peak (ATP $^{13}C_1{}^{15}N_1$) is not from ATP $^{13}C_5$ (e.g., a fully labeled ribose ring); that is, the resolution and accuracy are sufficient to separately account for the different neutron masses in the nuclei of ^{13}C and ^{15}N. This result unambiguously shows that some of the carbon and most of the nitrogen of the existing ATP pool were synthesized from glutamine in this experiment. In summary, this figure illustrates that it is practical to obtain simultaneously ATP structures with *eight* different metabolic "histories"; note that this biochemical information is gleaned by inspection of one metabolite from just one sample. Similar information exists for hundreds of other metabolites in the same spectrum (data not shown). Thus, far more than just pathway information is encoded in the isotopologue pattern: this spectrum contains information on the kinetics of multiple pathways interacting in the intact metabolic network of the cells. Unpublished figure courtesy of P. Lorkiewicz and T. Fan.

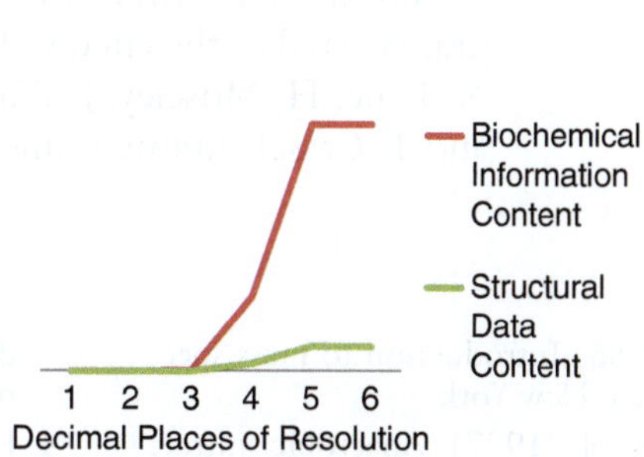

Fig. 25. Data and information content conveyed by MS. The figure assumes a molecule of 400 *m*/*z* and data is acquired with excellent accurate mass. Concepts conveyed by this figure are discussed in the text.

The green line illustrates that, in terms of chemical structure data—principally molecular formulae information—gains are not realized until the *m/z* resolution surpasses the third decimal place. There is considerable gain in molecular formula confidence with the fifth decimal place due to achievement of complete molecular formula based on the full count of protons, neutrons, and electrons while the sixth decimal place does not gain any more structural information. This green line also happens to represent the information content of MS for the Biomarker approach.

The red line in Fig. 25 describes the curve for stable isotope-labeled samples in the Pathway approach. Because biochemical pathway and network information is *encoded* in the isotopologue pattern (as illustrated by Figs. 18, 21, 22, 24, and refs. 2–4, 6–13), the information content is vastly higher. It follows that the red curve also describes HIT once sufficient resolution is reached.

This chapter has touched upon the key concepts of MS as it applies to metabolomics. However, perhaps the most important concept conveyed is that useful MS analysis is largely dependent on non-MS aspects, such as experimental design, in particular stable isotope encoding of pathways. Aspects of the experimental design (such as the use of stable isotope labeling) must maximally exploit the available MS resources, and vice versa. For the biologist, the analytical aspects should not be an afterthought, but rather an integral part of experimental design. Conversely, for the analytical chemist, intellectual engagement in the experimental design is increasingly a requirement in metabolomics.

Acknowledgments

The unpublished data shown here was supported in part by grants from NSF EPSCoR EPS-0447479, NIH 1R01CA118434-01A2, NCI R21CA133688, and the Susan G. Komen Foundation BCTR0503648 while the published data was supported by the grants listed in the cited publications. The author thanks T. Fan, A. N. Lane, H, Moseley, J. Winiike, P. Lorkiewicz, M. Arita, J. Goran, and T. Cassel, among numerous others, for helpful discussions.

References

1. Watson JT (1985) Introduction to mass spectrometry. Raven, New York
2. Fan TWM et al (1997) Anaerobic nitrate and ammonium metabolism in flood-tolerant rice coleoptiles. J Exp Bot 48(314): 1655–1666
3. Fan TW et al (2009) Altered regulation of metabolic pathways in human lung cancer discerned by (13)C stable isotope-resolved metabolomics (SIRM). Mol Cancer 8:41
4. Fan T et al (2005) Metabolomics-edited transcriptomics analysis of Se anticancer action in human lung cancer cells. Metabolomics J 1 (4):325–339
5. Aharoni A et al (2002) Nontargeted metabolome analysis by use of fourier transform ion

cyclotron mass spectrometry. OMICS 6 (3):217–234
6. Lane AN et al (2009) Isotopomer analysis of lipid biosynthesis by high resolution mass spectrometry and NMR. Anal Chim Acta 651: 201–208
7. Fan TW-M et al (2010) Stable isotope-resolved metabolomic analysis of lithium effects on glial-neuronal metabolism and interactions. Metabolomics 6(2):165–179
8. Lane AN et al (2009) Prospects for clinical cancer metabolomics using stable isotope tracers. Exp Mol Pathol 86(3):165–173
9. Lane AN, Fan TW, Higashi RM (2008) Stable isotope-assisted metabolomics in cancer research. IUBMB Life 60(2):124–129
10. Lane AN, Fan TW, Higashi RM (2008) Isotopomer-based metabolomic analysis by NMR and mass spectrometry. Methods Cell Biol 84: 541–588
11. Fan T et al (2008) Rhabdomyosarcoma cells show an energy producing anabolic metabolic phenotype compared with primary myocytes. Mol Cancer 7(1):79
12. Fan TWM, Higashi RM, Lane AN (2006) Integrating metabolomics and transcriptomics for probing Se anticancer mechanisms. Drug Metab Rev 38(4):707–732
13. Fan TWM, Lane AN, Higashi RM (2003) In vivo and in vitro metabolomic analysis of anaerobic rice coleoptiles revealed unexpected pathways. Russ J Plant Physiol 50(6): 787–793
14. Moseley HN (2010) Correcting for the effects of natural abundance in stable isotope resolved metabolomics experiments involving ultra-high resolution mass spectrometry. BMC Bioinformatics 11:139
15. Arita M (2003) In silico atomic tracing by substrate-product relationships in Escherichia coli intermediary metabolism. Genome Res 13 (11): 2455–2466
16. Arita M (2004) Computational resources for metabolomics. Brief Funct Genomic Proteomic 3(1):84–93
17. Arita M (2009) What can metabolomics learn from genomics and proteomics? Curr Opin Biotechnol 20(6):610–615
18. Cascante M et al (2010) Metabolic network adaptations in cancer as targets for novel therapies. Biochem Soc Trans 38(5): 1302–1306
19. Fan TWM, Lane AN, Higashi RM (2004) An electrophoretic profiling method for thiol-rich phytochelatins and metallothioneins. Phytochem Anal 15(3):175–183

Chapter 5

Metabolomic Applications of Inductively Coupled Plasma-Mass Spectrometry (ICP-MS)

Rob Henry and Teresa Cassel

Abstract

Inductively coupled plasma-mass spectrometry is a versatile technique for rapid multielement analysis of metabolomic samples. It allows analysis of elements in solution or solids at the major, minor, or trace component levels in a very wide range of sample matrices. Laser Ablation, Gas Chromatography, Liquid Chromatography, and Capillary Electrophoresis have been successfully interfaced to extend the analytical capability of the technique for the speciation of organometallic metabolites. The principles of the technique are described, with practical details, followed by illustrative examples in the metabolomics field.

Key words: Laser Ablation, Inductively coupled plasma, Mass spectrometry, Elemental analysis

1. Introduction

1.1. Inductively Coupled Plasma-Mass Spectrometry (ICP-MS)

ICP-MS was first introduced in the early 1980s as a rapid "dilute-and-shoot" technique for multielement analysis of samples in solution and has since been successfully developed to be the technique of choice for trace element analysis. Its success has been due mainly to the increasing requirement for the analysis of elements in solution at sub ng/mL (ppb) levels and below. ICP-MS today allows most of the elements in the periodic table to be analyzed in solution or directly as solids for major, minor, or trace components in a very wide range of sample types (1).

Other elemental analysis techniques include inductively coupled plasma-atomic emission spectroscopy (ICP-AES), introduced in the 1960s, which is limited to low ppb levels of detection in solution. Graphite furnace atomic absorption spectroscopy (GFAAS) allows sub-ppb detection limits for many elements, but it is a relatively slow technique.

Teresa Whei-Mei Fan et al. (eds.), *The Handbook of Metabolomics*, Methods in Pharmacology and Toxicology, DOI 10.1007/978-1-61779-618-0_5, © Springer Science+Business Media New York 2012

2. ICP-MS Optimization

2.1. Sample Introduction

Liquid or solid samples must first be converted into an aerosol of particles approximately <10 μm diameter, suitable for injection into the inductively coupled plasma (ICP).

2.2. Solution Analysis

Sample solutions may be natural liquids, solids dissolved in aqueous or organic phases, or eluants from chromatography. Before selection of the optimal sample introduction system, it is important to consider all aspects of the sample solutions, e.g., acidity, total dissolved solids (TDS), and matrix elements that may produce interferences on trace analytes. To analyze solutions, some type of nebulizer is used to generate an aerosol of the sample (Fig. 1). A concentric nebulizer is a "free-aspirating" nebulizer that generates a sample aerosol with a wide range of droplet sizes (2). The droplet sizes are dependent on the applied nebulizer argon pressure that must be optimized to maximize the production of small aerosol droplets prior to their injection into the plasma. Other nebulizers, e.g., V-groove, require the use of a peristaltic pump to deliver the solution to the ICP, in this case the speed of the pump must be also optimized to avoid either "starving" or "flooding" the nebulizer. Typical liquid sample flow rates for a concentric nebulizer are 0.2–1.0 mL/min and when using a peristaltic pumped system, consistent flow rates can be achieved that are less affected by different sample viscosities than free-aspiration.

The concentric glass nebulizer is easy to set up, is widely available, and requires no mechanical adjustment. However, it may be blocked when aspirating >0.2% TDS, and it is not resistant to aggressive acids

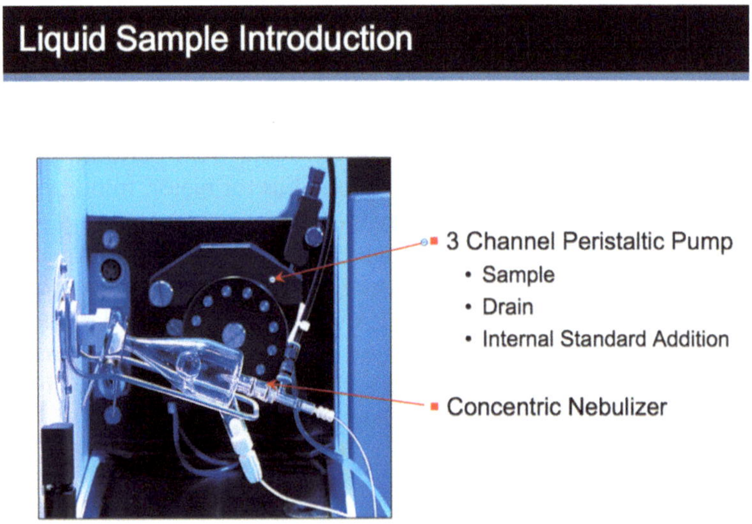

Fig. 1. An example liquid sample introduction system (ThermoFisher Scientific, with permission).

such as hydrofluoric acid (HF). Inert nebulizers are available for HF applications. Low flow nebulizers (0.05–0.2 mL/min) are also useful when sample size is limited but they are more susceptible to blockage.

Internal standards e.g., ^{6}Li, ^{45}Sc, ^{71}Ga, ^{89}Y, ^{103}Rh, ^{115}In, ^{159}Tb, ^{209}Bi cover most of the mass range and are normally added to compensate for signal intensity drift and/or matrix effects (signal suppression or enhancement). They are spiked into each standard and sample at the same concentration or added on-line using a third channel of the peristaltic pump, they mix with the sample in the spray chamber before entering the plasma. It is important to ensure that the internal standard used for correction is not present in the samples since the correction relies on having an identical concentration in all standards and samples.

Sample ionization in the ICP is most efficient when the mean droplet size of the sample aerosol is <10 μm, therefore a droplet sorting device (spray chamber) is used to condense the larger droplets and deliver the smallest to the plasma. When using a standard concentric nebulizer, only about 1% of the original sample aerosol is of optimal droplet size for the plasma, the remaining 99% is drained from the base of the chamber. In order to minimize memory effects between samples, the spray chamber should exhibit fast washout. Spray chambers are available in quartz or inert materials such as Teflon® or PEEK. Spray chambers may be temperature-controlled to reduce the effects of room temperature changes. Cooling the spray chamber to 3°C also reduces the water vapor pressure in the spray chamber resulting in lower water loading of the ICP, higher ionization efficiency and lower levels of oxide interferences in the mass spectrum (3).

Some applications are enhanced by the use of an additional mass flow controller (MFC) for controlled addition of specific gases into the spray chamber and ICP, e.g., methane, oxygen, helium, hydrogen, or nitrogen. (4).

Key instrument parameters for solution analysis sample introduction

1. Sample uptake tube:
   - (a) Free aspiration uptake—ensure that the tube is not blocked by observing and/or measuring the liquid flow rate.
   - (b) Peristaltic pump uptake—ensure that the pump tubing is in good condition, if not the signal will be unstable when compared with free aspiration.
2. Sample washout tube—ensure that the tube is not blocked or causing "pooling" in the spray chamber that would result in signal instability and drift.
   - (a) Internal Standard addition (if applicable)—when spiking all blanks, standards and samples ensure that the accuracy of the spike is consistent otherwise the correction calculation will produce inaccurate results.

   (b) If adding the Internal Standard on-line, ensure that the peristaltic pump tube is in good condition.
   (c) Depending on the sensitivity of the ICP-MS select a suitable concentration of internal standards to produce a low %RSD signal, 100,000–300,000 icps (integrated counts per second) is usually sufficient.
3. Peristaltic pump speed
   (a) When using free aspiration of the sample, ensure that the pump speed is sufficient to drain the excess sample effectively (see step 2).
   (b) When pumping the sample with or without internal standard, optimize the pump speed to maximize the signal and minimize the oxide interference formation (3).
4. Nebulizer gas flow—optimize the argon flow to maximize the signal for the elements of interest and minimize the oxide interference formation (3).
5. Nebulizer condition—ensure that it is not restricted or blocked by observing the liquid uptake.
6. Spray chamber condition—if it is not clean, it will not wash out the sample efficiently, which leads to memory effects, observe liquid flow in the drain tube. To clean immerse in 10% v/v nitric acid.
7. Gas and liquid connections—ensure that there are no leaks since an air leak will result in high oxide interference levels.
8. ICP torch condition—ensure that the torch is clean and that the sample injector is concentric in the torch, not damaged or melted at the tip.
9. Screen condition (if applicable)—should be clean and be mounted such that the torch is shielded from plasma RF coils.
10. Screen grounding (if applicable)—may be checked after plasma ignition by switching to "float" and observing a major loss of signal intensity.
11. ICP torch position—ensure that the horizontal and vertical position of the torch is aligned with the sample cone orifice to allow maximal ion extraction from the plasma. Ensure that the sampling depth is correct for the type of plasma used (hot or cold).

2.3. Solids Analysis: Laser Ablation ICP-MS (LA-ICP-MS)

The major advantage of laser sampling is the ability to analyze most solids directly for bulk elemental composition, spatial differentiation, and depth profiling (5). Accurate quantitative analysis is more difficult than for solution analysis due to the availability of suitable matrix matched standards. However, when standards are available, linear calibration graphs can be obtained over a wide concentration range (5). Unattended, automatic analysis is possible with LA-ICP-MS; however, the limiting factor is the number of samples that can be placed into the ablation cell.

Flat-top laser profiles are produced by current laser optics, enabling more efficient ablation and more accurate depth profile studies (6).

The coupling efficiency to opaque matrices has been greatly improved by utilizing UV lasers operating at 213 and 193 nm (7). A solid sample is ablated to form a dry aerosol by repetitively firing a laser focused at the sample surface enclosed in a gas tight cell. An argon or helium sweep gas flows at 0.5–1.5 L/min over the surface of the sample and is used to transport the aerosol to the ICP. Optimizing the ablation process includes the choosing the sample position, laser spot size, laser acquisition pattern, sweep gas flow rate, laser energy, and repetition rate (5). When ICP-MS is used with the Laser, the nebulizer and spray chamber glassware are removed and the dry aerosol generated in the laser sampling cell is delivered directly to the ICP torch injector.

Key parameters for laser ablation sample introduction

1. Sample position—the laser may be focused at the required starting point by using manual control of the x, y, z sample stage with a suitable lighting regime
2. Sample spot size and acquisition pattern.
   (a) Spot size—the size of the laser crater will affect the quantity of solid ablated (10 μm is typically the minimum); the larger the spot size, the greater the sensitivity as more sample material is ablated.
   (b) Acquisition pattern—single spots, multiple spots, lines, and raster patterns can be used for ablation and the same pattern can be repeated with a suitable focus change to extend the time of data acquisition. Single spots are usually used for feature analysis or depth profiling, whereas lines and raster patterns allow for bulk analysis and/or sample homogeneity experiments. The depth of the crater should be no more than 3 times the spot size to maintain efficient ablation of the sample.
3. Sweep gas flow rate—the sweep gas (usually Helium) flows across the surface of the sample and picks up the ablated particles and is mixed with the nebulizer gas before reaching the ICP. The sweep gas should be optimized in conjunction with the nebulizer gas flow. The nebulizer flow rate allows fine-tuning of the sensitivity once the optimal sweep gas flow is determined.
4. Laser energy—the laser energy control regulates the energy available at the sample surface and the energy required to ablate the sample efficiently depends on the sample type.

The depth of ablation per shot will affect the intensity of the signal produced. Therefore, the laser energy needs to be optimized for each sample matrix.

5. Laser repetition rate—the repetition rate (typically 10–20 Hz) is the number of laser shots per second arriving at the sample surface, and it determines the rate of sample ablation from the crater. When using a single spot, the depth of the crater is proportional to the total number of shots arriving at that spot until the laser is no longer in focus. When combined with the scan speed of the sample stage for lines and raster patterns, it determines the depth penetration during each scan.
6. Sample transfer tube—a flexible plastic tube (Tygon®) that may be replaced when contaminated. It transfers the sample through a switching valve, which also requires regular cleaning, to join the nebulizer gas before reaching the ICP.

Ion production

From the spray chamber, the aerosol passes rapidly into the central channel of the plasma, where it undergoes desolvation (in the case of liquids), vaporization, atomization, and finally ionization. The chemical nature of each element is determined by the number of protons (atomic number) in the nucleus. There are 211 isotopes of the natural elements; different isotopes of the elements contain the same number of protons with different numbers of neutrons. The isotopic abundance of each element is a factor that affects its relative sensitivity, i.e., ions per second of a specific isotope arriving at the detector. The natural isotopes and their abundances are shown in Fig. 2.

The specific isotopic "fingerprint" of multi-isotopic elements is also useful for confirming the presence of such elements in the sample and for identifying potential interferences (cf. Fig. 3).

The first ionization potential (IP) of each element is the number of electron volts (eV) required to release an electron from the outermost orbit of an atomic state to generate a singly charged ion (M^+). For example, lithium has two natural isotopes, with 6 and 7 atomic mass units (amu) consisting of 3 protons, 3 electrons, and 3 or 4 neutrons, respectively. After exciting one electron from each atom, Li^+ ions are formed at 6 and 7 amu that can be separated by a mass spectrometer. A mass spectrometer separates ions on a mass/charge (m/z) basis, so if two electrons were to be removed from each lithium atom, the resulting Li^{++} ions would appear in the mass spectrum at masses 3 and 3.5 amu potentially resulting in interferences on M^+ ions at those masses (in practice there are no nonradioactive elements at those masses).

The argon plasma produces an 8–10,000 degrees K temperature regime, at which temperature most samples are broken down to the atomic state and then transitioned from the atomic to the ionized state. The first ionization potential of argon is 15.8 eV and the high efficiency of the argon-based ICP source results in 80%

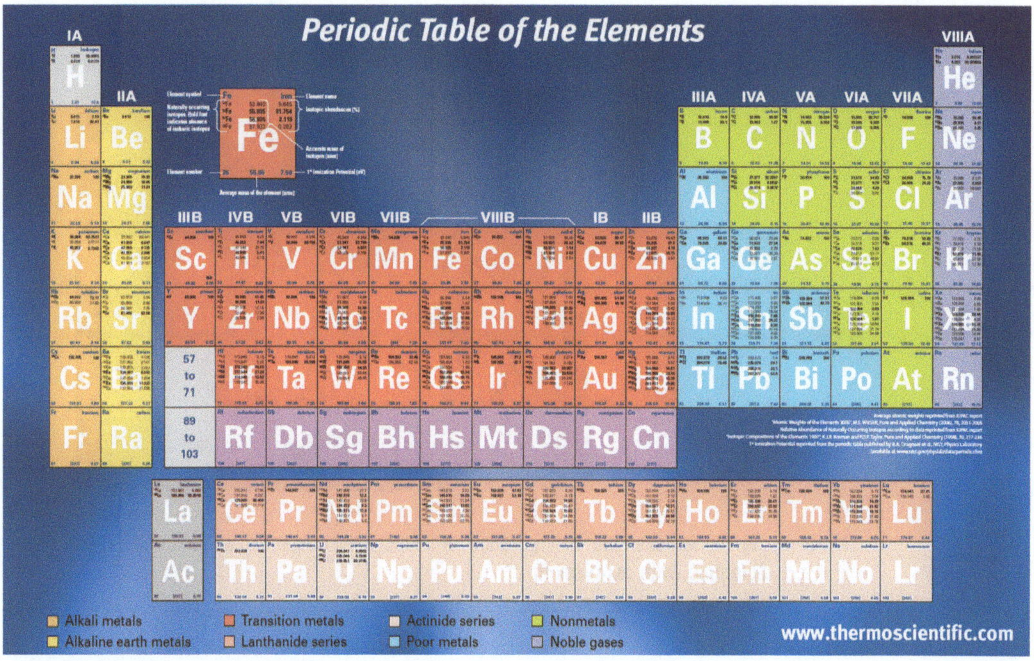

Fig. 2. Periodic table of the elements with distribution of naturally occurring isotopes and their abundance as well as the first ionization potential (ThermoFisher Scientific, with permission).

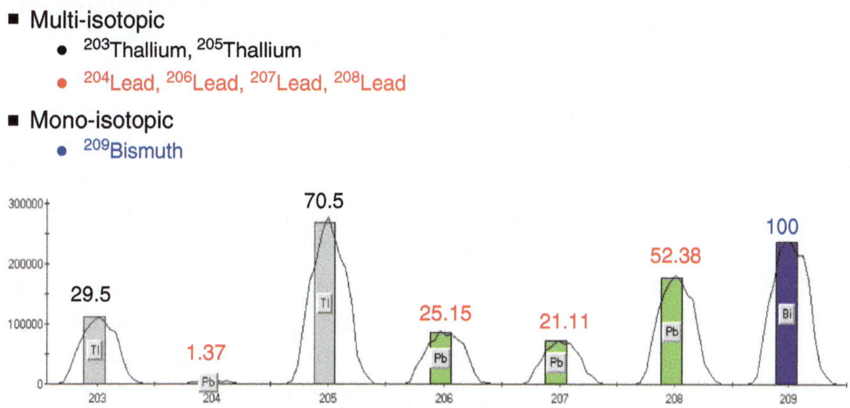

Fig. 3. Examples of the isotopic signatures of multi-isotopic elements thallium (Tl) and lead (Pb) and the monoisotopic element bismuth (Bi) (ThermoFisher Scientific, with permission).

of the elements being more than 75% ionized. The optimal temperature is achieved at approximately 12–14 mm from the load coil so the accurate positioning of the ICP relative to the mass spectrometer is very important. The great majority of elements entering the argon ICP form M^+ ions, resulting in a fairly simple mass spectrum even when many elements are present in the sample (1).

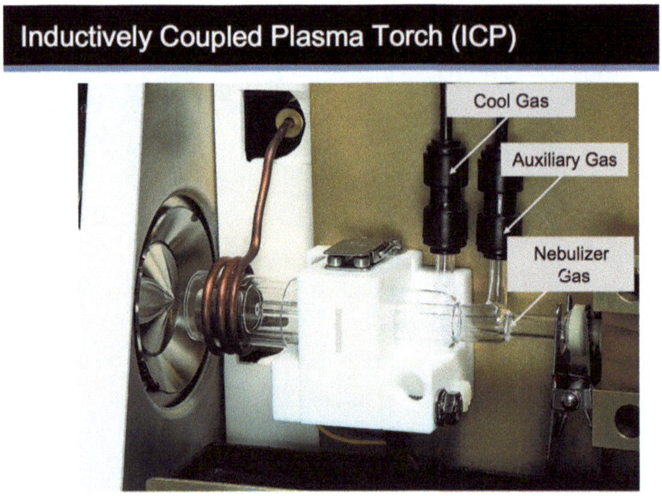

Fig. 4. An example configuration of inductively coupled plasma torch (ThermoFisher Scientific, with permission).

The standard torch used to contain the plasma comprises three concentric quartz tubes supplied with argon using MFCs for maximal plasma stability (Fig. 4):

1. 12–16 L/min argon to support the plasma and to prevent the outer quartz tube from melting.
2. Auxiliary gas, supplies argon at 0.7–1 L/min to allow optimal positioning of the plasma inside the torch. If the auxiliary gas flow is too high, the plasma will be unstable. If the auxiliary gas flow is too low, the tip of the injector will become hot and may "salt-out" the sample causing blockage and loss of signal or in the worst-case scenario melt the tip.
3. Nebulizer gas, the central tube (injector) delivers the sample aerosol to the plasma and "punches" the sample through the base of the plasma to form the central channel.

For applications where the HF is used for sample dissolution, a demountable torch system should be used. In this case the torch is quartz but the injector that is exposed to HF is corrosion resistant. A Teflon® insert seals the back of the torch and holds the injector of choice which may be alumina, sapphire, or platinum.

Standard ICP

Plasma formation can be explained by Fleming's Right Hand Rule (8), which describes the relationship between current flow, electrical field, and motion (cf. Fig. 5). The argon gas passes through the quartz torch at the axis of the load coil. The water-cooled load coil derives its power from an RF Generator and generates a radio-frequency field inside the torch. The oscillating

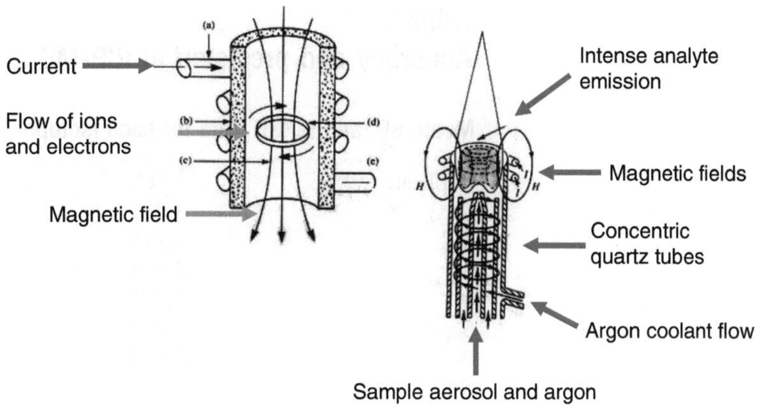

Fig. 5. Schematic of the argon plasma formation chamber (reproduced with permission of the Willard et al. (8)).

magnetic component of this field would not normally couple to an inert gas, but by passing a discharge from a Tesla coil into the argon, some Ar^+ ions are formed. This seeding of ions allows the RF magnetic field to couple with the argon and a cascade of Ar^+ ions are formed that result in a stable plasma inside the torch. A plasma is initially formed without nebulizer gas flow and has a toroidal shape. When the nebulizer gas flow is optimized, the sample stream is punched through the central channel of the plasma allowing the sample to be ionized (8).

High sensitivity ICP

Since the argon plasma consists of free Ar^+ ions and electrons sustained by an oscillating RF field and because the electrons are much more mobile than ions, they will follow much more closely the varying magnetic field from the RF coil. As a consequence, there is some charge separation within the plasma itself allowing it to act as a diode, which means that a small amount of the RF can be rectified. The net effect is that the plasma will be slightly positive (or negative) with respect to ground and the ions will be given a small extra acceleration. Another effect is that a small corona discharge is formed in the low-pressure region at the entrance to the mass spectrometer between the sample cone and the skimmer cone (see Sect. 3); it is thought that this is the region where some recombination reactions may take place (9).

By positioning a grounded screen between the RF source and the plasma, the amount of rectification in the plasma, the electrical discharge in the interface and consequently the number of recombinations can be reduced. A protective bonnet is also inserted between the RF coil and the screen to prevent any accidental grounding, which could cause the plasma to shut down. The screen may be used at low (~600 W) power (cool plasma) and high (~1,400 W) RF power (hot plasma) depending on the application.

Table 1
Accuracy and precision in ICP-MS

Mean, SD, and %RSD Data for each isotope

Replicate	^{235}U	^{238}U
1	3,749	1,044,856
2	3,718	1,030,898
3	3,734	1,031,154
4	3,704	1,029,351
5	3,719	1,029,117
X	3,725	1,033,075
S	16.9	6647.2
%RSD	0.45	0.64
Isotope ratios		
Replicate	$^{235}U/^{238}U$	$^{238}U/^{235}U$
1	0.00359	278.73874
2	0.00361	277.26463
3	0.00362	276.15056
4	0.00360	277.86526
5	0.00361	276.73497
X	0.00361	277.35083
S	0.000	1.002
%RSD	0.361	0.361

The result is improved sensitivity and lower detection limits in hot plasma mode, as shown in Table 1.

2.4. ICP-MS Accuracy and Precision

The accuracy and precision of ICP-MS data depends on many *user-defined* parameters:

1. Instrument tuning for sensitivity, background and stability.
2. How well polyatomic or isobaric interferences are corrected using an equation, or removed using a collision gas or high resolution.
3. How well the analyst prepares the standards (gravimetrically being the most accurate).
4. How closely the standard matrix matches that of the samples.
5. How well the internal standards (2.2) compensate for any drift or suppression during the data acquisition.
6. Whether external standard quantification (least accurate), standard additions or isotope ratio/dilution (most accurate) is used for calculation.
7. When using isotope ratios for quantification it is important to ensure that the pulse counting deadtime correction (3.4) is accurate and that the mass bias is calculated by analysis of a certified isotopic standard.

8. Total ion count rates (icps) achieved for each of the isotopes will affect the precision and hence the accuracy. When using Quadrupole-ICP-MS the dwell times used for each isotope combined with the number of averaged mass spectrometer sweeps and the number of replicates used to calculate the final answer. In the example (Table 1) for a 1 ng/L solution of depleted uranium each replicate was the average of 500 sweeps of the quadrupole with one point/peak data acquisition using a dwell time of 50 ms for the low count rate ^{235}U and 10 ms for the high count rate ^{238}U. By optimizing the dwell time it is possible to improve the counting statistics for low sensitivity isotopes such that the %RSDs closely match those for high sensitivity isotopes. Since the precision of the ratios is better than that of the individual isotopes it leads to improved accuracy when using isotope ratios for quantification.

Key parameters

1. Cool gas flow—usually 13–16 L/min, it is the major argon flow which prevents the outer cylinder of the torch from melting once the hot plasma has been formed.
2. Auxiliary gas flow—usually optimized between 0.7 and 1.0 L/min, it effectively moves the plasma within the confines of the torch and prevents the tip of the sample injector from melting.
3. Nebulizer gas flow—the gas flow for each nebulizer needs to be optimized to ensure that the sample is punched through the plasma where it can be efficiently ionized. Note that a high nebulizer flow rate will cool the central channel resulting in lower element sensitivity and high levels of interferences being observed, e.g., metal oxides.
4. Additional gas flow (if applicable)—when analyzing organic solutions oxygen should be added to burn off the excess carbon before it blocks the sample cone orifice. Other gases may be added to improve sensitivity (4).
5. ICP torch condition—the torch should be clean (soak in 10% v/v nitric acid) and not distorted by the heat of the ICP otherwise memory effects and poor sensitivity will be observed.
6. Screen condition (if applicable)—should be clean and be positioned such that it overlaps the RF load coil.
7. Screen grounding (if applicable)—the screen is "floated" during plasma ignition but grounded during normal operation. If the grounding is not functional significant sensitivity loss will be observed.
8. ICP torch position relative to the RF load coil—the ICP torch should be positioned in the RF load coil such that the injector

tip is set back (~5 mm) from the coil, i.e., the injector tip should not be inside the plasma.

9. RF Power—each element has a maximal hot plasma sensitivity at a specific RF Power setting (typically 1,000–1,600 W) but a compromise power setting is usually used to deliver reasonable sensitivity for each of the elements being analyzed. If only single element analysis is required the optimal power can be determined for each element. Cool plasma (550–600 W) has been used successfully for easily ionized elements e.g., Li, Na, K, Ca, Fe in simple matrices but due to the low temperature of the plasma many more interferences are observed.

3. Mass Spectrometer Optimization

3.1. ICP-MS Interface

The ions generated are injected into the first vacuum stage, which is formed by evacuating the volume between the sample and skimmer cones using a rotary vacuum pump (cf. Fig. 6). The pressure drops from atmospheric to <2 mbar. The high temperature of the plasma requires that the cones be efficiently cooled by a water chiller system set to ~20°C, otherwise the cones that are typically made from nickel, aluminum or platinum, would melt immediately. The geometrical design and positioning of the sample and skimmer cone is crucial to the efficiency of ion extraction and the orifices are typically 0.7–1 mm in diameter.

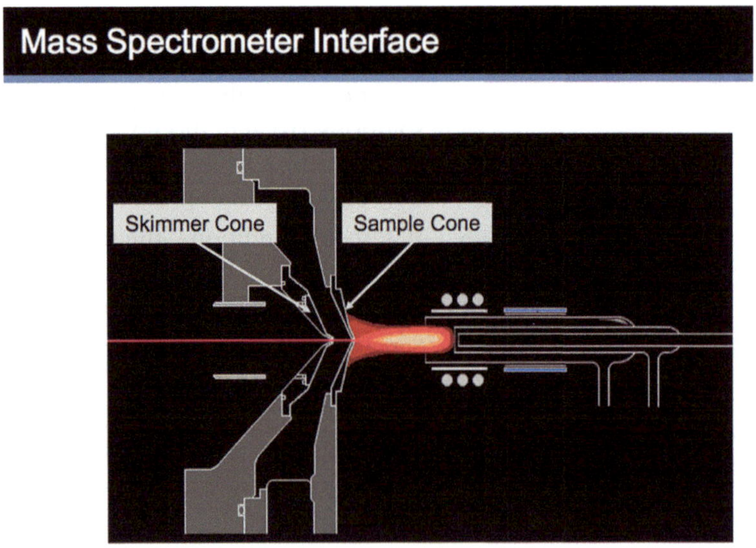

Fig. 6. ICP interface to mass spectrometer for ion detection (ThermoFisher Scientific, with permission).

The difference in temperature between the cooled sample cone and the plasma leads to the presence of a boundary layer at the surface of the cone. The shape and diameter of the sample cone orifice allows the boundary layer to be penetrated by the hot plasma gas. The reduction in pressure as the plasma gas passes through the sample cone gives rise to a rapid expansion of the gas. Inside the expansion region, the gas molecules reach supersonic speeds where they flow with non-turbulent, laminar motion. When the tip of the skimmer cone is placed in this region, the gas sampled will have a high component of motion in the axis of the instrument and the ion lenses are then used to control the motion.

The temperature regimes of the sample and skimmer cone may be designed to minimize deposition of sample matrix on the tips, which would otherwise compromise ion extraction and cause both short and long-term signal drift. The ICP torch also needs to be accurately aligned with the sample cone in the horizontal and vertical planes to ensure maximal ion sampling.

The distance of the sampling cone from the ICP torch (sampling depth), the auxiliary argon gas flow, and nebulizer gas flow all need be optimized in order to maximize the number of analyte ions being extracted into the mass spectrometer. For most applications an ICP torch sampling depth of 100–150 μm is optimal for ion extraction but other sampling depths can be used for specific applications such as for cool plasma. The effect of auxiliary gas flow was discussed previously. The nebulizer gas flow has a profound effect on performance, a low flow will result in low sensitivity since the plasma punch-through will not occur whereas too high a flow will increase the number of polyatomic interferences being formed due to cooling of the central ionization channel. In practice it is normal to fix the sampling depth and auxiliary gas flow and rely on the nebulizer alone for sensitivity and stability tuning.

Sample and skimmer cones should be "conditioned" by aspirating 300 ppm calcium in tap water for a few hours to "coat" the bare metal of new cones with oxide followed by retuning of the lenses, this process allows the cones to retain a consistent sensitivity over long periods of time. When cones need cleaning they should be sonicated in deionized water for a few minutes to remove matrix deposition but not the coating, followed by tuning after reinstallation.

Key parameters

1. ICP torch position relative to the sample cone.
   (a) Horizontal and Vertical—positions the sampling interface in line with the central channel of the ICP.
   (b) Sampling depth allows the maximal number of analyte ions to be extracted from the ICP.
2. Sample and skimmer cone mounting—ensure there are no air leaks.

3. Condition of sealing gasket(s)—to prevent air leaks.
4. Sample and skimmer cone orifice condition—depending on the sample matrix the cones will have a finite lifetime, when normal sensitivity cannot be met inspect the cones for matrix deposition and geometry, (clean or replace if necessary).
5. Expansion region vacuum (rotary pump oil condition)—if the normal vacuum is not achieved a lower sensitivity will result, inspect the rotary pump oil color regularly and change when recommended.

3.2. Ion Focusing: Standard Mode

In the high-vacuum lens region of the mass spectrometer, the pressure in the intermediate chamber is limited to $<10^{-4}$ mbar by the quantity of gas introduced through the skimmer cone. The mean free path of species in the plasma gas is sufficiently long for each species to move virtually independently to allow "tuning." The sampled ions may be accelerated and focused into the mass filter by lenses that consist of plates or tubes with precisely controllable DC voltages for attracting or repelling the ion beam. The gas sampled by the skimmer cone is comprised of neutrals, ions and electrons. The M^+ ions are selected by the use of electric potentials applied to plates placed within the chamber while neutrals and negative species are rejected; otherwise they would be seen as nonisotopic noise that would compromise detection of the target analytes at that mass.

Ion focusing: collision cell mode (CCT)

Modern ICP-MS systems may utilize some form of collision cell to reduce the significant levels of polyatomic species formed in the plasma by combination of matrix analytes, e.g., oxides, argides, nitrides and hydroxides (10). In this mode the ion optics use entry lenses to focus the M^+ ions into a multipole device which collimates the ion trajectory (cf. Fig. 7). The multipole rods are mounted inside a cylinder into which low flows of specific gases (e.g., cell gas 1) can be introduced. The cell is followed by a lens array between the cell and the mass analyzer.

The cell gas used and the lens voltages used for tuning will depend on the specific application and the target interferences. One mode of operation is known as kinetic energy discrimination (KED). In this mode the cell is pressurized with helium gas and the analyte and polyatomic ions enter the cell from the plasma with uniform kinetic energies. Polyatomic interfering species have larger cross sections than analyte ions of the same nominal mass and undergo more collisions before exiting the cell with much lower kinetic energy than the corresponding analyte ions. Applying an appropriate energy barrier e.g. +3 V between the cell and the mass analyzer will block the polyatomic ions from passing into the analyzer, whilst the analyte ions pass through for detection (Fig. 8).

Key parameters for standard and CCT modes

1. Tune for maximal sensitivity for the target analytes.

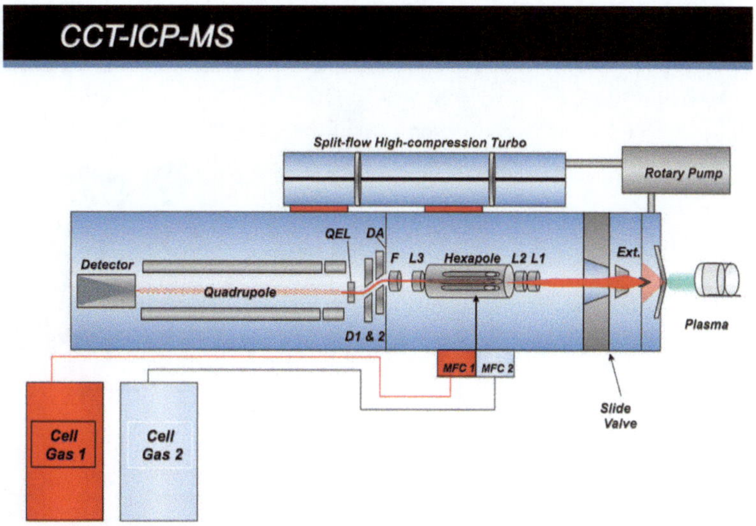

Fig. 7. Schematic of collision cell technology (CCT)-based ICP-MS (ThermoFisher Scientific, with permission).

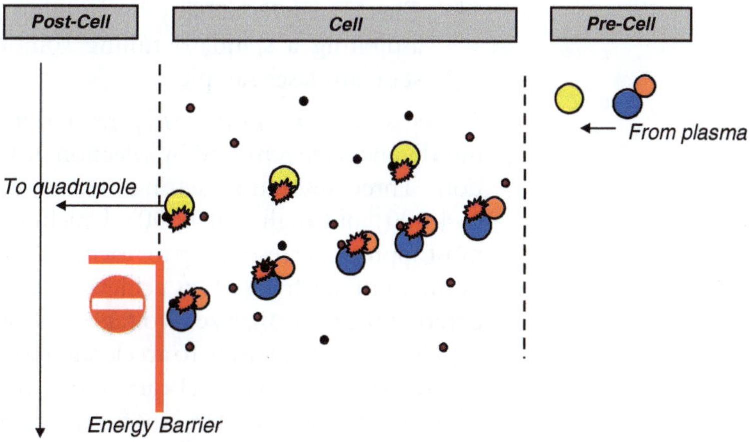

Fig. 8. The collision gas interacts with polyatomic ions to reduce their energy below the energy barrier, while interactions with monatomic ions do not attenuate their kinetic energy to below the energy barrier such that they enter the quadrupole and reach the detector. (ThermoFisher Scientific, with permission).

2. Check that interference levels are acceptable by observing the background signals for the analytes of interest and % oxide formation for elements such as Ce, U, Th.
3. Check that instrument background at 5 and 220 amu meet specifications, a low background count across the mass range is critical when trying to determine low concentrations of analytes, there should be no analyte signal in a normal ICP at masses 5 and 220.

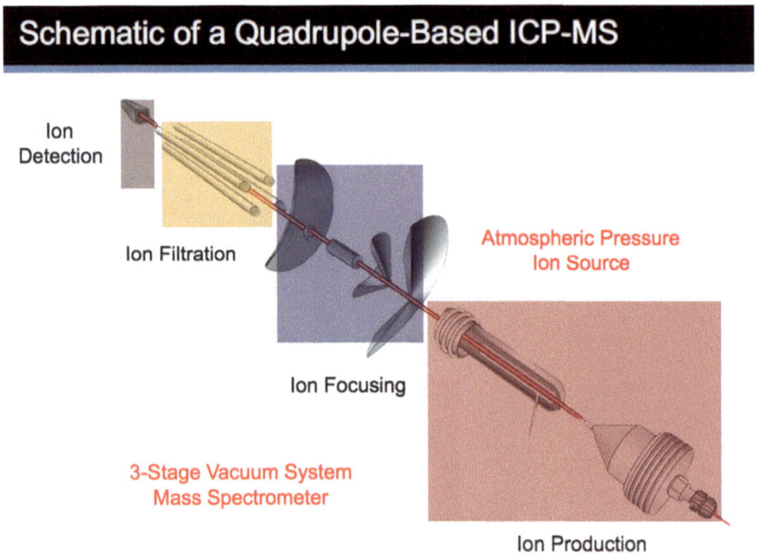

Fig. 9. Schematic of an example quadrupole-based ICP-MS (ThermoFisher Scientific, with permission).

4. Check analyte stability by running multiple replicates when aspirating a standard tuning solution or running a known standard laser sample.

Ion focusing: sector field mass spectrometer (high resolution ICP-MS) Interferences are removed by selection of an appropriate mass resolution. Three resolution settings are available low (300), medium (>4,000) and high (>10,000), which allow the user to select the most appropriate resolution for each isotope in a given matrix. The ion beam must be focused to achieve optimal signal intensity before entering the mass analyzer. Voltages on a set of cylindrical and quadrupole lenses are adjusted to accelerate and focus the ions to −8,000 V and shape the circular ion beam to pass through the rectangular slit. The extraction lens attracts ions from the plasma into the focusing lens that focuses the divergent ion beam onto the entrance slit through a quadrupole lens that shapes the beam to fit through the rectangular entrance slit. The same tuning parameters as described previously for quadrupole tuning are applicable, in addition to the optimization of each resolution to maximize interference removal.

3.3. Ion Separation: Quadrupole Mass Filter

The vacuum in this region should be $<3\times10^{-6}$ mbar to ensure maximal ion throughput. A quadrupole mass filter separates ions by passing the total ion beam through an oscillating electric field that filters ions of a specific mass/charge ratio (m/z) (cf. Fig. 9). A quadrupole consists of four rods, placed equidistant from each other. Ions move in response to an electric field and the force which moves them is proportional to the voltage so the ions move through the mass filter in response to an electric field.

The voltage and the frequency applied to the rods determine the path the ions will take through the mass filter such that only one mass has the correct acceleration speed to cycle all the way through the mass filter and will not be overlaid by an adjacent mass. The electrical conditions applied to the quadrupole determine the peak position (mass calibration) and the mass resolution (generally set to be 0.75 amu at 10% of the peak height) to maximize sensitivity and selectivity for each analyte.

Trace isotopes may occur at masses adjacent to matrix element peaks, so it is important that the trailing edges of those peaks are well controlled. The measure of this feature is known as abundance sensitivity, which measures the ratio between icps associated with the analyte mass M and the icps of at masses M^{+1} or M^{-1}. Typical abundance sensitivity values with standard plasma are 10^{-6} at the low mass side of the peak and 5×10^{-7} at the high mass side. Abundance sensitivity is controlled by optimizing the pole bias voltage (0 to +5 V) applied to the quadrupole, setting it more positive will reduce the low mass tail without a large drop in sensitivity. Using a screen narrows the M^+ ion energy spread and improves abundance sensitivity such that baseline resolution of adjacent isotopes is expected at lower pole bias settings.

Key parameters for quadrupole

1. Vacuum (sensitivity)—a poor vacuum will result in poor sensitivity as ions will be lost by collision with residual gas within the mass spectrometer.
2. Mass calibration (peak position)—a vital parameter that should be checked daily by analyzing a check standard containing elements across the mass range being used.
3. Mass resolution (peak width)—0.75 amu mass resolution at 10% peak height allows good separation of the isotopes while delivering high sensitivity.
4. Abundance sensitivity (pole bias setting)—poor abundance sensitivity will result in interferences from neighboring isotopes.

Ion separation: sector field mass spectrometer

After the focusing lenses, the analyte ions travel through a magnetic field inside a flight tube at high vacuum to avoid scattering by residual gas particles (cf. Fig. 10). The magnetic field, which is dispersive with respect to ion energy and mass, focuses all ions of a specific mass with diverging angles of motion from the entrance slit into the intermediate slit. After the magnetic sector, the ion beam passes an intermediate slit and enters the electrostatic analyzer (ESA). The ESA is a spherical deflection unit providing an electric field between two deflection plates. The electrical field bends and focuses the ions with respect to their energy onto the exit slit. The field is only dispersive with respect to ion energy ($1/2\ mv^2$). The energy dispersion of magnet and ESA are equal in magnitude

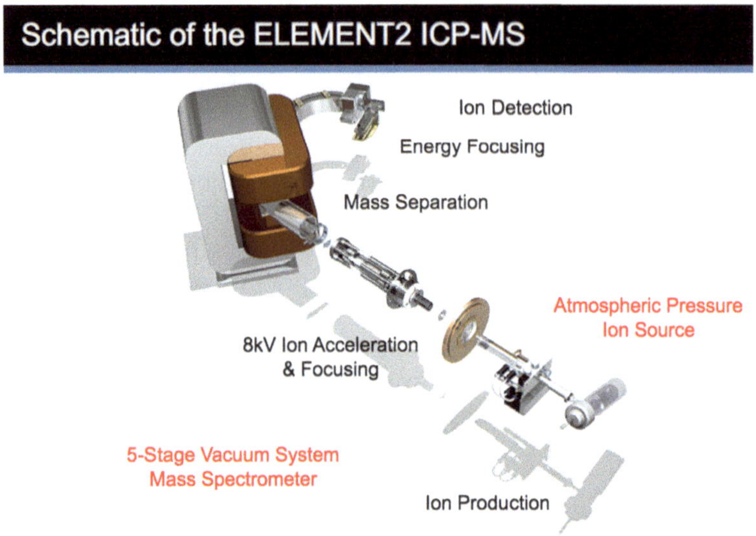

Fig. 10. Schematic of a magnetic sector-based ICP-MS (ThermoFisher Scientific, with permission).

but of opposite direction, therefore the magnet and ESA together focus both ion angles and ion energies but are dispersive for m/z, allowing user selected masses to be separated before striking the detector. After the ESA, two quadrupoles correct the focus and the beam rotation to align the beam into the exit slit. The same plasma parameters used for quadrupole mass spectrometers are applicable to each resolution.

3.4. Ion Detection

There are various types of ion detectors available but discrete dynode electron multipliers are usually used to improve counting efficiency (1). An M^+ ion striking the first dynode releases electrons, which are accelerated towards the next dynode which in turn releases more electrons. The electron cloud cascades down the body of the detector increasing at every dynode. The resulting electron cloud is counted as a single pulse at the base of the detector. The pulse counting (PC) mode is augmented by simultaneous extraction of an analog signal. The analog signal is the electron current measured approximately half way along the length of the detector and digitized into icps. All ion events are reduced to icps for each mass analyzed.

The operating voltages applied to electron multipliers are normally optimized such that a change in gain is not significantly affected by changes in applied voltage (the plateau region). To achieve good linearity between detector modes, cross calibration software monitors the PC and analog signals for each element found within a specific sensitivity range and calculates the conversion factor for each measured isotope. Since the detector is a volatile device, the cross calibration changes with time so it is best to cross calibrate on a regular basis depending on the concentrations of elements analyzed. Each detector has a finite lifetime, when the optimal plateau voltage reaches a specified level it needs replacing.

Ion detector deadtime

Since the arrival of ions at the detector is a random process, there will always be a small discrepancy between the number of ions arriving at the detector and the number counted by the detector. A compensating factor (deadtime) is introduced to correct for this that is related to the processing time of the electronic circuits. It is easy to determine the deadtime experimentally by measuring the isotope ratios of different concentrations of the same element such that one sample has an icps for the major isotope of <100,000 icps and another sample has ~1,000,000 icps, then adjusting the deadtime until the isotope ratio is equal for each concentration. The deadtime value (ns) will not change much over several weeks, however if running isotope ratio measurements it is recommended that the deadtime be optimized each day.

Key parameters for ion detection

1. Vacuum (sensitivity)
2. PC and Analog Voltage (sensitivity)
3. Deadtime (PC linearity)
4. Cross Calibration (PC and Analog linearity)

4. ICP-MS Applications in Metabolomics ("Metallomics")

4.1. Analytical Considerations

Selenium (Se) has low sensitivity due to its high ionization potential (IP = 9.75 eV). Its six isotopes have isotopic and polyatomic interferences ($^{40}Ar^{40}Ar$, $^{40}Ar^{37}Cl$, ^{78} and ^{82}Kr, etc.). All but the Kr can be effectively removed by the use of collision cell technology (CCT) or high m/z resolution. LC-ICP-MS has been used successfully for speciation (14, 15).

Arsenic (As) has low sensitivity due to its high ionization potential (IP = 9.81 eV). It is monoisotopic with a major polyatomic interference ($^{40}Ar^{35}Cl$). The interference can be effectively removed by the use of CCT or high resolution.

Copper is a sensitive element (IP = 7.73 eV) with only two isotopes. Potential polyatomic interferences include $^{40}Ar^{23}Na$ at mass 63. The interference can be effectively removed by the use of CCT or medium resolution. Because copper is used for many applications, blanks are often relatively high in copper, so care should be taken during sample and standard preparation.

Mercury has very low sensitivity due to its high IP (10.44 eV). Its seven isotopes all have isotopic and polyatomic interferences ($^{196 \text{ and } 198}Pt$, ^{204}Pb, $^{184}W^{17}OH$, $^{184}W^{16}O$, etc). Mercury also "sticks" to the sample introduction system resulting in poor wash-out and memory effects. 100 ppb gold, which forms an amalgam, is often added to all samples and rinse solutions to minimize the problem.

Zinc is a low sensitivity element (IP = 9.39 eV) that has five isotopes. It has isotopic and polyatomic interferences that include ^{64}Ni, ^{70}Ge, $^{67}Ba^{++}$, $^{68}Ba^{++}$. The polyatomic interferences can be effectively removed by medium resolution and are reduced by CCT. Zinc is a commonly used metal, so blanks are often relatively high in zinc. Care should be taken during sample and standard preparation.

Cadmium is a low sensitivity element (IP = 8.99 eV) with eight isotopes. It has isotopic and polyatomic interferences. ^{111}Cd is the recommended isotope, since it has the least number of potential interferences (MoO, ZrOH) that cannot be removed by high resolution and are reduced by CCT.

Manganese is very sensitive (IP = 7.43 eV) and monoisotopic. It has polyatomic interferences that can be effectively removed by the use of CCT or medium resolution.

Vanadium is very sensitive (IP = 6.74 eV) and essentially monoisotopic (^{51}V is 99.76 abundant). It has a major polyatomic interference ($^{16}O^{35}Cl$) that can be effectively removed by the use of CCT or medium resolution.

Iron is sensitive (IP = 7.87 eV) with four isotopes and has isotopic and polyatomic interferences (^{54}Cr, $^{40}Ar^{16}O$, $^{40}Ar^{17}OH$). These polyatomic interferences can be effectively removed by the use of CCT or medium resolution.

Iodine is a low sensitivity monoisotopic element (IP = 10.45 eV) but has few interferences.

Sulfur is a low sensitivity element (IP = 10.36 eV) with four isotopes and major water based interferences that can be effectively removed by the use of CCT or medium resolution.

Phosphorus is a low sensitivity monoisotopic element (IP = 10.49 eV) with a $^{14}N^{17}OH$ interference that can be effectively removed by the use of CCT or medium resolution.

Tin is sensitive (IP = 7.34 eV) with ten isotopes and few polyatomic interferences. ^{118}Sn or ^{120}Sn is usually selected for analysis.

Platinum has low sensitivity (IP = 9.00 eV) with six isotopes with few polyatomic interferences. ^{195}Pt is usually selected for analysis.

Chromium is sensitive (IP = 6.77 eV) with four isotopes and has isotopic and polyatomic interferences (^{54}Fe, $^{40}Ar^{12}C$, ^{50}V, ^{50}Ti). The polyatomic interferences can be effectively removed by the use of CCT or medium resolution. ^{52}Cr is usually selected for analysis.

Aluminum is a high sensitivity monoisotopic element (IP = 5.99 eV) with a few interferences that can be effectively removed by the use of CCT or medium resolution. Blanks are often relatively high in this common and abundant element, so care should be taken during sample and standard preparation.

4.2. Applications in Metabolomics

The use of ICP-MS as a technique for multielement analysis of metabolomic samples has been demonstrated in many applications over the past decade. It has provided rapid analysis of elements and element isotopes in solution or solids at the major, minor, or trace component levels in a very wide range of sample matrices. In many investigations, combinations of laser ablation, gas chromatography, liquid chromatography, and capillary electrophoresis have been successfully interfaced to extend the analytical capability of the technique to the determination of specific organometallic metabolites.

Our understanding of the metabolism of Se and As-containing compounds has been fundamentally advanced through the use of ICP-MS techniques. The technique for elemental analysis preceding ICP-MS was electrothermal atomic adsorption spectrometry (ETAAS). When speciation of elements (differentiation among organic and inorganic forms) becomes necessary, the use of ETAAS for quantification is hampered by differences in detection sensitivity to the various forms. The ICP-MS technique is superior in providing consistent sensitivity to all biologically relevant forms of Se in multiple matrices (11). In addition to the accurate quantification of multiple molecular forms of Se, ICP-MS techniques are effectively applied to the detection of multiple isotopes of Se. Due to the large number of stable isotopes of Se (see Sect. 1), isotopic enrichment (e.g., ^{77}Se) of metabolic tracers is practical. When such tracers are administered to biological systems, monitoring of metabolic products under enriched and natural abundance conditions provides insight into metabolic fluxes and transformations otherwise unattainable. Many examples of the utility of ICP-MS in performing Se speciation work are available.

- An increase in Se-77 due to a single dose of intrinsically Se-77-labeled yeast to human subjects was quantified to less than 1% of the total Se concentrations in plasma, urine, and feces (12).
- Using HPLC-ICP-MS, Suzuki et al. (13) compared the distribution and metabolism of selenite, labeled with ^{76}Se, and selenomehionine (SeMet), labeled with ^{77}Se, in rats under exactly identical biological and analytical conditions. The separation technique allowed quantification of the SeMet that remained intact and that of specific metabolites (e.g., selenosugars, trimethylselenonium ion). The isotopic ratios showed differences in uptake and distribution of the two forms of Se in various organs.

- Utilizing HPLC-ICP-MS, Larsen et al. (14) identified and quantified a number of selenoamino acids and selenonium metabolites (including a novel dimethylselenonium propionate) in yeast and halophytic *Chlorella* extracts.
- Fan et al. employed laser ablation-ICPMS (see below) to speciate selenoprotein profiles of crude protein extracts obtained from bird embryos and fish ovary inhabiting Se-laden agricultural drainage ponds (15). Such capability could be crucial to evaluating the ecotoxic role of Se incorporation into proteins in wildlife.

Plant metabolism of the nutritionally and toxicologically relevant elements Se and As has also been successfully investigated using ICP-MS. Separation techniques such as HPLC are again used to fractionate extracts and determine the proportion of biologically active compounds present. For example, the effects of fertilization with selenate in garlic on the distribution of Se-containing amino acids were determined by HPLC-ICP-MS (16). ICP-MS is particularly useful for investigating metabolic interactions of multiple elements. Size exclusion chromatography (SEC) was used to identify a high-molecular-weight entity containing both Se and most of the water soluble mercury found in the soybean plants (17). The metabolism of Se and As in plants was investigated with respect to contaminant exposure in nonhyperaccumulating plants (18). In this study, the investigators also made use of size exclusion and ion-pairing reversed phase liquid chromatography with ICP-MS to characterize the Se-rich fractions by molecular weight. Previously, Afton et al. (19) demonstrated the utility of these methods for separation of four specific Se species (selenite, selenate, selenomethionine, and selenocystine) and four arsenic species (arsenite, arsenate, monomethylarsenate, and dimethylarsenate).

As has been detected in many biomolecules by ICP-MS. Using cation exchange HPLC with ICP-MS, Sloth et al. (20) detected at least 23 different organic arsenic species in a scallop kidney. In subsequent work, anion exchange was used to separate inorganic As from all organic forms (21). Here, they used ICP-MS to quantify inorganic As in a variety of marine samples (fish, crustaceans, bivalves, and marine mammals), finding concentrations to be less than 1% of the total As content. Sloth and Larsen also showed the utility of gradient elution anion or cation exchange HPLC with ICP-MS to determine concentrations of nine arsenic species, both organic and inorganic, in human urine (22). In addition to the unknown arsenicals detected, the sum of the As species concentrations was found to be identical to the reference values for total As in the samples. Outside the animal model, concentrations of metals and metalloids often range over orders of magnitude from sample to sample. ICP-MS can be effectively applied in this type of research, as was shown by Ponthieu et al. (23) in their work using HPLC-ICP-MS to speciate As in landfill leachates. Using a cation exchange separation, the authors detected six arsenic species with a range of concentrations from 0.2 to 250 μg As L^{-1}.

The use of ICP-MS was recognized as a linchpin analytical method not only in the study of metal and metalloid species, but also of protein ligands involved in the metallome and the use of heteroelements to identify specific proteins, whether the element is naturally present or added as a tag (24). The described evolution in biological speciation has been recognized by others (25, 26) who point to epigenetics as an emerging application for ICP-MS. In this field, a variety of factors, including essential nutrients and environmental toxins such as Se and As (as described above), have been shown to affect individual incidence of heritable diseases. As interest in proteins associated with essential and toxic metals grows, the use of capillary and gel electrophoresis as tools for protein separation have been interfaced with the ICP-MS (27, 28). In the case of gel electrophoresis, laser ablation (see Sect. 2.3) is used to introduce bands of proteins separated on a gel matrix to the ICP-MS. Shi and Chance (29) review the use of ICP-MS in metalloproteomics and advocate the necessity of identifying protein-bound metals by ICP-MS in understanding the metabolic role of that protein in a biological system. In another review, Easter et al. (30) introduce vascular metallomics and compare analytical techniques, including ICP-MS, as they are applied to the role of trace metals in vasculature. Recently, Gonzalez-Fernandez et al. (31) have employed SEC, followed by reverse phase HPLC each coupled with ICP-MS to profile Cu-containing proteins in various organs of nonmodel animals. Such capability could be valuable towards environmental assessment of metal contamination. SEC-ICP-MS was also applied to speciating Fe and Zn binding ligands in cereal grain tissues (32), where the main ligand for Fe was phytic acid, while Zn was largely associated with peptides. This information could promote understanding of the relationship between Fe/Zn deficiencies and their chemical distribution in cereal grains.

5. Conclusions

ICP-MS is a very versatile and sensitive multielement analysis instrument that can be used effectively for simultaneous major, minor, and trace element analysis in complex biological matrices. Alternative sample introduction systems such as Laser Ablation, Gas Chromatography, Liquid Chromatography, and Capillary Electrophoresis have been successfully interfaced to solve specific analytical problems and provide insights into metabolome associated with metals and metalloids.

6. Resources

6.1. Sources of Equipment

ICP-MS

Thermo Fisher Scientific

http://www.thermo.com/com/cda/landingpage/0,2791,00.html

Agilent

http://www.chem.agilent.com/EN-Us/Products/instruments/ms/Pages/default.aspx

Perkin Elmer

http://las.perkinelmer.com/Catalog/CategoryPage.htm?CategoryID=ICP-Mass+Spectrometry

Laser Ablation New Wave Research

http://www.new-wave.com/1nwrProducts/LaserAblation.htm

Cetac

http://www.cetac.com/laser_ablation/

6.2. Standards

Thermo Fisher Scientific https://new.fishersci.com/wps/portal/CMSTATIC?LBCID=02177954&href=/Scientific/researchAnalytical/ProductsServices/Chemicals/sc_rea_Chemicals_052305_1158.jsp

Spex

http://www.spexcsp.com/crm/catalog/sid6cid1.html

VHG Labs http://www.vhglabs.com/Products/searchresults.php?standardsearch=d3A5WiswS1YyUnQ5Yng4ckNUbFVVb0VPU3Myc3IwWG4=

Inorganic Ventures http://www.vhglabs.com/Products/searchresults.php?standardsearch=d3A5WiswS1YyUnQ5Yng4ckNUbFVVb0VPU3Myc3IwWG4=

VWR

http://uk.vwr.com/app/Header?tmpl=/product_range/trace_analysis/icp_icpms.htm

NIST Laser Glass Standards

http://ts.nist.gov/measurementservices/referencematerials/index.cfm

6.3. Useful URLS, etc.

ICP-MS Handbook

http://www.amazon.com/Inductively-Coupled-Plasma-Spectrometry-Handbook/dp/0849323819

Journal of Analytical Atomic Spectrometry

http://www.rsc.org/Publishing/Journals/JA/

Spectroscopy

http://www.spectroscopymag.com/spectroscopy

US National Environmental Methods Index
http://www.nemi.gov/
PlasmaChem-L Mailing List
Open to anybody interested in any type of plasma chemistry
Send an e-mail to: "LISTSERV@LISTSERV.SYR.EDU" and in the body of the message type in: "SUBSCRIBE PLASMACHEM-L your firstname your lastname"
ELEMENT Users Mailing List
http://mail.library.ucsc.edu/mailman/listinfo/element
ELEMENT and Axiom specific users only
To be added to the list, send an e-mail to Rob Franks at "marchem@ucsc.edu"

Glossary

First ionization potential	(IP) of each element is the number of electron volts (eV) required to release an electron from the outermost orbit of an atomic state to generate a singly charged ion (M^+). This largely determines the ICP-MS sensitivity.
Inductively coupled plasma (ICP)	A confined plasma (qv) is maintained by energy input from a radiofrequency (rf) field. The plasma ionizes materials at the atomic level, which can then be analyzed by various detection modalities, including mass spectrometry.
ICPS integrated counts per second	
Laser ablation	Laser is an acronym for "light amplification by the stimulated emission of radiation." A laser produces a narrow, pulsed or continuous beam of monochromatic, coherent light in the visible, infrared (IR) or ultraviolet (UV) regions of the electromagnetic spectrum that delivers energy to where it is focused at the surface of the sample. For laser ablation the sample is contained in a sample chamber which has a window transparent to laser light. Argon or helium carrier gas is used to transport the sample particles produced by the ablation process to the argon plasma of the ICP-MS instrument.

Plasma	The fourth state of matter in which atoms are ionized to created a gas comprising free electrons and cations that interact over a substantial range. Plasmas are found in deep space, the sun, plasma screen monitors, as well as in laboratory conditions including ICP and in tokamaks. Such plasmas are created at very high temperature to maintain an ionized state.

References

1. Gray AL (1986) The evolution of the ICP as an ion source for mass spectrometry. J Anal At Spectrom 1:403–5
2. Gras L, Alvarez ML, Canals A (2002) Evaluation of new models for drop size distribution prediction of aerosols in atomic spectrometry: pneumatic nebulizers. J Anal At Spectrom 17:524–9
3. Zhu G, Browner RF (1988) Study of the influence of water vapour loading and interface pressure in inductively coupled plasma mass spectrometry. J Anal At Spectrom 3:781–9
4. Warburton E, Goenaga-Infante H (2007) Methane mixed plasma—improved sensitivity of inductively coupled plasma mass spectrometry detection for selenium speciation analysis of wheat-based food. J Anal At Spectrom 22:370–6
5. Pearce NJG, Perkins WT, Abell I, Duller GAT, Fuge R (1992) Mineral microanalysis by laser ablation inductively coupled plasma mass-spectrometry. J Anal At Spectrom 7(1):53–7
6. Mank AJG, Mason PRD (1999) A critical assessment of laser ablation ICP-MS as an analytical tool for depth analysis in silica-based glass samples. J Anal At Spectrom 14 (8):1143–53
7. Guillong M, Horn I, Gunther D (2003) A comparison of 266 nm, 213 nm and 193 nm produced from a single solid state Nd: YAG laser for laser ablation ICP-MS. J Anal At Spectrom 18(10):1224–30
8. Willard H, Merritt L, Dean J, Settle F (1981) Instrumental methods of analysis, 6th edn. Wadsworth, Belmont
9. Gray AL, Houk RS, Williams JG (1987) Langmuir probe potential measurements in the plasma and their correlation with mass-spectral characteristics in inductively coupled plasma mass-spectrometry. J Anal At Spectrom 2 (1):13–20
10. Koppenaal DW, Eiden GC, Barinaga CJ (2004) Collision and reaction cells in atomic mass spectrometry: development, status, and applications. J Anal At Spectrom 19(5):561–70
11. Gammelgaard B, Larsen EH (1998) Sensitivities of selenite, selenate, selenomethionine and trimethylselenonium ion in aqueous solution and in blood plasma—ETAAS compared with ICP-MS. Talanta 47(2):503–7
12. Sloth JJ, Larsen EH, Bugel SH, Moesgaard S (2003) Determination of total selenium and Se-77 in isotopically enriched human samples by ICP-dynamic reaction cell-MS. J Anal At Spectrom 18(4):317–22
13. Suzuki KT, Somekawa L, Kurasaki K, Suzuki N (2006) Simultaneous tracing of ^{76}Se-selenite and ^{77}Se-selenomethionine by absolute labeling and speciation. Toxicol Appl Pharmacol 217(1):43–50
14. Larsen EH, Hansen M, Fan T, Vahl M (2001) Speciation of selenoamino acids, selenonium ions and inorganic selenium by ion exchange HPLC with mass spectrometric detection and its application to yeast and algae. J Anal At Spectrom 16(12):1403–8
15. Fan TWM, Pruszkowski E, Shuttleworth S (2002) Speciation of selenoproteins in Se-contaminated wildlife by gel electrophoresis and laser ablation-ICP-MS. J Anal At Spectrom 17:1621–3
16. Larsen EH, Lobinski R, Burger-Meyer K, Hansen M, Ruzik R, Mazurowska L, Rasmussen PH, Sloth JJ, Scholten O, Kik C (2006) Uptake and speciation of selenium in garlic cultivated in soil amended with symbiotic fungi (mycorrhiza) and selenate. Anal Bioanal Chem 385(6):1098–108
17. Yathavakilla SK, Caruso JA (2007) A study of Se-Hg antagonism in Glycine max (soybean) roots by size exclusion and reversed phase HPLC-ICPMS. Anal Bioanal Chem 389(3):715–23

18. Afton SE, Catron B, Caruso JA (2009) Elucidating the selenium and arsenic metabolic pathways following exposure to the non-hyper-accumulating *Chlorophytum comosum*, spider plant. J Exp Bot 60(4):1289–97
19. Afton S, Kubachka K, Catron B, Caruso JA (2008) Simultaneous characterization of selenium and arsenic analytes via ion-pairing reversed phase chromatography with inductively coupled plasma and electrospray ionization ion trap mass spectrometry for detection applications to river water, plant extract and urine matrices. J Chromatogr A 1208(1–2):156–63
20. Sloth JJ, Larsen EH, Julshamn K (2003) Determination of organoarsenic species in marine samples using gradient elution cation exchange HPLC-ICP-MS. J Anal At Spectrom 18(5):452–9
21. Sloth JJ, Larsen EH, Julshamn K (2005) Report on three aliphatic dimethylarsinoyl compounds as common minor constituents in marine samples. An investigation using high-performance liquid chromatography inductively coupled plasma mass spectrometry and electrospray ionisation tandem mass spectrometry. Rapid Commun Mass Spectrom 19(2):227–35
22. Sloth JJ, Larsen EH, Julshamn K (2004) Selective arsenic speciation analysis of human urine reference materials using gradient elution ion-exchange HPLC-ICP-MS. J Anal At Spectrom 19(8):973–8
23. Ponthieu M, Pinel-Raffaitin P, Le Hecho I, Mazeas L, Amouroux D, Donard OF, Potin-Gautier M (2007) Speciation analysis of arsenic in landfill leachate. Water Res 41(14):3177–85
24. Szpunar J (2005) Advances in analytical methodology for bioinorganic speciation analysis: metallomics, metalloproteomics and hetero-atom-tagged proteomics and metabolomics. Analyst 130(4):442–65
25. Wrobel K, Caruso JA (2009) Epigenetics: an important challenge for ICP-MS in metallomics studies. Anal Bioanal Chem 393(2):481–6
26. Mounicou S, Szpunar J, Lobinski R (2009) Metallomics: the concept and methodology. Chem Soc Rev 38(4):1119–38
27. Becker JS, Lobinski R, Becker JS (2009) Metal imaging in non-denaturating 2D electrophoresis gels by laser ablation inductively coupled plasma mass spectrometry (LA-ICP-MS) for the detection of metalloproteins. Metallomics 1:312–6
28. Sonke JE, Salters VJ (2007) Capillary electrophoresis-high resolution sector field inductively coupled plasma mass spectrometry. J Chromatogr A 1159(1–2):63–74
29. Shi W, Chance MR (2008) Metallomics and metalloproteomics. Cell Mol Life Sci 65 (19):3040–8
30. Easter RN, Chan Q, Lai B, Ritman EL, Caruso JA, Qin Z (2010) Vascular metallomics: copper in the vasculature. Vasc Med 15(1):61–69
31. Gonzalez-Fernandez M, Garcia-Barrera T, Arias-Borrego A, Jurado J, Pueyo C, Lopez-Barea J, Gomez-Ariza JL (2009) Metallomics integrated with proteomics in deciphering metal-related environmental issues. Biochimie 91(10):1311–7
32. Persson DP, Hansen TH, Laursen KH, Schjoerring JK, Husted S (2009) Simultaneous iron, zinc, sulfur and phosphorus speciation analysis of barley grain tissues using SEC-ICP-MS and IP-ICP-MS. Metallomics 1:418–26

Chapter 6

Principles of NMR for Applications in Metabolomics

Andrew N. Lane

Abstract

In this chapter, the basic principles of high-resolution NMR relevant to metabolomics are reviewed, with an emphasis on practical aspects of experimental design, execution, and interpretation of the spectral data. This includes one- and two-dimensional NMR with isotope-editing techniques for metabolite identification, quantification, and positional isotopomer analysis. The principles of isotopomer analysis by NMR for pathway determination and flux analysis are introduced. These principles are illustrated with particular examples of simplified mixtures of common metabolites. Advanced approaches for speeding data acquisition, as well as additional experiments including prospects for three-dimensional NMR for ab initio identification of unknown metabolites, especially if metabolically labeled, are introduced.

Key words: High resolution NMR, Stable isotope editing, Positional isotopomer analysis, Metabolic pathways

1. Introduction

NMR is a versatile technique for identifying molecules, measuring their concentration, and obtaining atom-specific information about synthetic pathways. In this chapter, the basic principles of NMR relevant to metabolomics will be presented, followed by techniques for structure identification, determination, and concentration measurements. Finally, the analysis of positional isotope incorporation will be treated. For more detailed discussion of the NMR approach, there are numerous good textbooks that can be consulted (1–7).

1.1. Basic Principles of NMR

NMR is a form of spectroscopy like any other, in that the absorption of energy in the form of electromagnetic radiation is observed as a function of frequency. For this, there must be (at least) two separate energy states. In NMR, the difference in energy arises from the interaction of the magnetic moments of the nucleus with an

Teresa Whei-Mei Fan et al. (eds.), *The Handbook of Metabolomics*, Methods in Pharmacology and Toxicology, DOI 10.1007/978-1-61779-618-0_6,

external magnetic field. The magnetic moment depends on the nuclear spin, which is quantized; there are only certain allowed orientations of a nuclear spin with the direction of the applied magnetic field. The quantization and magnetic moment can be expressed according to:

$$\mu = \gamma hm/2\pi.Z \quad (1)$$

Here γ is the gyromagnetic ratio, h is Planck's constant and m is a quantum number whose values are determined by S, the spin quantum number. For $S=1/2$ m can take the values $\pm 1/2$, whereas for $S=1$, there are three possible values of m, $-1, 0, 1$.

For most nuclei of interest, the spin quantization permits only two orientations (the so-called spin 1/2 nuclei), which include ^{1}H, ^{3}H, ^{13}C, ^{15}N, ^{31}P, and ^{77}Se. Other nuclei such as ^{12}C have no magnetic moment, and therefore cannot be observed by NMR.

The spin makes the nucleus behave as a magnet, and thus the strength of the interaction of the nucleus with an applied magnetic field depends on the intrinsic spin properties of the nucleus in question. This is one of its major strengths, because ^{1}H, ^{13}C, ^{15}N, and ^{31}P all have very different magnetic moments (cf. Table 1).

Table 1
Magnetic properties of common biological nuclei

Nucleus	Spin	Relative γ	υ (MHz) at 14.1 T	Abundance (%)	Q
^{1}H	1/2	1	600	99.9	0
^{2}H	1	0.1536	92.16	0.1	0.29
^{12}C	0	0	0	98.9	0
^{13}C	1/2	0.251	151	1.07	0
^{14}N	1	0.072	43.29	99.63	2.04
^{15}N	1/2	−0.1	60.6	0.37	0
^{16}O	0	0	0	100	0
^{17}O	5/2	0.1355	81.31	0.038	−2.56
^{23}Na	3/2	0.2647	158.8	100	10.4
^{25}Mg	5/2	0.061	36.75	10	19.9
^{31}P	1/2	0.405	243	100	0
^{33}S	3/2	0.077	46.08	0.76	−6.78
^{39}K	3/2	0.0467	28.03	93.2	5.85
^{77}Se	1/2	0.191	114.8	7.63	0

Q is the quadrupolar coupling constant

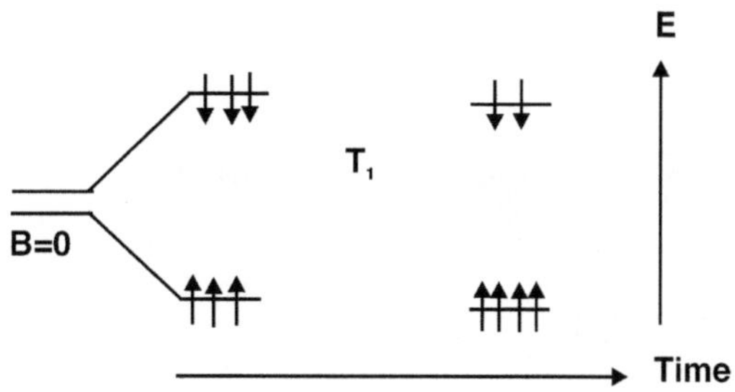

Fig. 1. Energy levels. In the absence of the magnetic field, the energy levels degenerate. Applying a magnetic field B splits the energy levels. Initially the populations of the lower and upper levels are equal, which is a nonequilibrium state. To reach thermal equilibrium, the spins must redistribute ("relax") and eventually reach a ratio of populations governed by the Boltzmann equation: $n_u/n_l = \exp \Delta E/kT$. The time taken to polarize the sample is determined by the spin–lattice relaxation time, T_1.

This in turn makes the energy difference for the nuclear orientation very different for these elements, so that NMR is actually a very effective elemental analyzer for low Z nuclei.

The magnetic field-induced separation of the energy levels for the nucleus gives rise to a differential population between the lower and upper energy levels, which is governed by the Boltzmann distribution (Fig. 1). The larger the energy difference, the greater is the population difference, which determines the sensitivity of the NMR experiment. It is easy to show for the Boltzmann distribution that the difference in population is given by:

$$\Delta p = n_t(1 - \exp \Delta E/kT)/(1 + \exp \Delta E/kT), \qquad (2A)$$

where p is the population, n_t is the total number of nuclei, ΔE is the energy difference between the lower and upper energy states, k is Boltzmann's constant and T is the absolute temperature. The energy difference is related to the resonant frequency by $\Delta E = h\boldsymbol{v}$ where h is Planck's constant. For a frequency of 600 MHz, and a temperature of 293 K, $h\boldsymbol{v}/kT = 9.85E-5$. Thus, this is in the high temperature limit, so the population difference is simply

$$\Delta p/n_t = \Delta E/2kT = hv/2kT \qquad (2B)$$

Thus, at 600 MHz, 293 K, the population difference amounts to around five parts per million.

At thermal equilibrium, the populations are described by (2). To excite the system, energy must be supplied at the frequency $\boldsymbol{v} = \Delta E/h$. The interaction of all of the individual magnets in the sample with the applied magnetic field gives rise to a net component along the field direction, conventionally assigned to z (Fig. 2). This interaction between B and the spin angular momentum of the nuclear magnets causes them to precess at their characteristic frequencies (also known as the Larmor frequency). The net magnetization

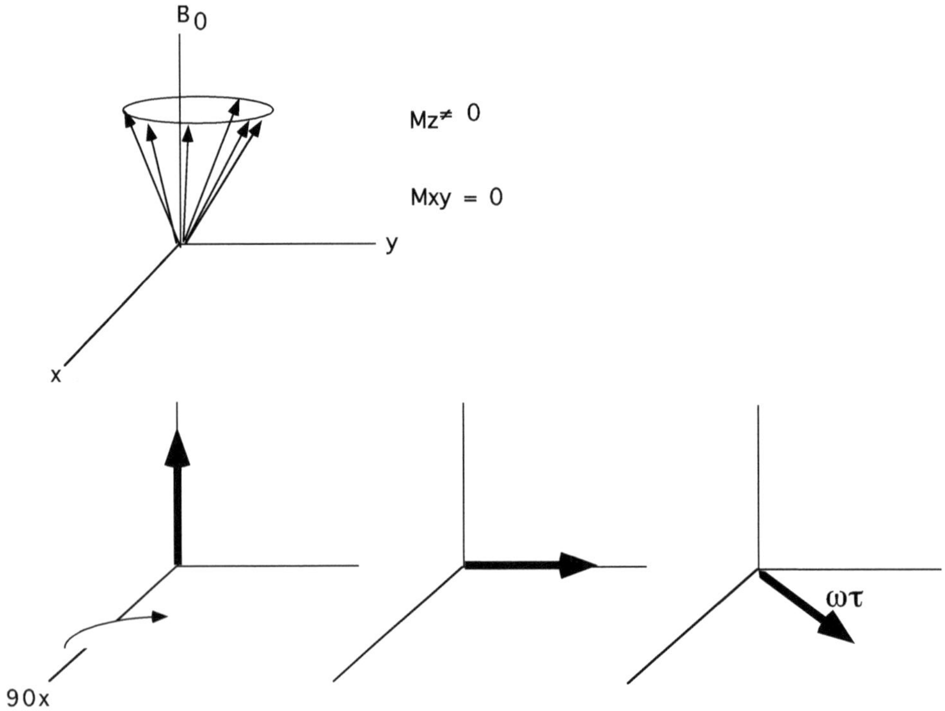

Fig. 2. Vector model. (**a**) Equilibrium Magnetization *Arrows* represent individual spins aligned along the magnetic field direction B_0, (*z*-axis) and at an angle theta. The smaller number of *arrows* aligned along $-z$ are not shown for clarity. The spins are precessing at the Larmor frequency ω, and maintain no phase coherence. Thus, the sum of the *x* and *y* components is zero. In contrast, the sum of the *z* components is the bulk magnetization, *Mz*. (**b**) Effect of a coherent pulse: rotation. The *thick arrow* represents the bulk magnetization (cf. (**a**)). The magnetic component of rf train propagating along the *x*-axis imposes a torque on *Mz*, causing it to rotate in the *y*–*z* plane. The angle of rotation depends on the product of the rf intensity and the duration of the pulse. If the pulse is terminated after 90° rotation, the magnetization continues to precess in the *x*–*y* plane at the Larmor frequency The angle of precession is then the product of the angular frequency ω and the time τ.

along z is $M_z = \Sigma m_{zi}$. Because there is no fixed phase relationship between the individually precessing spins, the magnetization along the *x* and *y* directions is zero. The excitation achieved by irradiating the sample with electromagnetic radiation in the radio frequency range, which applies a torque, and rotates the magnetization vector *M* around the propagation axis of the incoming radiation (Fig. 2). By adjusting the strength and duration of the radio frequency (i.e., delivering a pulse), the magnetization can be made to rotate through any desired angle. Rotation through 90° makes the magnetization align orthogonal to the main magnetic field, which has no component in this direction, Thus, it becomes possible to measure the value of *M* independent of the much more intense B_0.

The magnetization is measured indirectly. After rotation to the *y*-axis, the magnetization continues to precess at the Larmor frequency. This bulk magnetization will induce an emf in a nearby conductor, which can be amplified and detected easily. If the detector is placed along the *x*-axis, then as the vector rotates, the magnitude of the signal will oscillate:

$$S = S^0 \cos(\omega t).$$

By having a second detector orthogonal to the first one, a 90° out of phase signal is simultaneously detected, $S = S^0 \sin \omega t$

The sum of these components can be written

$$S = S^0(\cos\ \omega t + i\ \sin\ \omega t) = S^0 \exp i\omega t. \tag{3}$$

This signal does not persist forever as it is not at equilibrium. There are restoring force that will eventually return the magnetization to the *z*-axis. The loss of magnetization in the *x*–*y* plane is an exponential process, governed by a rate constant R_2, so the total signal becomes:

$$S(t) = \sum s_j^0 \exp(i\omega_j - R2j)t, \tag{4}$$

where the index j refers to individual spins, each having its own amplitude, Larmor frequency, and relaxation rate constant. This is called the free induction decay, or fid.

For more than a small number of spins, this is a very cumbersome equation, as demonstrated in Fig. 3. To convert the signal into the more familiar spectra (intensity vs. frequency), (4) can be Fourier transformed:

$$F(S) = 2a_0 \int \exp(i\Omega t)S(T). \tag{5}$$

This gives rise to two components, a real (cosine term) and imaginary (sine term) as follows:

$$2a_0(i\Delta\omega + R_2)/(\Delta\omega 2 + R_2^2). \tag{6}$$

The first term is the imaginary component and the second is the real component. The imaginary (sine) component has a dispersive line shape, and the real component has an absorptive (Lorentzian) line shape.

As $\Delta\omega = 2\pi\mathbf{v}$, the real part of (6) can be rewritten:

$$(a_0 L/2\pi)/[\Delta v^2 + L^2/4), \tag{7}$$

where $L = R_2/\pi$, R_2 is the damping constant in the free induction decay, and L is the width at half height.

Thus, three parameters are needed to describe an NMR peak, its frequency ($\mathbf{v}_0$), its width at half height, and its area.

1.1.1. Chemical Shift

The resonance frequency is directly proportional to the magnetic field strength, which makes comparing spectra recorded on different

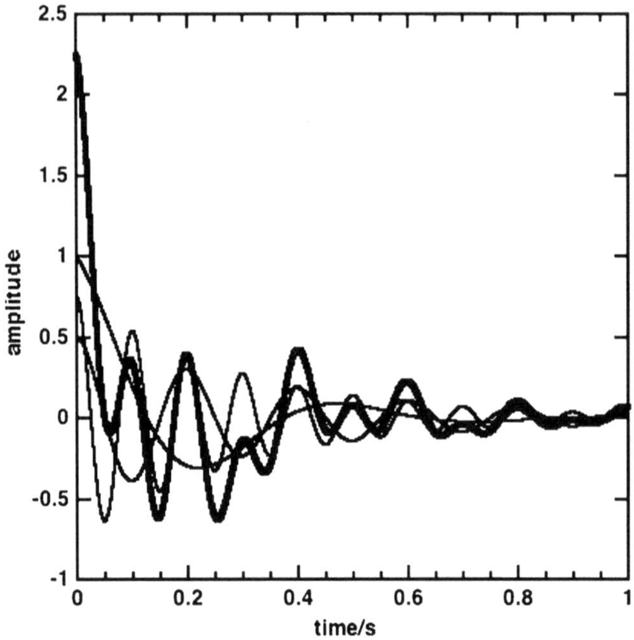

Fig. 3. Free induction decay. The figure is the superposition of three components with frequencies, amplitudes, and decay constants of 2 Hz, 1, 0.2 s; 5 Hz, 0.5, 0.4 s; 10 Hz, 0.75, 0.3 s, according to the equation $S(t) = a_0 \cos(\omega t)\exp(-R_2 t)$ The thick line is the sum of the three components.

instruments problematic. To overcome this limitation, the Larmor frequency is usually normalized to that of a standard, as follows:

$$\delta = 10^6(\upsilon - \upsilon_s)/\upsilon_s, \tag{8}$$

where δ is the chemical shift in ppm, $\boldsymbol{\upsilon}$ is the observed frequency of the peak in question, and $\boldsymbol{\upsilon}_s$ is the frequency of the standard. The chemical shift is strongly dependent on the chemical structure, and there are many tables of chemical shift compilations for various nuclei in a wide range of compounds (Table 2). This easy-to-measure parameter has long made NMR very valuable for structure identification in chemistry and biochemistry.

In order to compute such a scale, a reference compound must be used, preferably internally. There are several choices according to the nucleus being examined. For example, 2,2′ dimethylsilapentane-5-sulfonate (DSS), trimethylsilylpropionic acid (TSP), and tetramethylsilane (TMS) are all ^1H and ^{13}C chemical shift references that rely on the electropositive Si atom. When the methyl protons and carbons attached to the Si atom are assigned a chemical shift of zero, almost all biological metabolites appear at positive chemical shifts ("downfield").

The main differences between these compounds are solubility, pH dependence, and interference. DSS and TSP are both water-soluble compounds. DSS has no significant pH dependence, but

Table 2
Some relevant resources

Chemical shift compilations
Biological Magnetic Resonance Data Bank, BMRB: http://www.bmrb.wisc.edu/metabolomics/
Human Metabolome Database: http://www.hmdb.ca/
Fan et al. http://research.louisville.edu/metabolomics
Chemical shift referencing: http://www.bmrb.wisc.edu/ref_info/cshift.html
Hardware
NMR tubes and accessories
http://www.geocities.com/~shigemi/ (Shigemi susceptibility matched microtubes)
http://www.wilmad-labglass.com/index.jsp (Doty susceptibility plugs)
Norell https://www.nmrtubes.com/ (NMR tubes)
http://www.protasis.com/OMNMR/ (CAP microprobes)
Software sources
Chenomx NMR Suite; Targeted metabolomics software. http://www.chenomx.com/
iNMR (Swan NMR), NMR processing, and analysis software for Apple Macintosh computers. http://www.inmr.net/
Acorn NMR (NUTS), Basic NMR processing software for PCs. http://www.acornnmr.com/
ACD (Advanced Chemistry Development), http://www.acdlabs.com/ Comprehensive processing and analysis software; also MS and other spectroscopies
Biorad KnowItAll. Chemometrics, databases and NMR tools. www.knowitall.com/metabolomics
MestRe Nova: Windows-based processing and display software; http://www.mestrec.com/
Varian (VNMRJ) NMR processing and analysis tools. http://www.varianinc.com/cgi-bin/nav?products/nmr/software/vnmrj
Bruker Biospin. Amix databases and analysis tools http://www.bruker-biospin.com/amix.html
JEOL (Delta). NMR processing tools. http://www.jeol.com
Stable isotope sources
http://www.spectrastableisotopes.com/ (now incorporated into Cambridge Isotopes)
http://www.isotope.com/cil/index.html
http://www.sigmaaldrich.com/Area_of_Interest/Chemistry/Stable_Isotopes_ISOTEC_.html

does have proton resonances near 3 ppm that can overlap with resonances of important metabolites. Deuteriated forms of DSS and TSP are commercially available. The T_1 value of deuteriated DSS is substantially longer than the protiated form, which must be accounted for in quantitative analysis (see Sects. 1.1.4 and 2.2). TSP is pH sensitive near pH 4. TMS is soluble only in nonpolar solvents such as chloroform and can be used as an internal reference only for nonaqueous extracts. The methyl group of these compounds is set to zero in both the ^{1}H and ^{13}C dimensions. Note that the trimethyl peak has nine equivalent protons. It is also feasible to use endogenous metabolite resonances as internal shift standard, e.g., the well-resolved anomeric ^{1}H doublet of α-glucose at 5.22 ppm (pH-independent) or the ^{1}H singlet of phosphocholine at 3.22 ppm (negligible pH dependence).

$CDCl_3$ and CD_3OD are reasonable chemical shift references, but are not suitable concentration standards. For ^{31}P NMR, the choices are more limited because most compounds are pH-dependent. A commonly used external reference is methylene diphosphonate under defined conditions (100 mM Tris, pH 8.8) (8), though 85% phosphoric acid is also used. For absolute concentration determination by ^{31}P NMR, it is usually necessary to spike a sample with a known concentration of an appropriate stable phosphate compound such as AMP, or alternatively, use a compound whose concentration has been independently determined, such as by GC-MS (9). The external reference for ^{15}N is HNO_3 or liquid ammonia, neither of which is especially convenient. However, as ^{15}N is now almost always indirectly detected by attached protons, a more convenient reference approach is possible. The protons are referenced in the usual way using an internal standard such as DSS. The X nucleus is then referenced using the ratio γ_X/γ_H. As these are known with great accuracy, the chemical shift of the X nucleus at any given frequency can be calculated using this ratio. It is then a simple matter to convert that to an agreed external reference scale (10–14). The appropriate values have been tabulated in the BMRB (cf. Table 2).

1.1.2. Peak Area

The area of a peak represents the response of the amount of that nucleus present in the active volume of the receiver coil. For a mixture of compounds, the ratios of the peak areas are equal to the ratios of their concentrations, when corrected for the number of nuclei contained in each resonance. Thus, the area of a methyl group will be three times the area of a methine group within the same molecule. By including a compound at known concentration in the sample, the absolute concentration of the other components can be determined (see below).

1.1.3. Scalar Coupling

Although the area and chemical shift information are extremely valuable for structure identification and concentration determination, the existence of scalar coupling between magnetic nuclei brings additional information and also a mechanism that can be exploited or unambiguous structural characterization of covalent structures of molecules within a complex mixtures, and for isotopomer analysis (see below).

The scalar coupling is an electron nucleus interaction that is transmitted through covalent bonds and reflects bond order and strength. It decreases with the number of intervening bonds between the coupled nuclei. In general, the magnitude of the scalar coupling increases with increasing bond order and with decreasing length (cf. Table 3). The magnitude of the coupling constant is denoted J, and the number of bonds by a superscript to the left of J and the coupled pair of atoms as a subscript to the right of J. Thus, $^1J_{CH}$ and $^3J_{HH}$ represent the one-bond coupling between a ^{13}C and attached ^1H nucleus, and the three-bond

Table 3
Typical spin–spin coupling constants in metabolites

$^{3}J_{HH}$ 3–12	$^{1}J_{CH}$ 120–220	$\|^{2}J_{CH}\|$ 0–5	$^{3}J_{CH}$ 0–6	$^{1}J_{CC}$ 40–65
Molecule	C–X	$^{1}J_{CX}$/Hz	$^{2}J_{XH}$ $^{3}J_{XH}$/Hz	References
Lactate	C3–H3	127.5	C2–H3 4.55	(40)
	C2–H	146	C1–H3 4.49	This work
			H2–H3 6.99	This work
Alanine	CβH$_3$	128		(40)
	CαH	146		
Glutamine	CγH	131		This work
	CβH	131.6		
	CαH	147.3		
AMP	C8–H	216	N7–H8 11.1	(45)
	C2–H	203	N9–H8 7.9	
	C1′H	166.5	N1–H2 14.5	
	C2′H	150.9	N3–H2 14.5	
	C3′–H	152.6		
	C4′–H	150.9		
	C1′–C2′	42.2		
	C2′–C3′/ C3′–C4′	38.1		
UTP	C6–H	184.9		(46)
	C5–H	178.7		
UMP	C5–C6	66.9		(45)
Glucose	C1–Hα	169.5		(46)
	C1–Hβ	159.5		

coupling between two ^{1}H nuclei, respectively. It is because the scalar coupling is intramolecular that it is so useful for mixtures of compounds.

The scalar coupling is manifested as a splitting of a resonance. For the C–H fragment, the mutual scalar interaction causes the resonance of both the ^{13}C and the ^{1}H to split into two equal intensity components separated by the coupling constant *J*. For a CH_2, the carbon line is split into three components (triplet), with intensity ratios 1:2:1, and for CH_3, the resonance is split into four components (quartet) with intensity retains 1:3:3:1. For each case, the protons are always coupled to a single ^{13}C and are all doublets. The general rule is that for a nucleus scalar coupled to n equivalent nuclei, there will be $n + 1$ components in the resulting multiples, with intensity ratios given by Pascal's triangle (or the coefficients of the binomial expansion). Actually, more generally is that for m coupled spins, the number of multiplet components is 2^m, with equal intensity ratios. It is only the equivalence that makes the intensity ratios follow Pascal's triangle. Here, equivalence refers to the magnitude of the coupling constant. Such patterns provide information about the chemical nature of the resonance. A quartet immediately shows that the nucleus is scalar coupled to three equivalent nuclei. In metabolites, the homonuclear coupling patterns can become quite complex, owing to the possibility of a large number of coupling partners (consider the valine β proton which is scalar coupled to two methyls and the alpha proton, i.e., seven partners, giving a maximum number of multiplet components of $2^7 = 128$ lines, although in practice the methyl protons are equivalent). The splitting of a resonance automatically decreases the resolution and sensitivity of an experiment, as now the intensity is spread over several peaks (the sum of the components represent the area of the spin). For example, a doublet halves the peak height and effectively reduces the resolution by a factor of 2 (twice the number of peaks, components are separated by J).

As will be shown below, it is possible to exploit the various couplings between nuclei for structural identification and for isotopomer analysis. The scalar coupling is active between all of the common biological NMR nuclei, ^1H–^1H, ^1H–^{13}C, ^{13}C–^{13}C, ^1H–^{15}N, ^{13}C–^{15}N, ^{31}P–^1H, etc.

1.1.4. Relaxation

In the absence of a magnetic field, the population difference is zero; the energy levels degenerate (Fig. 1). The instant the sample is placed in a magnetic field, it must be in a nonequilibrium state, as under these conditions the equilibrium populations are determined by the Boltzmann distribution. Therefore, there must be a redistribution of spins between the upper and lower energy levels, i.e., the sample become polarized. As this requires an exchange of energy between the spins and their surroundings, the process of polarization takes a finite time. This time is characteristic of the spins themselves and is an exponential process governed by a rate constant R_1 (spin–lattice relaxation constant). The value of this constant is of practical importance as will be seen below.

Once a sample has been excited, a nonequilibrium state is created, and so it will relax back toward equilibrium. The z component of the magnetization steadily increases toward the equilibrium value as the Zeeman energy is regained. This is governed by the Bloch equation:

$$\mathrm{d}M_z/\mathrm{d}t = -R_1(M_z - M_z^0). \tag{9}$$

For a 90° rotation, the solution of this equation is:

$$M_z(t) = M_z{}^0(1 - \exp -R_1 D). \tag{10}$$

M_z^0 is the equilibrium magnetization and D is the time between excitation pulses.

Thus, the z component relaxes back to the equilibrium value exponentially. For a time $t = 1/R_1$, the restoration of the magnetization is 63%; for $2/R_1$, it is 86%; for $3/R_1$, it is 95%; and for $5/R_1$, it is >99%.

The spin–lattice relaxation rate has especial practical importance in optimal experimental design and for accurate quantitative analysis (see below). There is a second relaxation process that determines the appearance of the spectrum, called the spin–spin relaxation rate constant, denoted R_2. This determines the decay of the magnetization in the x–$y$plane and is related to the linewidth of resonances (cf. (7)). The origin of this process is dephasing of the initial coherence of the magnetization following the excitation pulse. This causes loss of magnetization in the x–y plane (and therefore in the detected signal) and can be faster than longitudinal relaxation. However, for small molecules, the R_2 and R_1 values are generally similar. The two become very different for large molecular weights (as in macromolecules) or where there is chemical exchange.

1.2. Sensitivity

As the rate of the transition in response to exciting electromagnetic radiation is proportional to Δp, (6.2) shows that the sensitivity is determined by the magnitude of the energy difference and the inverse of the temperature. The sensitivity is further proportional to the number of magnetic particles in the excitation region (n_t). This implies that maximum sensitivity is optimized by increasing the number of particles per unit volume (concentration) and maximizing the energy gap. The energy difference is determined by the strength of the interaction of the nuclear magnetic moment and the applied magnetic field, as expressed by $\Delta E = \gamma B_0$

B_0 is the strength of the applied magnetic field. γ is completely determined by the nuclear structure and is therefore not under experimental control. However, B_0 can be made very intense indeed, and as this determines in large measure the net sensitivity of NMR, has for many years been the driving force in NMR development.

The magnitude of γ (cf. Table 1) indicates that some nuclei are intrinsically more sensitive than others. In biological materials, the proton is by far the most sensitive nucleus owing to its high γ. Other common nuclei are intrinsically less sensitive, and also are present at much lower natural abundance (cf. Table 1). Therefore, for maximal sensitivity, the proton (^{1}H) is the nucleus of choice for detection of most purposes.

It has been shown that the integrated signal intensity, S, is approximately given by (15, 16):

$$S = kQ[\gamma B_0]^2 n.c.v/v_c, \tag{11}$$

where k is a constant that depends on the detector coil, temperature, and other electronics, Q is the detector coil quality factor (tuning), c is the solute concentration, v is the volume of the solute in the detection region, and v_c is the volume of the coil. v/v_c is also called the filling factor. The squared term arises because of the linear B_0 dependence of the populations, and the induced emf in detector is proportional to the rate of change of the magnetization, i.e., the Larmor frequency (Faraday's law of induction).

The rms noise depends on the square root of the frequency, i.e., $[\gamma B_0]^{0.5}$ (6), so that the net signal-to-noise ratio is given by:

$$\mathrm{SNR} = kQ[\gamma B_0]^{1.5}.n^{0.5}c.v/v_c. \quad (12)$$

Thus, all other things being equal, the SNR for an 18.8T magnet (800 MHz for ^{1}H) will be twice as large as that for an 11.75 T magnet (500 MHz for ^{1}H).

In pulsed NMR, the signal is coherent, so that the detected signal accumulates linearly with the number of fids, n. However, the noise accumulates as the square root of n. The SNR therefore increases only as $n^{0.5}$. Hence, to double the SNR, the acquisition time has to be increased fourfold. This is the law of diminishing returns.

The filling factor v/v_c is maximized by using thin-walled NMR tubes. Using a smaller diameter tube in a 5-mm probe (this is the outer diameter of the tube) reduces the filling factor and therefore the SNR. For example, a 3-mm tube in a 5-mm probe reduces v/v_c to $(3/5)^2 = 0.36$. Furthermore, the volume v is typically much smaller than the volume of material needed to fill the coil. This is because the solution/air interface creates a discontinuity in the magnetic susceptibility, which decreases the magnetic field homogeneity across the sample (see below). The active volume is typically <0.25 mL, in a 5-mm probe, but to achieve homogeneity, the solution is usually >0.6 mL. One solution to this waste of material (more than 50% is not detected) is to use susceptibility matched plugs or tubes such as Shigemi tubes, which have a plug of doped glass above and below the solution, allowing a substantial decrease in volume of solution (typically 0.3–0.33 mL) and a corresponding increase in concentration. In this geometry, the fraction of unused sample is <30% compared with >50%. The doping is used to match the susceptibility of the glass to that of the solvent used. Separate tubes or plug inserts are therefore required for different solvents, such as methanol or chloroform.

The value of Q depends on probe design, and also on how the coil interacts with the solution. Salty solutions effectively reduce Q, in large measure because the rf power is used in part to accelerate ions. The more ions, or other highly polar molecules, the less power is available for exciting the solute particle of interest. Indeed, it has been shown that the conductance of the solution is the critical parameter (17, 18). For this reason, nonaqueous solutions typically have a higher Q than salty aqueous solutions.

1.2.1. Cooled Probes and Other Circuitry

In recent years, a substantial improvement in signal-to-noise ratios has been obtained by recognizing that the main component of the noise term is thermal. Thus, if the primary coil and the preamp are cooled to low temperature (typically 25K), the thermal noise in the detection system is very greatly reduced. However, most metabolic NMR studies are conducted in the solution state, which is not compatible with 25K. In order to maintain the solution at say 293K, while cooling the coil to 25K, there has to be a thermal barrier between the two. This necessarily decreases the filling factor. However, the modern probe has managed to retain an acceptable filling factor while gaining immensely from the reduced thermal noise, such that sensitivity enhancements of three to fourfold for nonlossy samples are routinely achieved. This amounts to a time saving of about an order of magnitude and makes possible metabolomics studies on small amounts of tissue.

All of the above considerations apply strictly to signal-to-noise ratios, which refer to integrated peaks. The peak integrals are proportional to the number of nuclei detected, and so are essential for concentration determination. However, the area itself is not a measure of sensitivity, which is the ability to detect a signal above the noise. As NMR peaks are symmetrical Lorentzians, the peak area is proportional to the product of the peak height (h) and the width at half height (L). Indeed, the Lorenztian line shape is given by:

$$F(\upsilon) = [a_0 L/2\pi]/[\Delta\upsilon^2 + L^2]. \quad (13)$$

At the peak maximum, $\Delta\boldsymbol{\upsilon} = 0$, the height is $a_0/2\pi L$. Thus, anything that affects the width of the resonance also affects the peak height; a narrow resonance has a larger height than a broad resonance of the same area. Thus, a narrow peak will be detectable above the noise at lower concentrations than a broad peak. Furthermore, the resolution of the spectrum depends on peak width; two resonances separated by say 10 Hz will be well resolved if their widths are only 1 Hz wide, but would not be resolved if they are 10 Hz wide. Hence, there is a premium on ensuring that the resonances are as narrow as possible.

1.2.2. Microprobes and Automation

When sample is limited, such as from tissue biopsies, it is advantageous to concentrate the solution into a minimal volume and use a microcoil probe. Such probes are designed for very small amounts of solute, e.g., on the order μg or less material. For a metabolite of molecular weight 500, 1 μg is 2 nmol. When dissolved in 10 μL solvent, the solute concentration is of the order 200 μM. Coils designed for tubes with a 1 mm diameter are commercially available (cf. Table 2), which can be used in either flow or batch mode. The combination of a cooled coil and preamplifier on such microprobes promises to provide the ultimate in signal recovery for small amounts of material.

The active volume of a sample is always smaller than that of the sample volume needed to fill a cell and is determined by the coil height and sample diameter. Assuming a cylindrical geometry, the internal diameter of a tube, d_i, determines the cross-sectional area, so for a coil height, h_c, the active volume is $\pi h_c d_i^2/4$. For a 5 mm NMR tube, d_i is ca. 0.42 cm, and the coil height can be anywhere from 14 to 20 mm depending on the design. Assuming an average coil height of 16–18 mm, the sample volume is 0.22–0.25 mL. For a 3-mm tube, $d_i = 0.24$ cm, and the active volume is 0.074–0.083 mL. Smaller tubes are also available for special microprobes that have active volumes from 1 to 20 μL depending on the design. In all cases, however, the ratio of measured solution to that required to fill the detection volume is substantially less than 1, typically of the order 0.5 or less. There is also a trade-off between factors that govern sensitivity, ease of operation, and throughput.

There are several advantages of small sample volumes at high concentration; decreased contribution from solvent and other impurities, high magnetic field homogeneity over the sample and lower requirements for shimming, faster temperature equilibration, and where the salt concentration is high (as when dilute samples must be concerted by, e.g., lyophilization), better response of the probe, as salt effects decrease with decreasing radius.

The advantage of a flow design using a small sample volume is ease of automation, as the samples can be taken from a 96-well plate, for example, rapid thermal equilibration, and shimming is easier on a very small volume. With the flow cell, the sample height and diameter are always the same. Thus, some of the overhead from thermal equilibration and shimming are reduced in this automation mode, potentially giving rise to very high throughput, if the samples are very concentrated. Flow systems require hydraulics, so the push solvent should be the same as the sample solvent to avoid contamination. Also the wash cycle can be ultimately time-consuming as one usually wishes to minimize carryover from a previous sample. It is likely that with a flow system, 2 min is the minimum time for obtaining good quality, reproducible spectra, implying a throughput of up to perhaps 700 samples per day. Such a system is ideal for relatively abundant samples such as plasma or urine where 1D proton spectra can be recorded in a few acquisitions. For intrinsically weak samples, the flow approach has some disadvantages, including the ratio of the active volume to the minimal usable volume. The most sensitive approach currently seems to be a cryogenic (static) microprobe with an active volume of 2.5 μL, minimal volume of 5 μL under low salt conditions. Compared with a 5-mm cold probe, the 1-mm cold probe appears to deliver a threefold improvement in sensitivity (19). This latter can be achieved easily for proteins by membrane filtration, but for metabolic samples that have to be concentrated from large volumes, the salt concentration may become exceedingly high and affect chemical shifts or solubility. However, solvent-based extractions may alleviate this problem (see Chap. 2)

An alternative to flow automation is a robotic sample changer, which contains a number of preloaded standard NMR tubes. With these systems, the sample changing overhead including loading, shimming, finding solvent peak positions, etc. is of the order 2–5 min depending in the sample. The ability to record a spectrum in a few seconds seems of little utility under these circumstances.

1.2.3. Digitization

Although the primary signal is an induced emf in the receiver coil, all modern NMR is digital. The primary signal has to be converted to a digital signal, which is achieved using a fast ADC, typically with 16 bits resolution. The resolution of the spectrum is determined by the length of time that the fid is measured. The raw resolution is simply 1/at where at is the acquisition time in seconds. Thus, to resolve two features differing in frequency by ^{1}H, the acquisition time must be at least 1 s. As small metabolites have narrow lines, inadequate digitization will result in artificial line broadening, and therefore lower resolution. Suppose that a spectrum is acquired with a spectral width of 5,000 Hz using 16,384 complex data points. Then 8,192 points are real, and the acquisition time is 1.64 s, giving a raw digital resolution of 0.61 Hz/point. The intrinsic line width may be <0.5 Hz, but without sample spinning, the residual magnetic inhomogeneity is likely to be of the order 1 Hz.

1.2.4. Sample Sensitivity

NMR is often regarded as a relatively insensitive technique, compared with other forms of spectroscopy and mass spectrometry. In part, this is a consequence of the very low population differences (cf. (6.2)), so that in effect only 1 in 10^4 or fewer nuclei are detected (0.1%). In fact, this is comparable to the ionization efficiency in many MS techniques (20) (see Chap. 4). The important practical parameter for sensitivity is how much material is needed to obtain a spectrum of the desired signal-to-noise ratio in a given amount of experimental time.

This depends on the set up. For a regular NMR sample in a 5-mm tube with an autosampler, the time taken to introduce the sample, equilibrate, lock, and shim is about 3–4 min. This is considerably less on a flow system using small volumes, where the time is 1–2 min. For strong samples such as many biofluids, a small number of acquisitions are adequate to obtain high signal-to-noise ratios even for many dilute components.

With a 5-mm cold probe operating at 600 MHz for protons, a concentration of 1 μM in the active volume can yield a 1D proton spectrum with a signal-to-noise ratio of 10 in 30 min acquisition. Using Shigemi tubes, with a volume of 0.35 mL, this is equivalent to

0.35 nmol solute. By using microflow probes (active volume <10 μL) and concentrating the sample, it may be possible to achieve a higher sensitivity and reduce the lower limit to perhaps 0.1 nmol with current technology. This can be compared with optical spectroscopy. For a very strongly absorbing solute having an absorption coefficient of 100 mM^{-1} cm^{-1}, for a 1 cm pathlength an absorbance of 0.1 is 1 μM. For a microcell of volume 0.1 mL, this equates to 0.1 nmol. For more typical biological aromatic chromophores, $\varepsilon < 10$ mM^{-1} cm^{-1}, implying a sensitivity limit of the order 1 nmol. Of course the measurement time is much less for optical spectroscopy.

In direct infusion nanospray MS where flow rates are < 1 μL/min, the amounts of material consumed during measurement are typically of the order pmol to fmol, though under ideal conditions as little as several attomoles consumption has been reported by several groups for obtaining useful spectra (see Chap. 4 for a detailed discussion of MS sensitivity).

1.2.5. Alternative Data Acquisition Techniques

The Fourier transform method is highly robust and is the default method on all spectrometers. However, the linear sampling in time in principle is wasteful, as much of the time may be spent sampling noise. This is especially pronounced in sparse spectra. Alternative sampling techniques can be used that in effect spend most of the time sampling signal rather than noise. This of course requires some prior knowledge. One technique is to use the Hadamard transform, in which only a select subset of resonances is excited, making use of the fast waveform generators on modern spectrometers. The pulse program is supplied with a preassembled list of frequencies, so that only metabolites that have these frequencies within a narrow bandwidth are excited (21). Thus, within a complex mixture, this would be a means of spectral editing. As the method can be very fast (a 2D can be recorded in less than 1 min for strong samples) (21–23), a series of selected metabolites could be monitored in a short period.

Nonuniform sampling is another means to achieve increased sensitivity per unit time by reducing the number of points that must be sampled. Depending on the sampling profile, which may need some tailoring to different cases, the nonlinear sampling technique, which may concentrate relatively more point near the start of the fid (maximize sensitivity), but still sample late in the fid (for high resolution) (24–27). For certain 2D experiments, notably HSQC, time savings of a factor of 3–6-fold over conventional sampling may be achieved (24–26).

An obvious limitation on the overall speed of acquisition is the need to allow the system to return to thermal equilibrium, which for protons in metabolites can be quite long as T_1 values vary from 1 to more than 5 s. The SOFAST method used in macromolecular NMR relies on efficient spin diffusion from a reservoir of on-excited protons to those of interest (e.g., the amide protons in ^{15}N HMQC) (28).

However, this is not effective for small metabolites where spin diffusion is very inefficient. An alternative is ASAP in which unused magnetization along the *z* direction can act as a reservoir for the spins that are being monitored. This requires a mechanism to transfer magnetization from the reservoir to the observed spins. One approach is to use TOCSY in scalar coupled systems (29). For example, in a natural abundance HSQC, only 1% of the hydrogen atoms attached to carbon are being observed, so the other 99% can act as a reservoir. The active spin system can then be repeatedly excited, limited only by the acquisition time and the time to transfer from the reservoir. Time savings of the order 6–10-fold may be achieved in favorable cases. However, for weak samples that require extensive signal averaging, the reservoir may also deplete, and the quantitative aspects are likely to be compromised owing to the variable efficient of the TOCSY transfer for different spin systems.

For higher dimensional NMR experiments (3D, 4D, etc.), the conventional FT approach is very time-consuming because the various time domains must be sampled sequentially. Thus, a 3D HSQC-TOCSY experiment might take 24 h or more even with two scans per increment (i.e., selecting the most intense compounds). With projection-reconstruction and GFT methods, the sampling can be greatly reduced, either by collecting a relatively small number of 2D planes at different angles in the 3D cuboid (PR) or by incrementing the indirect time dimension in lock step (GFT) (30–32). This essentially reduces the dimensionality, so that a 3D experiment can be recorded in a fraction of the time it takes for the full 3D experiment (33–36). To date, these approaches have been applied primarily in the structural genomics field, but there may be useful applications also in metabolomics (see below).

1.2.6. Linearity/Dynamic Range

Many forms of spectroscopy have limited dynamic range. The Beer–Lambert Law typically limits the dynamic range in optical absorbance spectroscopy to around 2 decades (e.g., absorbance of 0.01–2) before serious nonlinearity ensues. Similarly, the dynamic range for most fluorometric observations is limited at the upper end by inner filter effects, and at the lower end by dark current.

In NMR, the relationship between signal area and number of nuclei is strictly linear; only relaxation effects influence the response. The dynamic range within a sample is high and is ultimately set by the capacity of the linear amplifiers and the ADC dynamic range. Most spectrometers now use 16 bit digitizers, or a maximal range of 65,536. To ensure adequate digitization of the most intense signal and the noise, the effective dynamic range is about 16,000:1. As with most techniques, quantifying weak features in the presence of nearby strong ones is difficult; in metabolomics samples, the within-sample dynamic range is more like <5,000:1.

1.2.7. Lock Circuitry and Solvents

Modern spectrometers usually are set up to lock on ^{2}H signals either from the solvent, or from a molecule in a concentric tube. Although the field drift of a good superconducting magnet can be very low (<^{2}H/h), long acquisitions on weak samples of small molecules can still be affected because the intrinsic linewidths are very narrow. The lock is used to eliminate the effect of field drift. D_2O is a particularly good solvent for this purpose for two reasons. First, the concentration of deuterium is very high (110 M in neat solvent), and secondly, because the T_1 values are quite short, which means that the lock signal does not saturate easily. It provides a strong signal that can be used for gradient auto shimming.

Other deuterated solvents are less amenable, both because the deuterium signal is present at a lower concentration and because the T_1 values tend to be long. Thus, d_4-methanol (72.5 M methyl deuterons) is a good solvent for many organic compounds, but requires care because there will be two deuterated signals, one from the methyl group and the other from the hydroxyl deuteron exchanging with residual moisture. Careful adjustment of the value of z_0 and phase is therefore essential. Furthermore, the lock power needs to be kept low to avoid saturating the signal (long T_1) and shielding as much as possible from pulsed filed gradients, which interfere with the lock and its slow recovery can cause loss of the lock during acquisition. Deuterated chloroform is even worse because of its lower concentration (12.3 M) and rather long T_1.

1.3. Data Processing

1.3.1. Zerofilling

The resolution can be automatically increased a factor of 2 by adding an equal number of zeros to the end of the fid; increasing the data table from 16,384 points by adding 16,384 zeroes will increase the resolution to 0.305 Hz/point for a spectral width of 5 kHz. In effect, this first zero fill compensates for the discarding of the imaginary (dispersive) signal. Additional zero fills improve peak definition, but do not increase the real spectral resolution.

1.3.2. Linear Prediction

Linear prediction is a way of increasing the resolution of a spectrum by extending the length of the fid. Instead of merely padding with zeroes (see above), the fid is extended with an oscillating damped function. Typically, a fid is extended once or perhaps twice by this process, which can take some adjustment. It is most successful where the signal-to-noise ratio is high, and the fid is truncated, as occurs with long T_2 values. This is especially useful in 2D experiments in the indirect dimension where time constraint makes acquiring data for as long as $3T_2$ (i.e., when the signal decays to 5% of its initial value) impractical. For example, a heteronuclear 2D experiment might extend to a $t_{1\max}$ of only 10–15 ms or less, even though the T_2 values are >100 ms. This gives a severely truncated fid in t_1, which requires processing to avoid artifacts like sinc wiggles (see below) and limits the resolution in *F*1 to ca. 50 Hz (assuming 1 zero fill). Linear prediction to 2–4 time the length of the fid, plus a zero fill, would improve the resolution 4–8-fold and also require a different processing function that makes use of all of the directly acquired signal.

1.3.3. Apodization

The issue of truncation can be important with metabolites because of the long T_2 values. A truncated fid is equivalent to multiplying the time domain by a boxcar function, so that the data do not smoothly approach zero. As the Fourier transform assumes an infinite time function, this abrupt transition shows up as high frequency ripples in the frequency domain. It is easy to show that the Fourier transform of a rectangular function (cf. a pulse) is a sinc function ($\sin x/x$), which can extend over wide ranges of frequencies and even be mistaken for spectra features in some instances. A simple solution is to multiply the fid by a smooth monotonically decreasing function that reaches zero at the end of the fid. This apodization (removal of the feet) abolishes sine wiggles, at the expense of an increase in linewidth as the decreasing function accelerates the natural decay in the time domain, just like a shorter T_2 value. The integral is preserved, however, if the first point is unity. Functions such as exponential decays and half Gaussians fulfill all of the requirements nicely.

1.3.4. Resolution Enhancement/SNR Improvement

Apodization functions such as the exponential and Gaussian weighting also suppress noise at the end of the time domain, without affecting the integrated signal. Therefore, they also increase the SNR. The optimal SNR enhancement is obtained using a matched filter, i.e., that causes the time domain to decay twice as fast as the raw data, doubling the linewidth. It is also possible to enhance the resolution, by multiplying the time domain by an increasing function. Optimally this would be an exponential that increase at the same rate that the fid decays, clearly impossible for a mixture in which there are wide variations in T_2 values. Although this certainly can enhance resolution by decreasing time widths (but having no influence on the extent of multiplets arising from scalar coupling), it also produces a severely truncated fid, and this introduces sinc wiggles in the transform. This can be alleviated by using a peaked function, which enhances the early part of the fid but smoothly approaches zero at the end of the fid. Shifted Gaussians or shifted sine-squared functions perform well under these circumstances. Because the first point is not multiplied by unity, the resulting peak does have negative lobes and integration of the peaks is less reliable. Furthermore, the greater the resolution enhancement, the lower the resulting SNR. On balance, for the most part resolution enhancement is rarely needed for extracts, but may be valuable in in vivo NMR, where line broadening from magnetic inhomogeneity can be quite substantial.

1.3.5. Area Determination

There are two common ways for determining the area of a peak. The first, implemented in all commercial software, is called integration.

As the points are equally spaced, the height of the point times the digital resolution is the area of a rectangular strip. Hence, summing up the areas of these strips across the peak approximates the area of the entire peak. In fact for symmetric peaks (as in a Lorentzian or Gaussian line shape), and with adequate digitization, this approach is very accurate. The main problem is noise and exactly where to start and stop the limits of the integration. This may become a significant problem in crowded spectra, especially as Lorentzian peaks have rather broad "wings," or where the baseline is distorted. Obviously as the peak height is being measured, this must be with respect to the baseline at zero. For this reason, it is imperative to ensure that the baseline is flat, and that there is no DC offset, which will add to all integrals. The second approach is to fit the line shape to a theoretical function, usually a Lorentzian (the theoretical line shape) with perhaps an admixture of Gaussian to account for instrumental imperfections or in tissue NMR chemical shift heterogeneity. As both Lorentzian and Gaussian line shapes are analytical, it is straightforward to use a least squares fitting routine to deconvolute overlapping spectra to recover the peak parameters (frequency, half widths, and area, for example). An additional advantage is that baseline distortions can also be modeled. As a theoretical function is being used, it is imperative for accurate areas that the peaks are indeed symmetric and approximate to Lorentzians. In large measure, certainly for analysis of high-resolution spectra of extracts, this depends mainly on adequate shimming both of the radial and especially the higher order *z* shims. The latter can often be simplified using computer-controlled gradient autoshimming. This further puts a premium on using good quality NMR tubes and constant column height from sample to sample so that reproducible shimming can be ensured. As most of the area is near the base of the resonance, which is where the tube imperfections and shimming distortions can be most severe, it is important to have good line shapes when peak fitting is used.

2. NMR Analysis of Metabolites

2.1. Information Content

The commonest NMR experiments in metabolomics are one-dimensional NMR spectra. The issues that determine the quality of the spectrum, other than the sample preparation, have been discussed above. However, there are numerous ways in which 1D NMR spectra can be acquired to extract or display information.

2.1.1. ^{1}H NMR

This is used routinely because of the high innate sensitivity, and because most biological molecules are proton-rich. For many purposes then, ^{1}H NMR is used for detection in metabonomics, as well as most 2D methods. However, owing to solvent peaks, and in biofluids, the presence of paramagnetic agents, and macromolecules, quantitative information can be difficult to obtain because of the need to suppress these undesired signals. Solvent and solute suppression techniques can leave the baseline distorted, or intensities distorted via differential relaxation effects. Furthermore, the chemical shift range of protons is relatively narrow, making 1D NMR spectra very crowded.

For samples dissolved in D_2O, solvent suppression is not a difficult problem, as presaturation with a weak rf field from the transmitter is sufficient. Furthermore, most extraction procedures remove macromolecule components, so that solute suppression is not required. For direct detection of biofluids, however, solvent suppression is very important, and a number of techniques have been proposed. Watergate (37) is one of the simplest and most robust techniques that uses pulsed field gradients to dephase the water signal. It requires calibrating only the excitation pulse and setting of the carrier on resonance with the water (though optimization of the gradient field strength can improve the suppression significantly). The degree of suppression is very high, so that even dilute samples can be routinely recorded in H_2O solution. The main disadvantages are the nonuniform excitation across the spectrum and the loss of signal intensity of resonances near to the water. An alternative, WET (38) uses gradients and relaxation to achieve a similar effect. It requires more optimization, but performs better than Watergate near to the water frequency. The extended delay in the pulse train does, however, cause loss of some exchangeable protons. A significant advantage, however, is that it can be used for multiple frequency suppression. The 1D NOESY experiment (39) is also used which is robust, but can require more optimization than Watergate and generally gives lesser suppression.

All of these techniques suppress the water resonance, but do not suppress the solute peaks. In biofluids, especially plasma or CSF, the content of protein and lipids is very high, and these broad, poorly resolved components often mask the small molecules of interest. These components can be suppressed using differential spin–spin relaxation properties; the metabolites have very sharper resonances, whereas the macromolecules have short T_2 values. Thus, a spin-lock, or more usually, a CPMG pulse train causes loss of magnetization of the macromolecular components faster than those of the small metabolites; CPMG train of 100–200 ms are often needed to reduce the macromolecular components to the baseline, which also causes a significant attenuation of the metabolites. As T_2 values differ for various metabolites, quantification needs a correction analogous to that used for T_1 saturation:

$$M(\text{obs}) = M(\text{true})\exp(-R_2 D), \tag{14}$$

where R_2 is the spin–spin relaxation rate constant and D is the spin-echo period. The 180 C pulses in the CPMG train must be spaced close together to avoid artifacts from the scalar couplings in the majority of metabolites. Under these conditions, the pulse train approaches a spin-lock condition. As described below, the macromolecular component signals can be retained by exploiting the differential translation diffusion rates of large and small molecules. In the stimulated gradient echo technique, small, fast diffusing molecules are smeared out, whereas the more ponderous macromolecules retain their magnetization for longer periods. This can be extended to two dimensions to separate molecules based on their translation diffusion coefficients and resonance frequency (40–42).

2.1.2. ^{13}C NMR

For targeted metabolomic approaches, it can be advantageous in some instances to use direct detection of other nuclei. Direct detection of ^{13}C is commonly used for in vivo NMR (see Chap. 11), but also in extract work. The major advantage of direct detection is that all carbons are detected, not only those that have a directly attached proton. This includes the carbonyls that are common in biological materials and the quaternary carbons typically found in ring systems. The other reason for detecting carbon directly is to measure the effect of ^{13}C–^{13}C scalar coupling in enriched samples, for isotopomer analyses (see below).

The sensitivity of direct detection is very much less than for inverse (proton) detection because of its smaller γ ($\gamma_H/\gamma_C=4$) and its low natural abundance (1.1%). The former gives a sensitivity advantage by virtue of the high population of the protons (fourfold) and the high Larmor frequency, inducing a larger emf in the receiver coil. If an INEPT-reverse INEPT scheme is used, the proton detection improvement in SNR over direct detection is $(\gamma_H/\gamma_X)^{5/2}=32$ fold for ^{13}C. However, the raw carbon sensitivity can be enhanced by two different mechanisms, namely the NOE (dominated by attached protons) or by polarization transfer from an attached proton. These do not improve the signal intensity of carbonyl quaternary carbons noticeably, thereby significantly negating the advantage of ^{13}C detection. The NOE is maximally $1+\gamma_H/2\gamma_C$ for enhancement of threefold. The polarization transfer by INEPT utilizing the scalar coupling between ^{13}C and ^{1}H depends on the magnitude of the coupling constant, as $\sin \pi Jt$. This is a maximum when $t=1/2\,J$, and for a fixed time t, is somewhat variable for different values of J. For aliphatic C–H, J is typically 120–130 Hz, for anomeric C–H is 160–180 Hz, and for aromatic systems, typically >180 Hz. Thus, setting $t=3.125$ ms (optimal for $J=160$ Hz), the transfer variation amounts to approximately 0.92 ($J=120$ Hz) to 1 ($J=160$ Hz). The maximum enhancement by INEPT is fourfold. The NOE is also rather variable, depending on solution conditions and the presence of paramagnetic relaxation agents. Thus, compared with proton detection, carbon detection with INEPT is at least eightfold less sensitive (or a factor of 64 in measurement time).

Although the one-bond coupling constants are typically large, it is possible to detect carbon ^{13}C by long-range interactions to protons on adjacent carbons, where the two- or three-bond coupling constant is <10 Hz. This is the basis of the HMBC experiment, or for rare spins, long-range HSQC (see below). The enhancement is also proportional to the number of detected protons, so a methyl group is three times as sensitive as a methine group.

2.1.3. ^{15}N NMR

^{15}N NMR is much preferred over ^{14}N NMR, even though the abundances are 0.37 and 99.63%, respectively, because for ^{14}N $I = 1$, whereas for ^{15}N $I = 1/2$.

As γ_H/γ_N is about 10 for ^{15}N, there is a very large advantage to ^1H detection over direct ^{15}N detection, which in fact is rarely carried out. Because the incidence of ^{15}N–^{15}N bonds in biological molecules is rare, long-range detection of ^{15}N by ^1H is straightforward using HSQC-type experiments, which provide a sensitivity enhancement over nitrogen detection with INEPT of at least 30-fold (900-fold in measurement time) (see below). It should be noted also that γ_N is negative, which gives rise to a large, negative NOE enhancement for small molecules (up to −4), but which is substantially smaller than the gain from polarization transfer by scalar coupling (tenfold enhancement).

Using INEPT, the same considerations apply as for ^{13}C, with two main provisos. The one-bond coupling $^1J_{NH}$ is in the range 80–100 Hz depending on the hybridization of the nitrogen. For sp^2, it is generally in the 90–95 Hz range as in amide bonds. However, in order to observe the proton, it is necessary to work either in light water, or in a dry aprotic solvent, as otherwise the proton exchanges with solvent protons, or in the case of D_2O, with deuterons. These are not generally suitable for detection. Furthermore, even in light water, the directly attached hydrogen may exchange rapidly with solvent protons, leading to extreme line broadening or complete disappearance of the signal. In the limit of fast exchange on the chemical shift timescale, the average shift will be dominated by the very high concentration of water protons (>100 M). It is possible to slow down the exchange of even amino protons by going to low pH and low (ca. 5°C) temperature, under which conditions HSQC and HSQC TOCSY experiments can be made to work (43, 44). Such experiments do require additional effort to suppress the intense water signal. An alternative is to make use of the longer range couplings to hydrogen attached to adjacent carbons such as in the fragment N–CH or NCCH (two- and three-bond couplings, respectively). Under these conditions, one can work in D_2O. As the two- and three-bond coupling constants are relatively small (<10 Hz), a long delay is needed in the HSQC experiments, or the order 100 ms. However, as the T_2 values are long, this is not a serious impediment. Indeed, in nucleotides, the two-bond coupling between ring nitrogen and H8 (purines) or H6, H5 (pyrimidines) can be substantial (45), making this experiment rather attractive for following ^{15}N incorporation into nucleotides in growing cells, for example (and see below).

2.1.4. ^{31}P NMR

^{31}P is essentially 100% abundant (cf. Table 1), and $\gamma_H/\gamma_P = 2.5$, which for proton detection compared with INEPT gives a maximal enhancement of fourfold. Furthermore, ^{1}H will not detect inorganic phosphate or phosphates other than the αP in NDP and NTP. ^{1}H detection is always long range (three bonds for biological samples). For abundant phosphorylated metabolites such as inorganic phosphate, NAD+/NADH and the major nucleotides such as ATP and UTP, and UDP-sugars, direct detection is an attractive option. Indeed, for ATP the chemical shift of the β and γ phosphates is strongly dependent on the degree of saturation with Mg, and the chemical shift of inorganic phosphate and phosphomonoesters is strongly pH-dependent. Indeed, this property is exploited extensively for monitoring intracellular pH by in vivo ^{31}P NMR (1).

Nevertheless, for extracts, where high-resolution spectra are obtained, the concentration and behavior of a wider range of phosphorylated metabolites is of considerable interest (8), and for which proton detection methods become attractive for selection, resolution, and identification.

2.2. Concentration Determination

The signal in NMR is proportional to the number of nuclei in the active volume, v, defined by the receiver coil (cf. Fig. 1). As this a fixed value, the number $n = c.v$

Where c is the concentration of the solute being measured. As (11) showed, the measured signal also depends on the details of the spectrometer and the particular probe present; for a given spectrometer, one can write the signal as:

$$S = kcv, \quad (15A)$$

where k is a constant that includes all of the spectrometer responses.

Thus, the concentration is not an absolute measurement. However, if one includes within the sample a molecule of known concentration (a spike), the relative signal is simply

$$S_1/S_2 = c_1/c_2. \quad (15B)$$

Hence if c_2 is known, the value of c_1 can be readily determined.

As the chemical shift of the resonances is also not absolute, but is defined with reference to an agreed standard, it is customary to include an appropriate chemical shift standard such as DSS or TSP. This can also act as a concentration reference.

For a single acquisition, the concentrations determined by (14) are correct to high accuracy (determined by resolution and SNR). However, for many metabolites, the SNR in a single scan is inadequate for quantification, so signal averaging is needed. It can be shown that the optimal SNR is achieved when the repetition rate is 1.27 T_1, assuming a 90° excitation pulse width (2). However, in a complex mixture, there will be a rather large range of T_1 values, e.g., from <1 s to as high as 7 s (39, 46–48). So either one must choose a repetition rate that is five times the longest T_1 (i.e., 35 s), or one must deal with saturation effects.

The observed signal under conditions of rapid acquisition (90° pulse) is:

$$M_{\mathrm{obs}} = M^0(1 - \exp D/T_1). \tag{16}$$

M^0 is the true equilibrium magnetization and D is the recycle time. Figure 4 shows the value of M_{obs} as a function of D for four representative T_1 values. If one were to choose a repetition time D of $2 \times 1.27 = 2.54$ s (i.e., 1.27 times the median T_1 value) for optimal sensitivity, the recovery would be 99, 92, 71, and 39% for the T_1 values of 0.5, 1, 2, 5 s, respectively. Clearly, unless the saturation is accounted for, this could produce substantial errors in determination of concentrations for many metabolites.

Figure 4b shows the time needed to active a given SNR for different repetition rates for the 4 T_1 values. The minimum is at 1.27 $T_1 = 2.54$ s for $T_1 = 2$ s as expected, at which point the magnetization recovers only 70%. For 90% recovery, the repetition time is 4.6 s, which requires an experimental time of only 16% longer than the optimal pulse rate for sensitivity, compared with a factor of twofold for >99% recovery. Clearly, fast repetition rates are very inefficient, as the degree of saturation is so high that the overall experimental time becomes very long, and the experiments are not quantitative.

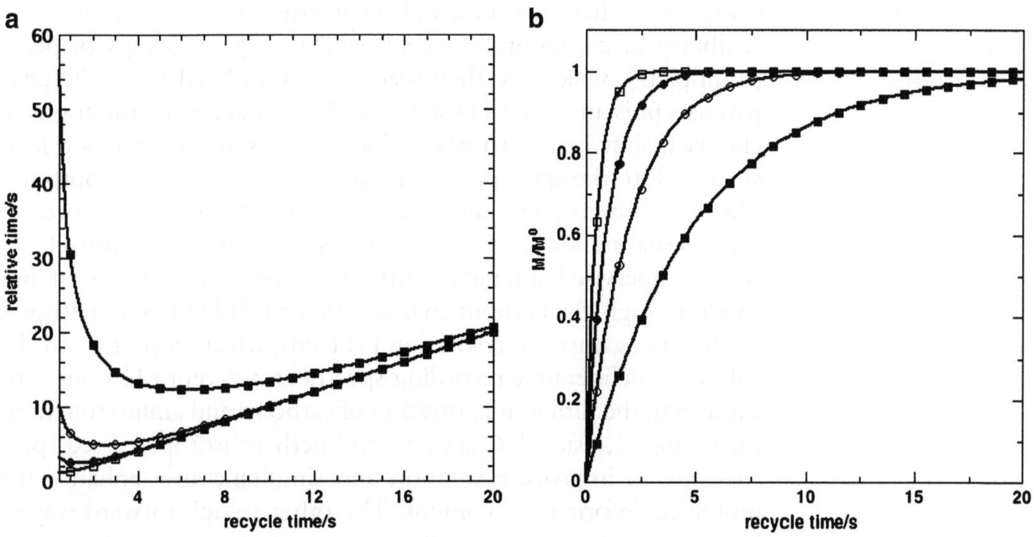

Fig. 4. Saturation factors. The extent of recovery of *Mz* was calculated as a function of recycle time (relaxation delay + acquisition time) for four different T_1 values: 0.5 s (*open square*), 1 s (*filled circle*), 2 s (*open circle*), 5 s (*filled square*), assuming a 90° excitation pulse and exponential relaxation according to (10). (**a**) Dependence of steady state magnetization on recycle time for four T_1 values. (**b**) Relative time needed to maintain given SNR as a function of recycle time D for four T_1 values. Time = D/f^2 where f is M^0/M.

Extracting the information from NMR spectra is a combination of experience and access to convenient software tools and databases. For 1D NMR, the primary information available in a metabolomic study is the peak position and area. There have been many approaches to automate the extraction of usable information, depending on the kind of study. In earlier studies in which the spectra were primarily to be used for diagnostic purposes, the emphasis was on automatic measurement of differences between spectra. As spectra alignment of NMR is quite difficult. Owing to variability in chemical shifts due to overlap, pH, and ionic strength, one approach has been to degrade the spectral resolution by binning. Different degrees of sophistication have been applied (e.g., variable width binning); the basic premise is that a bin of sufficient width preserves the integral (concentration) characteristics and is less likely to be affected by small changes in peak position This approach tends to eliminate any scalar coupling information present, therefore making identification of the metabolites less reliable. To alleviate this problem, guesswork (experience) followed by spiking with an authentic compound is commonly used. Changes in spectral regions are then tabulated, and the resulting data matrices (e.g., concentration vs. treatment) are subjected to any one of a number of multivariate statistical analyses. A commonly used approach is Principal Components Analysis (PCA) (49), which is now being superseded by partial least squares (50–52). These various approaches differ as to whether they are supervised or unsupervised. Details can be obtained from a number of reviews (53–59).

An alternative approach developed at Chenomx (39) and elsewhere eschews binning and retains the full spectral resolution. A library of compounds is converted to digital groups of peaks (multiplets), which are then scaled and translated to fit the peak patterns present in the 1D spectra. This can allow for variations in chemical shift owing to pH and salt effects and produces a least squares fit to the appropriate region of the spectrum. The output is a list of assigned metabolites and their concentrations (referenced to the internal standard DSS). This is termed a targeted approach. As this is a supervised, interactive procedure, it is, at least at present, not suited to high-throughput analysis. As with all 1D-based methods, it runs up against the resolution problem, which in part might be solved by deliberately recording spectra at different pH values (by exploiting the differential titration of carboxyl and amino functions for example), using ^{13}C spectra, and perhaps isotope-edited spectroscopy to improve resolution and simultaneously enhance the biological information content. The other straightforward way to improve resolution drastically is to use two or more frequency dimensions, as described below.

3. Multidimensional NMR: Increasing Resolution and Information Access

3.1. 2D NMR

The resolution in spectroscopy is determined by the ratio of the peak widths and the separation between them. For small molecules, the peak width depends both on the molecular size via to rotational correlation time and on the spectrometer frequency; the linewidth decreases with slightly increasing frequency for small molecules. The rotational correlation time is determined also by solution viscosity and temperature. The separation increases linearly with increasing frequency. However, as the magnetic field strength is increased, more metabolites tend to become observable because of increased sensitivity as well as increased resolution.

An alternative to increasing the magnetic field strength is to spread the signals across a plane instead of along a line. This can give rise to a very large increase in resolution for the same magnetic field strength, and in addition, provide new information or at least easier access to information that is difficult to obtain from crowded 1D NMR spectra.

All 2D experiments fundamentally use the same principles, and indeed are highly modular. The execution of a 2D experiment requires creating a second frequency dimension, which is achieved indirectly. This is done by recording a series of 1D NMR spectra, which differ from one another systematically by incrementing a time interval. This incremental time interval then defines the second time domain analogous to that in the directly detected fid. Thus, a Fourier transform with respect to the second time domain will also produce a second frequency domain, generally orthogonal to the directly detected frequencies. The size of the time increment in the indirect dimension is simply 1/SW, which is detected by the expected frequency range of resonances. This can be as small as 100 Hz for a J-resolved experiment (see below) to 30 kHz for ^{13}C.

The basic 2D NMR experiment comprises a relaxation period followed by an excitation pulse, an incremented period t_1, followed by a mixing pulse, and finally the acquisition period (cf Fig. 5). During the period t_1, the excited spins evolve under the chemical shift, scalar coupling, and any other relevant interactions. For different values of t_1, a different nonequilibrium state is produced, and the spins evolve under the shift and coupling to different degrees. The maximum value of t_1 (i.e., the number of increments) has to be chosen to ensure that the evolution is sufficiently long to sample the interaction being studied. The value of $t_{1\max}$ also determines the resolution in the indirect dimension; this represents the acquisition time. Thus, if the interaction being examined is the three-bond scalar coupling between two protons, the relevant interaction strength is $^3J \approx 5$–10 Hz. As the evolution varies as $\sin \pi J t_1$, it is clear that to sample such a

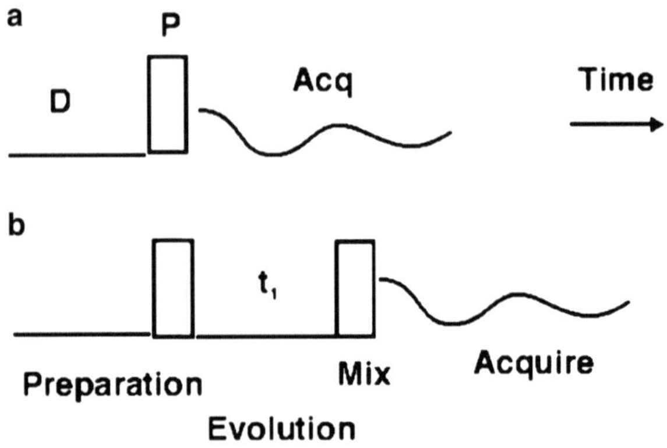

Fig. 5. Pulse sequence diagram. Such diagrams represent the sequence of events in an NMR experiment. The *rectangle* (*P*) denotes a pulse of specified duration (usually microseconds) calibrated to produce a rotation of the bulk magnetization of 90 or 180° with a particular phase. *D* is a delay (relaxation period) and Acq is the acquisition period (free induction decay). (**a**) Simplest one-pulse experiment. For proton NMR, a weak rf field may be applied during *D* at a specific frequency, e.g., to saturate a solvent resonance. (**b**) Generic 2D experiment. The preparation period comprises a relaxation delay and an excitation pulse. During the incrementable period t_1, the excited spin system evolves, and magnetization exchange occurs via scalar or dipolar interactions for example. For detection, the coupled system is mixed with a final observation pulse, and then detected during the free induction decay. The experiment is repeated for increasing values of t_1 to produce a series of 1D spectra. This 2-pulse experiment describes a simple COSY, and also a T_1 experiment ("saturation recovery").

coupling adequately needs a period t_1 of the order $1/2J = 50–100$ ms, which gives a resolution of 10–20 Hz without zero filling. In contrast, if the scalar interaction is between ^{13}C and the attached protons, where $J \approx 30$ Hz, $1/2J = 16.7$ ms and the sampling time needs to be only about 3.5 ms. This of course would give a very poor resolution of 280 Hz/point.

For the purposes of assignments, there needs to be usable databases of 2D spectra recorded of standards. Such databases are only now being established (40) (see Chap. 7).

3.1.1. NMR Experiments

There are two main classes of 2D NMR experiments in common use (cf Table 4). Those that make use of the dipolar interaction (NOESY, ROESY) and those that make use of the scalar interaction. In general, the latter is of most use in mixtures of small molecules as in principle, intermolecular dipolar interactions can occur, which are absent with scalar coupling. However, the dipolar experiments are used extensively in natural products NMR to determine stereochemistry.

The scalar experiment can be further subdivided into two main domains, the homonuclear experiments (primarily $^1H–^1H$ interactions) and the heteronuclear interactions, which usually utilize the scalar coupling between a proton and a second magnetic nucleus

Table 4
Commonly used NMR experiments in metabolomics

Experiment	Type	Action	Use
Presat	1D proton	1D, suppress solvent	Routine 1D NMR
CPMG	1D proton	T_2 filter	Suppresses broad peak
DOSY	1D proton	Spin echo filter	Suppress narrow peaks
Watergate	1D proton	Gradient-based water suppression	Solvent suppression
Wet	1D proton	Gradient-based water suppression	Solvent suppression
JR	1D proton	Pulsed water suppression	Solvent suppression
NOESY-presat	1D proton	Water suppression	Solvent suppression
X observe	1D X (^{13}C, ^{15}N ^{31}P etc.)	Usually decouple ^1H May be gated to avoid NOE	Direct observation of non-X nuclei
Xobs + NOE	1D X	Usually decouple ^1H	Direct observation of non-X nuclei with NOE. Not compatible with INEPT
INEPT	1D X	Polarization transfer from ^1H via J	Sensitivity enhancement by γ_H/γ_X
1D HS/MQC	1D H	Detects H attached to X by scalar coupling (1–3 bonds)	X-edited proton Isotope enrichment
2D J-resolved	2D proton	Separates *J* coupling from shift	Improved resolution, scalar information about peaks
(DQF-) COSY	2D proton	Correlates proton shifts via scalar coupling (2–4 bonds). Antiphase multiplets	Covalent connectivity network, assignments
TOCSY	2D proton	Correlates proton shifts via scalar coupling (2–4 bonds). In phase multiples	Covalent connectivity network, assignments
2Q-COSY (Inadequate)	2D protons, 2D carbon	Scalar coupling single quantum correlated with 2Q frequencies	Assignments, no diagonal.
NOESY	2D proton	Dipolar interactions; proximity	Assignments, conformation. Positive or negative size-dependent

(continued)

Table 4 (continued)

Experiment	Type	Action	Use
ROESY	2D proton	Dipolar interactions; proximity	Assignments, conformation. Always positive
HMQC/HSQC	2D ^{1}H–X	Correlates X with ^{1}H shifts	Assignments; indirect X–X scalar interactions
HSQC-TOCSY	2D ^{1}H–X	Correlates X with ^{1}H shifts in network	Assignments
HCCH-TOCSY or HCCH-COSY	2D ^{1}H–H edited via ^{13}C–^{13}C coupling	Correlates X with ^{1}H shifts in network filtered through X–X coupling	Assignments of labeled compounds
HCACO, HCCO	2D/3D correlation	Correlate Hα shifts with Cα and carbonyl carbon shift via one-bond scalar couplings	Assignment of labeled compounds

such as ^{13}C, ^{15}N, or ^{31}P. The commonest versions of these experiments are discussed below. To illustrate the spectral appearance, a common sample has been used that comprises a mixture of UDP, ATP, ADP, AMP, Lysine, lactate, natural abundance glutamine, and ^{13}C/^{15}N glutamine, dissolved in PBS, pH 7.2, lyophilized, and redissolved in D_2O. DSS was added as a chemical shift reference. The one-dimensional proton spectrum is shown in Fig. 6a.

3.1.2. Homonuclear 2D NMR

The three most commonly used 2D homonuclear NMR experiments used in metabolomics research are J-resolved, COSY, and TOCSY. Each one correlates proton frequencies in the two dimensions.

Methods Based on Scalar Couplings

The J-resolved experiment actually separates the chemical shift from the scalar coupling information of a given resonance, and it is not actually orthogonal (though projections can be made to be so). As multiples may spread over as much as 50 Hz, the resulting overlap severely increases the complexity of the 1D NMR spectrum. However, by effectively rotating the multiplet structure onto the second dimension, the projection of the spectrum produces a proton-decoupled proton spectrum comprising singlets only, with enhanced resolution. Furthermore, the coupling information such as multiplicity is now easily read from the second dimension (Fig. 6b). This information in conjunction with the chemical shift is very valuable for confirming metabolite identification (60–63).

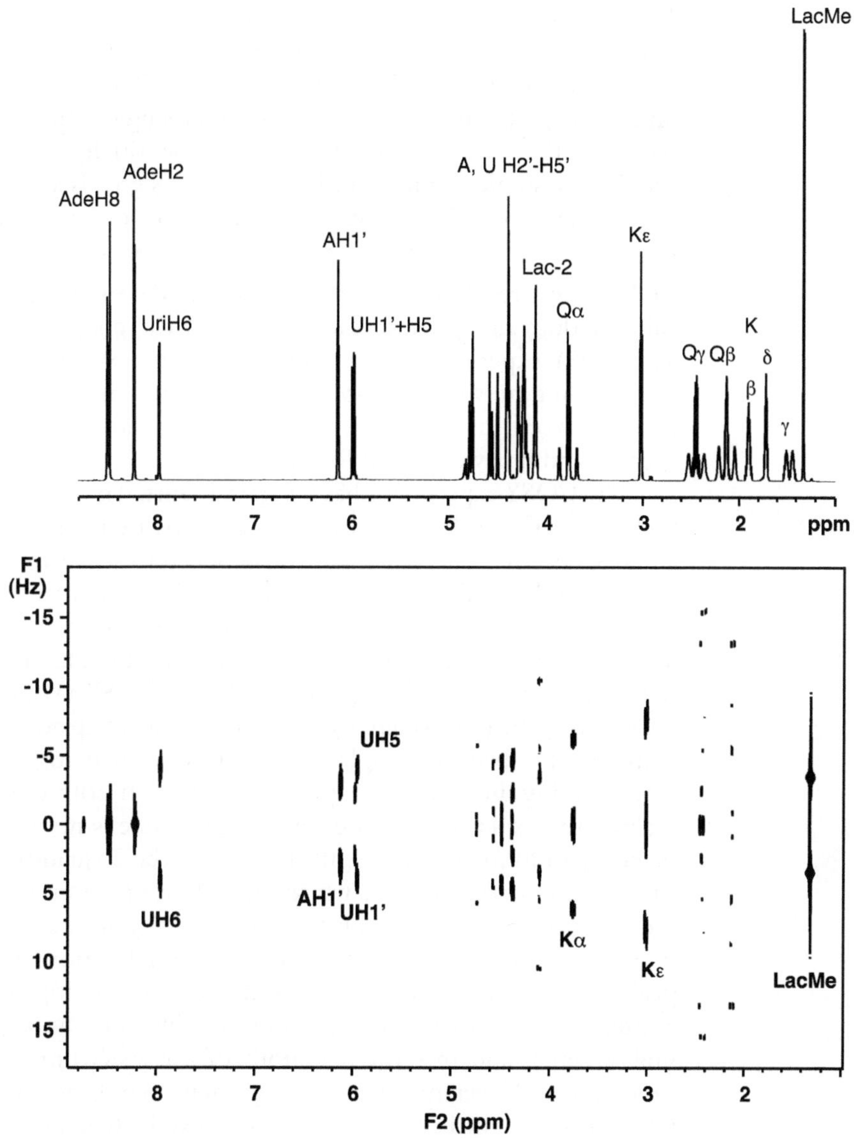

Fig. 6. J-resolved experiment. The spectrum was recorded at 800 MHz on a 5-mm HCN probe at 20°C. The sample comprised a mixture of mM UDP, mM ATP, mM ADP, mM AMP, mM L-Lysine, mM D-lactate, mM natural abundance L-glutamine, and mM uniformly enriched $^{13}C/^{15}N$ glutamine. The sample was dissolved in 0.1 M NaCl, 20 mM Na phosphate, pH 7.2, lyophilized, and redissolved in D_2O. DSS (mM) was added as a chemical shift reference. (**a**) 1D NMR spectrum. (**b**). 2D J resolved spectrum. The acquisition time in t_2 was 1 s, and the acquisition time in t_1 was 0.78 s. Experimental time was 25 min.

This is one of the simplest 2D experiments and can be performed very rapidly. A series of spin-echo 1D spectra is acquired as a function of t_1, which is incremented so as to sample the range of couplings to a given multiplet. A complex multiplet might span 30 Hz, so the spectral width in *F1* is usually set to be 50–100 Hz, i.e., increments of 10–20 ms. As one wants to resolve coupling of

1–15 Hz, the value of t_{1max} needs to be up to 500 ms, which still implies a small number of increments $n = 32$–64. Assuming an acquisition time plus relaxation delay of ca. 2 s for each fid, the minimal experimental time for $n = 32$ and a single scan is only 64 s. Note that this requires rather high intrinsic sensitivity, i.e., a SNR of >100 for a single acquisition. However, the signal is also decaying during the t_1 period; even with T_2 values of the order 0.5–1 s, for a t_{1max} of 0.5 s, the signal decays to 20–50% of its initial value.

COSY. The J-resolved experiment separates the multiples from the shift. It does not provide the partners in the coupling network. The COSY experiment (COrrelated SpectroscopY) directly shows the coupling network in a spin system. Because it selects the coupling network, the resulting patterns reflect individual molecular species, and it is well suited for mixtures.

The COSY experiment has several variants. The original experiment gave rise to line shapes that are a mixture of the absorptive and dispersive components, so that the spectra are usually displayed in magnitude mode, i.e., positive, and with substantial resolution enhancement to make the peaks narrow. This causes a significant loss in sensitivity and also makes integration difficult. An alternative, the so-called double quantum-filtered COSY (DQF-COSY) creates 2-quantum coherence between scalar-coupled spins and converts this back to single quantum coherence for detection. The resulting line shapes are pure absorption in both dimensions, making the experiment phase-sensitive, so there is no need to use severe resolution enhancement. A bonus of the 2-quantum filter is that it suppresses singlets, which by definition cannot create 2-quantum states. There is a performance penalty, in the 2-quantum filter decreases the net sensitivity by 1/2. Furthermore, the cross-peak fine structures (which represent the scalar multiplets) are in antiphase, which makes integration more difficult (the actual integral is zero), and in crowed regions of the spectrum, can cause cancelation. Nevertheless, for assignment purposes, the DQF-COSY experiment is very valuable, as it explicitly generates cross-peaks between scalar-coupled spins up to four bonds apart, which for the most part is protons on adjacent carbons in a molecular fragment. Thus, it is possible to trace out a carbon backbone in metabolites (Fig. 7).

As there is no penalty for maintaining high resolution in t_2, relatively long acquisition times (e.g., at least 0.5 s) are used. In the indirect dimension, generally an acquisition time of 50 ms is adequate, so that with a recycle time of 2 s (relaxation delay plus acquisition time), a total of 256 complex pair, and eight acquisitions per increment, the experimental time is around 2 h. This will be sufficient for strong samples or very abundant metabolites (i.e., present at >0.1 μmol in the NMR tube). Weaker samples require proportionately longer total acquisition times.

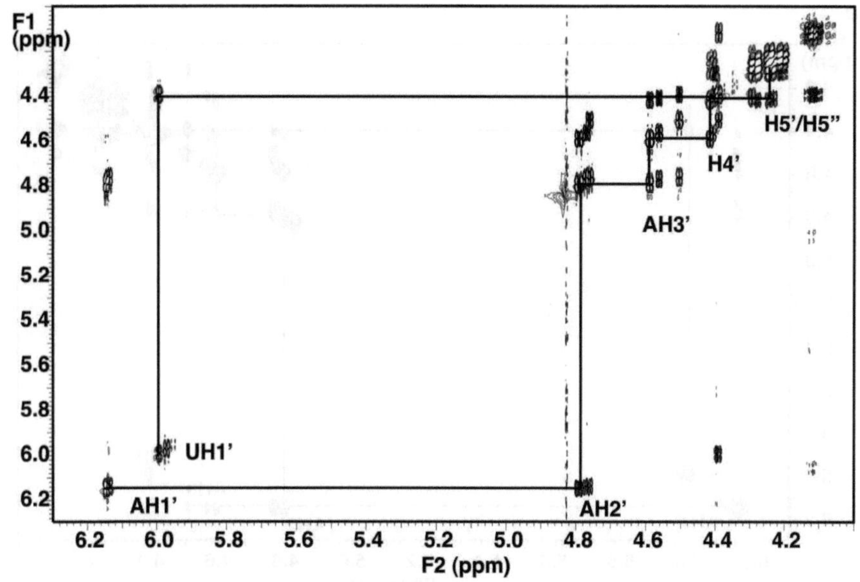

Fig. 7. DQF COSY. The same sample as in Fig. 6 was used and recorded under the same physical conditions. The acquisition times in t_2 and t_1 were 0.32 s and 50 ms, respectively. The data set was recorded in 2.3 h. The data were processed using 8,182 × 2,048 points, with mild resolution enhancement using a shifted Gaussian function in both dimensions.

TOCSY

As the name suggests, Total Correlation Spectroscopy not only correlates protons having a direct scalar coupling through two–four bonds as in COSY, but also protons with mutual scalar coupling, as in the molecular fragment CH_A–CH_B–CH_C–CH_D. Whereas the COSY spectrum will have cross-peaks connecting H_A with H_B, H_B with H_C, and H_C with H_D, the TOCSY experiment will in addition show cross-peaks between H_A and H_C, H_D and H_B with H_C and H_D. Thus, the resulting pattern can be used to trace out the carbon backbone in metabolites. Thus, entire molecular connectivities can be traced out. This experiment is intrinsically more sensitive than DQF-COSY as it does not have a p-filter, and the components of the cross-peaks are all in-phase and absorptive. It does automatically make the 2D spectra more complex than DQF-COSY, and it is not always possible to discriminate based on peak intensity alone whether a cross-peak is a three-bond coupling or a longer range interaction. For this, a series of TOCSY with different mixing times would be needed, which requires rather a large amount of NMR time. Alternatively, as the cross-peak patterns at a given mixing time are highly characteristic of the compound, library matching of the patterns generally gives rise to unambiguous identification (Fig. 8).

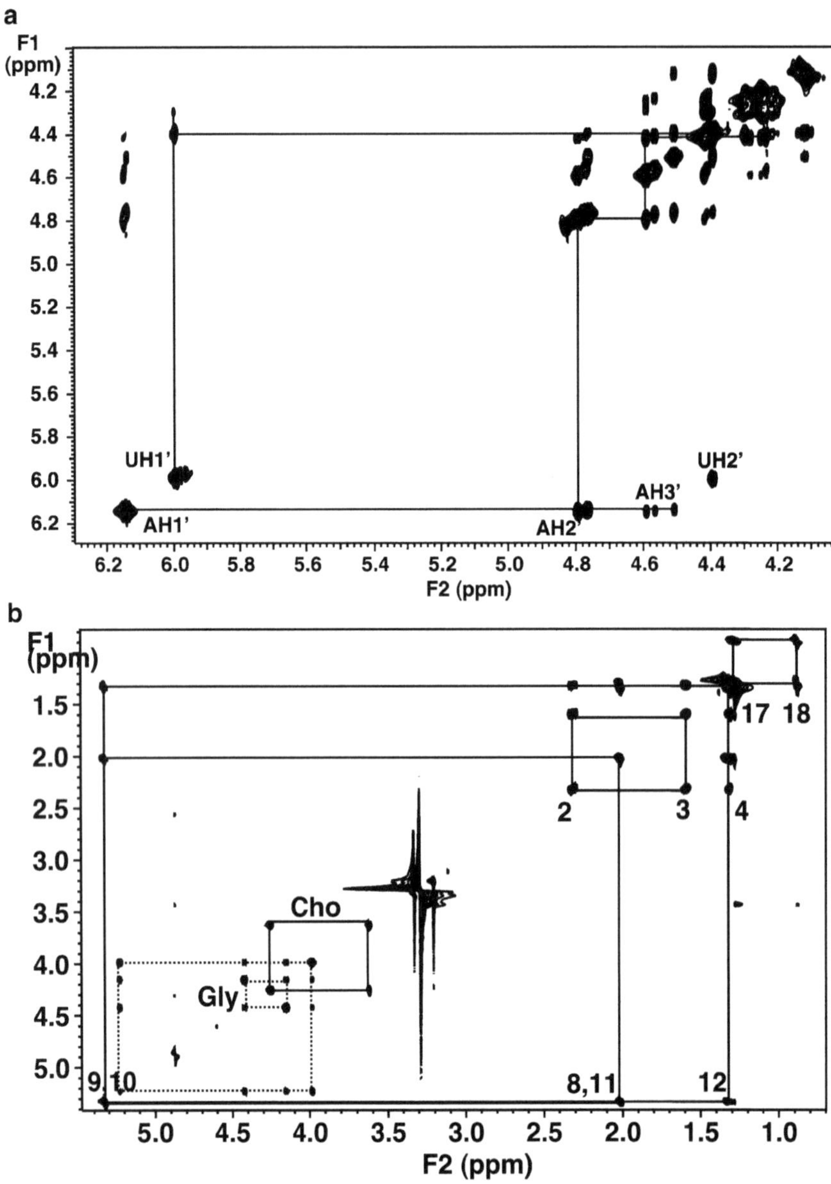

Fig. 8. TOCSY. (**a**) The same sample as in Fig. 6 was used and recorded under the same physical conditions. The acquisition times in t_2 and t_1 were 0.32 s and 50 ms, respectively. The data set was recorded in 2.3 h. The spin-lock strength was 8.6 kHz for a duration of 50 ms, using MLEV-17. The data were processed as 8,192 × 2,048 complex points, with an unshifted Gaussian apodization function in both dimensions. The SNR compared with DQF-COSY (Fig. 7) Ha–Hb 284:1 vs. 45:1. (**b**) TOCSY spectrum of DOPC in d_4-methanol recorded at 18.8 T with a mixing time of 50 ms. The spectrum was apodized using unshifted Gaussians in both dimensions, and 0.5 Hz line broadening exponential.

COSY and TOCSY together unambiguously trace out the covalent connectives in molecular fragments, which together with ^{13}C or other heteronuclear 2D experiments generally provide complete assignment of structures (see below)

The TOCSY experiment differs from the COSY experiment essentially by the mixing period. In lieu of free precession, the spins are locked along the *x*- (or *y*-) axis in the rotating frame by the application of a weak B_1 field. The spins now precess around this new field direction (that is orthogonal to B_0). The strength of this field is usually 8–10 kHz (corresponding to a pulse width of 25–30 μs) and may be active for up to ca. 100 ms. During the spin-lock period, the scalar-coupled spins, which now effectively have the same chemical shift, exchange magnetization at a rate determined by their coupling constants. The degree of exchange is then determined by the duration of the spin-lock. As this is under experimental control, it is possible to map out the coherence transfer in a coupling network by monitoring the cross-peak intensity as a function of the mixing time. The determination of the spin-lock strength requires an additional calibration, although with amplifiers in the linear range the pulse width can be simply calculated from the calibration at a higher power level. A choice also has to be made for the duration of the spin-lock. The strength is largely set by the characteristics of the probe and the separation (in Hz) between scalar-coupled spins. The spin-lock strength needs to be substantially larger than this separation. For many metabolite mixtures and currently used magnetic field strengths, 8–10 kHz B_1 is sufficient. The duration needs to be long enough for coherence transfer, which is of the order $1/2J$. A short mixing time (e.g., 20 ms) favors directly coupled spins with average coupling constant on the 4–8 Hz range. Longer mixing times (ca 100 ms) are needed to transfer coherence among spins having small coupling constants (<2–4 Hz) and spin systems containing multiple steps such as long aliphatic side chains in, e.g., lysine or alkyl chains of fatty acids. A reasonable compromise for general analysis seems to be about 50 ms. Very long mixing times (100 ms or longer) while mixing large spin systems lose sensitivity by relaxation in the rotating frames and may also affect probe performance if a strong spin-lock is used, due to heating effects. This is particularly severe in salty solutions and can lead to smearing of cross-peaks.

Heating effects are less obvious in nonionic samples, such as in d_4-methanol. This is a good solvent for polar lipids such as cholesterol and phospholipids, as extracted from cells (triglycerides are extracted by less polar solvents such as chloroform). Figure 8b shows a TOCSY spectrum of a standard Dioleylphosphatidlycholine (DOPC), which is a major unsaturated lipid in mammalian cell membranes. The connectives clearly resolved the three glycerol carbons protons from the two choline methylene groups. The acyl chain moieties show connectivities for the terminal methyl to the essentially bulk CH_2 position, and for the C2–C3–C4. Most saturated PL appear rather similar, differing only in the size of the bulk CH_2 resonance according to the chain length. However, unsaturated lipids, as DOPC, show additional resonances due to the HC = CH moiety, which can often be placed according to its position in the chain using the TOCSY (and DQF COSY) connectivity plus HSQC (Fig. 11c). Thus, in principle it is possible to estimate both average chain length and degree of unsaturation of a phospholipid extract. The differentiation of the headgroups and acyl chain moieties is valuable also for isotopomer analysis to complement the higher chemical resolution obtainable by mass spectrometry (cf. Chap. 4).

The overall experimental time requirements for TOCSY are similar to those of COSY, so for a reasonably strong sample, a good quality TOCSY experiments can be acquired in about 2 h, and proportionately longer where the less abundant metabolites need to be sampled.

2-quantum COSY. Prior to indirect detection methods (see below), establishing the carbon backbone in small molecules was difficult. For abundant samples, a technique called INADEQUATE (for Incredible Natural Abundance Double Quantum Detection Experiment) was developed (64, 65), which correlates carbon shifts through crate of 2-quantum coherence via scalar coupling, at natural abundance. This is a very insensitive technique, as at natural abundance the probability of finding adjacent ^{13}C atoms is only 1 part in 10^4. However, a feature of this experiment is that for direct connectivities, there is no diagonal. This is rather valuable for compounds where many of the nuclei have rather similar chemical shifts, and thus produce a very crowded COSY or TOCSY spectrum, such as for sugars. The technique can be applied to proton spectroscopy (therefore being very sensitive). The experiment correlates single quantum frequencies with 2*Q* frequencies that are disposed about a pseudo skew diagonal. The directly scalar-coupled spins are separated either side of this pseudo diagonal and correlate with successive spins in a network. In addition, in the complex spin topologies of sugars and many other metabolites, a further set of peaks, so-called remote peaks, are observed. These arise from the effects of mutual coupling between spins in a network, in which at least one partner directly coupled pair of spins is coupled to another resolved spin. This makes it possible to identify coupling partners even in crowed regions of the spectrum, as shown in Fig. 9. For example, remote peak (ellipses) connect H1′ with H3′ and H2′ with H4′, and they show up at the sum of the chemical shift on *F*1 and at the common spin shift in F2 (e.g., for ATP $\delta H1' + \delta H3' = 6.12$ ppm + 4.56 ppm = 10.68 ppm, $\delta H2' = 4.77$ ppm). This shows that in a crowded region, the 2D spectrum may resolve peaks that are difficult to see in the TOCSY or COSY (cf. Fig. 7 and 8), as shown by the resolution of the ATP, ADP, and AMP peaks. A further set of peaks can arise where there is equivalence, as in CH_2 and CH_3 resonances. These peaks are found at the 2-quantum frequency (i.e., in *F*1) of the equivalent spins and at the frequency of the scalar-coupled spin in *F*2. Thus, for A_2X, the equivalence peak for A_2 is at ω_X, $2\omega_A$.

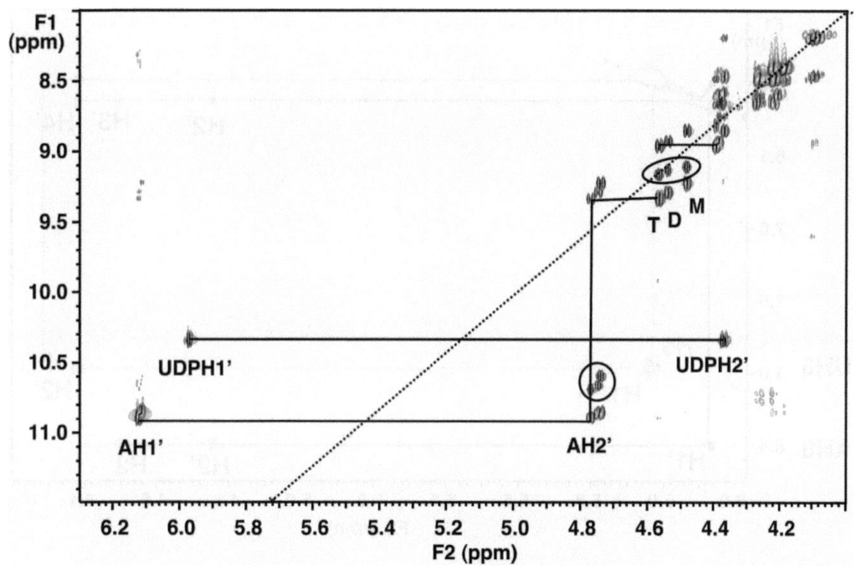

Fig. 9. DQ COSY (^{1}H inadequate). The same sample as in Fig. 6 was used and recorded under the same physical conditions. The acquisition times in t_2 and t_1 were 0.32 s and 40 ms, respectively. The data set was recorded in 2.3 h. The skew diagonal is shown as a *dotted line*.

Because there is a fixed delay of $1/2J$ (usually set to about 50 ms), there are additional T_2 losses compared with COSY, but for small molecules this is often not a serious limitation. The line shapes are mixed absorptive and dispersive in *F2*, and there is no fine structure in *F1*. As the indirect dimension is the 2-quantum frequency scale, the spectral width in *F1* is up to twice as large as in *F2*, so more increments may be needed to obtain adequate digitization.

ROESY/NOESY

ROESY and NOESY rely on dipolar interactions between spatially adjacent spin and provide the major information for conformation analysis in macromolecule. For metabolomics, the dipolar interactions are less extensively used as they are relatively less sensitive than their scalar counterparts, and usually one is interested more in identification and quantification rather than conformation. However, where unknown spin systems appear in spectra, these experiments are sometimes useful for identification purposes, because magnetization transfer is independent of the number of intervening bonds. For molecules where the product $\omega\tau = (5/4)^{0.5} \approx 1.12$, the homonuclear NOE intensity is zero. At this point, the NOE changes sign from positive (small molecules) to negative (large molecules). For a Larmor frequency of 600 MHz, this corresponds to a rotational correlation time τ of about 0.3 ns. τ depends on the size of the molecules, temperature, and solvent; in a mixture of metabolites, some species will have weak NOES, and indeed, the signs of the NOE cross-peak can differ for different molecules in the samples. For very small molecules, the maximum size of the

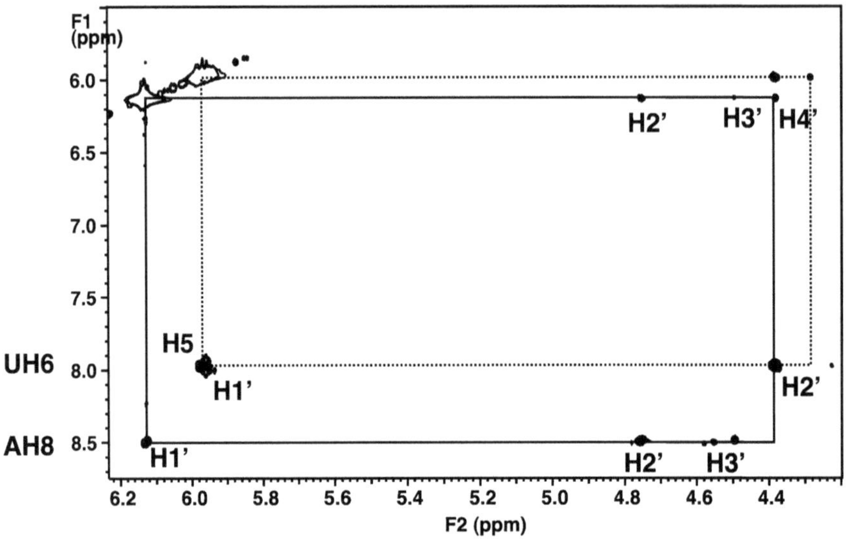

Fig. 10. NOESY. The same sample as in Fig. 6 was used and recorded under the same physical conditions. The acquisition times in t_2 and t_1 were 0.32 s and 46 ms, respectively. The data set was recorded in 6.3 h. The NOEs are $<1\%$ of the diagonal peak. Diagonal peaks are positive, cross-peaks are negative (positive NOEs). *Box* denotes NOEs from the H8 of the Ade to the sugar protons. The *dotted box* denotes connections from UH6 to the neighboring H5 and the sugar protons.

NOE is 0.5. In the rotating frame experiment (ROESY), the cross-relaxation occurs under the influence of a weak spin-lock field (typically 4 kHz), as in the TOCSY experiment. Now the magnetization exchange occurs at essentially zero field, so the ROE is always positive (opposite in sign to diagonal peaks), and the transfer rate is twice as high as in the NOESY experiment.

It is also necessary to choose an appropriate mixing time. For maximum sensitivity, this should be of the order T_1 in the NOESY experiment (longer mixing times lead to loss of cross-peak intensity), and in ROESY as the rates are faster, of the order $T_1/2$. Much shorter mixing times are used for conformational analysis. Figure 10 shows a NOESY spectrum of the test mixture recorded with a mixing time of 1 s. This shows positive NOEs for the base protons of the three adenine nucleotides with H1′ and H2′, but not from H2, indicating an antiorientation of the base with respect to the sugar ring. NOEs for UDP H6 with the nearby H5, H1′, and H2′ protons are shown in the dashed box. The base-H1′ and H2′ cross-peaks show that indeed the bases and sugars are connected, which is not visible by simple proton–proton scalar connectivity and also indicates that in this case, the bases are anti with respect to the sugar.

DOSY

The DOSY (Diffusion Ordered Spectroscopy) experiment separates molecules according to their translational diffusion coefficients. The diffusion coefficient can be measured by gradient-stimulated spin echoes. During the application of a magnetic field gradient along a particular axis, rapidly moving molecules experience a wide range of field strengths, which affect their Larmor frequency, and therefore smear out the resonance on detection. In contrast, a slowly moving molecule experiences a single magnetic field during the gradient period, and so its magnetization is effectively refocused. Thus, very small molecules are rapidly dephased and are not detected after a relatively short delay, whereas large molecules are detected. This is the basis of suppression the metabolites in favor of the lipoprotein moieties in, for example, plasma samples (41, 62). By extending the concept to two dimensions, a representation of the diffusion coefficient at each frequency is obtained, which provides physical information, rather than chemical information, about the molecules so resolved.

3.1.3. Heteronuclear 2D NMR

The simplest 2D heteronuclear experiments are probably those that simply correlate the X nucleus frequency with that of the directly attached proton, for which there are three main variants. The oldest form, Hetcor, detects the X nucleus directly. As this suffers greatly in sensitivity compared with detecting the attached proton, it is no longer used. The proton detection methods, HMQC and HSQC, are much preferred. For routine work, there is little to choose between the two, though HSQC is now used because of some advantages for spectral editing. The INEPT sequence is convenient to tune for multiplicity, so that an HSQC experiment can be used to discriminate in a straightforward manner between CH, CH_2, and CH_3, for example, as they can be made to differ in sign.

HSQC or HMQC correlate an X nucleus frequency with that of a proton, via the scalar coupling between the two nuclei, as shown in Fig. 11. The sensitivity compared with the directly detected correlation experiment (Hetcor) is proportional to $(\gamma_H/\gamma_X)^3$ ignoring relaxation effects and variable transfer efficiencies. The latter depend on the value of the one-bond coupling constant, which is significantly variable for C–H bonds. For example, the $^1J_{CH}$ of methyl group in alanine and lactate is about 127 Hz, whereas for the methine CH it is ca. 145 Hz. Anomeric sugar CH have $^1J_{CH}$ of around 160–170 Hz, and aromatic CH typically have $^1J_{CH}$ in the range 180 Hz and higher (cf Table 3). Thus, in a single experiment, the transfer efficiency cannot be optimized for all groups simultaneously, which calls for two separate experiments each with a $^1J_{CH}$ setting optimized for aliphatic or aromatic/anomeric protons. Recording two spectra increases the total experimental time needed, and absolute quantification is only possible if the coupling constants are known. However, with a setting of $J = 140$ Hz (or a delay in the INEPT period of around 3.6 ms), the variation in the INEPT transfer for coupling constant in the range 120–160 Hz is only 2.5%. A greater distortion of intensity (peak volumes) may arise from the relaxation delay. Such spectra are usually recorded with relatively short acquisition

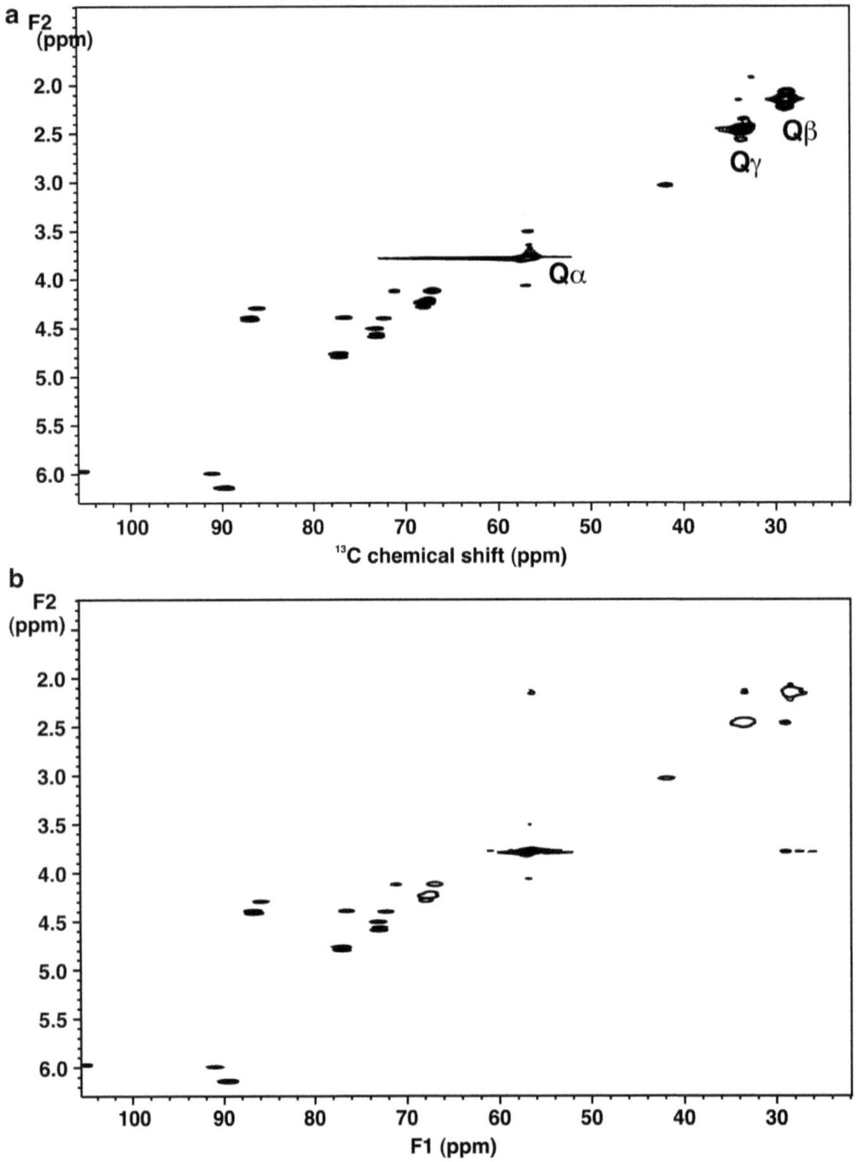

Fig. 11. ^{13}C–^{1}H HSQC. The same sample as in Fig. 6 was used and recorded under the same physical conditions. The acquisition times in t_2 and t_1 were 0.14 s and 14 ms, respectively, using the gradient selected HSQC experiment (gHSQC), at 18.8 T. (**a**) Regular HSQC. (**b**) Refocused, edited HSQC. *Open peaks* are CH_2, *closed peaks* are CH. Total experimental times were 1 h each. (**c**) Spectrum of DOPC same as in Fig. 8. The acquisition times were 150 and 10.2 ms in t_2 and t_1, respectively; total experimental time was 3.6 h.

time in t_2 owing to the active X-decoupling. An acquisition time of <0.15 s is commonly used which limits the resolution to 6.7 Hz/point (or 3.3 Hz/point after 1 zero filling) in *F*2. To improve overall sensitivity, the spectra are often acquired with quite short relaxation delays, less than 1.5 s. Under these conditions, the ^{1}H, whose T_1 values determine the net magnetization transfer, are significantly

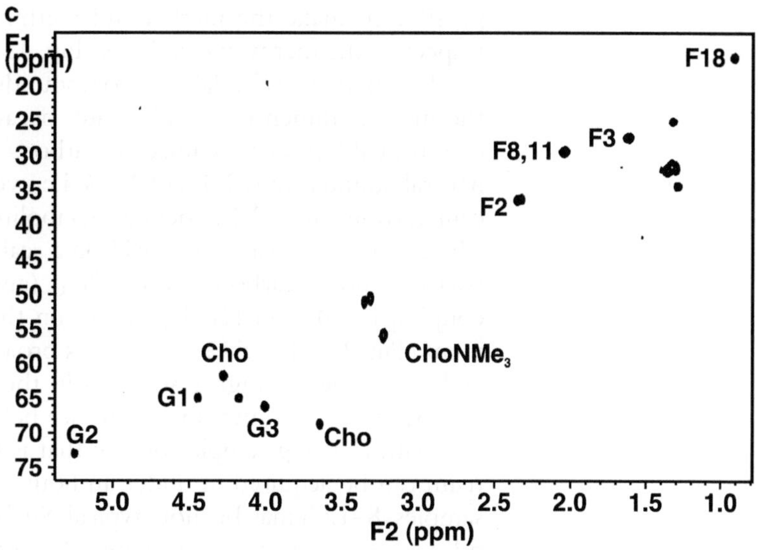

Fig. 11. (continued)

saturated, which can distort intensities if not accounted for in any relative quantification. ^{13}C decoupling efficiency also may affect the intensities. For large spectral widths, and at high magnetic field strength, the offset from the decoupler frequency can be quite high at the edge of the spectrum. Even with high bandwidth composite decoupling schemes, incomplete decoupling may occur for resonances far from the decoupler frequency, which results in decreased peak intensity compared with well-decoupled resonances. Peak height measurements can thus be compromised. Indeed, the choice of decoupler scheme becomes important for small molecules where the linewidths are intrinsically small, as high bandwidth decoupling schemes such as GARP are less efficient in decoupling than narrow bandwidth schemes like WALTZ. The effects of this are discussed in detail in Chap. 7 and for quantification in (66).

Decoupling also may affect the sample temperature, especially for salty extracts, and thus chemical shifts. This is less significant in organic solvent extracts. For example, methanol d_4 extracts are generally less salty than PCA or TCA extracts, and HSQC spectra perform better, as shown in Fig. 11c. The spectrum is of DOPC recorded at 18.8 T optimized for the aliphatic region (the unsaturated carbons resonate at about 132 ppm), i.e., with ^{13}C offsets of about 7,000 Hz at the extremities of the spectrum. Even at low resolution in the ^{13}C dimension ($t_1 = 10$ ms), the protiated carbons are well resolved, including to some extent the bulk CH_2 region at 1.32/32 ppm.

The INEPT transfers in the HSQC spectrum can also be used to edit the spectra according to multiplicity due to the number of attached protons. Thus, by incorporating additional delays, it is possible to make the methyl and methine carbons inverted with respect to the methylene carbons (Fig. 11b).

For mixtures of unlabeled compounds, moderate resolution in the indirect dimension is adequate, because all peaks are singlets (the probability of two adjacent carbons in the same molecule at natural abundance is 1.1% of 1.1%, i.e., very low). However, adjacent carbons in a ^{13}C-enriched metabolite may be simultaneously labeled, in which case there will be a scalar coupling between the two (or more) carbons with a $^{1}J_{CC}$ (and possible longer range coupling) of 40–60 Hz depending on the functional group fragment (Fig. 1). This gives rise to peak broadening at low resolution, and at sufficiently high resolution in the indirect dimension, the C–C splitting becomes observable see below (Fig. 17b).

With a strong sample (or one that is highly enriched), a spectrum can be acquired in under an hour, though for limited tissue samples, 8–12 h may be more typical. Such an experiment can make full use of the proton sensitivity inherent in an inverse detection cold probe.

The HSQC experiment is an editing experiment; only protons scalar coupled to an active X nucleus can generate the coherences to be detected. Thus, in a mixture in which ^{15}N has been supplied, all peaks that contain ^{15}N can be selected, or those molecules enriched in ^{13}C can be selectively detected (see below). For many purposes, the 1D ^{13}C-edited proton spectrum is sufficient (Fig. 17a), which has the obvious advantage of speed.

These experiments are routinely used for ^{13}C or ^{15}N editing of enriched samples, i.e., to visualize specifically those metabolites that have become enriched. Using the same approach is valuable for selecting only the phosphorylated metabolites. Here the ^{31}P is at natural abundance, but as the majority of the phosphorylated compounds are sugars, the spectrum can be complicated. Selecting only phosphorylated compounds using the three-bond coupling constant (usually a CH_2 attached to the phosphate group) can lead to the identification of a large number of compounds in a cell extract (8, 67)). Here the three-bond coupling is in the range 5–7 Hz, so the HSQC INEPT period needs to be tuned appropriately, typically in the range 15–20 Hz (cf Fig. 13).

HSQC-TOCSY

The 2D version of this 3D experiment is an X-edited proton TOCSY and selects for molecules containing scalar-coupled protons, at least one of which is ^{13}C. This experiment is often recorded as a ^{1}H–^{13}C correlation (equivalent to a projection of the 3D experiment), so that each ^{13}C site shows interactions with its directly bonded proton (HSQC) and to other protons that are scalar coupled to that proton, as in the molecular fragment Ha–^{13}C–^{12}C–Hb. Magnetization is transferred between Ha and Hb via isotropic mixing (TOCSY), filtered through the ^{13}C. At natural abundance, this experiment shows all correlations, and

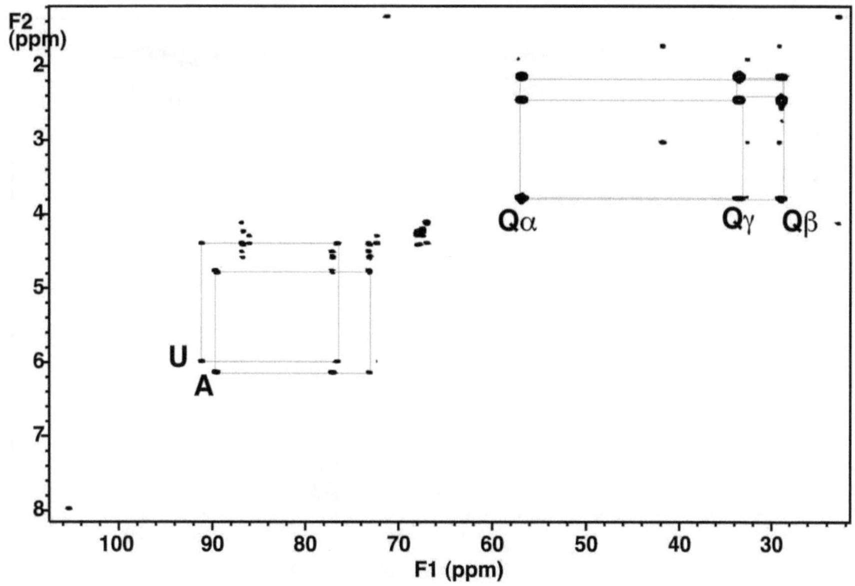

Fig. 12. ^{13}C–^{1}H HSQC-TOCSY. The HSQC-TOCSY experiment was recorded at 18.8 T as in Fig. 6, using a 50 ms TOCSY mixing time at $B_1 = 8.55$ kHz. The acquisition times in t_2 and t_1 were 0.34 and 0.014 s, respectively, with a total experimental time of 2 h.

therefore does not show extensive editing in ^{13}C, though it is useful for structure identification as the ^{13}C chemical shifts are recorded in addition to the ^{1}H shifts (68, 69). For isotopomer analysis, it is very effective where a relatively small number of ^{13}C sites are substantially enriched, as those fragments are very much more intense than the background natural abundance, as shown in Fig. 12. Even an enrichment of a few percent gives rise to a very large increase in signal intensity over background. Since a complete set of scalar correlations from ^{13}C to ^{1}H is observed in Fig. 11, the identity of these metabolites is readily determined. HSQC-TOCSY is also valuable for discerning metabolites whose resonances fall in a crowded spectral region. For example, phosphorylated sugars are typically difficult to resolve, but with ^{31}P editing, only the phosphorylated compounds are detected, and with the TOCSY relays, it is practical to identify these metabolites more reliably (70). Figure 13 shows a ^{31}P–^{1}H TOCSY and a ^{31}P–^{1}H HSQC-TOCSY experiment of the test mix. As only ATP, ADP, and ADP are phosphorylated, only these compounds were selected in these experiments. As the mixing time of the TOCSY sequence is increased, coherence is transferred beyond the H′H5″ to first H4′, then H3′ and H2′ by 80 ms.

HCCH-TOCSY

This is a two-dimensional proton correlation experiment in which protons attached to an NMR-active heteronucleus, e.g., ^{13}C, are correlated via magnetization transfer between scalar-coupled ^{13}C

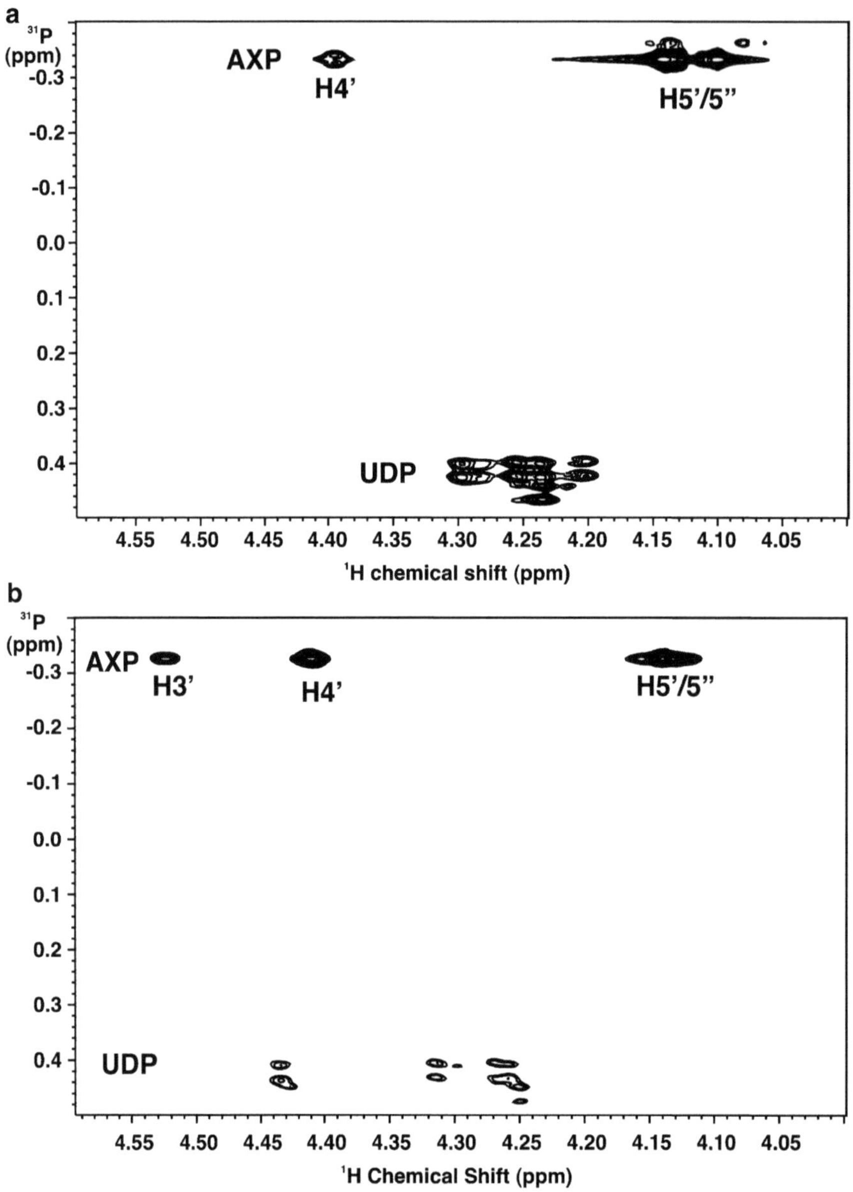

Fig. 13. ^{31}P–^{1}H HSQC-(TOCSY). The same sample as in Fig. 6 was used and recorded under the same physical conditions, expect using a 5 mm triax HCP probe. (**a**) The HSQC spectrum was recorded in 2 h using a Δ delay of 15 ms. (**b**) The HSQC-TOCSY spectrum was recorded in 2 h using a Δ delay of 15 ms, and an isotropic mixing time of 80 ms. The ^{31}P chemical shifts were arbitrarily referenced to zero ppm in the center of the spectrum.

nuclei such as in the fragment H–^{13}Ca–^{13}Cb–H. Magnetization is transferred between Ca and Cb using isotropic mixing (TOCSY). This editing experiment therefore detects only molecular fragments of this kind where both carbons in the same molecule are labeled, whereas molecules in which either Ca or Cb only are labeled are not detected (69). As shown in Fig. 14, only the labeled glutamine shows up in this

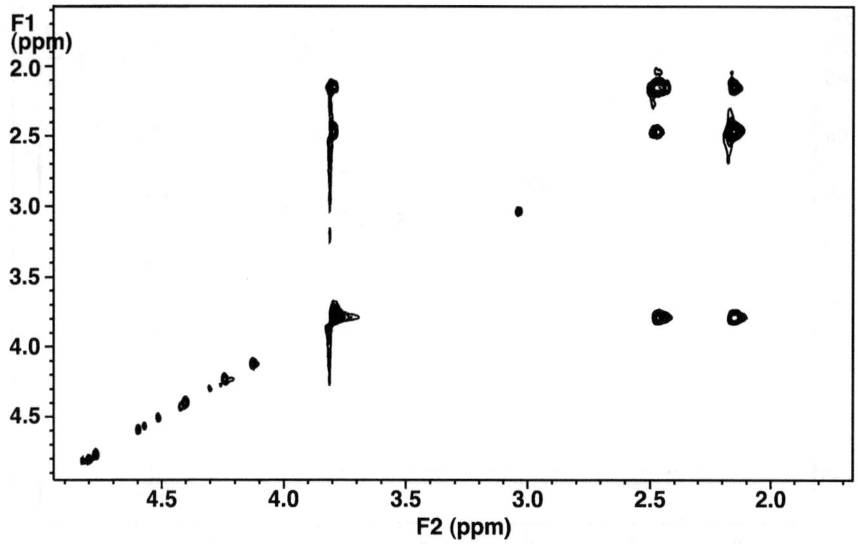

Fig. 14. ^{13}C–^{1}H HCCH-TOCSY. The HCCH-TOCSY experiment was recorded at 18.8 T as in Fig. 6, using a 15 ms isotropic carbon mixing time at 8 kHz, centered at 50 ppm. The acquisition times in t_2 and t_1 were 0.4 and 0.042 s, respectively.

spectrum, as the concentration of all the other species present in the mixture is essentially 0.01% of the uniformly labeled Gln.

HMBC and Long-Range HSQC

The HSQC-based experiments generally detect ^{13}C to which there is a directly attached proton through the large one-bond coupling. As such, the carbons that do not have a directly attached proton are not detected, which includes the functionally important carbonyl groups and quaternary carbons. In principle, one could simply tune the INEPT delay to a value commensurate with the two- or three-bond couplings, typically <10 Hz to adjacent CH, such as in the fragment O = C–CH–CH–. This is largely achieved using the HMBC experiment, which has a long delay to allow evolution of the two or three-bond C–H coupling and pulses to suppress the one-bond interaction. This latter is imperfect owing to the variation on $^{1}J_{CH}$ (cf. Table 3). An example is shown in Fig. 15. The two carbonyl groups of the glutamine are distinguishable, with one coupling more strongly to the Ha and the other coupling more strongly to the Cγ position. The numerous peaks in the aromatic region correspond to interactions between H8 and H2 of the three adenines with the quaternary carbons of the purine ring system.

For ^{15}N, the simple long-range HSQC is often more straightforward, because the ^{15}N nucleus is comparatively rare and there are no intervening magnetic nuclei. Thus, a fragment of the kind N–CH is particularly suited to this kind of detection. In some instance, the quaternary nitrogen atoms in an aromatic ring display two-bond N–H couplings in the 5–10 Hz range (45), making this a very sensitive experiment (68) (and see below).

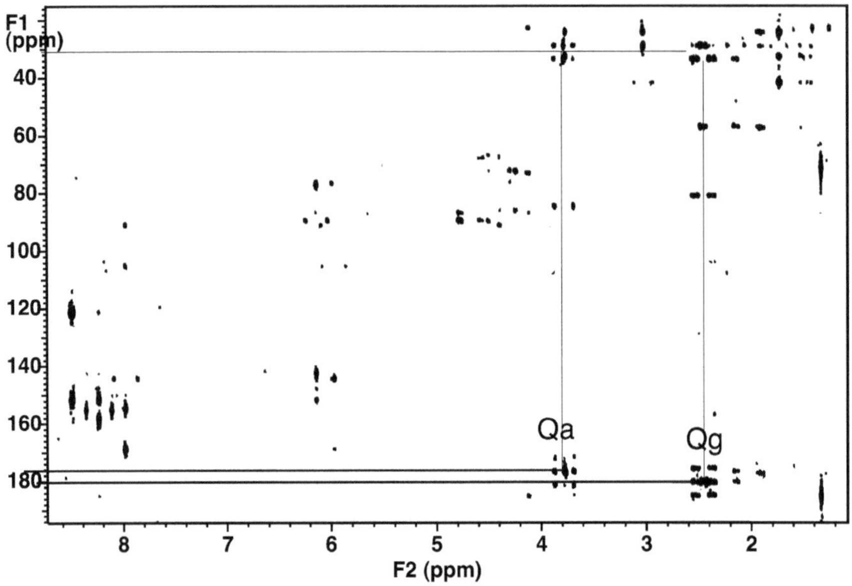

Fig. 15. ^{13}C–^{1}H HMBC. The HMBC experiment was recorded at 18.8 T as in Fig. 6, with the ^{13}C carrier centered at 100 ppm. The acquisition times in t_2 and t_1 were 0.34 and 0.012 s, respectively, with a total experimental time of 4.5 h.

3.1.4. 2D Integration

Integration in 1D is straightforward and poses few problems other than overlap. In 2D the integration is of a volume, which can be achieved readily by the same methods as for 1D, i.e., adding up the intensity at each point within a defined region of integration (e.g., a box or ellipse). However, the meaning of the resulting integral depends on the nature of the experiment and is affected by numerous additional factors. In the simple HSQC or HMQC where isolated spin pairs give rise to the cross-peak, the volume integral is proportional to the amount of the spin pair observed and is affected by relaxation rate constants in the same ways as the 1D integral described above (cf. (6.15)). Note that for HSQC, the relevant relaxation time is that of the protons, as this supplies the reservoir of magnetization. The second factor is the transfer function, which for HSQC is determined by the magnitude of $^{1}J_{CH}$ (and see above), and the number of protons attached to ^{13}C. The third factor is broadband decoupling efficiency during the direct acquisition period. This is a function of offset from the carrier and the particular decoupling scheme that is used. For large offsets (especially at high magnetic field strengths), the decoupling efficiency can be quite poor. For relative abundances of CH-vectors within a molecule or comparing molecules in a mixture, this can be quite accurate, as described in Chap. 7.

Homonuclear 2D integration is more complex. Although the peak volume in the NOESY or ROESY experiment, if normalized to the diagonal peak at a mixing time of zero, does provide information about the cross relaxation rate constant and thence internuclear distances (2, 7), the same approach is not commonly used for scalar experiments like COSY or TOCSY. Indeed, in the DQF-COSY experiment, because the multiplet components are in antiphase, the volume integral of the cross-peak is zero. In contrast, the cross-peaks are in phase in the TOCSY experiment, However, the transfer function is relatively complex, especially for extended spin systems, and the variation of the three-bond coupling is substantial compared with the median value. Therefore, it is not commonly used for assessing relative concentrations of different molecules in a mixture. However, as will be shown below, it is very valuable for determining the relative abundances of isotopomers within a molecules as here one compares the volume of the labeled and unlabeled components in a given cross-peak.

3.1.5. 3D NMR Experiments

3D NMR experiments were introduced first to macromolecular analyses using homonuclear methods (71). It quickly became clear that a much greater variety of experiments could be designed if several nuclei were included for the various dimensions (5). Furthermore, polarization transfers by INEPT from a proton to the directly attached ^{13}C or ^{15}N is very efficient for even quite large molecules, leading to high sensitivity. The separation of signals from different nuclei into the various dimensions enabled the assignment of protein backbones, side chains ($^{13}C + ^{15}N$) (5), and related experiments for nucleic acids ($^{13}C + ^{31}P$) (72–77).

For metabolites, few 3D NMR experiments have been applied, in part because the 2D experiments have been adequate for most purposes, especially where 2D planes of 3D experiments can be recorded rather quickly, and the majority of the ones useful for metabolomics require high enrichment with, e.g., ^{13}C. Full 3D experiments are comparatively time-consuming. However, recent developments have made it possible to record 3D experiments in the time traditionally taken for 2D, with an increased requirements for postacquisition processing (cf. GFT methods (32, 78)). One of the most complex sets of common metabolites is the phosphosugars (e.g., G6P, F6P, FDP, and the nucleotide conjugates UDP-Glc, etc.), as these tend to have very similar spectra that do not always resolve well in 2D NMR. To be sure, abundant sugars can be readily selected using a ^{31}P filter (i.e., only those metabolites that are phosphorylated are observed), and observation of ^{13}C in the sugar moiety is then straightforward. In a 2D ^{31}P-edited HSQC, the presence of ^{13}C labeling would be manifest as $^{1}J_{CH}$ splittings in the ^{1}H dimension; a splitting of 120–160 Hz would identify that carbon as being labeled. Nevertheless, this is an area where 3D NMR might be profitably used for identification of phosphorylated sugars in a complex mixture. TOCSY-HSQC and HCP 3D NMR experiments would be able to resolve a large number of labeled metabolites, providing they have sufficient concentration.

4. Stable Isotopomer Analysis

4.1. Pathways

The techniques described above can be applied to any complex mixture of compounds, and the resolving power is often sufficient to identify and quantify a large number of compounds. For metabolic flux analysis, however, one is also interested in the flow of atoms through metabolic pathways, as this is where the information about metabolic regulation resides. However, as the intracellular environment is maintained near to steady states, concentrations of intermediary metabolites do not change greatly under external perturbations, and to determine fluxes, it is essential to be able to measure rate of change of concentrations. Thus, for a quasi steady state condition, it is necessary to introduce a label that can be used to monitor the fate of a supplied precursor during its myriad metabolic transformations. Stable isotope labeling offers one such possibility, because with the appropriate choices the labeled atoms can be monitored by NMR and by mass spectrometry. This is analogous to the use of radioisotope tracers, with the differences that in stable isotope analysis, the labeled atoms are generally >98% enriched. The true power of stable isotope labeling with NMR detection is that it is atom-specific, rather than molecule or group-specific, so that no chemical or physical degradation is necessary to determine the position of isotopically enriched atoms in the target molecules. Because the labeled precursor is supplied as a pulse, it is possible to follow the fate of the individual precursor atoms during metabolic transformation as a function of time, even while the system is in a chemical steady state. This is how flux information can be obtained. From a detailed time course, specific absolute fluxes can be calculated, often with the aid of modeling (cf. Chaps. 8–11). Analysis of the isotopomer distributions themselves can often be used to delineate the relative importance of alternative pathways to an observed intermediate.

Consider the simple pathway:

$$Glc_0 \leftrightarrow Glc_i \leftrightarrow X \leftrightarrow Pyr \leftrightarrow Lac_i \leftrightarrow Lac_0$$

The black box approach would be to measure the changes in the extracellular glucose as a function of time, and the appearance of lactate on the medium. For this scheme, the rate of production of lac(o) equals the rate of glucose depletion in the extra cellular space, and in the steady state, and glucose decreases exponentially, while lactate would build up and eventually plateau out. In practical terms, because the medium volume greatly exceeds the cellular volume, the secreted lactate and the glucose concentrations represent the total amounts (per unit volume). However, if there are other possible source molecules present, and in eukaryotic stems this is inevitably the case, the production of lactate does not have to equal the rate of glucose consumption. Indeed, if the cells are growing, the glucose consumption is likely to exceed the lactate production as carbon is diverted into alternative produces, such as biomass.

In the slightly more complex scheme:

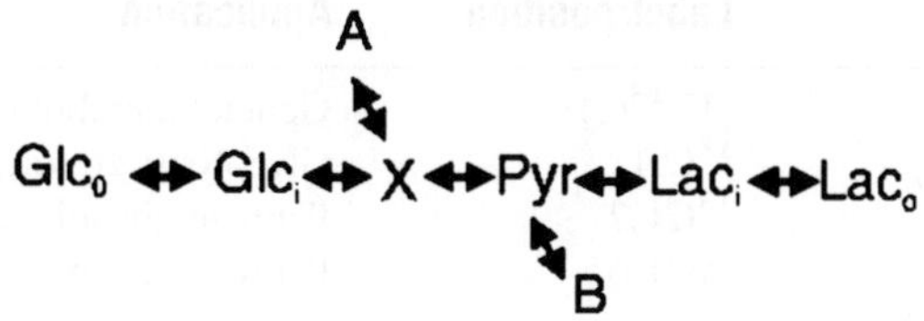

A and B represent alternative sources and products from the glycolytic pathway. Under these conditions, it is important to determine how much of the consumed glucose is converted into the observable lac(o) without using tracer methods. However, suppose that the glucose is labeled with ^{13}C, then any lactate that was synthesized using this carbon will be different from lactate that was produced from other, unlabeled sources such as A or B. By monitoring the consumption of ^{13}C glucose and the appearance of ^{13}C lactate, it is possible to determine the faction of glucose consumed that is converted to lactate. Furthermore, the unlabeled lactate is easy to distinguish from the labeled lactate by ^{1}H or ^{13}C NMR (see below), and each isotopomeric form can be individually quantified. Hence, the information content about relative flux through different parts of a metabolic network can be determined by using isotopic tracers. The mathematical treatment of such data can be done by metabolic flux analysis (Chap. 8) and metabolic control analysis (Chaps. 9 and 10).

In the remainder of this chapter, we will concentrate mainly on ^{13}C as the stable isotope label, but the principles can be generally applied to other magnetic nuclei such as ^{15}N, ^{77}Se, and ^{31}P. Fortunately, there are many commercially available ^{13}C- and ^{15}N-labeled metabolic precursors that can be used to probe different parts of metabolism as shown in Table 5.

4.2. Effect of a Magnetic Stable Isotope

As ^{13}C is a magnetic nucleus, whereas ^{12}C is not, a ^{13}C NMR experiment recorded at natural abundance with proton decoupling will consist of a series of singlets, one for each carbon atom. However, if a molecule is enriched in ^{13}C, adjacent carbons may couple and give rise to splitting in the same manner as the ^{1}H spectrum. The one-bond ^{13}C–^{13}C coupling constants are typically in the range 40–50 Hz. Thus, for a fully enriched precursor molecule, terminal carbons will appear as doublets and internal carbons as triplets or possibly double doublets. With sufficient resolution, longer range couplings may become observable. The splitting from the ^{13}C–^{13}C coupling forms the basis of isotopomer analysis by ^{13}C NMR. In a mixture of labeled and unlabeled molecules, the details of the observed patterns reflect the abundances of the various

Table 5
Commonly used and commercially available stable isotope-labeled precursors

Source	Label/position	Application
Glucose	[U-^{13}C] ^{13}C-1 ^{13}C1,2 ^{13}C1,6	General metabolism; surveys Glycolysis; glycogen synthesis; TCA Pentose phosphate + glycolysis Pentose phosphate + glycolysis
Glutamine	[U-^{13}C] $^{13}C_5{}^{15}N_2$	Glutaminolysis; amino acid metabolism, TCA; nucleotide biosynthesis
Glutamine	$^{15}N_2$	Nitrogen metabolism
Serine	[U-^{13}C]	Serinolysis; amino acid metabolism
Glycine	^{13}C/^{15}N	1-carbon metabolism
Arginine	^{13}C/^{15}N	Urea cycle, NOS
Palmitic acid, octanoic acid	[U-^{13}C]	Fatty acid oxidation; lipid biosynthesis
Acetate	^{13}C1/^{13}C2 [U-^{13}C]	Fatty acid biosynthesis; TCA Fatty acid biosynthesis; TCA

isotopomers (and see below). Figure 16 shows the eight possible ^{13}C isotopomeric states for lactate. The unlabeled isotopomer (I) is invisible by NMR. The singly labeled species II–IV are distinguishable as their carbon resonances are singlets, and because the carbonyl C2 and C3 chemical shifts are very different, are independently observable. The three doubly labeled isotopomers (V–VII) are either doublets (V, VI) or a singlet (VII). The final, fully labeled species gives doublets for C1 and C3, and a triplet (or double doublet as the two $^{1}J_{CC}$ values are significantly different for coupling involving a carbonyl or a methyl group). By definition, this approach does not detect the unlabeled species, so the total enrichment of the metabolite pool cannot be determined.

For example, the biosynthesis of Gln/Glu and GAB has been studied extensively by ^{13}C NMR in live brains (79–81). These five-carbon molecules have 32 possible isotopomeric states for ^{13}C. Programs have been written to analyze the resulting complexity.

An alternative to ^{13}C observe is ^{1}H indirect detection, which is inherently more sensitive. The interaction of a ^{1}H with the directly bonded ^{13}C gives rise to a splitting of 120–200 Hz, depending in the bond order. This is easily detectable in a proton experiment, as the ^{13}C splitting creates satellite peaks (cf. Fig. 16). As one now detects both the ^{12}C and ^{13}C atoms simultaneously, it is possible to measure the absolute fractional enrichment at each position. For example, in the

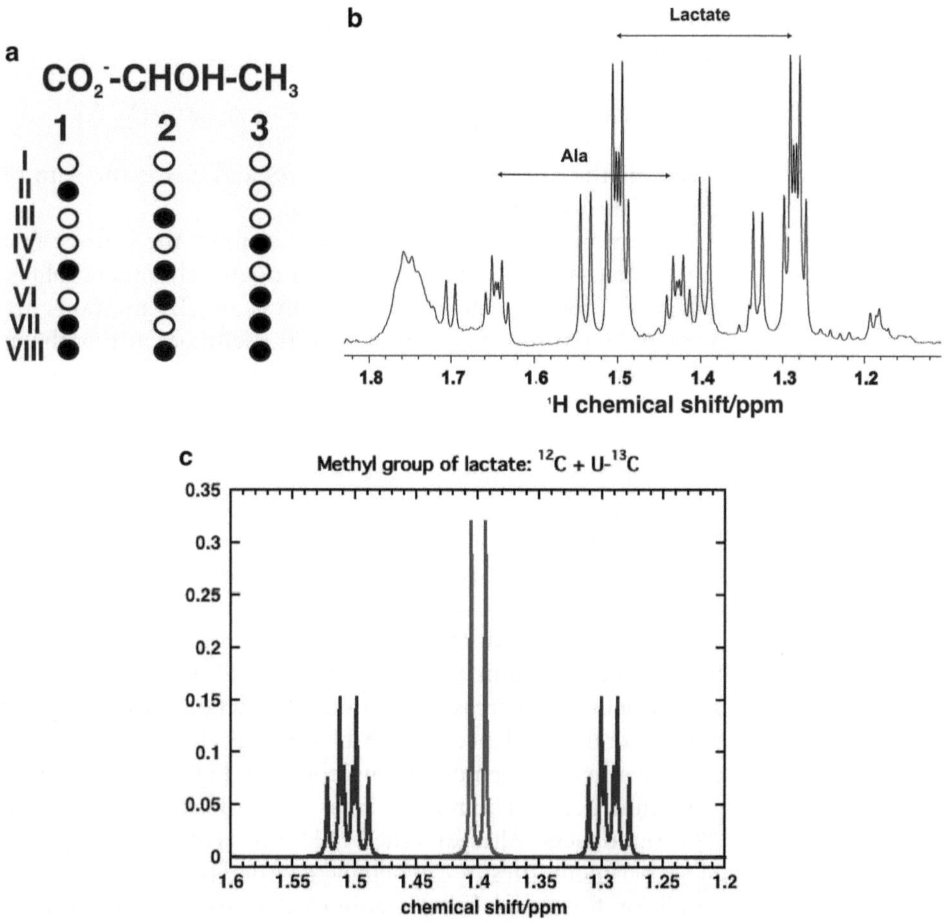

Fig. 16. ^{13}C isotopomers of lactate. (**a**) Possible isotopomers. *Open circles* denote ^{12}C, *filled circles* ^{13}C. All eight isotopomers are distinguishable by NMR (see text) (**b**) Methyl region of an extract of cells grown in the presence of [U-^{13}C]-glucose. The satellite peaks either side of the lactate methyl doublet at 1.4 ppm and the alanine methyl doublet at 1.54 ppm show the scalar coupling between the CH_3 protons with the neighboring CH (three-bond coupling), the neighboring ^{13}C (two-bond heteronuclear coupling), and the 3-bond heteronuclear coupling to the carboxyl carbon atom. This pattern demonstrates that the lactate molecule contains three ^{13}C atoms. (**c**) Simulation of the lactate methyl resonance using coupling constants of $^{3}J_{HH} = 7$ Hz, $^{1}J_{CH} = 127$ Hz, $^{2}J_{CH} = {}^{3}J_{CH} = 5$ Hz.

test sample containing both ^{12}C and ^{13}C glutamine, integration of the 1D spectrum gave $47 \pm 0.5\%$ enrichment at the β and γ positions. Because of the overlap in the Hα region, the 1D integration was inaccurate for Hα. However, this is resolved in 2D TOCSY and can be completely specified (see below).

The fine structure of the proton spectrum reflects all significant couplings, and in this case, the lactate was labeled at all three positions as first demonstrated by Lloyd et al. (82). If one uses ^{13}C-1 and ^{13}C-2 glucose, the lactate becomes labeled at different positions, and the appearance of the satellites is quite different.

Further, the ^{13}C produces a small, but measurable and in fact practically useful, isotope shift from the attached protons.

$$\text{Fractional isotope abundance: } F = A(\text{sats})/(\textstyle\sum \text{A}). \quad (17)$$

A(sats) is the area of the satellite peaks and ΣA is the sum of the areas of the satellite and central peaks.

For molecules such as lactate and alanine, the isotope fraction can be determined in 1D spectra. For many other metabolites, the spectra are too crowded for such analysis, so 2D methods may be needed. Here proton detection is most useful because of the inherent sensitivity and the ability to determine positional isotope distributions from individual cross-peaks. A particularly simple approach is to use the TOCSY experiment, with no X nucleus decoupling (which destroys the isotope information).

4.3. 2D Detection

For screening purposes, the 1D HSQC experiment is very valuable for selecting those metabolites which are enriched with ^{13}C, although what is observed really reflect the abundance of ^{13}C atoms, i.e., the product of the metabolite concentration times the fractional enrichment at the detected site. However, even a modest 10% enrichment increases the effective concentration nearly tenfold over natural abundance. Figure 17 shows a 1D HSQC spectrum of the test mixture, demonstrating the very high enrichment of the glutamine peaks. The relative areas of the peaks reflect the relative ^{13}C abundances. Although the 1D HSQC is the first increment of a 2D experiment, these are generally recorded under rather saturating condition for speed. For screening where some quantitative information is desired, a longer relaxation delay might be used. As the experiment is very sensitive, it requires very little experimental time and is comparable to that of a conventional 1D ^{1}H experiment.

The HSQC spectrum shows only the relative abundance of ^{13}C at each protiated carbon atom, and this will be weighted by the abundance times the fractional enrichment at that position. Within a molecule, the intensities of the various resonances should then reflect their relative enrichments, as the carbons all have the same concentration; only the number of attached protons needs to be accounted for. However, where there are mixed isotopomers, this cannot provide a detailed picture of the isotopomer distribution, and of course cannot provide information about labeling of carbonyl carbons. One solution is to work at high resolution in the carbon dimension, such that any ^{13}C–^{13}C couplings are resolved, and this gives the isotopomer distribution in the same way as a 1D ^{13}C observe spectrum does (see above), with the additional correlation C–H information.

For example, to acquire an HSQC spectrum with a spectral width of 100 ppm, or 20 kHz at 18.8 T, 1,000 points (resolution = 20 Hz/point) are needed to resolve the C–C couplings into doublets and triplets, etc. This is shown in Fig. 17b. However, with linear

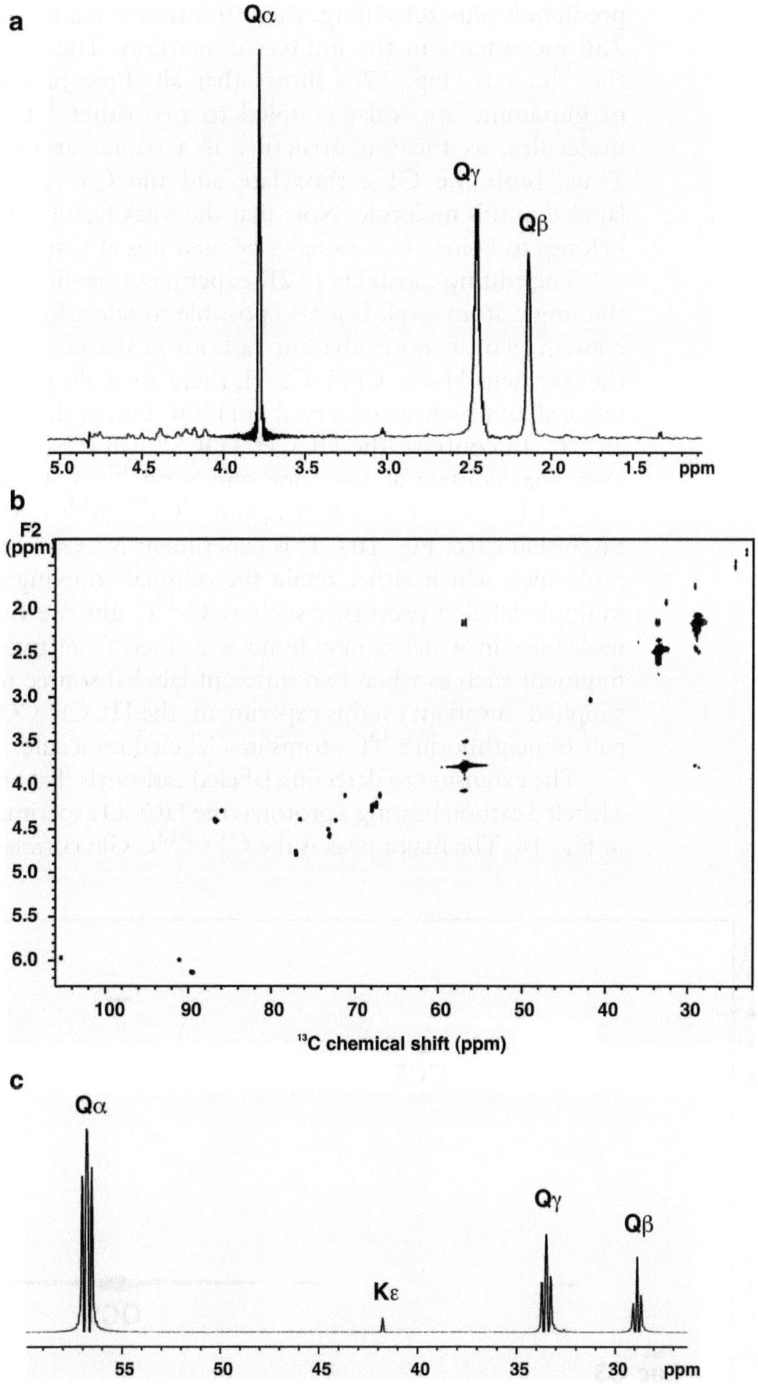

Fig. 17. 1D HSQC and HR-HSQC. HSQC recorded on the test mixture as a 1D spectrum and as a high-resolution spectrum in *F*1. (**a**) 1D HSQC equivalent to a ^{13}C-edited ^{1}H spectrum. (**b**) 2D high-resolution HSQC with 1,024 increments and extended to 4,096 point for transformation, giving a resolution of 11 Hz/pt in *F*1, with a total experimental time of 3.8 h. (**c**) ^{13}C*F*1 Projection of the Gln region in (**b**) showing triplet fine structure due to 1-bond ^{13}C–^{13}C couplings. Sums of couplings are 100 Hz (C2), 91 Hz (C4), and 82 Hz (C3) corresponding to about 41 Hz for $^{1}J_{C2C3}$ and $^{1}J_{C3C4}$, 50 Hz for $^{1}J_{C2C1}$, and 50 Hz for $^{1}J_{C4C5}$.

prediction plus zerofilling, the resolution is readily achieved with 256 increments in the indirect dimension. The projection onto the ^{13}C axis (Fig. 17c) shows that all three protiated carbons of glutamine are scalar coupled to two other ^{13}C in the same molecules, as the fine structure is a triplet at this resolution. Thus, both the C1 carboxylate and the C5 carbonyl are ^{13}C labeled in this molecule. Note that the weak feature at 44 ppm that belongs to lysine εC is a singlet because it is at natural abundance.

The editing capability of 2D experiments is shown by HSQC at the single atom level. It is also possible to select for molecules that contain two or more adjacent carbons in the same molecule. For the fragment H–Ca–CbH–Cc–H, there are eight possible isotopomers, all of which are observed in HSQC except the one containing all ^{12}C. In contrast, the HCCH TOCSY will select those isotopomers that contain at least one one-bond ^{13}C–^{13}C coupling, i.e., ^{13}Ca^{13}Cb^{12}Cc, ^{12}Ca^{13}Cb^{13}Cc, and ^{13}Ca^{13}Cb^{13}Cc, which are distinguishable (cf Fig. 10). This experiment is useful for editing for molecules, which either retain the original coupling patterns in a multiple-labeled precursor such as U-^{13}C glucose or Gln, or for molecules in which a new bond is formed from two ^{13}C-labeled fragment such as when two different labeled source molecules are supplied. A variant on this experiment, the HCCH COSY picks out pair of neighboring ^{13}C atoms in a labeled molecule.

The extension to detecting labeled carbonyls that are attached to a labeled carbon bearing a proton is the HCCO experiment, as shown in Fig. 18. The major peak is the C1 of ^{13}C Gln correlating with the

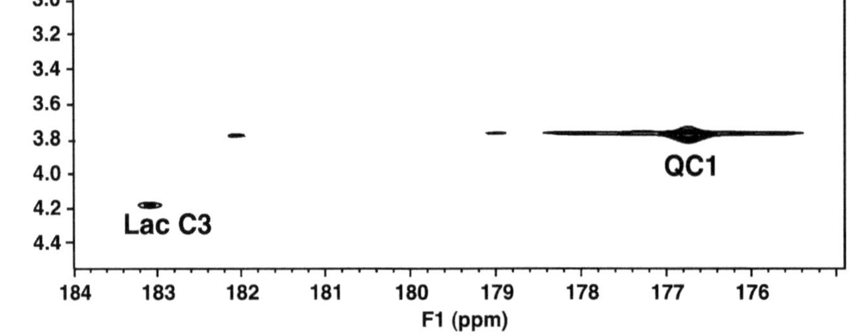

Fig. 18. Two-dimensional HACACO experiment. The spectrum of the test mix was acquired as a 2D plane correlating H with the carbonyl frequency in a gradient selected HACACO 3D experiment. The spectrum was recorded in 40 min (eight acquisitions per increment). The SNR of the Gln carbonyl signal was 384.

Hα as expected. As the relevant ^{13}C–^{13}C and ^{13}C–^{1}H one-bond coupling constants are large, the sensitivity of the experiment is high.

Clearly, such experiments are very valuable for picking out specific labeled metabolites in a complex sea of metabolites that are unlabeled or partially labeled and help with the assignment and identification of particular active pathways under the chosen experimental conditions (68).

Although these experiments show that ^{13}C is incorporated at specific positions in identifiable metabolites, it does not give the degree of enrichment. For this, it is necessary to be able to observe separately the different isotopomers, including those that are not labeled. The proton experiment is straightforward in this regard, as the ^{13}C satellites are completely resolved from the protons attached to ^{12}C (see above). In two dimensions, the same principle applies, but now it is possible to distinguish among all of the possible isotopomers, at least in principle. Thus, for a fragment of the kind HCCH, the scalar-coupled protons give rise to cross-peaks in COSY or TOCSY at the coordinates of the respective chemical shifts. If both carbons are ^{13}C, then each proton has two satellite peaks displaced by $^{1}J_{CH}/2$, and in the COSY or TOCSY spectrum, they will be correlated, giving rise to a square pattern. This is shown in Fig. 19. The ^{13}C glutamine shows cross-peaks at the expected positions for coupling between Hα, Hγ, and Hβ, due to the presence of the unlabeled glutamine present. These peaks are surrounded by a square of satellite peaks for the uniformly labeled Gln present and is easily seen in both the COSY and the TOCSY spectra (Fig. 19a, b). The short mixing time TOCSY makes the appearance of the spectrum similar to that in the COSY where single step transfers only are possible. The main difference is the appearance of the fine structure. In practice, the antiphase fine structure of the Gln α−β cross-peak leads to partial cancelation, especially of the broader ^{13}C satellite peaks, whereas the TOCSY cross-peaks are in phase and show substantially higher sensitivity. With a longer mixing time (50 ms, Fig. 19c), the α−γ cross-peaks show up strongly and fully resolved from the α−β cross-peak. Thus, the satellite peaks involving β and γ can be assessed in a clear region of the spectrum rather than close to the diagonal as in COSY. Figure 19d shows the patterns obtained in the 2-quantum COSY experiment. The remote α−γ correlation peaks show clearly the isotopomer pattern; such peaks may be useful in otherwise very crowded spectra or where cross-peaks are close to the diagonal.

The relative intensities of the central peak (unlabeled) and the satellite peaks reflect the different abundances of the isotopomers. In the present case, there are only two isotopomers present, unlabeled and labeled at all carbons, and the volumes of the satellite peaks (sum of the points in the square) are essentially equal to that of the central peak, as expected as this is a 50:50 mixture. It is notable that this spectrum shows that all three protiated carbons are either labeled or unlabeled in the same molecules.

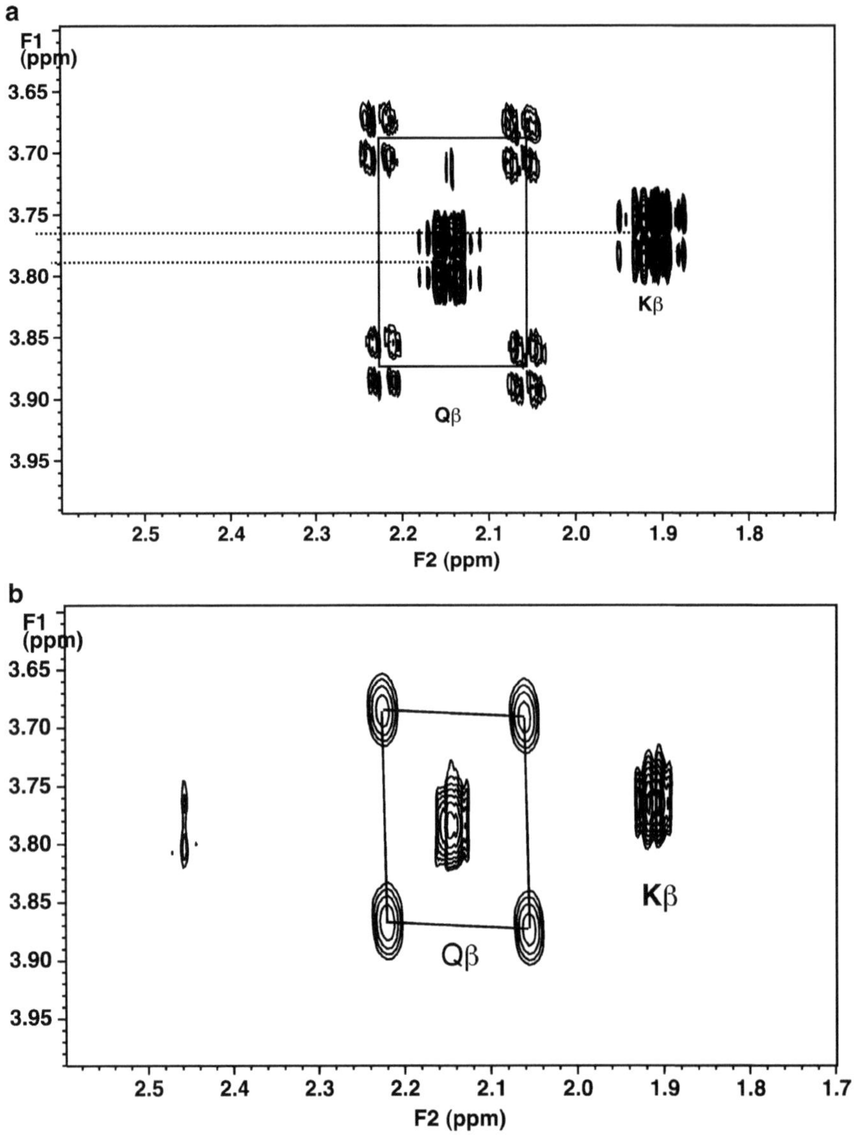

Fig. 19. Isotopomers in Gln. The glutamine C2,C3,C4 region of the test mix is shown to indicate the splitting patterns. Acquisition times were 0.58 and 0.05 s in t_2 and t_1, respectively. The mixing pulse was MLEV17 for the TOCSY, at a B_1 field strength of 8 kHz. (**a**) DQF-COSY. (**b**) 25 ms TOCSY. (**c**) 50 ms TOCSY. (**d**) Inadequate. The ^{13}C isotope shift in the spectra is approximately 0.01 ppm. Each experiment was recorded in 2.3 h.

However, the synthesis of Glu or Gln in vivo involves transamination or reductive amidation of 2-oxoglutarate, which is the result of oxidative decarboxylation of isocitrate. Thus, the labeling pattern of Glu and Gln depends on the source of ^{13}C supplied, how many times the citric acid cycle has turned, and the relative importance of anaplerotic reactions including glutaminolysis and pyruvate carboxylase activity. The scrambling at the succinate partially randomizes label in the two halves of succinate through to OAA, and this gives rise to a variety of possible isotopomers of

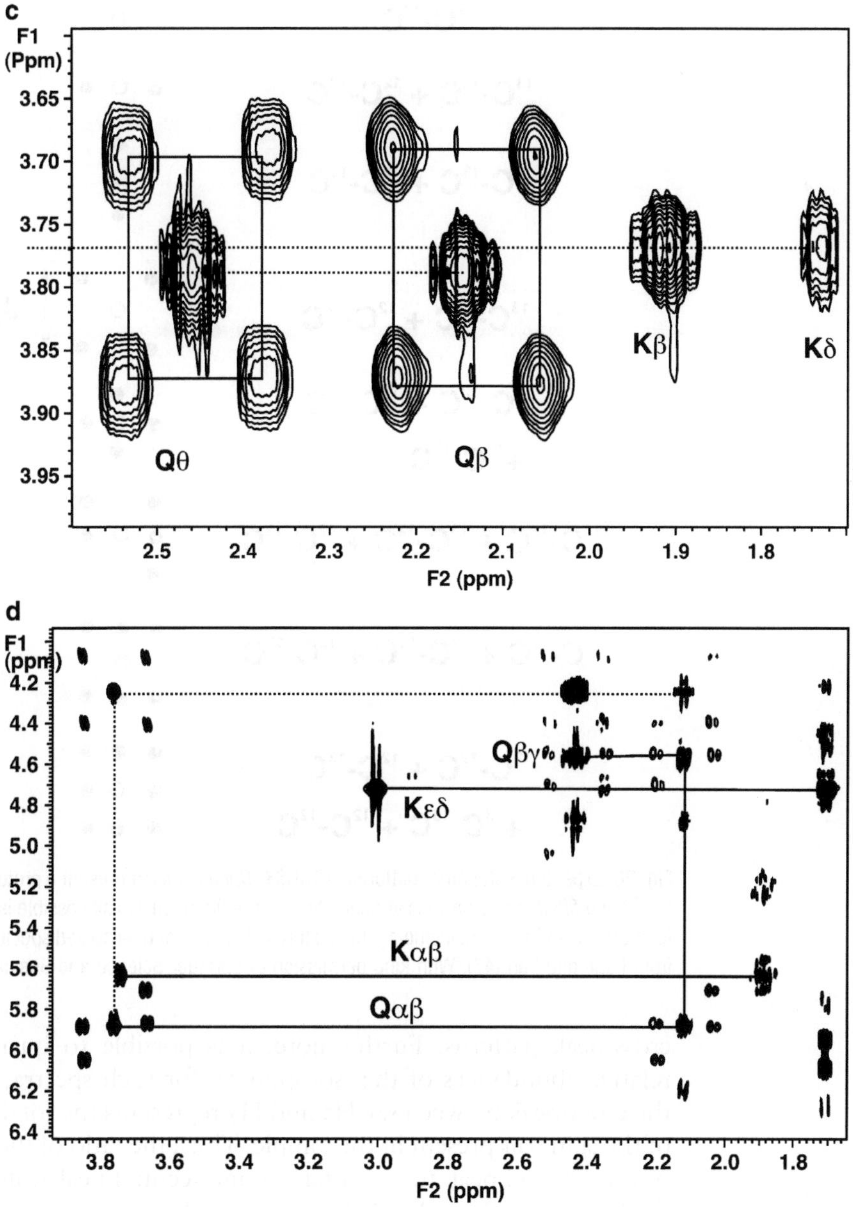

Fig. 19. (continued)

2-oxogutrate. Thus, it s possible to obtain different amounts of label at all of the positions of the observed Glu. The possible TOCSY patterns for isotopomer distributions are shown in Fig. 20. This demonstrates how it is possible to distinguish between a molecule in which two adjacent carbons are labeled in the same molecule, or whether there is a mixture of two isotopomers with either one or the other carbon labeled. The extension to multiple carbons is trivial. This shows the power of the 2D NMR approach for identifying the positional isotopomers, simply by examining

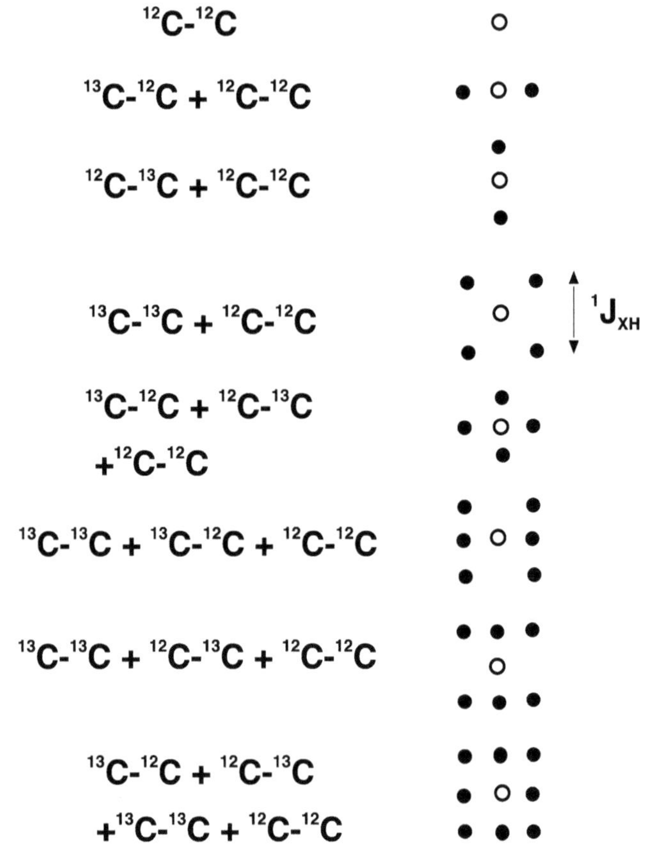

Fig. 20. Expected isotopomer patterns in TOCSY. *Open circles* represent a proton attached to ^{12}C and *filled circles* protons attached to ^{13}C. The figure shows all possible isotopomers for a CHa–CHb fragment, including the mixtures of labeled and unlabeled species (Figure 3 from Lane and Fan (47), With kind permission of Springer Science and Business Media.

cross-peak patterns. Furthermore, it is possible to quantify the relative abundances of the isotopomers for such spectra, because the cross-peak between say Hα and Hγ represents the total amount of the spin pair present in the sample. Thus, the ratio of the volume of the $^{12}C^{12}C$ peak to the total volume (central peak+satellites) is the fraction of the unlabeled isotopomer. By volume integration of the various satellites, it is possible to obtain an accurate estimate of the fraction of each form present.

Because the transfer function in TOCSY is the same for each component of the cross-peak, when taking ratios, the details of the function cancel out, leaving only the abundances. However, 2D spectra are usually recorded under conditions where there is substantial signal saturation. This will give rise to an error if the various components relax at different rates. The protons attached to ^{13}C relax faster than those attached to ^{12}C, so the raw ratio overestimates the enrichment with ^{13}C. To some extent, this is offset in TOCSY because the differential relaxation during the

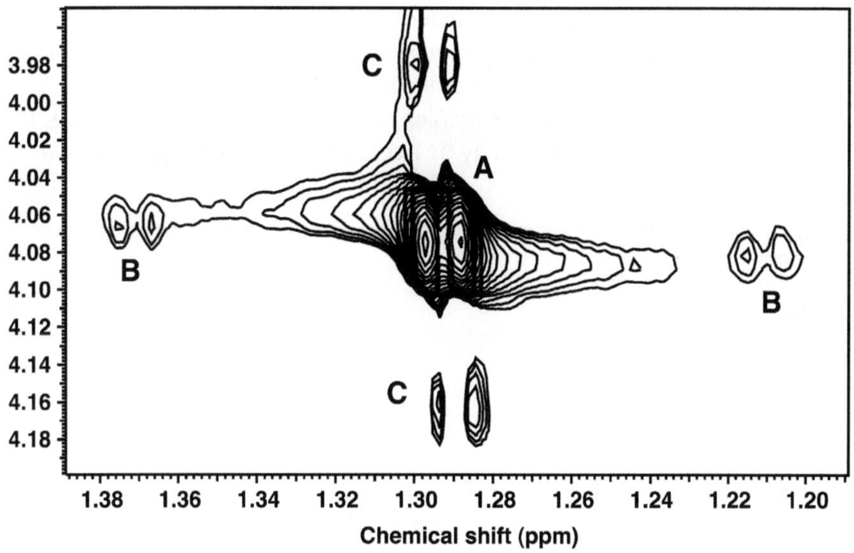

Fig. 21. Natural abundance satellite peaks in lactate. Sodium lactate was dissolved in 100 mM KCl, 10 mM sodium phosphate, pH 7, lyophilized, and redissolved in D_2O to give a final concentration of 2.3 mM. TOCSY spectrum was recorded at 20°C at 18.8 T with a mixing time of 50 ms, a spin-lock field strength of 8 kHz, and acquisition times of 0.34 and 0.05 s in t_2 and t_1, respectively. The figure shows the unlabeled and two natural abundance satellites cross-peaks. The spectrum was recorded in 2 h. The peaks labeled as A, B, and C correspond to ^{12}C2–^{12}C3, ^{12}C2–^{13}C3, and ^{13}C2–^{12}C3 isotopomers, respectively (Figure 4, from Lane and Fan (47), With kind permission of Springer Science and Business Media).

spin-lock period has the opposite effect to that of the longitudinal relaxation (40, 46, 47). We have found that using a recycle time of 2 s, the error from differential relaxation is quite small. The error can be reduced to essentially zero by correcting the volumes using known T_1 values for ^{12}C and ^{13}C.

The sensitivity of the TOCSY-based method is determined by the usual considerations, but in also the satellite intensity is spread over several components, which reduces the relative volume of each one. In principle, decoupling in one or the other dimension would increase the sensitivity of the satellites by a factor of 2 (and overall resolution), but at the expense of loss of information about position. Figure 21 shows a TOCSY spectrum of a lactate standard recorded on 2.3 mM lactate. The satellite peaks are each at 12.6 μM lactate, i.e., a dynamic range of 200:1 compared with the central peak. The cross-peaks appear in a cross formation (Fig. 21), verifying that what is observed is a mixture of three isotopomers, namely fully unlabeled (central peak) and the two singly labeled isotopomers. The doubly labeled isotopomer would be present at 1% of the peaks, and they lie below the noise level. Integrating the peaks showed a ^{13}C label at $1.2 \pm 0.2\%$, without any correction for differential relaxation. This compares favorably with the expected 1.1%. Thus, the intrinsic accuracy is acceptable for most purposes.

Depending on the ^{13}C source, the TOCSY cross-peaks routinely can be used for following glucose carbons into different ribonucleotides, nucleobases, amino acids, lactate, fatty acids in phospholipids, glycerol metabolites, and quantifying individual positions with good accuracy and precision.

The same principles can be applied to ^{15}N labeling, though for some atoms, it may be necessary to work in light water to detect the

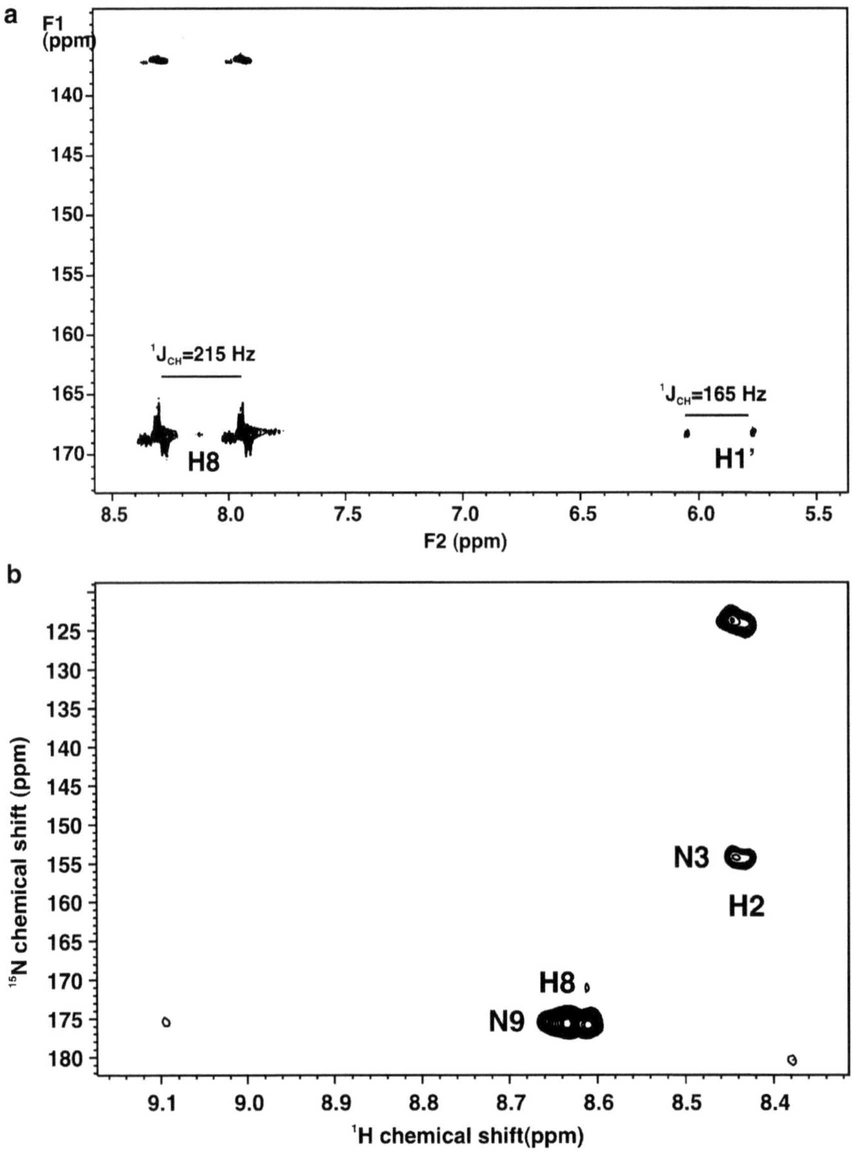

Fig. 22. $^{13}C/^{15}N$ HSQC of GTP. (**a**) 2.2 mM $U^{15}N,^{13}C$ GTP in D_2O 20°C 14. 1 T The ^{15}N–^1H HSQC spectrum was recorded in 1.7 h with acquisition times of 1 s in t_2 and 80 ms in t_1 in 1.7 h. The was no decoupling during t_2, allowing the ^{13}C and ^{15}N coupling to be observed in the proton dimension. The $^1J_{CH}$ between H8 and C8 is 281 Hz. The optimum delay in the HSQC for the two-bond coupling between H8 and the N7, N9 was 15 Hz. The two-bond couplings constant are 7.6 Hz for H8–N9 and 11.4 Hz for H8N7 (45). (**b**) TCA extract of MDMAMB231 cells grown in the presence of 5 mM ^{12}C glucose and 5 mM U-[$^{13}C,^{15}N$]-glutamine. The ^{15}N of the amido group of Gln enters the ring positions shown in the long-range HSQC spectrum, using an INEPT delay of 15 ms.

attached proton. It turns out that in nucleotides, the two-bond N–H coupling is quite large (8–11 Hz in purines) which means that nitrogen incorporation into nucleotides (e.g., from glutamine) can be easily detected in D_2O, as is shown in Fig. 22. In this instance, the ^{13}C coupling to the H8 is also observed (as well as to the H1′) as the molecule is doubly labeled. This shows that in a complex mixture, a simple 2D experiment could be used to select for molecules that are labeled with ^{15}N, as well as ^{13}C. This is exemplified further in the extract of breast cancer cells grown in the presence of $^{15}N/^{13}C$ glutamine (Fig. 20b), which shows the expected nitrogen position labeled from ^{15}N Gln as source. An example of double labeling from two independent sources has been described for rice coleoptiles fed with ^{15}N ammonia and ^{13}C acetate, and following the double label into GAB (44).

5. Conclusions

NMR is a very high information content spectroscopic technique that can provide unambiguous structure identification of known compounds and give valuable clues to the identity of unknowns. It is also a quantitative technique with an intrinsically high dynamic range. Furthermore, it is one of the few methods that can give quantitative positional isotopomer information, and for this, it is the method of choice. As stable isotope analyses are the key to following atoms through pathways, the use of NMR would seem to be essential. The major drawback of the technique remains its relatively low sensitivity when compared with mass spectrometry, though it holds its own with most other forms of spectroscopy. In fact, NMR becomes even more powerful when combined with mass spectrometry, as the two approaches can provide complementary as well as overlapping information, which both extends the range of compounds that can be analyzed, as well as improves the reliability of identification and quantification. We have promoted the use of the joint platform for metabolic studies for many years (9, 46, 69, 83, 84).

Acknowledgments

This work was supported in part by grants from the Susan G. Komen Foundation BCTR0503648, NIH Grant Number RR018733 from the National Center for Research Resources, NSF EPSCoR EPS-0447479, and the Brown Foundation.

Glossary

Apodization	Removal of the feet. A manipulation of the free induction decay (FID) to ensure that the time domain smoothly approaches zero at the end to avoid truncation artifacts (sinc wiggles).
Bloch equations	Classical dynamical equations that describe the time dependence of the *x,y,z* components of the magnetization, viz: $$\mathrm{d}Mz/\mathrm{d}t = \omega_1 My - (Mz - M^0)/T_1,$$ $$\mathrm{d}Mx/\mathrm{d}t = -(\omega - \omega_0)My - Mx/T_2,$$ $$\mathrm{d}My/\mathrm{d}t = (\omega - \omega_0)Mx - My/T_2$$ ω_0 is the Larmor frequency (qv), T_1 and T_2 are the relaxation times (qv), and ω_1 is the strength of the applied radiofrequency field.
Chemical shift	Relative resonant frequency, defined (in ppm) as 10^6 $(\nu_{obs} - \nu_{ref})/\nu_{Fref.}$ Depends on chemistry such as type of atom, nearest neighbors, bonding, and therefore is characteristic of local functional groups. It is also very sensitive to inductive effects from nearby ionizable groups such as carboxyls and amino functions.
Coherence	NMR is a coherent form of spectroscopy because a pulse excites all spins, and the bulk magnetization (resultant) is rotated en mass to a defined axis. The magnetization vector continues to precess in phase. Dephasing will occur due to spin–spin relaxation (qv), resulting in a loss of phase coherence. Magnetization is the observable in NMR and is a single quantum coherence. Other coherences can be created between interacting pairs (or higher order) of spins in which there is a coherence (e.g., phase) between the interacting spins. This is used extensively in multiple quantum spectroscopy where different orders of coherence can be generated through scalar coupling. For a pair of spins, both double and zero quantum coherence can be created, in which the components rotate in the same sense (2-quantum state)

	or in opposite direction (zero quantum state). These have distinct phase properties that can be selected by gradient or phase cycling.
Correlation time	Time taken for a property to decay to $1/e$ of its initial value. Usually refers to rotational correlation time, which is related to the size and shape of a molecule, and defines the timescale for reorientation of a molecule by random processes.
COSY	COrrelation SpectroscopY. Usually refers to correlation of resonances of scalar-coupled nuclei. Used for determining through-bond interactions within a covalent network. Defines molecular fragments via proton–proton connectivity.
CPMG	Carr Purcell Meiboom Gill spin-echo pulse sequence consisting of a train of alternating 180° pulses orthogonal to the initial exciting pulse separated by a tunable delay. This compensates for imperfections of the 180° pulse and effectively refocuses magnetization along a defined axis. As such, it is suitable for accurate measurement of T_2. If the delay D is short, evolution of scalar couplings is suppressed, allowing recording of in-phase spectra of scalar-coupled spin systems. Used in metabonomics for suppressing macromolecule signals in biofluids.
Coupling constant	Interaction strength between two scalar-(through-bond) coupled magnetic nuclei. The scalar coupling constant (denoted J) is a measure of nuclear interactions transmitted through the bonding network. Three-bond J values provide information on the torsion angle.
Dipolar coupling	Interaction between magnetic nuclei via dipole–dipole interactions. This depends on the inverse sixth power of the internuclear separation, and the intrinsic magnetic strength of the two nuclei.
FID-free induction decay	Rotating magnetization induces a voltage in the receiver coil (magnetic induction) which decays exponentially by *relaxation processes.* The time-dependent voltage is digitized and converted into a frequency response by

Fourier transformation (qv). The two signals in quadrature are:

$$S(\text{real}) = a_0 \exp(-t/R_2)\cos(\omega t),$$

$$S(\text{imaginary}) = a_0 \exp(-t/R_2)\sin(\omega t).$$

Fourier transform (FT) — Mathematical trick for converting one periodic function into another function. In NMR, the raw data comprise an exponentially decaying sum of cosinusoidal functions. The FT converts time into frequency. The decaying part of the signal becomes manifest as a broadening of the resonance. The FT of a single resonance is:

$$\text{Re}\left[a_0 \int \mathrm{d}t \exp(-i\Omega t)\exp(i\omega - 1/T)t\right]$$

$$= (2a_0/T)/((\Omega-\omega)^2 + 1/T^2)$$

width at half height $L = 1/\pi T$
T is the decay time constant (also called "T_2")

Gyromagnetic ratio — γ is a property of nuclei that determines the strength of the nuclear magnetic moment and is characteristic for each isotope. The fundamental frequency is proportional to the product of γ and the applied magnetic field strength.

GFT NMR — G-matrix Fourier transform NMR. A projection method that reduces dimensionality by incrementing indirect time dimension in lock step (cf Accordion spectroscopy) allowing a large saving in NMR time for higher dimensional experiments. Functionally equivalent projection-reconstruction methods.

HMQC — Heteronuclear Multiple Quantum Coherence. Formation of multiple quantum coherence via scalar coupling between nuclei, e.g., C–H or N–H, occurs in any multipulse experiment. The coherence common evolution of the coupled spins is not directly observable, but its effects are detectable on reconversion to SQC. Such experiments are commonly used in inverse detection of low γ nuclei. MQC also has different relaxation properties (involves terms at higher frequencies) than SQC.

HSQC — Heteronuclear Single Quantum Coherence. Homologue of HMQC, but only single

	quantum coherences are selected. This experiment requires more pulses than HMQC, but has more favorable relaxation properties and is the experiment of choice for ^{15}N–H systems.
HSQC-TOCSY and HMQC-TOCSY	Combination of two experiments that can be used in 3D mode or as 2D. The former correlates a heteronucleus (e.g., ^{13}C with the directly attached proton, and other protons that are in the same molecular fragment). This is useful for assignments of compounds in complex mixtures when some atoms are enriched or otherwise rare (e.g., ^{15}N in amino or amido compounds or ^{31}P in phosphorylated compounds). HCCH-TOCSY specifically selects for two or more directly bonded heteroatoms such as ^{13}C in molecular fragments of the type HC–CH, and the protons are correlated with one another. This experiment edits complex spectra and shows where multiply labeled compounds retain their bonds, or if new bonds are formed between labeled compounds.
INADEQUATE	Incredible Natural Abundance Double Quantum Transfer Experiment. This experiment, developed for tracing carbon networks in small molecules at natural abundance with ^{13}C detect, has been improved to proton detection, and as the two-quantum COSY, for proton correlations over three bonds.
INEPT	Insensitive Nuclei Enhanced by Polarization Transfer. Magnetization from an abundant high γ spin is transferred to one of low γ by transfer through scalar coupling. The enhancement is equal to γ_A/γ_B and is governed by a rate $\sin \pi J\Delta$ where Δ is the delay time. Typically achieved using a pulse sandwich comprising a 90° pulse on the high γ nucleus, followed by a delay $\Delta = 1/2J$ and then simultaneous 90° pulses on the two coupled nuclei. Refocusing of chemical shift evolution is often included using a 180° pulse on both nuclei at $\Delta/2$.
Inverse detection	Detection of a "weak" X nucleus (low γ) via a strong nucleus (usually ^{1}H) usually via INEPT. Usually applies to proton detection of ^{13}C, ^{15}N. Requires scalar coupling

	between the X nucleus and the ^{1}H atom, generally (but not exclusively) by one bond. The sensitivity enhancement (SNR) possible is given by the ratio $(\gamma_H/\gamma_X)^{5/2}$. This is >300 fold for ^{15}N.
Isotopomers	Are versions of the same compound in which differ by the distribution of isotopes of each element. In a 3-carbon compounds such as lactate, there are eight possible stable isotopomers (^{12}C and ^{13}C) corresponding to ^{12}C-3, ^{13}C-3, and three each of ^{12}C-1^{13}C-2, and ^{13}C-1^{12}C-2. In NMR, these correspond to eight distinguishable compounds. In mass spectrometry, there are only four mass isotopomers $m0$, $m+1$ $m+2$ and $m+3$ because the three isotopomers of $m+1$ and $m+2$ have identical mass.
Larmor frequency	Fundamental rotation frequency of the spins produced by the torque produced by the external magnetic field acting on the spin magnetic moments (qv). The Larmor frequency depends on the magnetic field strength and the intrinsic magnetic moment (qv) of the spin.
Magnetic moment	Protons and neutrons have the property of spin. As these are particles having charged components, they must have a magnetic moment (i.e., behave as magnets). Some nuclei have an imbalance of protons and neutrons, such that the nuclear spins are not all paired, leaving a net magnetic moment. The strength of the magnetic moment is a fundamental nuclear property, that is described by the gyromagnetic ratio, which is related to the effective distribution of spinning charge in the nucleus (in the classical picture).
NOE	Nuclear Overhauser Enhancement. Increase in magnetization of a spin when the magnetization of a neighboring spin is perturbed from equilibrium. The NOE depends on r^{-6} and is therefore the primary source of distance information within a molecule.
NOESY	Nuclear Overhauser Enhancement SpectroscopY- 2D experiment to measure NOE effects.
Relaxation time	Characteristic time for the return of bulk magnetization to the equilibrium value.

	Comes in two main flavors, T_1-spin–lattice relaxation and T_2, spin–spin relaxation. T_1 is the relaxation time that described return of *z*-magnetization and is a process that is associated with changes in enthalpy. T_2 is a loss of phase coherence among spins in the *x*–*y* plane and is an entropic process.
Rotating frame	Larmor frequencies are in the 100s of MHz and vary by a few tens of kHz for similar spins. It is convenient to remove this high frequency rotation from consideration by working in a frame rotating at the Larmor frequency. In this frame, the spins appear stationary.
ROESY	Rotating frame Overhauser Enhancement SpectroscopY. ROEs are positive for all molecular correlation times. Exchange has opposite sign, and so this experiment is useful for distinguishing exchange reactions from dipolar interactions.
Scalar interactions	Through-bond interactions, nuclei interact via bonding electrons, which transmit the information about nuclear spin state through the covalent network. This gives rise to the coupling constant (qv) which is a measure of the interaction strength.
Spin	Property of particles that has a classical analog (a spinning top has spin angular momentum, etc.). In the original Schrödinger wave mechanics, there were only three quantum numbers and no spin. Spin arises naturally as a consequence of a relativistic treatment of wave mechanics (cf. P.A.M. Dirac). Spin is also quantized; only discrete values are possible. For the common case, the spin quantum number is 1/2, i.e., there are but two spin states (up and down, α and β). Magnetic nuclei are also referred to as spins.
TOCSY	Total Correlation Spectroscopy. Also known as HOHAHA. Provides (scalar) correlations within an entire spin system. Especially useful for identification of compounds in mixtures, and also for quantitative analysis of isotopomer distributions.
Zeeman energy	Is the energy of the interaction of a magnetic moment due to a spin with the external magnetic field.

References

1. Gadian DG. NMR and its applications to living systems. 2nd ed. Oxford: Oxford University Press.; 1995. p. 283.
2. Ernst RR, Bodenhausen G, Wokaun A. Principles of nuclear magnetic resonance in one and two dimensions. Oxford: Clarendon Press; 1990.
3. Sanders JKM, Hunter BK. Modern NMR spectroscopy. A guide for chemists. Oxford: Oxford University Press; 1987.
4. Claridge TDW. High-resolution NMR techniques in organic chemistry. San Diego: Elsevier; 1999.
5. Cavanagh J, Fairbrother WJ, Palmer AG, Skelton AGNJ. Protein NMR spectroscopy principles and practice. San Diego: Academic; 1996.
6. Homans SW. A dictionary of concepts in NMR. In: Dwek RA, editor. Biophysical techniques. Oxford: Clarendon Press; 1992.
7. Pochapsky TC, Pochapsky SS. NMR for physical and biological scientists. New York: Taylor & Francis; 2007.
8. Gradwell MJ, Fan TWM, Lane AN. Analysis of phosphorylated metabolites in crayfish extracts by two-dimensional H-1-P-31 NMR heteronuclear total correlation spectroscopy (heteroTOCSY). Anal Biochem. 1998;263 (2):139–49.
9. Fan TWM, Higashi RM, Lane AN, Jardetzky O. Combined use of H-1-NMR and GC-MS for metabolite monitoring and invivo H-1-NMR assignments. Biochim Biophys Acta. 1986;882(2):154–67.
10. Wishart DS, Bigam CG, Yao J, Abildgaard F, Dyson HJ, Oldfield E, Markley JL, Sykes BD. 1H, 13C and 15N chemical shift referencing in biomolecular NMR. J Biomol NMR. 1995;6 (2):135–40.
11. Zhang HY, Neal S, Wishart DS. RefDB: a database of uniformly referenced protein chemical shifts. J Biomol NMR. 2003;25(3):173–95.
12. Harris RK, Becker ED, De Menezes SMC, Goodfellow R, Granger P. NMR nomenclature. Nuclear spin properties and conventions for chemical shifts—(IUPAC recommendations 2001). Pure Appl Chem. 2001;73 (11):1795–818.
13. Edzes HT. Determination of the resonance frequency ratio of the P-31 and H-1-NMR resonance shift standards 85-percent orthophosphoric acid and tetramethylsilane. Magn Reson Chem. 1992;30(9):850–4.
14. Wishart DS, Bigam CG, Yao J, Abildgaard F, Dyson HJ, Oldfield E, Markley JL, Sykes BD. H-1, C-13 and N-15 chemical-shift referencing in biomolecular NMR. J Biomol NMR. 1995;6(2):135–40.
15. Hoult DI. NMR receiver—description and analysis of design. Prog Nucl Magn Reson Spectrosc. 1978;12:41–77.
16. Hoult DI, Richards RE. Signal-to-noise ratio of nuclear magnetic-resonance experiment. J Magn Reson. 1976;24(1):71–85.
17. Kelly AE, Ou HD, Withers R, Dotsch V. Low-conductivity buffers for high-sensitivity NMR measurements. J Am Chem Soc. 2002;124(40):12013–9.
18. Lane AN, Arumugam S. Improving NMR sensitivity in room temperature and cooled probes with dipolar ions. J Magn Reson. 2005;173(2):339–43.
19. Aramini JM, Rossi P, Anklin C, Xiao R, Montelione GT. Microgram-scale protein structrue determonation by NMR. Nat Methods. 2007;4:491–3.
20. Siuzdak G. The expanding role of mass spectrometry in biotechnology. San Diego: MCC Press; 2003.
21. Kupce E, Freeman R. Two-dimensional Hadamard spectroscopy. J Magn Reson. 2003;162 (2):300–10.
22. Kupce E, Freeman R. Fast multi-dimensional Hadamard spectroscopy. J Magn Reson. 2003;163(1):56–63.
23. Kupce E, Freeman R. Frequency-domain Hadamard spectroscopy. J Magn Reson. 2003;162(1):158–65.
24. Mobli M, Maciejewski MW, Gryk MR, Hoch JC. Automatic maximum entropy spectral reconstruction in NMR. J Biomol NMR. 2007;39(2):133–9.
25. Hyberts SG, Heffron GJ, Tarragona NG, Solanky K, Edmonds KA, Luithardt H, Fejzo J, Chorev M, Aktas H, Colson K, Falchuk KH, Halperin JA, Wagner G. Ultrahigh-resolution H-1-C-13 HSQC spectra of metabolite mixtures using nonlinear sampling and forward maximum entropy reconstruction. J Am Chem Soc. 2007;129(16):5108–16.
26. Rovnyak D, Hoch JC, Stern AS, Wagner G. Resolution and sensitivity of high field nuclear magnetic resonance spectroscopy. J Biomol NMR. 2004;30(1):1–10.
27. Schmieder P, Stern AS, Wagner G, Hoch JC. Quantification of maximum-entropy spectrum reconstructions. J Magn Reson. 1997;125 (2):332–9.
28. Schanda P, Kupce E, Brutscher B. SOFAST-HMQC experiments for recording two-dimensional heteronuclear correlation spectra of proteins within a few seconds. J Biomol NMR. 2005;33(4):199–211.

29. Kupce E, Freeman R. Fast multidimensional NMR by polarization sharing. Magn Reson Chem. 2006;45(1):2–4.
30. Moseley HNB, Riaz N, Aramini JM, Szyperski T, Montelione GT. A generalized approach to automated NMR peak list editing: application to reduced dimensionality triple resonance spectra. J Magn Reson. 2004;170(2):263–77.
31. Constans A. GFT NMR proves its structural genomics mettle. Scientist. 2005;19(23):40.
32. Kim S, Szyperski T. GFT NMR, a new approach to rapidly obtain precise high-dimensional NMR spectral information. J Am Chem Soc. 2003;125(5):1385–93.
33. Mishkovsky M, Kupce E, Frydman L. Ultrafast-based projection-reconstruction three-dimensional nuclear magnetic resonance spectroscopy. J Chem Phys. 2007;127 (3):034507.
34. Freeman R, Kupce E. Distant echoes of the accordion: reduced dimensionality, GFT-NMR, and projection-reconstruction of multidimensional spectra. Concepts Magn Reson A. 2004;23A(2):63–75.
35. Kupce E, Freeman R. Fast multidimensional NMR spectroscopy by the projection-reconstruction technique. Spectroscopy. 2004;19 (10):16–20.
36. Kupce E, Freeman R. Projection-reconstruction technique for speeding up multidimensional NMR spectroscopy. J Am Chem Soc. 2004;126(20):6429–40.
37. Piotto M, Saudek V, Sklenar V. Gradient-tailored excitation for single-quantum NMR-spectroscopy of aqueous-solutions. J Biomol NMR. 1992;2(6):661–5.
38. Smallcombe SH, Patt SL, Keifer PA. WET solvent suppression and its applications to LC NMR and high-resolution NMR spectroscopy. J Magn Reson Ser A. 1995;117(2):295–303.
39. Weljie AM, Newton J, Mercier P, Carlson E, Slupsky CM. Targeted profiling: quantitative analysis of H-1 NMR metabolomics data. Anal Chem. 2006;78(13):4430–42.
40. Fan TW, Lane AN. Structure-based profiling of metabolites and isotopomers by NMR. Prog NMR Spectrosc. 2008;52:69–117.
41. Lindon JC, Nicholson JK, Everett JR. NMR spectroscopy of biofluids. In: Annual reports on NMR spectroscopy, Vol. 38. San Diego: Academic; 1999, p. 1–88.
42. Daykin CA, Foxall PJD, Connor SC, Lindon JC, Nicholson JK. The comparison of plasma deproteinization methods for the detection of low-molecular-weight metabolites by H-1 nuclear magnetic resonance spectroscopy. Anal Biochem. 2002;304(2):220–30.
43. Fan TWM. Metabolite profiling by one- and two-dimensional NMR analysis of complex mixtures. Prog Nucl Magn Reson Spectrosc. 1996;28:161–219.
44. Fan TWM, Higashi RM, Frenkiel TA, Lane AN. Anaerobic nitrate and ammonium metabolism in flood-tolerant rice coleoptiles. J Exp Bot. 1997;48(314):1655–66.
45. Ippel JH, Wijmenga SS, de Jong B, Hues HA, Hilbers CW, de Vroom E, van de Marel CA, van Boom JH. Heteronuclear scalar couplings in the bases and sugar rings of nucleic acids: their determination and application in assignment and conformational analysis. Magn Reson Chem. 1996;34:S156–76.
46. Lane AN, Fan TW, Higashi RM. Isotopomer-based metabolomic analysis by NMR and mass spectrometry. In: John HWD, Correia J, editors. Biophysical tools for biologists. San Deigo: Academic; 2007. p. 18.
47. Lane AN, Fan TW. Quantification and identification of isotopomer distributions of metabolites in crude cell extracts using 1H TOCSY. Metabolomics. 2007;3:79–86.
48. Weljie AM, Newton J, Mercier P, Carlson E, Slupsky CM. Targeted profiling: quantitative analysis of 1H NMR metabolomics data. Anal Chem. 2006;78(13):4430–42.
49. Dieterle F, Ross A, Schlotterbeck G, Senn H. Metabolite projection analysis for fast identification of metabolites in metabonomics. Application in an amiodarone study. Anal Chem. 2006;78(11):3551–61.
50. Beger RD, Schnackenberg LK, Holland RD, Li DH, Dragan Y. Metabonomic models of human pancreatic cancer using 1D proton NMR spectra of lipids in plasma. Metabolomics. 2006;2(3):125–34.
51. Lopez-Diez EC, Winder CL, Ashton L, Currie F, Goodacre R. Monitoring the mode of action of antibiotics using Raman spectroscopy: investigating subinhibitory effects of amikacin on *Pseudomonas aeruginosa*. Anal Chem. 2005;77(9):2901–6.
52. Kind T, Tolstikov V, Fiehn O, Weiss RH. A comprehensive urinary metabolomic approach for identifying kidney cancer. Anal Biochem. 2007;363(2):185–95.
53. Wold S. Pattern-recognition by means of disjoint principal components models. Pattern Recogn. 1976;8(3):127–39.
54. Wold S. Cross-validatory estimation of number of components in factor and principal

components models. Technometrics. 1978;20 (4):397–405.

55. Trygg J, Holmes E, Lundstedt T. Chemometrics in metabonomics. J Proteome Res. 2007;6(2):469–79.

56. Kettaneh N, Berglund A, Wold S. PCA and PLS with very large data sets. Comput Stat Data Anal. 2005;48(1):69–85.

57. Trygg J, Wold S. O_2-PLS, a two-block (X-Y) latent variable regression (LVR) method with an integral OSC filter. J Chemom. 2003;17 (1):53–64.

58. Trygg J, Wold S. Orthogonal projections to latent structures (O-PLS). J Chemom. 2002;16(3):119–28.

59. Wold S, Trygg J, Berglund A, Antti H. Some recent developments in PLS modeling. Chemometr Intell Lab Syst. 2001;58(2):131–50.

60. Viant MR. Improved methods for the acquisition and interpretation of NMR metabolomic data. Biochem Biophys Res Commun. 2003;310(3):943–8.

61. Lin CY, Viant MR, Tjeerdema RS. Metabolomics: methodologies and applications in the environmental sciences. J Pestic Sci. 2006;31 (3):245–51.

62. Nicholson JK, Foxall PJD, Spraul M, Farrant RD, Lindon JC. 750-Mhz H-1 and H-1-C-13 NMR-spectroscopy of human blood-plasma. Anal Chem. 1995;67(5):793–811.

63. Mutzenhardt P, Guenneau F, Canet D. A procedure for obtaining pure absorption 2D J-spectra: application to quantitative fully J-decoupled homonuclear NMR spectra. J Magn Reson. 1999;141(2):312–21.

64. Bax A, Freeman R, Frenkiel TA, Levitt MH. Assignment of C-13 NMR-spectra via double-quantum coherence. J Magn Reson. 1981;43 (3):478–83.

65. Bax A, Freeman R, Frenkiel TA. An NMR technique for tracing out the carbon skeleton of an organic-molecule. J Am Chem Soc. 1981;103(8):2102–4.

66. Lewis IA, Schommer SC, Hodis B, Robb KA, Tonelli M, Westler WM, Suissman MR, Markley JL. Method for determining molar concentrations of metabolites in complex solutions from two-dimensional H-1-C-13 NMR spectra. Anal Chem. 2007;79(24):9385–90.

67. Fan TWM, Lane AN. Identification of glycerophosphorylcholine in Mussel ovarian extracts by 2-dimensional nuclear-magnetic-resonance. Anal Biochem. 1992;206(2):251–5.

68. Fan TW-M, Lane AN. NMR-based stable isotope resolved metabolomics in systems biochemistry. J Biomol NMR. 2011;49:267–80.

69. Fan TW-M, Kucia M, Jankowski K, Higashi RM, Ratajczak MZ, Ratajczak J, Lane AN. Proliferating Rhabdomyosarcoma cells shows an energy producing anabolic metabolic phenotype compared with primary myocytes. Mol Cancer. 2008;7:79.

70. Gradwell MJ, Fan TWM, Lane AN. Analysis of phosphorylated metabolites in crayfish extracts by two-dimensional 1H-31P NMR heteronuclear total correlation spectroscopy (hetero TOCSY). Anal Biochem. 1998;263 (2):139–49.

71. Oschkinat H, Griesinger C, Kraulis PJ, Sorensen OW, Ernst RR, Gronenborn AM, Clore GM. 3-Dimensional NMR-spectroscopy of a protein in solution. Nature. 1988;332 (6162):374–6.

72. Ramachandran R, Sich C, Grune M, Soskic V, Brown LR. Sequential assignments in uniformly C-13- and N-15-labelled RNAs: the HC(N, P) and HC(N, P)-CCH-TOCSY experiments. J Biomol NMR. 1996;7 (3):251–5.

73. Richter C, Reif B, Worner K, Quant S, Marino JP, Engels JW, Griesinger C, Schwalbe H. A new experiment for the measurement of (n)J (C, P) coupling constants including (3)J(C4(i) ('), P-i) and (3)J(C4(i)('), Pi + 1) in oligonucleotides. J Biomol NMR. 1998;12 (2):223–30.

74. Wu ZR, Tjandra N, Bax A. P-31 chemical shift anisotropy as an aid in determining nucleic acid structure in liquid crystals. J Am Chem Soc. 2001;123(15):3617–8.

75. Clore GM, Murphy EC, Gronenborn AM, Bax A. Determination of three-bond (1)H3′-P-31 couplings in nucleic acids and protein nucleic acid complexes by quantitative J correlation spectroscopy. J Magn Reson. 1998;134 (1):164–7.

76. Luy B, Marino JP. H-1-P-31 CPMG-correlated experiments for the assignment of nucleic acids. J Am Chem Soc. 2001;123 (45):11306–7.

77. Sich C, Ohlenschlager O, Ramachandran R, Gorlach M, Brown LR. Structure of an RNA hairpin loop with a 5′-CGUUUCG-3′ loop motif by heteronuclear NMR spectroscopy and distance geometry. Biochemistry. 1997;36 (46):13989–4002.

78. Szyperski T, Atreya HS. Principles and applications of GFT projection NMR spectroscopy. Magn Reson Chem. 2006;44:S51–60.

79. Goddard AW, Mason GF, Appel M, Rothman DL, Gueorguieva R, Behar KL, Krystal JH. Impaired GABA neuronal response to acute benzodiazepine administration in panic disorder. Am J Psychiatry. 2004;161(12):2186–93.

80. Patel AB, de Graaf RA, Mason GF, Rothman DL, Shulman RG, Behar KL. The contribution

of GABA to glutamate/glutamine cycling and energy metabolism in the rat cortex in vivo. Proc Natl Acad Sci U S A. 2005;102 (15):5588–93.

81. Mason GF, Petersen KF, de Graaf RA, Kanamatsu T, Otsuki T, Rothman DL. A comparison of C-13 NMR measurements of the rates of glutamine synthesis and the tricarboxylic acid cycle during oral and intravenous administration of 1-C-13 glucose (vol 10, pg 181, 2003). Brain Res Protoc. 2003;11(2):143.

82. Lloyd SG, Zeng HD, Wang PP, Chatham JC. Lactate isotopomer analysis by H-1 NMR spectroscopy: Consideration of long-range nuclear spin-spin interactions. Magn Reson Med. 2004;51(6):1279–82.

83. Fan TWM, Lane AN, Shenker M, Bartley JP, Crowley D, Higashi RM. Comprehensive chemical profiling of gramineous plant root exudates using high-resolution NMR and MS. Phytochemistry. 2001;57(2):209–21.

84. Fan TWM, Lane AN, Pedler J, Crowley D, Higashi RM. Comprehensive analysis of organic ligands in whole root exudates using nuclear magnetic resonance and gas chromatography–mass spectrometry. Anal Biochem. 1997;251(1):57–68.

Chapter 7

Novel NMR and MS Approaches to Metabolomics

Ian A. Lewis, Michael R. Shortreed, Adrian D. Hegeman, and John L. Markley

Abstract

Identifying and quantifying metabolites in complex biological samples is one of the most challenging aspects of metabolomics. Recently, several important advances in databases, software, instrumentation, and laboratory techniques have greatly simplified the most laborious tasks of metabolite identification and have made quantification more reliable. These technological advances have made bioanalytically oriented studies a feasible alternative to the statistics-based methods commonly used for metabolomics. We discuss the tools that have become most important in our own research and comment on emerging technologies that may play an important role in future studies. In addition, we provide practical guidelines for designing studies and give the step-by-step protocols used in our lab for sample preparation, metabolite identification, and accurate quantification of molecules.

Key words: Bioanalytical metabolomics, BMRB (BioMagResBank), extraction methodology, identification, informatics resources, mass spectrometery, MMCD (Madison Metabolomics Consortium Database), NMR spectroscopy, quantification, rNMR, software

1. Bioanalytical Metabolomics

All metabolomics studies involve elements of natural products chemistry, analytical chemistry, and statistics. The degree to which each of these elements is weighted influences experimental design and the type of data that is ultimately derived from a study. Currently, most metabolomics investigations emphasize statistics. Spectroscopic data derived from these studies are deciphered by using sophisticated multivariate tools, and potential biomarkers are identified on the basis of their statistical significance (1). Although multivariate analyses are effective for classifying samples, they do not provide a transparent mechanism for identifying and quantifying individual metabolites.

Teresa Whei-Mei Fan et al. (eds.), *The Handbook of Metabolomics*, Methods in Pharmacology and Toxicology, DOI 10.1007/978-1-61779-618-0_7, © Springer Science+Business Media New York 2012

Bioanalytical metabolomics is an emerging strategy that emphasizes comprehensive metabolite assignment, accurate measures of concentration, and transparent data analyses that minimize the use of statistics. Although these characteristics are similar to traditional metabolism research (2, 3), bioanalytical metabolomics differs from traditional studies in scope. Unfractionated biological samples contain hundreds (NMR) to thousands (MS) of observable signals. Whereas traditional methods restrict analyses to a few predetermined metabolites, bioanalytical metabolomics attempts to identify and quantify all of the observable signals. Until recently, this type of comprehensive metabolite profiling was too labor intensive to be practical in routine analyses. However, the tools and techniques discussed in this chapter have dramatically simplified the laborious aspects of data analysis and have made bioanalytical metabolomics a practical alternative to statistics-based studies.

2. Sample Preparation

Consistent sample preparation is an important component of bioanalytical metabolomics. Although a wide variety of techniques are effective (Chap. 2), no protocol is appropriate for all metabolites. Extraction conditions, such as solvent temperature and hydrophobicity, directly affect the molecules that can be identified and quantified in a study. Aqueous solvents extract hydrophilic molecules; nonpolar solvents extract hydrophobic metabolites; harsh conditions (acids, bases, and boiling) promote unwanted chemistry at labile functional groups; gentle conditions (cold methanol-water) are less effective for denaturing proteins. In short, every procedure alters one's perception of in vivo metabolism. The goal is to find a reproducible method that preserves the metabolites relevant to a particular study. In this section, we present some general guidelines for minimizing technical error and provide the sample preparation protocol we use for routine NMR-based metabolomics studies of aqueous metabolites. A more extensive discussion of sample preparation is found in Chap. 2.

2.1. Methods for Minimizing Technical Error

Metabolite concentrations observed in tissue extracts and biological fluids can vary considerably across a dataset. These sample-to-sample differences originate from both natural variability and technical error. Whereas biological variance is essential for interpreting metabolic differences between samples, technical error is simply an obstacle to meaningful data analysis. Although there are many sources of error in metabolomics studies, the main contributors are inconsistent sample preparation and technical shortcomings in analytical equipment (e.g., resonance overlap, ion suppression, and imprecision in peak picking). Careful experimental design can control these sources of error.

Extraction solution conditions. Variation in the amount biological material used to prepare each sample is one of the primary sources of technical error in metabolomics. Inconsistency at this level is directly proportional to quantitative error in the final analysis. Sample-to-sample differences also affect solution conditions (osmolarity, pH, etc.) of the extraction buffer and analytical medium. These second-order effects alter the extraction efficiencies of sparingly soluble compounds and complicate data analysis.

A direct method for controlling variation in sample size is to aliquot tissues on the basis of mass. This approach is most effective in studies involving large sample sizes and becomes increasingly error-prone as sample size diminishes. Animal tissues can be weighed directly on an analytical balance whereas plant samples generally require prior lyophilization to standardize water content. An alternative strategy, which is appropriate for cell cultures, is to prepare samples with uniform optical density and aliquot samples on the basis of volume. We have found this method to be less consistent, but considerably more convenient, than centrifuging cell suspensions and aliquotting samples on the basis of mass.

The volume of solvent present in the extraction medium can also contribute to technical error, particularly in extractions involving volatile organic solvents or high temperatures. Solvent loss due to evaporation can be minimized by using sealed reaction vials. We have found 22-mL screw-top vessels to be convenient for parallel extractions; they allow 16 or more samples to be incubated, centrifuged, filtered and lyophilized simultaneously with conventional laboratory instrumentation.

Preparation of analytical solutions. Solution conditions in the analytical medium are another major contributor to technical error. Salinity, pH, and the concentrations of metal ions affect the sensitivity of NMR spectrometers and the efficacy bioinformatics-based resonance assignments. The strategy for standardizing these conditions is analogous to the methods used for standardizing extractions; samples need to be prepared with a consistent solute to solvent ratio.

The most reliable method for ensuring consistent analytical conditions is to analyze raw extracts without any additional sample preparation. Unfortunately, metabolites present in unconcentrated extracts are generally too dilute for NMR analyses. Furthermore, extractions typically employ ^{1}H-containing solvents, which are another potential source of error in NMR analyses (e.g., spectral overlap, radiation damping, and receiver overflow resulting from incomplete solvent suppression). Consequently, NMR-based studies often prepare analytical solutions from dried extracts dissolved at relatively high concentrations in perdeuterated solvents. Though necessary, this strategy introduces some additional complications into sample preparation and data analysis.

We employ two strategies for preparing dried extracts: (1) dissolving all samples in a fixed volume of solvent and (2) preparing solutions on a mass to volume basis. Of the two approaches, the fixed volume method is preferable, because it requires the least amount of sample handling. In studies involving easily standardized extractions, the fixed volume approach yields technical error of less than 5% in our hands. The alternative mass-to-volume approach is appropriate for studies involving large samples (>40 mg extract) with major sample-to-sample differences in salinity. In these cases, we prepare analytical solutions from dried extracts dissolved in 8–17 μL of perdeuterated solvent per mg of sample.

Titrating pH in analytical solutions. Rigorous pH control is an essential component of bioanalytical metabolomics. All of the existing tools for bioinformatics-based metabolite identification and resonance assignment require samples to match the solution conditions used in the public databases (4). Minor deviations in pH (0.01) alter NMR chemical shifts and pH-dependent exchange broadening alters the intensities of metabolites that are near their pK_a. These effects can have a significant impact on the amount of time required to assign spectra and the reliability of quantities analyses.

In our experience, simply adding a buffer to the analytical medium (up to 25 mM HEPES) is insufficient for controlling pH to the degree required for automated resonance assignment. Each sample must be hand titrated using a pH meter equipped with a small electrode. We adjust sample pH using concentrated acid or base (~1 M DCl or ~1M NaOD) to minimize titration-related volume changes. For a trained technician, titrating 400 μL sample to 7.400 ± 0.004 requires about 3 min. Although titration is tedious, it saves considerable time overall because it allows labor-intensive data analysis to be replaced with automated resonance assignments.

Internal standards. The use of internal standards is one of the simplest means of ensuring data quality. Although highly reproducible data can be collected without an internal standard, small changes in NMR line shape, sample dilution, and salt concentration affect the intensities of NMR signals. Standards control for these variables and allow biologically relevant variation to be distinguished from technical error. Furthermore, clever use of internal standards allows one to calculate metabolite concentrations relative to the amount of starting material.

Our strategy is to extract 400 mg of dry weight tissue in 16 mL of water containing 167 μM of an internal standard. This approach allows us to relate metabolite concentrations observed in the NMR tube to the dry weight of the tissue. We typically use HEPES or MES as an internal standard because these compounds have multiple peaks that are well isolated from biological resonances in 2D

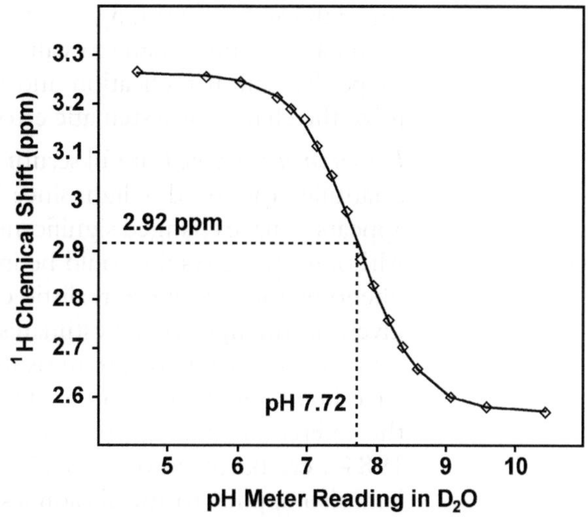

Fig. 1. The ^{1}H chemical shifts of several HEPES peaks are pH sensitive and can be used as in internal pH reference. The titration curve was generated from a HEPES buffered saline solution (290 mOsm) in D_2O. The *dotted lines* indicate the observed pK_a of HEPES as an uncorrected meter reading in D_2O.

^{1}H–^{13}C NMR spectra. HEPES is convenient because it acts as an internal pH indicator (Fig. 1), but MES is probably a better concentration reference because of its lower pK_a. Neither of these compounds would be suitable for 1D ^{1}H or 2D homonuclear ^{1}H experiments because their resonances overlap with those of many biological compounds.

Although we have only applied the internal standard normalization strategy to aqueous extractions, the principle should be applicable to other types of extractions. In some cases, biological internal standards may already be present in the data. Plants grown in MES buffer, for example, accumulate MES proportionally to their dry mass (5, 6). Non-metabolized biological internal standards are extremely useful provided that their normal in vivo concentrations can be calculated.

Entropy in sample order. Metabolite signals observed in either NMR or MS spectra can be influenced by the order of sample analysis. In the case of NMR data, systematic changes in shimming over the course of many samples results in different (usually worse) line shape. While these variations can, in theory, be corrected by normalization to an internal standard, data should always be collected in a random order to minimize systematic error. Furthermore, all NMR and MS data should be collected with technical replicates. Although technical replication is routine in the MS world, the NMR community has tended to avoid technical replication on the grounds that NMR yields high technical reproducibility. While NMR analysis can be made extremely reproducible through careful shimming, we have found that data collected with automated sample changers can have considerable variation in line shape. Technical replication and randomized sample order minimize the chance of systematic errors.

Errors in error bars. Careful scrutiny of the various studies that have quantified the speed of light since 1676 indicates that the value of *c* appears to have changed significantly over the last few centuries (7). Although these results could be interpreted as an exciting physical phenomenon, the more realistic explanation is that the error bars given on the light speed estimates were too low. Misleading error estimates are not unique to measurements of universal constants. In a landmark 1984 paper, Stuart Hurlbert showed that about half of the inferential statistics published in ecology between 1960 and 1984 were based on questionable data replication (8). This problem also applies to metabolomics. Confusing technical replicates with biological replicates grossly misrepresents real biological variation and will inevitably lead to erroneous interpretations of statistical tests. Biologically meaningful investigations require careful experimental design with respect to replication. Although Hurlbert's paper was written for ecology, his recommendations for experimental design are directly applicable to the design of metabolomics experiments. Mehta et al. have also published a review on this topic that addresses the problems encountered in high-throughput studies (9).

2.2. Protocol for Extracting High-Abundance Aqueous Metabolites

The majority of research topics encountered in our laboratory involve studies of highly abundant water-soluble metabolites. The protocol presented here is a general method for preparing samples that is suited to NMR-based assays of amino acids, sugars, polyamines, polyols, and other thermally stable molecules found at high abundance in tissue extracts. We prefer this protocol because it is easy to parallelize, produces low technical error with relatively high yields, and results in a similar complement of NMR-observable metabolites from a wide variety of samples (6). The disadvantages of the protocol include its specificity to hydrophilic molecules and poor recovery of thermally unstable compounds (e.g., ATP, and other phosphorylated intermediates). However, many of the highly abundant metabolites found in tissue extracts are thermally stable and suitable to this preparation method. Of the amino acids we have observed, only glutamine (which undergoes thermal conversion to pyroglutamate) is significantly degraded.

1. Cryogenically homogenize tissue in a ball mill or mortar and pestle.
2. Lyophilize homogenized samples for 24 h.
3. Aliquot 400 mg dry weight tissue samples into 22-mL screw-top reaction vessels.

4. Add 16 mL of boiling ddH_2O containing 167 μM HEPES or MES. HEPES or MES is used as an internal concentration reference and will have a final concentration of 1–5 mM in the final NMR analysis solution (depending on the volume of D_2O used).
5. Suspend sealed sample vials in a boiling water bath for 7.5 min.
6. Cool samples on ice for 10 min and then centrifuge reaction vials in a swinging bucket centrifuge for 30 min at 1,000 × *g*.
7. Harvest supernatant and pressure filter the mixture through glass wool to remove any remaining particulate matter.
8. Microfilter the metabolite extract with a 3 kDa molecular weight cutoff spin concentrator to remove soluble proteins. Microfilters must be thoroughly washed prior to this step to remove glycerol from the membrane surface. We wash 25-mL spin concentrators by running 100 mL of water through the filters prior to use; even this amount of washing leaves detectable levels of glycerol in the final sample.
9. Lyophilize the metabolite filtrates to a dry powder.
10. Dissolve dried metabolite powder in a fixed volume of NMR solvent (D_2O containing 500 μM DSS and 500 μM NaN_3). We use 800 μL for most tissues, but this volume is dependent the salinity of the tissue. The object with this step is to concentrate samples as much as possible without leaving a precipitate or generating excessively high salt concentrations (which will be evident from long 90° NMR pulse lengths). All samples related to a study must be prepared using the same volume of solvent.
11. Titrate samples with concentrated acid or base (~1 M DCl or ~1M NaOD) to a pH of 7.400 ± 0.004.

3. Resources for NMR- and MS-Based Metabolomics

Traditional methods for identifying and quantifying molecules rely on visual inspection of data and hand assignment of signals. Although this approach is effective when applied to simple mixtures, it is too labor intensive to be practical for comprehensive analysis of complex biological extracts. Modern bioanalytical metabolomics relies on bioinformatics, databases of metabolite standards, and specialty software, to make comprehensive analyses a more tractable challenge. Recent developments in these tools have dramatically improved the efficiency and reliability of analyses and have made bioanalytical metabolomics an increasingly popular research strategy. In this section, we focus on the tools we have found most effective in our own research; a more complete listing of useful resources can be found in Table 1.

Table 1
List of freely accessible metabolomics resources

Standards Initiative
Metabolomics Standards Initiative (http://msi-workgroups.sourceforge.net/)
Small molecule databases
ChemIDplus (http://chem.sis.nlm.nih.gov/chemidplus)
Human Metabolome Database (www.hmdb.ca)
Madison Metabolomics Consortium Database (http://mmcd.nmrfam.wisc.edu)
Metlin (http://metlin.scripps.edu)
PubChem (http://pubchem.ncbi.nlm.nih.gov)
Metabolic pathway databases
BioCyc (www.biocyc.org)
ExPASy (www.expasy.ch/cgi-bin/search-biochem-index)
KEGG (www.genome.jp/kegg)
Reactome (www.reactome.org)
TAIR (www.arabidopsis.org)
UM-BBD (http://umbbd.msi.umn.edu)
Laboratory Information Management Systems (LIMS)
Sesame LIMS (www.sesame.wisc.edu)
SetupX (http://fiehnlab.ucdavis.edu/projects/binbase_setupx)
NMR and MS databases
BioMagResBank (BMRB) (www.bmrb.wisc.edu)
Human Metabolome Database (www.hmdb.ca)
Madison Metabolomics Consortium Database (http://mmcd.nmrfam.wisc.edu)
Mass Spectrometry Database Committee (www.ualberta.ca/~gjones/mslib.htm)
NIST Chemistry WebBook (http://webbook.nist.gov/chemistry)
NMR metabolomics database of Linkoping (http://www.liu.se/hu/mdl/main)
NMRShiftDB (http://www.nmrshiftdb.org)
NMR Data Analysis software
MetaboMiner (http://wishart.biology.ualberta.ca/metabominer/)
rNMR (http://rnmr.nmrfam.wisc.edu/)

3.1. Databases and Bioinformatics

For NMR-based studies, one of the most important advances in recent years has been the introduction of three libraries of experimental data collected on pure metabolite standards. Although several commercial and public NMR libraries have been in existence for years, the previous databases were either not curated, contained data collected under a variety of conditions (10), or were not focused on biologically relevant molecules (11). Furthermore, all of the earlier resources were restricted to 1D NMR data. In the last few years, the Madison Metabolomics Consortium (MMC), the Human Metabolome Project (HMP), and Bruker have expended considerable resources on collecting NMR data of standard compounds. These libraries are distinct from their predecessors in that they were collected under defined conditions, include a wide variety of NMR experiments and, in the case of the MMC and HMP data, are freely available. Between the MMC and HMP, spectra of about 1,000 metabolites are freely available over the Web. These data have made it possible to replace many of the time-consuming steps of metabolite identification and resonance assignment with bioinformatics and have paved the way for quantitative NMR-based metabolomics.

For MS-based researchers, the state of experimentally derived data libraries is more complicated. GC-MS researchers enjoy a high degree of standardization with respect to commercial instruments, instrumental settings, retention time reporting, and mass fragmentation. As a result, several large, high-quality libraries (e.g., NIST Standard Reference Database) are available as well as specialized metabolomics libraries (e.g., BinBase from Oliver Fiehn's laboratory). LC-MS has yet to achieve the same level of standardization enjoyed by GC-MS. As a result, experimental libraries of LC-MS-observed retention times, exact masses, and fragmentation patterns are of more limited use. None the less, the HMP has made a considerable effort in standardizing data collection and reporting of LC-MS data and has collected spectra of about 2,000 metabolites.

BioMagResBank (*BMRB*). The BMRB has served the NMR community for many years as the world repository of NMR data related to proteins and nucleic acids (12, 13). Recently, the BMRB expanded its archives to include spectra of small molecules collected under standardized conditions (14, 15). The defining characteristics of the BMRB for metabolomics are as follows: the data are freely available, data entries are curated, all of the solvent and NMR spectral parameters are clearly defined, and the raw spectral data (in addition to peak-picked and processed spectra) can be downloaded. Having the raw spectral data at hand is important because it allows spectra of standards to be overlaid over extracts for hand verification of metabolite assignments.

Currently, the BMRB contains more than 7635 NMR spectra of 1070 unique compounds collected by the MMC. These data were tailored to tissue-based metabolomics analyses in the design of their solvent conditions (D_2O, pH 7.400 $\pm$ 0.004, 50 mM $NaPO_4$ for water soluble metabolites; $CDCl_3$ for organic soluble metabolites) and have shown to be useful for identifying metabolites in complex ^1H–^{13}C NMR spectra of a variety of extracts (6). Although all of the data currently available from BMRB have been contributed by the MMC, the BMRB and HMP are working toward incorporating the extensive HMP archives into the BMRB.

The BMRB offers several bioinformatics tools to enhance its function as a data repository. In contrast to the tools offered by the Human Metabolome Database (HMDB) and Madison Metabolomics Consortium Database (MMCD), which are best suited to broader queries of the metabolite literature, the BMRB tools are primarily designed to make all of the archived data easily accessible.

An NMR peak query provides a rapid means of locating standards. Similarly, MS tools allow researchers to translate exact masses into molecular formulae or locate records on the basis of monoisotopic masses. In summary, the BMRB provides an extensive collection of freely available, high-quality NMR data coupled with an efficient query system. The BMRB database is available over the Web at www.bmrb.wisc.edu.

HMDB. The HMDB was officially launched in January, 2007 and currently holds the honorable distinction of being the world's largest repository of NMR and MS data collected under standardized conditions relevant to metabolomics (16). As the name implies, the HMP's main focus is human metabolism. To this end, the Canadian group has amassed a prodigious database related to the biological significance, metabolic pathways, and physical properties of metabolites found in humans. The centerpiece of the HMDB is their collection of experimentally acquired MS and NMR data. Although there is approximately 30% overlap between the data collected by the MMC and HMP, the datasets were collected with different purposes in mind. The HMDB's main focus is biological fluids, whereas the MMCD is aimed at analysis of tissue extracts. These different foci provide flexibility to the metabolomics community with respect to experimental design.

The HMDB offers a number of browsing and bioinformatics tools for accessing their data and searching the literature. One of the most useful HMDB features is their "metabocard," a single Web page containing approximately 90 data fields summarizing all of the HMDB information related a particular compound. This feature provides an efficient mechanism for learning about your recently identified metabolites. Similar to the MMCD, the HMDB provides direct links to other databases containing information relevant to a metabolite of interest. The links lead to a multitude of other resources specific to the metabolite in question. Although the HMDB also offers several bioinformatics tools for querying the database with experimental MS or NMR data, we have found the main advantage of the database to be in browsing the metabolomics literature. The HMDB is unquestionably the most powerful resource available to the metabolomics community for this purpose. The HMDB is available over the Web at http://www.hmdb.ca.

MMCD. The MMCD was initially developed as an in-house tool for identifying metabolites. The MMCD was released to the public in late 2006 as a bioinformatics resource for both MS and NMR based metabolomics (4). In its first year of operation the MMCD received 91,000 visitors from around the globe. Public interest in the MMCD stems from its collection of 20,000 small molecules of biological interest gathered from electronic databases and the scientific literature. These data include the following: chemical formula, names and synonyms, structure, physical properties, NMR and MS data on pure compounds (when available), NMR chemical shifts determined by empirical and theoretical approaches, calculated isotopomer masses, information on the presence of the metabolite in different biological species, and extensive links to other databases.

In contrast to the HMDB, which excels at browsing metabolite data, the main advantage of the MMCD is in its bioinformatics capabilities. For identifying metabolites by name, the text search engine has a large collection of synonyms and automatically allows for fuzzy text matching. Users can also enter database ID numbers from a variety of other public resources (e.g., KEGG and CAS). For structure-based searches, the MMCD allows queries by molecular formula, string representation (e.g., SMILES and INCHI) or common structure files (e.g., .mol and .pdb). Alternatively, the structure can be drawn directly into a molecular graphics window. Users can combine as many as six structural criteria in a logical fashion to further refine the searches.

Perhaps the most powerful attributes of the MMCD are its metabolite assignment tools. Users can upload experimental NMR or mass spectra for bulk queries of the database. The NMR-based searches compensate for differences in magnetic field strength and filter search results on the basis of the overall patterns in the submitted peaks. NMR-based queries average about 95% sensitivity and 4% false discovery when analyzing 2D ^{1}H–^{13}C HSQC spectra of pure compound mixtures (4). Although the MMCD's performance is diminished by chemical shift variation in real biological extracts, it is still one of the most effective automatic NMR-based metabolite identification tools in the public domain.

For mass-based searches, the MMCD is primarily designed for identifying metabolites by exact mass, although the MMCD can also handle LC-MS, and MS/MS data. Users can specify the ionization mode, mass accuracy, carbon and nitrogen isotopic composition and allow for common adducts. Experimental LC-MS and MS/MS peak lists can be uploaded directly either as flat text files or in JCAMP-DX format for batch queries. Although sensitivity and false discovery rates are harder to estimate for MS based queries, MMCD users can expect between one and three matches for each mono-isotopic mass entry. As with most mass based queries, the efficacy of the search engine is primarily dictated by the mass accuracy and the mass range being queried. MMCD's main advantage for MS queries is that it allows users to restrict mass queries to known metabolites by using the biological filter provided under the miscellaneous search engine.

We recently upgraded the MMCD server and software to match heavy user traffic and will continue to expand the resource as demand increases. Currently, users can expect metabolite assignments on ^{1}H–^{13}C HSQC spectra in less than 2 s per spectrum. The MMCD is available over the Web at http://mmcd.nmrfam.wisc.edu.

3.2. Laboratory Information Management Systems

Laboratory information systems (LIMS) are a convenient means of organizing the large volume of data produced by metabolomics studies. Ideally, a LIMS should track every procedure that has been performed and capture all of the information known about a given sample. In addition to improving record keeping, a well designed LIMS should also make repetitive data entry tasks more efficient. Although LIMS can be helpful in many smaller settings, they are particularly useful for large-scale projects requiring the coordination of multiple investigators. In this section, we describe Sesame, a freely available LIMS system used by our laboratory.

We initially developed Sesame as a versatile Web-based LIMS to support both small and large-scale structural genomics projects (14, 17). In this application, Sesame has been adopted by a number of laboratories around the world and has proved indispensable to our own research. Although older versions of Sesame could be used for metabolomics, the LIMS was not well adapted to the requirements of small molecule studies. In response to this, we developed "Lamp," a new module for Sesame specifically for metabolomics. Lamp is divided into two subparts: one section manages data related to small molecule standards; the other is devoted to tracking information related to biological samples. The standards section captures the source of the standard, the amount of material remaining, the storage location, the investigators who have used the standard to prepare samples, the protocol used to prepare the standard. In addition, Lamp captures NMR spectra, chromatograms, MS data, and other instrumental data. The section of Lamp devoted to biological samples was designed to ensure that the LIMS captured all of the requisite information outlined by the metabolomics standards initiative (18). These entries include metadata (e.g., species, tissue, sex, age, environmental conditions, etc.), extraction protocols, NMR/LC/MS data, and results derived from any given study.

One of the most useful features of Sesame is its flexibility. The LIMS is built on a Java platform, and its Web-based format makes it accessible to any computer with Internet access. Furthermore, users can modify the existing format, design their own data fields, and create lab-specific protocols. Although the platform was designed to give everyone equal access to data, project managers can restrict access according to the needs of their own applications. The flexibility of this system allows pertinent information from databases, bench scientists, laboratory instrumentation, and software packages to be seamlessly integrated in a single interface.

Another useful feature of Sesame is its ability to track and read barcodes. Beyond the obvious application of identifying samples by bar code, the system allows specific actions to be linked to a barcode scanner. This is particularly useful in repetitive tasks such as performing inventories of standards. The Sesame LIMS is freely available from http://www.sesame.wisc.edu.

3.3. Software for NMR Data Analysis

Bioanalytical NMR-based metabolomics studies often require more than a thousand resonances assignments. Currently, this is a laborious task that is subject to human error and is difficult to document. Chemical shifts of many metabolites are subject to unpredictable variations resulting from uncontrolled differences in solution chemistry between samples. Consequently, resonances assigned in one spectrum cannot be transferred directly to other spectra. Although there are several effective software tools for identifying metabolites in complex NMR data (e.g., MMCD, metaboMiner, Chenomx, Bruker Amix, and BioRad KnowItAll), none of the existing tools were designed for assigning resonances across multiple spectra. As a result, every spectrum must be assigned individually. Using existing software tools, this task can require weeks of visual data inspection.

To make comprehensive NMR data analysis more feasible, we developed an open source software (rNMR) (19) written for the R statistical software environment. rNMR operates on a fundamentally different principle from existing NMR tools; rather than assigning peaks, rNMR extracts user-defined regions of interest (ROIs) from spectra. Unlike peak lists, which are static summaries containing limited information, ROIs contain all of the NMR data present with a defined set of chemical shift ranges and can be visually inspected. rNMR displays ROIs extracted from hundreds of samples side-by-side, and allows users to dynamically manipulate the size and placement of ROIs while simultaneously visualizing all of the NMR data related to an assignment. This strategy allows thousands of resonances to be visually inspected in a few minutes. Moreover, rNMR allows users to correct assignment errors at any stage of an analysis by simply adjusting the bounds of the affected ROI. Because all resonance assignments are made within the context of a defined chemical shift range, rNMR enforces consistent resonance assignments across hundreds of samples while maintaining flexibility to variations in chemical shift.

In addition to simplifying resonance assignment procedures, rNMR also makes quantitative analyses more transparent. Quantitative algorithms are based directly on the ROI data displayed to users, and the underlying NMR data behind any data point can be examined by simply clicking on the appropriate ROI. Because rNMR generates quantitative data on the fly from raw NMR spectra and a table containing the boundaries of each ROI, any rNMR analysis can be replicated by other researchers.

We initially developed rNMR as an in-house tool to solve practical problems encountered in our own research. Since its initial development, rNMR has expanded to include a broad range of peak picking, data visualization, and metabolite assignment tools that simplify data analysis. In addition, rNMR's architecture and licensing (general public license version 3) give users the freedom to customize and redistribute the program. The rNMR program, extensive help documentation, instructional videos, compiled standards data from the BMRB, and example datasets are available free of charge from http://rnmr.nmrfam.wisc.edu.

4. Mass Spectrometry Methods for Identifying and Quantifying Metabolites

Metabolomics researches fall into two categories: those who use mass spectrometry (MS), and those who wish that NMR had the sensitivity of MS. Although the respective advantages of NMR and MS are well known, it is worth mentioning that despite the clear superiority of MS with respect to detection limit, MS has two fundamental challenges: nonuniform ionization efficiencies and translating identified masses into specific metabolites.

Direct analysis of metabolic extracts by MS has been reported (20, 21), but MS analysis typically requires some form of fractionation to reduce ionization artifacts. Traditionally, this is handled by online coupling of liquid (LC) or gas chromatograph (GC) with the mass spectrometer. GC-MS is used extensively for profiling nonpolar compounds and derivatives of some polar molecules (22, 23). Many of the technical challenges associated with GC-MS based research have been resolved, but LC-MS is becoming increasingly popular for metabolomics analyses because of its compatibility with a wider range of biological compounds (24–30). The topics addressed in this section cover several new LC-MS compatible methods that have made identifying and quantifying metabolites a more tractable problem. A detailed overview of mass spectrometry methods is given in Chap. 4.

Quantification with selective isotope labeling. The analytical precision of ESI-MS is primarily limited by two related variables: ionization efficiency and matrix effects (31). Ionization efficiency, or the percent of a molecular species that is ionizable, depends on a number of instrumental factors, molecular characteristics and solution conditions. Instrumental factors, particularly pressure and temperature at the ion source, are difficult to control and can produce significant run-to-run and day-to-day variations. Matrix effects, which occur when ions other than the target compound compete for charge, are also problematic because minor changes in the matrix can have a pronounced effect on ionization efficiency. Although chromatography can reduces these problems, observed peak intensities in metabolomics studies are inevitably influenced by factors other than metabolite concentrations (32).

One method for improving the quantitative performance of MS is to relate observed signals to isotopically labeled (^{2}H, ^{13}C, ^{15}N, or ^{18}O-substituted) internal standards for each of the target molecules. Some care should be taken with ^{2}H labeled compounds to ensure that labels are limited to nonlabile atoms and that the perdeuterated positions do not interact with the chromatographic columns (perdeuteration can lead to chromatographic shifts) (33, 34). The main advantage of internal isotopic standards is that they coelute with their unlabeled counterparts and thus can be used to normalize variation in ionization efficiency and matrix effects. In practice, this entails dividing peak intensities (or volumes) of unlabeled compounds by the intensities of the corresponding labeled standards. Accurate concentrations of the unlabeled compounds can then be calculated by multiplying the normalized signals by the known concentrations of the standards. The primary disadvantage of this approach is that an isotopically labeled standard is needed for every compound of interest, which becomes difficult in comprehensive studies because of the price (~$100/mg) and potential unavailability of labeled standards.

There are several alternatives for larger-scale projects in which absolute quantification can be replaced by relative abundance. One method involves in vivo isotopic labeling of a control sample using an economical substrate (e.g., *Escherichia coli* grown on U–^{13}C glucose or acetate). A fixed amount of the labeled mixture produced in vivo is added to each of the test samples, and the relative abundances of metabolites are computed by comparing the signal from labeled molecules to their corresponding unlabeled counterparts (24, 29, 35, 36). This strategy works well for most small free living organisms (yeast, bacteria, and tissue cultures) and is applicable to some whole plants. However, the approach is limited in mammals because of the difficulty in achieving uniform isotopic labeling and the prohibitive expense.

An alternative strategy for calculating relative abundances of metabolites is to use selective chemistry to isotopically label molecules containing a particular functional group (Fig. 2) (37–41). The general strategy for the selective chemistry approach is similar to the in vivo approach in that an isotopically-labeled control mixture is used as a concentration reference sample for a series of test samples. Quantification based on selective chemistry requires each test mixture to be derivatized in the same manner as the isotope-labeled control. To distinguish between molecules originating from the test and control mixture, test samples are derivatized with unlabeled reagents (natural abundance levels of isotopes), whereas control mixtures are derivatized with isotopically labeled reagents. The "heavy" control mixtures are then mixed with "light" test samples creating a composite mixture. When analyzed, the heavy and light derivatives coelute from the LC-column and appear in the mass spectrum as pairs of peaks with a mass-shift equal to the difference in mass of the two isotopic labels (Fig. 3). The ratio of peak areas or intensities for each pair can then be used to compute the relative metabolite abundances in each of the test samples.

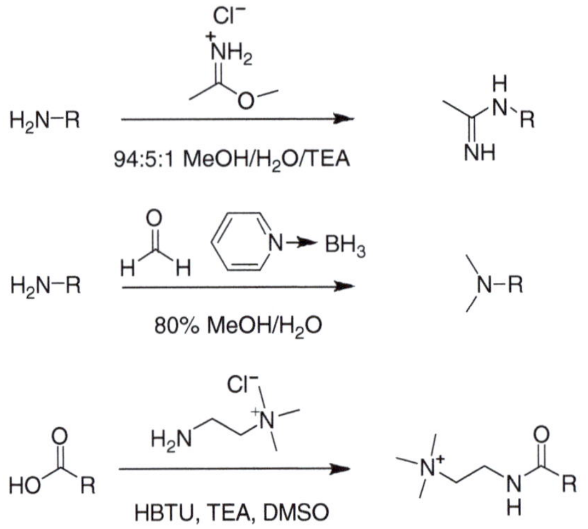

Fig. 2. Isotopic labeling chemistry under different reaction conditions. Isotopic shifts resulting from differential labeling of amines with (*top*) methylacetimidate, where a 2 Da shift is produced from the two ^{13}C atoms; (*middle*) formalin, where primary amines acquire two ^{13}C methyl groups to produce a 2 Da shift, and (*bottom*) cholamine, where ^{2}H on all three methyl groups produce a 9 Da shift. (Abbreviations: MeOH, methanol; TEA, triethanolamine; HBTU, 2-(1H-benzotriazole-1-yl)-1,1,3,3-tetramethyluronium hexafluorophosphate; and DMSO, dimethyl sulfoxide).

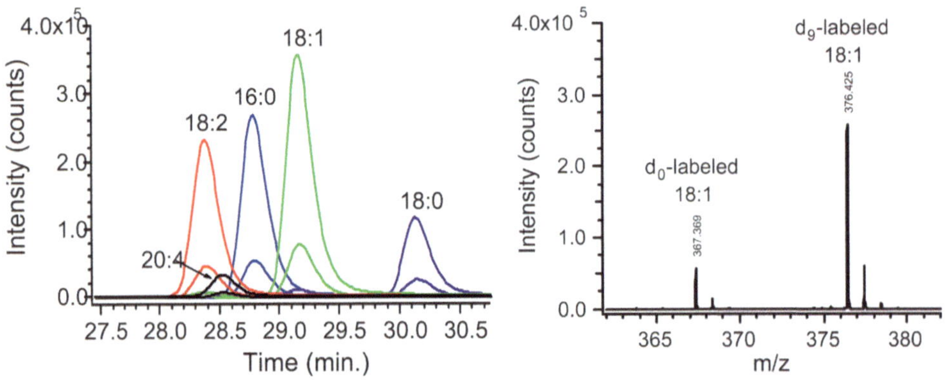

Fig. 3. Representative extracted ion chromatograms and a mass spectrum for cholamine-labeled fatty acids (1). Light and heavy labeled fatty acids coelute from reverse phase LC (*left*) and are easily distinguished by MS by their characteristic 9 Da shift (*right*). Amines labeled as shown in Fig. 2 yield analogous results.

The selective chemistry approach to quantification offers a number of advantages to the metabolomics community. Most importantly, it improves quantitative precision by normalizing variations in detection sensitivity resulting from ionization suppression (42–44) and variability in retention time between runs (34). This is possible because the "light" and "heavy" metabolites coelute within a single run and therefore have identical retention times and are electrosprayed from identical solution conditions. A second benefit of using a derivatization reagent is that it can help identify a metabolite by indicating the presence of a certain functional group.

By employing a number of labeling strategies, one can target various classes of compounds. Furthermore, well-designed labeling reagents can improve chromatographic separation, enhance detection sensitivity and yield low coefficients of variation (37–39, 45). Although it is too early to judge the efficacy of this approach in metabolomics settings, selective chemistry promises to be a powerful, cost-effective, tool in the MS metabolomics arsenal.

Isotope constrained formula assignments. High-resolution MS spectra of tissue extracts contain hundreds to thousands of peaks. Assigning identities to each of these features is far from trivial. Although common metabolites can be identified by GC-MS using the well developed commercial libraries, these libraries are of little use for novel compounds. Furthermore, existing LC-MS/MS literature (primarily from the HMDB) is of limited utility because of the large platform-dependent variability present in LC-MS systems. Currently, LC-MS analysis and novel compound identification require more extensive analytical techniques than those used for GC-MS.

One analytical strategy that can be used for identifying metabolites is to calculate elemental compositions of mass peaks obtained from high accuracy mass measurements. This approach is only feasible for compounds of low molecular weight and requires very high mass accuracy estimates, such as those obtained via FT-ICR MS (Chap. 4). Unique molecular formula assignments of compounds less than 250 amu typically require a mass accuracy of 3 ppm. As mass increases, or mass accuracy decreases, the number of matching formulas balloons exponentially.

Computational and experimental constraints can be used to reduce the number of possible formulas for higher molecular weight species. Both natural abundance isotopic distribution (46) and heuristically-derived limits on elemental composition (47) are effective means of constraining molecular assignments. A more experimental approach is to create mixtures of uniformly substituted isotopomers and measure the mass shift associated with isotopic labeling (48). For example, a spectrum can be collected for a mixture of unlabeled, fully ^{13}C labeled, and fully $^{15}N/^{13}C$ labeled versions of a molecule. Mass shifts observed in the spectrum of this mixture can then be used to calculate the number of carbon and nitrogen atoms present in a compound, and these, in turn, can be used to restrict the number of possible formula assignments (49). Such empirically-determined constraints greatly simplify molecular formula calculations and allow unique formula assignments to be made at much higher mass values (Fig. 4).

Metabolomics applications of the isotopically-constrained formula assignment method require uniform isotopic labeling. As mentioned previously, in vivo ^{15}N and/or ^{13}C isotopic labeling is relatively straightforward and cost-effective in small free

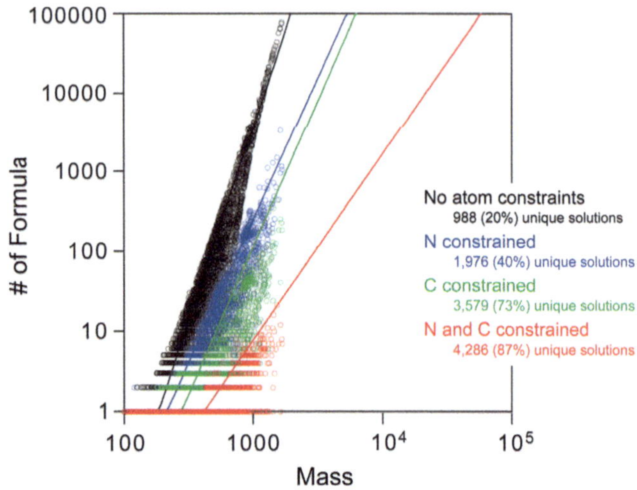

Fig. 4. Number of calculated formulae with and without nitrogen and carbon constraints for 4,918 unique formulae derived from the BMRB database assuming mass accuracy of ±3 ppm.

living organisms or tissue cultures (50). However, some care should be taken to ensure that metabolites are uniformly labeled. Partial labeling results in excessive spectral complexity resulting from the various partially substituted isotopomers. We have recently added several computational resources to the BMRB as a tool for researchers who are interested in using isotope constrained assignments (49).

5. NMR Methods for Identifying and Quantifying Metabolites

Although NMR is a relatively insensitive technique when compared to MS, NMR-based analyses enjoy several advantages over MS. Specifically, NMR peak intensities scale proportionally with concentration, NMR is sensitive to a wide variety of metabolite structures, and NMR analyses require little to no sample preparation. Although NMR has become a popular tool for statistics-based metabolomics, NMR-based bioanalytical studies are relatively rare because of practical challenges in data analysis. However, the bioinformatics and software tools discussed in Sect. 3 have largely eliminated these practical constraints.

In this section, we discuss several alternative strategies for collecting quantitatively reliable NMR data that can be used for bioanalytical metabolomics. A unifying theme of the techniques presented here is that they provide a mechanism for separating overlapped NMR signals. Overlapped signals, such as those found in 1D ^{1}H spectra of biological extracts, scale proportionally to the total overlapped spectral density and can neither be assigned nor quantified (6).

Although 1D ^{1}H NMR is a reproducible chemometrics tool (51), bioanalytical studies require well-defined spin systems for resonance assignments and isolated peaks for quantification (6). Currently, there are three general strategies for producing the sufficiently sparse spectra required for quantitative studies: mathematical deconvolution of spectra, multidimensional NMR, and selective pulse sequences (see Chap. 6 for a detailed description of NMR principles and methodologies).

5.1. Mathematical and Statistical Methods

As a rule, signals correlate very well with themselves. Not surprisingly, various peaks from the same compound are highly covariant across multiple spectra. The Nicholson laboratory recognized this several years ago and formalized the use of covariance matrices to group resonances of various compounds (52). This approach has the advantage of allowing investigators to use 1D ^{1}H NMR spectra, the fastest and most sensitive NMR experiment, and still provide a mechanism for dispersing resonances from individual compounds. However, the covariance approach does not provide a mechanism for quantification. As a result, quantitative estimates of peaks identified through covariance are still rooted in the dubious metric of overlapped 1D ^{1}H signals.

An alternative approach developed by Weljie et al. is to fit overlapped signals with modeled peaks and base quantitative estimates on the modeled data (53). Resonance deconvolution has been used for decades in a wide variety of traditional NMR studies and is a well established method for separating overlapped peaks. The curve fitting method introduced by Weljie, A.M. et al. is probably the most reliable approach for quantifying metabolites from overlapped 1D ^{1}H NMR data and has become the preferred strategy for many bioanalytically oriented researchers. However, resonance deconvolution is a finicky hand-manipulated process whose performance is affected by the skill of the person operating the software. A commercial implementation of Weljie's method, Chenomx, removes some of this uncertainty. However, Chenomx is dependent upon matching metabolites with one of the standards present in their commercial library and thus can be ineffective for some compounds. In addition, Chenomx is expensive and only supports 1D NMR analyses. Despite these disadvantages, resonance deconvolution is a viable method for deriving quantitative information from overlapped NMR spectra and may be an attractive alternative to researchers who are constrained to using 1D NMR.

5.2. Multidimensional NMR Methods

One of the most effective methods for mitigating problems associated with resonance overlap is to use one of the myriad of multidimensional NMR experiments that have been developed by bimolecular NMR spectroscopists (Chap. 6). In contrast to other methods for separating overlapped resonances discussed here, multidimensional NMR has the significant advantage of contributing empirically determined structural information about the observed resonances. This is of no small consequence to bioanalytical metabolomics studies, which must differentiate between many structurally similar metabolites.

Several groups have applied multidimensional NMR to metabolomics (5, 54–56), but practical challenges have made this technique unpopular for routine studies. 2D pulse sequences require longer acquisition times, are less quantitatively robust, are prone to data artifacts, and require more NMR expertise than traditional 1D spectroscopy. In this section, we provide guidelines for mitigating these problems and discuss the trade-offs of various multidimensional NMR strategies.

Resolution versus sensitivity. Two categories of 2D NMR have proven effective in metabolomics: ^{1}H–^{1}H homonuclear and ^{1}H–^{13}C heteronuclear experiments. These categories have several inherent trade-offs that must be considered in the experimental design phase of any bioanalytical metabolomics study. Homonuclear proton experiments are more sensitive because of the 100% natural abundance of ^{1}H and its favorable magnetogyric ratio. However, metabolite signals in ^{1}H–^{1}H experiments occupy a narrow bandwidth (roughly 10 ppm), and most ^{1}H–^{1}H pulse sequences produce multiple signals from each resonance (i.e., symmetrical cross-peaks, and diagonal peaks). The low bandwidth and signal redundancy result in resonance overlap problems. In contrast, ^{1}H–^{13}C sequences offer superior separation of metabolite signals because of carbon's larger bandwidth (roughly 180 ppm) and because most ^{1}H–^{13}C pulse sequences produce fewer signals per metabolite. Although modern ^{1}H-detected ^{13}C experiments are significantly more sensitive than the traditional direct detection methods used in 1D–^{13}C experiments, the low natural abundance of carbon (1.1%) limits metabolite investigation in unlabeled samples. The lower sensitivity of ^{1}H–^{13}C experiments can be partially mitigated by concentrating NMR samples (we prepare samples at up to 10 × higher concentrations than found in vivo) or by isotopically enriching samples. However, sample limitation and biological constraints often make concentration or isotopic enrichment unfeasible. As a result, many NMR-based studies must either choose high sensitivity experiments at the cost of increased spectral overlap, or better signal separation at the cost of lower sensitivity. The correct choice is governed by the biological goals of a study, the amount of material that can be obtained, the concentrations of target metabolites, and the complexity of the mixture being investigated.

Additional practical considerations may influence the decision between 2D homonuclear ^{1}H and heteronuclear ^{1}H–^{13}C experiments. Studies involving 2D ^{1}H–^{1}H experiments require considerably longer NMR acquisition times to adequately resolve metabolite signals. In addition, chemical shift variations are more problematic in ^{1}H–^{1}H spectra because ^{1}H shifts are more affected by solution conditions than ^{13}C shifts. Consequently, bioinformatics-based assignments of ^{1}H–^{1}H data are less reliable, and metabolite identifications are more ambiguous. On the other hand, ^{1}H–^{13}C analyses at natural abundance ^{13}C levels requires 40 mg of metabolites per NMR sample (roughly 400 mg starting material). If sufficient starting material can be obtained for a single representative sample, then we recommend using ^{1}H–^{13}C analysis of a concentrated sample for metabolite identification purposes. These assignments can then be transferred to ^{1}H–^{1}H data for analyses of more dilute test samples. For investigators who are new to 2D NMR, we recommend learning the metabolite identification and quantification process using a biological model that allows all samples to be analyzed via ^{1}H–^{13}C HSQC (heteronuclear single quantum coherence) or HMQC (heteronuclear multiple quantum coherence). This recommendation is based on the relative ease of assigning and quantifying ^{1}H–^{13}C data.

Metabolite identification. The introduction of the BMRB, MMCD, and HMDB databases has dramatically reduced the length of time required to assign NMR spectra. These resources allow researchers to submit peak lists from experimental data and return a list of possible metabolite identifications. Currently, the results of these queries must be verified by overlaying spectra of standards (available from www.bmrb.wisc.edu) onto a representative extract. Step-by-step instructions for validating resonance assignments are given below. Although our methods may be adapted to some 1D NMR applications, the procedures described here primarily refers to the analysis of 2D ^{1}H–^{13}C or ^{1}H–^{1}H NMR spectra. As mentioned above, we have found that 2D ^{1}H–^{13}C HSQC data are easier to assign than ^{1}H–^{1}H experiments and recommend that new investigators learn the assignment process with ^{1}H–^{13}C data.

5.2.1. Protocol for Metabolite Identification

1. Collect a high-resolution sensitivity enhanced ^{1}H–^{13}C HSQC spectrum (e.g., Varian pulse sequence gHSQC) of a representative sample. This will likely require 512–2,048 increments in the indirect dimension, four scans, and as long an acquisition time as the decoupling strategy allows. The goal of the initial spectrum is to produce one high-quality, unambiguous dataset with minimal peak overlap to be used for metabolite identification purposes. It is virtually impossible to resolve all of the signals, but most aliphatic signals are dispersed in 1,028 indirect increments. It is important to match the sample's solvent conditions to those used by either the MMC or HMDB because bioinformatics-based assignments require predictable peak locations.
2. After a high quality spectrum has been collected, process the data with the minimum appropriate window function (excessive line broadening will mask J-coupling), reference the

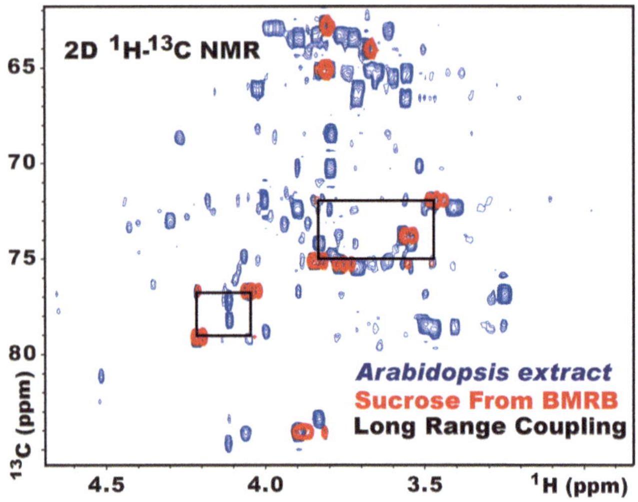

Fig. 5. Two-dimensional ^{1}H–^{13}C HSQC NMR spectrum of sucrose from the BMRB (*red*) overlaid onto an aqueous whole-plant extract from *Arabidopsis thaliana* (*blue*). *Black boxes* indicate long-range proton carbon couplings used to validate the assignment.

chemical shifts, peak-pick the data, and submit the peak list to the MMCD, HMDB, or BMRB. Accurate chemical shift referencing is critical for bioinformatics-based assignments.

3. Bring the experimental data into rNMR (19) for analysis (rNMR supports conversions of data in Bruker, Varian, or NMRpipe formats to the Sparky format used by rNMR) and download spectra of the possible matches from either the HMDB or BMRB. We have converted most of the BMRB ^{1}H–^{13}C HSQC and ^{1}H–^{1}H TOCSY standards to Sparky format, and these data can be downloaded in bulk from http://rnmr.nmrfam.wisc.edu.

4. Overlay the spectra of each potential metabolite onto your high resolution spectrum of the representative extract. Reliable metabolite assignments must have all of the correct ^{1}H and ^{13}C chemical shifts, correct peak multiplicities, and intense peaks should show long-range ^{1}H–^{13}C coupling consistent with the standard (Fig. 5). Some tolerance can be given for chemical shift variation (± ~0.025 ppm), provided that all of the other criteria are fulfilled. A few resonances are more variable than others. Specifically, malate, citrate, and a number of aromatic resonances can have considerable variation despite careful pH titration. Ambiguous metabolite assignments can be checked by adding pure standards to the extract; correct assignments will show increases in peak intensity proportional to the amount of standard added.

The metabolite identification protocol outlined here will provide reliable assignments in most cases, but this method of analysis is not unequivocal. Important assignments (i.e., those that are

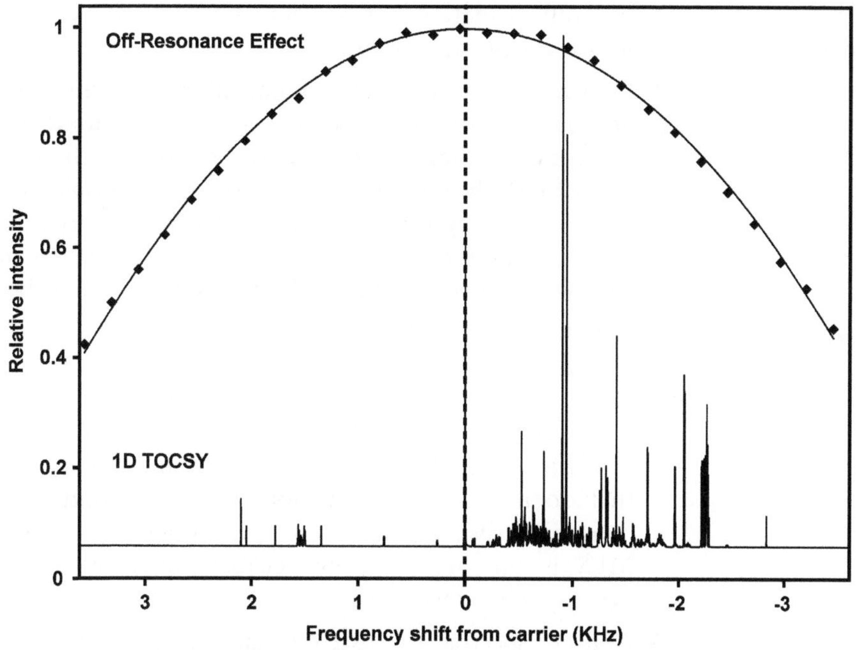

Fig. 6. Off-resonance effects are one of the many factors that can influence peak intensities observed in NMR experiments. In this example, the intensities in ^{1}H–^{1}H TOCSY were measured as a function of ^{1}H frequency offset. The peak intensity is highest when the peak is closest to the transmitter frequency and lowers as the transmitter is tuned to higher or lower frequencies.

shown to have significant changes between groups) should be validated by an independent analytical technique.

Calculating molar concentrations from 2D NMR spectra. Multidimensional pulse sequences have significant quantitative problems resulting from off-resonance effects, incomplete resonance transfer, complex relaxation pathways, decoupling artifacts and mixing times. These variables make peak intensities (and volumes) an unreliable metric for quantification (Fig. 6). Several laboratories are developing more quantitatively reliable versions of common bimolecular NMR pulse sequences (57–59). Unfortunately, these efforts have yet to produce experiments that are sufficiently robust for bioanalytical metabolomics. However, we have developed a practical approach to metabolite quantification that allows researchers to use any NMR pulse sequence. The basic feature of our method is that we do not control quantification through pulse sequence design. Instead, we relate observed peak intensities to those of mixtures of pure standards of known concentration. Differences in relaxation rates and shimming are controlled by normalizing observed metabolite signals to an internal standard. The metabolite quantification strategy described here and the fast data collection method described in the next section are the components of our fast metabolite quantification (FMQ by NMR) approach, which is the basis of all of our laboratory's routine metabolomics work.

5.2.2. Metabolite Quantification Protocol

1. Identify all metabolites present in an extract (see *Protocol for metabolite identification*).
2. Prepare three mixtures containing all of the identified metabolites at 2, 5, and 10 mM. Although standardized metabolite intensities are linear well beyond the range of these standards (±20-fold), the concentrations of standards should be adjusted to match the approximate range of expected concentrations. Mixtures should be prepared at high volume to minimize weighing errors. All standards and extracts should be titrated to pH 7.400 ± 0.004.
3. Include 5 mM of an internal standard in all of the standards mixtures and extracts to serve as an internal concentration reference. For ^{1}H–^{13}C NMR studies, we recommend HEPES or MES because both compounds have multiple isolated peaks that do not overlap with biological compounds. HEPES is convenient because it acts as an internal pH indicator, but MES is probably a more reliable concentration reference because of its lower pK_a.
4. Collect spectra of extracts and concentration reference samples under identical NMR acquisition conditions at the same time using the same instrument. Every sample, including the concentration reference samples, should be collected twice to produce two technical replicates for each sample. The sample order should be randomized. Each test sample should have at least three (preferably many more) independent biological replicates. From a statistical perspective, it is much better to have many independent biological replicates than to analyze many metabolites (large alpha corrections, such as Bonferroni correction, must be made in studies that use multiple comparisons).
5. Measure the peak intensities (area for 1D, peak height for 2D) of nonoverlapped peaks from extracts and the concentration reference samples. Although peak area is a robust metric in 1D NMR, we have found 2D peak volumes to be considerably less reliable than peak heights when used in this procedure (regardless of the NMR analysis software).
6. Normalize signals observed in each spectrum to the average signal of the dispersed HEPES (MES) peaks. Raw intensities can be used without normalization, but any variations in salt concentration (or paramagnetic relaxation agents) between samples will be erroneously interpreted as differences in metabolite concentrations. If samples and standards are osmotically identical, then normalization is undesirable because it introduces some technical error. However, many NMR probes are highly salt sensitive, and even the standards may show strong nonlinear effects of salt. If in doubt, it is better to normalize to the internal standard and accept a small increase in technical error.

7. Average normalized peak intensities across technical replicates.
8. Regress normalized peak intensities of the standards to produce a concentration versus peak intensity equation for each dispersed signal.
9. Calculate the observed concentrations for each normalized peak in the test samples using the equations derived from the standards samples.
10. Average concentration estimates across all dispersed peaks from each molecule.

The protocol described here produces concentration estimates with as little as 2.7% technical error from complex 2D NMR spectra (Fig. 7.) (6). The main disadvantage of this approach is its dependence on standards, many of which are unavailable or are

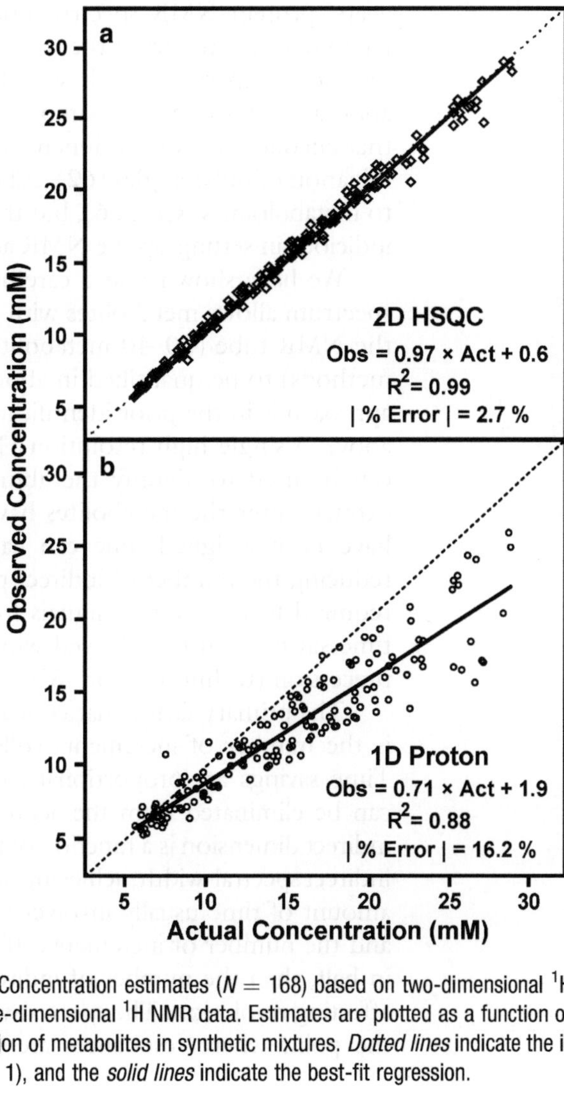

Fig. 7. (**a**) Concentration estimates ($N = 168$) based on two-dimensional ^{1}H–^{13}C HSQC and (**b**) one-dimensional ^{1}H NMR data. Estimates are plotted as a function of the known concentration of metabolites in synthetic mixtures. *Dotted lines* indicate the ideal regression (slope 1), and the *solid lines* indicate the best-fit regression.

prohibitively expensive to use in the quantities required for this procedure. If the requisite standards can be obtained, however, then this strategy produces reliable quantitative information from most of the existing NMR pulse sequences. Moreover, the internal concentration references we use to control for differences in longitudinal (T_1) relaxation, and other variations between samples, can be introduced early in the sample preparation process to relate observed signal intensities to biologically relevant concentrations.

Fast multidimensional experiments. Although multidimensional NMR has seen qualitative applications to metabolomics for many years (5, 54–56), very few studies have used the technique for quantitative purposes. One reason for this is that multidimensional NMR spectra take longer to collect than 1D ^{1}H NMR spectra, although the long acquisition times of 2D experiments have been somewhat exaggerated in the metabolomics community. Over the years, protein NMR spectroscopists have developed a wealth of techniques for reducing the requisite acquisition times of multidimensional experiments. These techniques range from mathematical approaches for nonlinear sampling of data (60), to pulse sequences that encode the indirect dimensions using gradients (61) and optimization of pulse angles (62). All of these techniques are applicable to metabolomics (Chap. 6), but the easiest way to save time is to be judicious in setting up the NMR acquisition parameters.

We have shown that a carefully adjusted 2D ^{1}H–^{13}C HSQC spectrum allows metabolites with concentrations over ~500 μM in the NMR tube (30–40 metabolites using our sample preparation methods) to be quantified in about 10 min (6). The secret to our approach is in the prior identification of compounds. As discussed above, a single high-resolution HSQC of a representative sample can be used to identify the abundant metabolites present in an extract. After the metabolites have been identified and the peaks have been assigned, one can capitalize on the assignments by reducing the number of indirect points and time to the minimum required to resolve two signals from each target molecule. These time savings can be achieved while maintaining high quantitative precession (technical error ~3%) (6).

The primary factor that contributes to lengthy 2D experiments is the number of increments collected in the indirect dimension. Time savings are proportional to the number of increments that can be eliminated from the acquisition. Because resolution in the indirect dimension is a function of the number of increments and the indirect spectral-width, achieving adequate resolution in the minimal amount of time usually involves trimming both the spectral-width and the number of increments. If the indirect spectral-width is cut in half, then the number of indirect points can be halved without affecting resolution. The spectral-width can be reduced well beyond the point where resonances are no longer contained within the

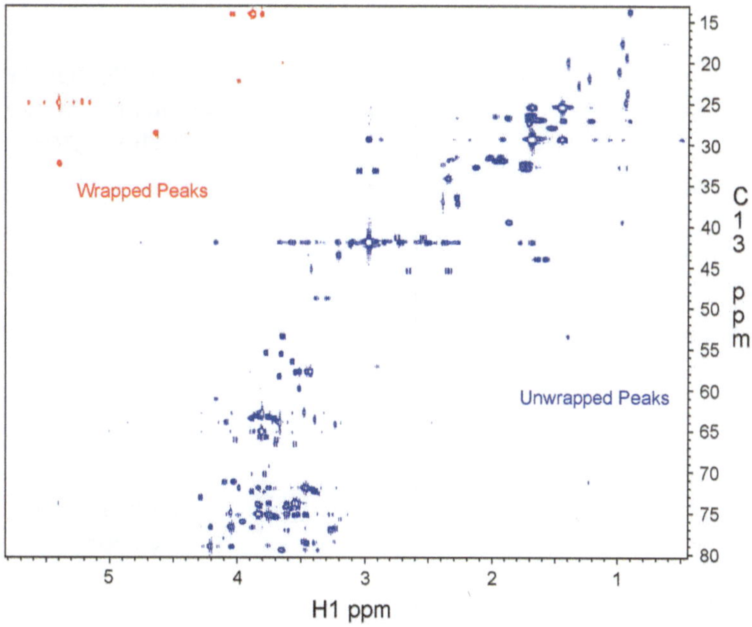

Fig. 8. Quantitative $^{1}H-^{13}C$ HSQC NMR spectrum of a synthetic mixture of 26 metabolites. The spectral width in the indirect dimension was reduced to allow for shorter acquisition times. *Blue peaks* are in their correct locations, whereas *red peaks* have been wrapped into the top of the spectrum from their normal downfield positions.

spectral window. Resonances with signals outside of the spectral-width will wrap back into the spectral window with a chemical shift that is equal to their original shift plus or minus a multiple of the spectral-width (Fig. 8). In more extreme cases, resonances may be wrapped multiple times. If the original chemical shifts and the spectral-width are known, then a heavily wrapped spectrum can be unwrapped by using simple arithmetic. Spectral folding may result in undesirable overlap between analytically important signals, but overlap can often be alleviated with small adjustments of the indirect carrier frequency. As discussed above, off resonance effects play a major role in observed peak intensities. After acceptable settings for the spectral-width, number of increments, and the transmitter offset have been found, it is critical that these values be kept constant across all of the test samples and standards.

5.3. Selective NMR Methods

Selective NMR is a back to the future idea revived from the early days of protein NMR. Although selective experiments have been largely outdated in protein NMR by modern multidimensional pulse sequences, the technique is appropriate for targeted metabolic studies. Selective NMR works by carefully sculpting the excitation pulse to cover a narrow bandwidth. This, in combination with other sequences such as TOCSY, allows individual spin systems to be isolated from amazingly complex mixtures (Fig. 9).

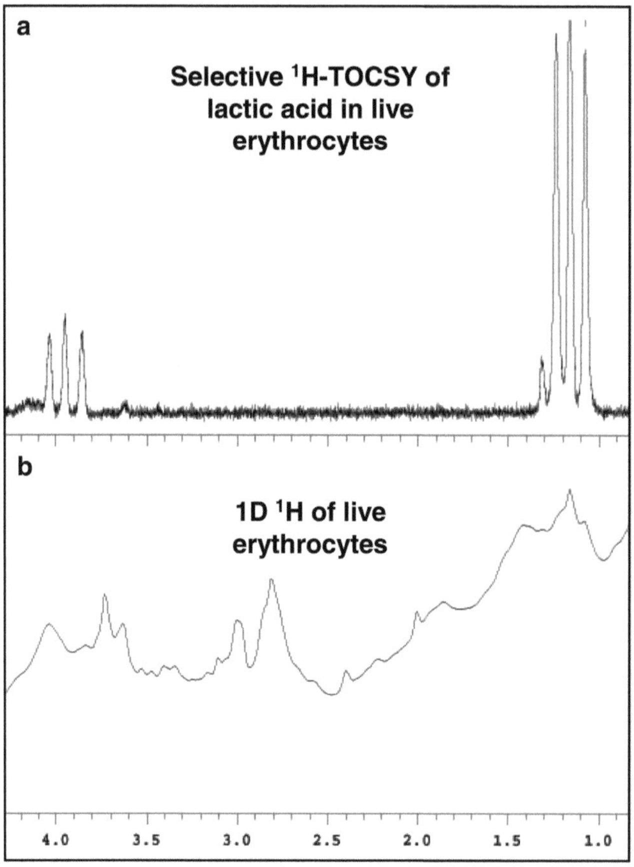

Fig. 9. (**a**) Selective 1D ^1H–^1H TOCSY for lactate in live red blood cells. (**b**) Standard 1D ^1H NMR spectrum of the same sample. Cells were labeled with [U–^{13}C]-glucose, the triplet-like splitting observed in the TOCSY arises from [U–^{12}C]-lactate (center peak) and fully labeled [U–^{13}C]-lactate (two satellite peaks).

Similarly, the technique can be used to selectively remove overpowering resonances from a spectrum. Dan Raftery's group first introduced the idea to the metabolomics community by showing that signals from minor components of honey could be accurately isolated and quantified without being influenced by the large glucose and fructose signals (63). One of the most powerful aspects of the selective TOCSY is that data can be collected very quickly (~1 min per spectrum). For studies requiring accurate quantification of a few metabolites in complex mixtures, this is one of the fastest NMR techniques available.

One must keep a few practical considerations in mind when using selective pulse sequences. Selective experiments require hand tuning of the excitation pulse, and this tuning may change from sample to sample if the target metabolite is subject to chemical shift variation. Secondly, selective experiments lose their time advantage in studies involving multiple metabolites. After the number of target metabolites reaches about ten, then a full 2D ^{1}H–^{1}H TOCSY or ^{1}H–^{13}C HSQC is more efficient and does not require hand manipulation of the pulses between experiments. However, if a study only calls for analysis of a few molecules, then selective TOCSY is one of the best tools for the job.

6. Future Prospects

Technological advances of recent years have dramatically increased the efficiency with which metabolites can be identified and accurately quantified. High quality empirical libraries, bioinformatics-based spectral assignment tools, improved analytical software, and practical methods for identifying and quantifying NMR and MS signals in complex spectra have taken the field a step closer to the automation enjoyed by mainstream bioanalytical methods. Despite these advances, bioanalytical metabolomics is still in its early development and is far from capitalizing fully on state-of-the-art NMR and MS technology. A significant proportion of signals in every study go unassigned, bioinformatics tools suffer from unacceptable false discovery rates, quantification requires ad hoc correction of quantitatively unreliable data, and specialized expertise is required to collect, analyze, and interpret data. Finding practical solutions to these problems is paramount to bioanalytical metabolomics and is a promising area for future technology development.

Acknowledgments

This work was supported by the National Center for Research Resources of the National Institutes of Health under grant P41 RR02301; I.A.L. was the recipient of a fellowship from the NHGRI 1T32HG002760.

Glossary

1D	One-dimensional
2D	Two-dimensional
Bioanalytical metabolomics	Comprehensive quantitative analysis of metabolites in complex biological samples

HSQC	Heteronuclear single quantum correlation
MS	Mass spectrometry
NMR	Nuclear magnetic resonance

References

1. Lindon JC, Holmes E, Nicholson JK. Metabonomics in pharmaceutical R&D. FEBS J. 2007;274:1140–51.
2. Radda GK, Seeley PJ. Recent studies on cellular metabolism by nuclear magnetic resonance. Annu Rev Physiol. 1979;41:749–69.
3. Shulman RG, Brown TR, Ugurbil K, Ogawa S, Cohen SM, den Hollander JA. Cellular applications of 31P and 13C nuclear magnetic resonance. Science. 1979;205:160–6.
4. Cui Q, Lewis IA, Hegeman AD, Anderson ME, Li J, Schulte CF, Westler WM, Eghbalnia HR, Sussman MR, Markley JL. Metabolite identification via the Madison Metabolomics Consortium Database. Nat Biotechnol. 2008;26:162–4.
5. Fan TW, Lane AN, Shenker M, Bartley JP, Crowley D, Higashi RM. Comprehensive chemical profiling of gramineous plant root exudates using high-resolution NMR and MS. Phytochemistry. 2001;57:209–21.
6. Lewis IA, Schommer SC, Hodis B, Robb KA, Tonelli M, Westler WM, Sussman MR, Markley JL. Method for determining molar concentrations of metabolites in complex solutions from two-dimensional ^{1}H–^{13}C NMR spectra. Anal Chem. 2007;79:9385–90.
7. Brown LM, Pais A, Pippard AB. Twentieth century physics. New York: American Institute of Physics Press; 1995.
8. Hurlbert SH. Pseudoreplication and the design of ecological field experiments. Ecol Monogr. 1984;54:187–211.
9. Mehta T, Tanik M, Allison DB. Towards sound epistemological foundations of statistical methods for high-dimensional biology. Nat Genet. 2004;36:943–7.
10. Steinbeck C, Krause S, Kuhn S. NMRShiftDB-constructing a free chemical information system with open-source components. J Chem Inf Comput Sci. 2003;43:1733–9.
11. Sadtler P. Sadtler Standard NMR Spectra N.M.R. Chemical Shift Index. Philadelphia: Sadtler Research Laboratories, PA (proton and carbon-13 spectra); 1967.
12. Seavey BR, Farr EA, Westler WM, Markley JL. A relational database for sequence-specific protein NMR data. J Biomol NMR. 1991; 1:217–36.
13. Doreleijers JF, Mading S, Maziuk D, Sojourner K, Yin L, Zhu J, Markley JL, Ulrich EL. BioMagResBank database with sets of experimental NMR constraints corresponding to the structures of over 1400 biomolecules deposited in the Protein Data Bank. J Biomol NMR. 2003;26:139–46.
14. Markley JL, Anderson ME, Cui Q, Eghbalnia HR, Lewis IA, Hegeman AD, Li J, Schulte CF, Sussman MR, Westler WM, Ulrich EL, Zolnai Z. New bioinformatics resources for metabolomics. Pac Symp Biocomput. 2007;12:157–68, 17990487.
15. Ulrich EL, Akutsu H, Doreleijers JF, Harano Y, Ioannidis YE, Lin J, Livny M, Mading S, Maziuk D, Miller Z, Nakatani E, Schulte CF, Tolmie DE, Kent Wenger R, Yao H, Markley JL. BioMagResBank. Nucleic Acids Res. 2008;36:D402–8.
16. Wishart DS, Tzur D, Knox C, Eisner R, Guo AC, Young N, Cheng D, Jewell K, Arndt D, Sawhney S, Fung C, Nikolai L, Lewis M, Coutouly MA, Forsythe I, Tang P, Shrivastava S, Jeroncic K, Stothard P, Amegbey G, Block D, Hau DD, Wagner J, Miniaci J, Clements M, Gebremedhin M, Guo N, Zhang Y, Duggan GE, Macinnis GD, Weljie AM, Dowlatabadi R, Bamforth F, Clive D, Greiner R, Li L, Marrie T, Sykes BD, Vogel HJ, Querengesser L. HMDB: the Human Metabolome Database. Nucleic Acids Res. 2007;35:D521–6.
17. Zolnai Z, Lee PT, Li J, Chapman MR, Newman CS, Phillips Jr GN, Rayment I, Ulrich EL, Volkman BF, Markley JL. Project management system for structural and functional proteomics: sesame. J Struct Funct Genomics. 2003;4:11–23.
18. Sansone SA, Fan T, Goodacre R, Griffin JL, Hardy NW, Kaddurah-Daouk R, Kristal BS, Lindon J, Mendes P, Morrison N, Nikolau B, Robertson D, Sumner LW, Taylor C, van der Werf M, van Ommen B, Fiehn O. The metabolomics standards initiative. Nat Biotechnol. 2007;25:846–8.
19. Lewis IA, Schommer SC, Markley JL. rNMR: open source software for high-throughput NMR-based bioanalytical chemistry. Magn Reson Chem. 2009;47:S123–6.
20. Vaidyanathan S, Rowland JJ, Kell DB, Goodacre R. Discrimination of aerobic

endospore-forming bacteria via electrospray-Ionization mass spectrometry of whole cell suspensions. Anal Chem. 2001;73:4134–44.
21. Aharoni A, Ric de Vos CH, Verhoeven HA, Maliepaard CA, Kruppa G, Bino R, Goodenowe DB. Nontargeted metabolome analysis by use of Fourier transform Ion cyclotron mass spectrometry. OMICS. 2002;6:217–34.
22. Koek MM, Muilwijk B, van der Werf MJ, Hankemeier T. Microbial metabolomics with gas chromatography/mass spectrometry. Anal Chem. 2006;78:1272–81.
23. Fiehn O, Kopka J, Dormann P, Altmann T, Trethewey RN, Willmitzer L. Metabolite profiling for plant functional genomics. Nat Biotechnol. 2000;18:1157–61.
24. Wu L, Mashego MR, van Dam JC, Proell AM, Vinke JL, Ras C, van Winden WA, van Gulik WM, Heijnen JJ. Quantitative analysis of the microbial metabolome by isotope dilution mass spectrometry using uniformly ^{13}C-labeled cell extracts as internal standards. Anal Biochem. 2005;336:164–71.
25. Want EJ, O'Maille G, Smith CA, Brandon TR, Uritboonthai W, Qin C, Trauger SA, Siuzdak G. Solvent-dependent metabolite distribution, clustering, and protein extraction for serum profiling with mass spectrometry. Anal Chem. 2006;78:743–52.
26. Wang W, Zhou H, Lin H, Roy S, Shaler TA, Hill LR, Norton S, Kumar P, Anderle M, Becker CH. Quantification of proteins and metabolites by mass spectrometry without isotopic labeling or spiked standards. Anal Chem. 2003;75:4818–26.
27. von Roepenack-Lahaye E, Degenkolb T, Zerjeski M, Franz M, Roth U, Wessjohann L, Schmidt J, Scheel D, Clemens S. Profiling of Arabidopsis secondary metabolites by capillary liquid chromatography coupled to electrospray ionization quadrupole time-of-flight mass spectrometry. Plant Physiol. 2004;134:548–59.
28. Tolstikov VV, Fiehn O. Analysis of highly polar compounds of plant origin: combination of hydrophilic interaction chromatography and electrospray ion trap mass spectrometry. Anal Biochem. 2002;301:298–307.
29. Lafaye A, Labarre J, Tabet JC, Ezan E, Junot C. Liquid chromatography-mass spectrometry and 15N metabolic labeling for quantitative metabolic profiling. Anal Chem. 2005;77:2026–33.
30. Dalluge JJ, Smith S, Sanchez-Riera F, McGuire C, Hobson R. Potential of fermentation profiling via rapid measurement of amino acid metabolism by liquid chromatography-tandem mass spectrometry. J Chromatogr A. 2004;1043:3–7.
31. Stokvis E, Rosing H, Beijnen JH. Stable isotopically labeled internal standards in quantitative bioanalysis using liquid chromatography/mass spectrometry: necessity or not? Rapid Commun Mass Spectrom. 2005;19:401–7.
32. Roy SM, Anderle M, Lin H, Becker CH. Differential expression profiling of serum proteins and metabolites for biomarker discovery. Int J Mass Spectrom. 2004;238:163–71.
33. Yang WC, Mirzaei H, Liu XP, Regnier FE. Enhancement of amino acid detection and quantification by electrospray ionization mass spectrometry. Anal Chem. 2006;78:4702–8.
34. Pan CL, Kora G, Tabb DL, Pelletier DA, McDonald WH, Hurst GB, Hettich RL, Samatova NF. Robust estimation of peptide abundance ratios and rigorous scoring of their variability and bias in quantitative shotgun proteomics. Anal Chem. 2006;78: 7110–20.
35. Birkemeyer C, Luedemann A, Wagner C, Erban A, Kopka J. Metabolome analysis: the potential of in vivo labeling with stable isotopes for metabolite profiling. Trends Biotechnol. 2005;23:28–33.
36. Mashego MR, Wu L, Van Dam JC, Ras C, Vinke JL, Van Winden WA, Van Gulik WM, Heijnen JJ. MIRACLE: mass isotopomer ratio analysis of U-13C-labeled extracts. A new method for accurate quantification of changes in concentrations of intracellular metabolites. Biotechnol Bioeng. 2004;85:620–8.
37. Lamos SM, Shortreed MR, Frey BL, Belshaw PJ, Smith LM. Relative quantification of carboxylic acid metabolites by liquid chromatography-mass spectrometry using isotopic variants of cholamine. Anal Chem. 2007;79:5143–9.
38. Shortreed MR, Lamos SM, Frey BL, Phillips MF, Patel M, Belshaw PJ, Smith LM. Ionizable isotopic labeling reagent for relative quantification of amine metabolites by mass spectrometry. Anal Chem. 2006;78:6398–403.
39. Yang WC, Adamec J, Regnier FE. Enhancement of the LC/MS analysis of fatty acids through derivatization and stable isotope coding. Anal Chem. 2007;79:5150–7.
40. Regnier FE, Julka S. Primary amine coding as a path to comparative proteomics. Proteomics. 2006;6:3968–79.
41. Berry KA, Murphy RC. Analysis of cell membrane aminophospholipids as isotope-tagged derivatives. J Lipid Res. 2005;46:1038–46.
42. Sterner JL, Johnston MV, Nicol GR, Ridge DP. Signal suppression in electrospray ionization Fourier transform mass spectrometry of multi-component samples. J Mass Spectrom. 2000;35:385–91.

43. Constantopoulos TL, Jackson GS, Enke CG. Effects of salt concentration on analyte response using electrospray ionization mass spectrometry. J Am Soc Mass Spectrom. 1999;10:625–34.
44. Annesley TM. Ion suppression in mass spectrometry. Clin Chem. 2003;49:1041–4.
45. Guo K, Ji C, Li L. Stable-isotope dimethylation labeling combined with LC-ESI MS for quantification of amine-containing metabolites in biological samples. Anal Chem. 2007; 79:8631–8.
46. Kind T, Fiehn O. Metabolomic database annotations via query of elemental compositions: mass accuracy is insufficient even at less than 1 ppm. BMC Bioinforma. 2006;7:234–44.
47. Kind T, Fiehn O. Seven golden rules for heuristic filtering of molecular formulas obtained by accurate mass spectrometry. BMC Bioinforma. 2007;8:105.
48. Rodgers RP, Blumer EN, Hendrickson CL, Marshall AG. Stable isotope incorporation triples the upper mass limit for determination of elemental composition by accurate mass measurement. J Am Soc Mass Spectrom. 2000;11:835–40.
49. Hegeman AD, Schulte CF, Cui Q, Lewis IA, Huttlin EL, Eghbalnia H, Harms AC, Ulrich EL, Markley JL, Sussman MR. Stable isotope assisted assignment of elemental compositions for metabolomics. Anal Chem. 2007; 79:6912–21.
50. Beynon RJ, Pratt JM. Metabolic labeling of proteins for proteomics. Mol Cell Proteomics. 2005;4:857–72.
51. Dumas ME, Maibaum EC, Teague C, Ueshima H, Zhou B, Lindon JC, Nicholson JK, Stamler J, Elliott P, Chan Q, Holmes E. Assessment of analytical reproducibility of 1H NMR spectroscopy based metabonomics for large-scale epidemiological research: the INTERMAP study. Anal Chem. 2006;78:2199–208.
52. Holmes E, Cloarec O, Nicholson JK. Probing latent biomarker signatures and in vivo pathway activity in experimental disease states via statistical total correlation spectroscopy (STOCSY) of biofluids: application to HgCl2 toxicity. J Proteome Res. 2006;5:1313–20.
53. Weljie AM, Newton J, Mercier P, Carlson E, Slupsky CM. Targeted profiling: quantitative analysis of 1H NMR metabolomics data. Anal Chem. 2006;78:4430–42.
54. Fan TW. Metabolite profiling by one- and two-dimensional NMR analysis of complex mixtures. Prog Nucl Magn Reson Spectrosc. 1996;28:161–219.
55. Viant MR. Improved methods for the acquisition and interpretation of NMR metabolomic data. Biochem Biophys Res Commun. 2003;310:943–8.
56. Kikuchi J, Shinozaki K, Hirayama T. Stable isotope labeling of *Arabidopsis thaliana* for an NMR-based metabolomics approach. Plant Cell Physiol. 2004;45:1099–104.
57. Peterson DJ, Loening NM. QQ-HSQC: a quick, quantitative heteronuclear correlation experiment for NMR spectroscopy. Magn Reson Chem. 2007;45:937–41.
58. Koskela H, Kilpelainen I, Heikkinen S. Some aspects of quantitative 2D NMR. J Magn Reson. 2005;174:237–44.
59. Heikkinen S, Toikka MM, Karhunen PT, Kilpelainen IA. Quantitative 2D HSQC (Q-HSQC) via suppression of J-dependence of polarization transfer in NMR spectroscopy: application to wood lignin. J Am Chem Soc. 2003;125:4362–7.
60. Hyberts SG, Heffron GJ, Tarragona NG, Solanky K, Edmonds KA, Luithardt H, Fejzo J, Chorev M, Aktas H, Colson K, Falchuk KH, Halperin JA, Wagner G. Ultrahigh-resolution (1)H-(13)C HSQC spectra of metabolite mixtures using nonlinear sampling and forward maximum entropy reconstruction. J Am Chem Soc. 2007;129:5108–16.
61. Shrot Y, Frydman L. Spatially resolved multidimensional NMR spectroscopy within a single scan. J Magn Reson. 2004;167:42–8.
62. Ross A, Salzmann M, Senn H. Fast-HMQC using Ernst angle pulses: an efficient tool for screening of ligand binding to target proteins. J Biomol NMR. 1997;10:389–96.
63. Sandusky P, Raftery D. Use of selective TOCSY NMR experiments for quantifying minor components in complex mixtures: application to the metabonomics of amino acids in honey. Anal Chem. 2005;77:2455–63.

Chapter 8

Metabolic Flux Analysis

Tae Hoon Yang

Abstract

In modern metabolomics, cellular reactions are observed as an integrated and networked system, termed as the metabolic network, instead of individual enzymatic reactions. Based on the metabolic network quantitated in terms of fluxes which are the rates at which materials are processed through the metabolic pathways, functional and regulatory activities of cells can be understood in its entirety. Typically, a realistic metabolic network which comprises catabolic and anabolic pathway fluxes of cells represents an underdetermined system from a stoichiometric viewpoint. This yields the intracellular fluxes that cannot be calculated from other fluxes measured. In order to determine those fluxes, ^{13}C labeling information is most frequently applied. This involves mathematical models that compute distributions of fluxes together with experimental tools for ^{13}C labeling analysis.

In this regard, understating the modeling techniques that aim the metabolic flux analysis using ^{13}C isotopomer analysis is one central issue of metabolomics. Therefore, we describe the principle of different modeling strategies of the metabolic flux analysis in this chapter. First, we introduce the stoichiometry-based approach which is the foundation of the ^{13}C-based approaches. Further to this, the modeling aspect of ^{13}C-based approaches and related tools such as computer-aided optimal design of ^{13}C labeling experiments and numerical computation of fluxes from measured ^{13}C labeling states of metabolic products are treated. Also, the mathematical and statistical background is provided, which are relevant to the modeling of ^{13}C-based metabolic flux analysis.

Key words: Metabolic Flux Analysis, Isotopic Labeling, Modeling

1. Introduction

An important and novel aspect of studying metabolism is considering cellular reactions as an integrated and networked system instead of individual enzymatic reactions. Thus, the notion of a metabolic network is centrally important for understanding functional and regulatory activities of cells in their entirety (1). Various experimental, mathematical, and computational tools have been developed for understanding structural and quantitative aspects of metabolic networks. Hereto, the biochemical reaction steps connecting a set of input and output components within the network, i.e., metabolic pathways, have to be expressed using adequate physical quantities.

Teresa Whei-Mei Fan et al. (eds.), *The Handbook of Metabolomics*, Methods in Pharmacology and Toxicology,
DOI 10.1007/978-1-61779-618-0_8, © Springer Science+Business Media New York 2012

To this end, the so-called "metabolic flux" is applied, which describes the rate at which material is processed through a metabolic pathway defined in the network (2). When the metabolic network is quantified in terms of fluxes, issues of design, control, and optimization of bioprocesses involved in metabolic and genetic engineering can also be considered. Such approaches have proven useful for understanding functional and regulatory activities of cells, the targeted optimization of industrial production strains, and physiological studies emerging in the medical and pharmaceutical areas (1, 3–5). In this sense, developing a method for accurate quantification of fluxes in vivo is vitally important for biological engineering science (1, 6, 7). Flux analysis and regulation are complementary problems. Some aspects of metabolic control theory are presented in Chaps. 9 and 10.

To determine metabolic fluxes, mathematical models incorporating experimental tools are required to compute their distributions, since they are not all directly measurable. Typically, a realistic metabolic network that comprises catabolic and anabolic pathway fluxes of cells represents an underdetermined system from a stoichiometric viewpoint. Therefore, additional constraints have to be imposed to quantify the fluxes. The general strategies (8, 9) are as follows:

1. Introduce additional balances, e.g., cometabolite balances such as NAD(P)H and/or ATP
2. Introduce linear programming with a biological objective function or
3. Conduct isotopic tracer experiments, e.g., using ^{13}C-labeled substrates and nuclear magnetic resonance spectroscopy (NMR) or mass spectrometry (MS)

The strategy (3) allows fluxes to be determined through pathways most extensively and precisely. Owing to progress in NMR and MS techniques, this ^{13}C-based metabolic flux analysis (^{13}C MFA) has been successfully applied to different classes of prokaryotes such as bacteria, eukaryotic cells, and mammalian cells as evidenced by numerous recent publications (10–16) Thus, ^{13}C MFA has replaced the conventional stoichiometry-based MFA, although stoichiometry is still necessary for ^{13}C MFA as it is an extension of the stoichiometric MFA. An important difference is that the additional balances of cometabolites are not used in ^{13}C MFA because they are susceptible to producing erroneous results (17).

In this chapter, the concepts of metabolic pathway flux modeling are addressed that inform the MFA. We briefly describe the methodology of the stoichiometry-based MFA, an essential part of ^{13}C MFA. Further, the modeling aspect of ^{13}C MFA and related tools such as computer-aided optimal design of ^{13}C labeling experiments and numerical computation of fluxes from measured ^{13}C labeling states of metabolic products are treated. Also, the mathematical and statistical backgrounds are provided, which are relevant to ^{13}C MFA modeling.

Mathematical notations used in this chapter are as follows. A symbol appearing in bold type refers to an array, i.e., row vectors, column vectors, or matrices. Typically, a matrix is represented by a bold capital letter such as "**B**," while a vector is denoted by a bold lowercase letter such as "**b**." If not specified, the vectors are in a column format, e.g., $\mathbf{b} = (b_1, b_2, \ldots, b_n)^{\mathrm{T}}$, where "$b_i$" denotes a scalar element of "**b**," the superscript "T" is the transpose of the row array $(b_1, b_2, \ldots, b_n)$, and "n" is the length of "**b**." Bold numbers also denote column vectors, i.e., "**0**" is the column vector or matrix whose entries are zeros, e.g., $\mathbf{0} = (0, 0, \ldots, 0)^{\mathrm{T}}$ and "**1**" is the column vector whose entries are ones, e.g., $\mathbf{1} = (1, 1, \ldots, 1)^{\mathrm{T}}$. A matrix in text is formulated using commas and semicolons as the row and column separators, respectively. Hence, a 2 × 3 matrix **A** whose first row is $(0, 0, 0)$ and second is $(1, 2, 3)$ appears as $\mathbf{A} = (0, 0, 0; 1, 2, 3)$.

2. Stoichiometric Metabolic Flux Analysis

A stoichiometric MFA model consists of a linear algebraic equation system of material balances. It typically assumes stationary or quasi-stationary states for intracellular metabolite pools. This means the pools do not change over the time the experiment takes place. This assumption obviously holds true in a continuous culture and, with some care, in the exponential phase of a batch culture or in a batch-fed culture with slow variations in the input feed (1, 18).

For an intracellular metabolite with p incoming and q outgoing reactions, its balance can be set up as:

$$\sum_{i=1}^{p} (\boldsymbol{v}_{\mathrm{in},i} s_i) - \sum_{j=1}^{q} (\boldsymbol{v}_{\mathrm{out},j} s_j) = 0 \quad (1)$$

The v_{in} denotes incoming fluxes, v_{out} are outgoing fluxes, and s is the stoichiometric coefficient of each particular reaction. The stoichiometric coefficient indicates how many moles of the metabolite are converted from reactants (s_i) and into products (s_j) for which the balance is set up. All fluxes are physiologically constrained such that $\boldsymbol{v}_i = \{\boldsymbol{v}_i \in \Re | \boldsymbol{v}_i \geq 0\}$. For instance, suppose the metabolites A, B, and C are converted into a metabolite D and D into metabolites E, F, and G where the stoichiometry of the reactions are $v_{\mathrm{in},1}$: A → D, $v_{\mathrm{in},2}$: 2B → D, $v_{\mathrm{in},3}$: C → 2D, $v_{\mathrm{out},1}$: D → E, $v_{\mathrm{out},2}$: D → 2F, $v_{\mathrm{out},3}$: 3D → G (Fig. 1).

According to (1), the flux balance set up around the pool of metabolite D is:

$$(\boldsymbol{v}_{\mathrm{in},1} + \boldsymbol{v}_{\mathrm{in},2} + 2\boldsymbol{v}_{\mathrm{in},3}) - (\boldsymbol{v}_{\mathrm{out},1} + \boldsymbol{v}_{\mathrm{out},2} + 3\boldsymbol{v}_{\mathrm{out},3}) = 0 \quad (2)$$

Since the balance region of (2) is set up for metabolite D, we are only interested in how many moles of D are converted from each reactant and into each product, which is represented by the corresponding stoichiometric coefficient.

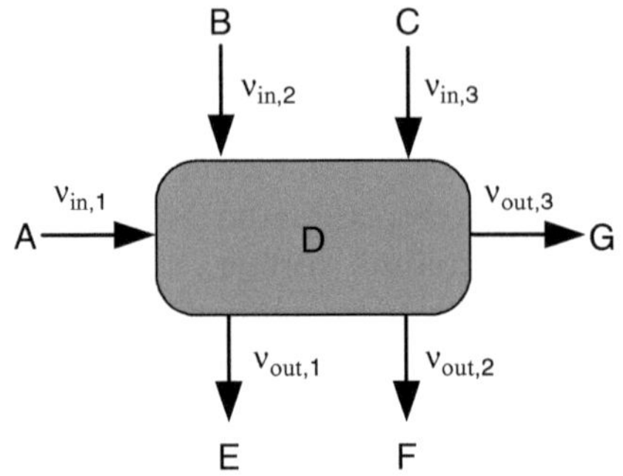

Fig. 1. Metabolic fluxes around the balance region of a metabolite pool. A, B, C, D, E, F, and G are certain metabolites; $v_{in,i}$ are incoming and $v_{out,i}$ are outgoing fluxes from the pool of metabolite D.

2.1. Solution by Stoichiometric MFA

Once balances such as (2) have been set up for all metabolites defined in the metabolic network, we get a system of linear equations. The system can be formulated using a matrix notation such that:

$$\mathbf{S}\boldsymbol{\nu} = \mathbf{0} \tag{3}$$

S is the stoichiometric matrix and the vector $\boldsymbol{\nu}$ is the flux variables. When none of $\boldsymbol{\nu}$ is measurable, (3) is a homogeneous system having at least the trivial solution of $\boldsymbol{\nu} = \mathbf{0}$. In practice, the flux variables consist of unmeasurable intracellular fluxes $\boldsymbol{\nu}_{\text{intra}}$ and measurable extracellular fluxes $\boldsymbol{\nu}_{\text{extra}}$, and the system is nonhomogeneous. Therefore, one can reformulate (3) using the following matrix form:

$$\mathbf{S}_{\text{intra}}\boldsymbol{\nu}_{\text{intra}} + \mathbf{S}_{\text{extra}}\boldsymbol{\nu}_{\text{extra}} = \mathbf{0} \tag{4}$$

Denoting $\mathbf{S}_{\text{intra}}$ and $\mathbf{S}_{\text{extra}}$ stoichiometric matrices correspond to $\boldsymbol{\nu}_{\text{extra}}$ and $\boldsymbol{\nu}_{\text{intra}}$, respectively. Considering components of $\boldsymbol{\nu}_{\text{extra}}$ are associated with measurement errors, this linear problem (4) can be reformulated by introducing an error term such that:

$$\mathbf{S}_{\text{extra}}\boldsymbol{\nu}_{\text{extra}} = -\mathbf{S}_{\text{intra}}\boldsymbol{\nu}_{\text{intra}} + \boldsymbol{\varepsilon} \tag{5}$$

Here, the vector $\boldsymbol{\nu}_{\text{extra}}$ and $\boldsymbol{\nu}_{\text{intra}}$ have dimensions of $q \times 1$ and $n \times 1$ and the matrix $\mathbf{S}_{\text{intra}}$ and $\mathbf{S}_{\text{extra}}$ have dimensions of $m \times n$ and $m \times q$, respectively. Hence, n equals the number of unknown fluxes, q equals the measured fluxes, and m is the number of balance equations. The error term $\boldsymbol{\varepsilon}$ associated with $\boldsymbol{\nu}_{\text{extra}}$ is assumed to be normally distributed with expectation vector **0** and its covariance matrix $\boldsymbol{\Sigma}$ such that: $\boldsymbol{\varepsilon} \in N(\mathbf{0}, \boldsymbol{\Sigma})$.

The linear problem (5) can be formulated using the covariance-weighted least-squares concept, allowing the function to be minimized:

$$\min_{\boldsymbol{\nu}_{\text{intra}}} f(\boldsymbol{\nu}_{\text{intra}}), \quad f = \frac{1}{2}(\mathbf{S}_{\text{extra}}\boldsymbol{\nu}_{\text{extra}} + \mathbf{S}_{\text{intra}}\boldsymbol{\nu}_{\text{intra}})^{\mathrm{T}}(\mathbf{S}_{\text{extra}}\boldsymbol{\Sigma}\mathbf{S}_{\text{extra}}{}^{\mathrm{T}})^{-1} \times (\mathbf{S}_{\text{extra}}\boldsymbol{\nu}_{\text{extra}} + \mathbf{S}_{\text{intra}}\boldsymbol{\nu}_{\text{intra}}) \tag{6}$$

According to the first-order optimality condition, the gradient of the objective function f becomes zero at the solution $\hat{\boldsymbol{\nu}}_{\text{intra}}$ (19), that is:

$$\nabla f = \mathbf{S}_{\text{intra}}{}^{\text{T}}(\mathbf{S}_{\text{extra}}\boldsymbol{\Sigma}\mathbf{S}_{\text{extra}}{}^{\text{T}})^{-1}(\mathbf{S}_{\text{intra}}\hat{\boldsymbol{\nu}}_{\text{intra}} + \mathbf{S}_{\text{extra}}\boldsymbol{\nu}_{\text{extra}}) = 0 \quad (7)$$

Solving (7) for $\hat{\boldsymbol{\nu}}_{\text{intra}}$ results in:

$$\begin{aligned}\hat{\boldsymbol{\nu}}_{\text{u}} = -&\left(\mathbf{S}_{\text{intra}}{}^{\text{T}}(\mathbf{S}_{\text{extra}}\boldsymbol{\Sigma}\mathbf{S}_{\text{extra}}{}^{\text{T}})^{-1}\mathbf{S}_{\text{intra}}\right)^{-1} \\ \times\ &\mathbf{S}_{\text{intra}}{}^{\text{T}}(\mathbf{S}_{\text{extra}}\boldsymbol{\Sigma}\mathbf{S}_{\text{extra}}{}^{\text{T}})^{-1}\mathbf{S}_{\text{extra}}\boldsymbol{\nu}_{\text{extra}}\end{aligned} \quad (8)$$

This is the solution of the linear least-square problem (6). Note that the unique solution for $\boldsymbol{\nu}_{\text{intra}}$ is only available if and only if the rank of the system matrix $\text{rank}(\mathbf{S}_{\text{intra}}) \geq n$ and thus the matrix $\mathbf{S}_{\text{intra}}{}^{\text{T}}(\mathbf{S}_{\text{extra}}\boldsymbol{\Sigma}\mathbf{S}_{\text{extra}}{}^{\text{T}})^{-1}\mathbf{S}_{\text{intra}}$ is invertible. Here, $(\mathbf{S}_{\text{intra}}{}^{\text{T}}(\mathbf{S}_{\text{extra}}\boldsymbol{\Sigma}\mathbf{S}_{\text{extra}}{}^{\text{T}})^{-1}\mathbf{S}_{\text{intra}})^{-1}\mathbf{S}_{\text{intra}}{}^{\text{T}}(\mathbf{S}_{\text{extra}}\boldsymbol{\Sigma}\mathbf{S}_{\text{extra}}{}^{\text{T}})^{-1}$ is the so-called Moore–Penrose pseudoinverse in covariance-weighted form. Assuming that $\hat{\boldsymbol{\nu}}_{\text{intra}}$ is unbiased and normally distributed gives the covariance of the estimate $\hat{\boldsymbol{\nu}}_{\text{intra}}$ as follows (20):

$$\boldsymbol{\Sigma}_{\hat{\boldsymbol{\nu}}_{\text{intra}}} = \left(\mathbf{S}_{\text{intra}}{}^{\text{T}}(\mathbf{S}_{\text{extra}}\boldsymbol{\Sigma}\mathbf{S}_{\text{extra}}{}^{\text{T}})^{-1}\mathbf{S}_{\text{intra}}\right)^{-1} \quad (9)$$

Using the stoichiometry-based MFA technique, the immeasurable intracellular fluxes can be determined from measured extracellular fluxes. However, unique flux determination is possible only if the flux measurements are nonredundant and determined (9, 21, 22).

2.2. Overdetermined System

If $\text{rank}(\mathbf{S}_{\text{intra}}) < m$, the system is called redundant, i.e., overdetermined. In a redundant system, consistency is not given a priori status (1, 8, 23). A redundant system contains the so-called balanceable fluxes in $\boldsymbol{\nu}_{\text{extra}}$. These balanceable fluxes must be detected and corrected to render the system consistent (23). As described in van der Heijden et al. (23), the redundant matrix **R**, for which $\mathbf{R}\boldsymbol{\nu}_{\text{extra}} = \mathbf{0}$ always holds, is given by:

$$\begin{aligned}\mathbf{R} = \mathbf{S}_{\text{extra}} - \mathbf{S}_{\text{intra}}&\left(\mathbf{S}_{\text{intra}}{}^{\text{T}}(\mathbf{S}_{\text{extra}}\boldsymbol{\Sigma}\mathbf{S}_{\text{extra}}{}^{\text{T}})^{-1}\mathbf{S}_{\text{intra}}\right)^{-1} \\ \times\ &\mathbf{S}_{\text{intra}}{}^{\text{T}}(\mathbf{S}_{\text{extra}}\boldsymbol{\Sigma}\mathbf{S}_{\text{extra}}{}^{\text{T}})^{-1}\mathbf{S}_{\text{extra}}\end{aligned} \quad (10)$$

Only if the system is not redundant, the matrix **R** equals the zero-matrix and thus $\mathbf{R}\boldsymbol{\nu}_{\text{extra}} = \mathbf{0}$ holds automatically. The rank of the redundant matrix rank(**R**) gives the degree of redundancy. The redundancy matrix can be used to correct possible inconsistency among the measurements in the vector $\boldsymbol{\nu}_{\text{extra}}$. Suppose that **R** is not the zero-matrix and thus the system is redundant. By removing the dependent rows in **R**, we get the reduced redundancy matrix $\mathbf{R}_{\text{RED}}$ (refer to the Gauss–Jordan elimination in Sect. 3.1.2. The dependent rows can be detected by the use of the reduced row echelon form of **R**!). The occurrence of inconsistency yields $\mathbf{R}_{\mathrm{RED}}\boldsymbol{\nu}_{\mathrm{extra}} \neq \mathbf{0}$. Therefore, the measurements values in $\boldsymbol{\nu}_{\mathrm{extra}}$ have to be corrected into $\boldsymbol{\nu}_{\mathrm{extra,corr}}$ by calculating the deviations $\boldsymbol{\delta}$ using:

$$\mathbf{R}_{\mathrm{RED}}\boldsymbol{\nu}_{\mathrm{extra,corr}} = \mathbf{R}_{\mathrm{RED}}(\boldsymbol{\nu}_{\mathrm{extra}} - \boldsymbol{\delta}) = \mathbf{0} \tag{11}$$

The $\boldsymbol{\delta}$ is estimated by solving the following linear least-squares problem such that:

$$\min_{\boldsymbol{\delta}} \frac{1}{2}(\mathbf{R}_{\mathrm{RED}}(\boldsymbol{\nu}_{\mathrm{extra}} - \boldsymbol{\delta}))^{\mathrm{T}}(\mathbf{R}_{\mathrm{RED}}\boldsymbol{\Sigma}\mathbf{R}_{\mathrm{RED}}{}^{\mathrm{T}})^{-1}(\mathbf{R}_{\mathrm{RED}}(\boldsymbol{\nu}_{\mathrm{extra}} - \boldsymbol{\delta})) \tag{12}$$

Analogously to (8), the solution of (12) that satisfies the first-order optimality is given by:

$$\hat{\boldsymbol{\delta}} = (\mathbf{R}_{\mathrm{RED}}{}^{\mathrm{T}} \cdot (\mathbf{R}_{\mathrm{RED}}\boldsymbol{\Sigma}\mathbf{R}_{\mathrm{RED}}{}^{\mathrm{T}})^{-1}\mathbf{R}_{\mathrm{RED}})^{-1} \times \mathbf{R}_{\mathrm{RED}}{}^{\mathrm{T}}(\mathbf{R}_{\mathrm{RED}}\boldsymbol{\Sigma}\mathbf{R}_{\mathrm{RED}}{}^{\mathrm{T}})^{-1}\mathbf{R}_{\mathrm{RED}}\boldsymbol{\nu}_{\mathrm{extra}} \tag{13}$$

Assuming that $\hat{\boldsymbol{\delta}}$ is unbiased and normally distributed, its covariance matrix results in (20):

$$\boldsymbol{\Sigma}_{\hat{\boldsymbol{\delta}}} = (\mathbf{R}_{\mathrm{RED}}{}^{\mathrm{T}}(\mathbf{R}_{\mathrm{RED}}\boldsymbol{\Sigma}\mathbf{R}_{\mathrm{RED}}{}^{\mathrm{T}})^{-1}\mathbf{R}_{\mathrm{RED}})^{-1} \tag{14}$$

Moreover, assuming that errors associated with $\boldsymbol{\nu}_{\mathrm{extra}}$ and $\boldsymbol{\delta}$ are identical, then $\boldsymbol{\Sigma} = \boldsymbol{\Sigma}_{\hat{\boldsymbol{\delta}}}$. Consequently, (13) can also be formulated as:

$$\hat{\boldsymbol{\delta}} = \boldsymbol{\Sigma}\mathbf{R}_{\mathrm{RED}}{}^{\mathrm{T}}(\mathbf{R}_{\mathrm{RED}}\boldsymbol{\Sigma}\mathbf{R}_{\mathrm{RED}}{}^{\mathrm{T}})^{-1}\mathbf{R}_{\mathrm{RED}}\boldsymbol{\nu}_{\mathrm{extra}} \tag{15}$$

Now $\boldsymbol{\nu}_{\mathrm{extra,corr}}$ can be obtained by subtracting $\hat{\boldsymbol{\delta}}$ from $\boldsymbol{\nu}_{\mathrm{extra}}$, rendering the system consistent.

2.3. Underdetermined System

In case the matrix $\mathbf{S}_{\mathrm{intra}}$ is rank deficient, i.e., rank($\mathbf{S}_{\mathrm{intra}}$) < n, and thus the system is underdetermined, the unique solutions are not available for all entries of $\boldsymbol{\nu}_{\mathrm{intra}}$. To answer the question of which entries have nevertheless unique solutions, one can formulate the general solution of (6) by the linear combination of (8) with the null space (8) of the system matrix $\mathbf{S}_{\mathrm{intra}}$.

$$\hat{\boldsymbol{\nu}}_{\mathrm{intra}} = -(\mathbf{S}_{\mathrm{intra}}{}^{\mathrm{T}}(\mathbf{S}_{\mathrm{extra}}\boldsymbol{\Sigma}\mathbf{S}_{\mathrm{extra}}{}^{\mathrm{T}})^{-1}\mathbf{S}_{\mathrm{intra}})^{-1}\mathbf{S}_{\mathrm{intra}}{}^{\mathrm{T}}(\mathbf{S}_{\mathrm{extra}}\boldsymbol{\Sigma}\mathbf{S}_{\mathrm{extra}}{}^{\mathrm{T}})^{-1} \times \mathbf{S}_{\mathrm{extra}}\boldsymbol{\nu}_{\mathrm{extra}} + \mathrm{null}(\mathbf{S}_{\mathrm{extra}}) \cdot \beta \tag{16}$$

The null($\mathbf{S}_{\mathrm{intra}}$) denotes the rational basis for the null space obtained from the reduced row echelon form of $\mathbf{S}_{\mathrm{intra}}$ and $\boldsymbol{\beta}$ a vector containing arbitrary nonzero values. Accordingly, the ith element of $\boldsymbol{\nu}_{\mathrm{intra}}$ is uniquely estimable if and only if the ith row of null($\mathbf{S}_{\mathrm{intra}}$) entirely consists of zeros. Further details of the MFA approach to an underdetermined metabolic network are described in Klamt et al. (8).

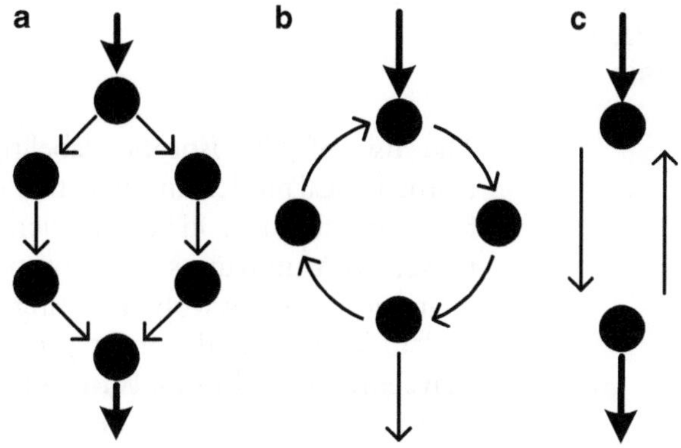

Fig. 2. Typical situations of limited MFA solely based on the stoichiometric balances: parallel pathways without any related flux measurement (**a**); certain metabolic cycles (**b**); bidirectional reaction steps (**c**); ➔: measurable fluxes; →: immeasurable fluxes (18).

2.4. Limitations in Stoichiometric MFA Models

In most cases, there are more unknown reactions than the number of balance equations. Therefore, a model solely based on stoichiometry is typically underdetermined. Consequently, the stoichiometry-based MFA is strongly limited and fails in many situations encountered in realistic networks, illustrated in Fig. 2 (18, 24–26).

To overcome this, additional constraints are required as mentioned in this chapter's introduction. The strategy (1) to introduce additional balances can be successful if all reactions that produce and consume cometabolites and ATP maintenance processes are fully known. This approach is practically complicated due to often unclosed NAD(P)H/NAD(P)-balances (18, 27, 28), for example. This presence of transhydrogenase activity reversibly transfers a hydride ion equivalent between NADH and NADPH and futile cycles, like that present in anaplerotic reactions.

For the strategy (2) that introduces a biological objective function, mostly using linear programming techniques for obtaining solutions, the choice of an appropriate objective function is crucial. Optimality criteria often used are maximizations of cometabolites productions (29, 30) or growth rate (31). However, this method is still not sufficient to solve the problems inherent to the metabolite balancing techniques and cannot give a unique solution of fluxes (9, 32).

In contrast, the use of stable isotope labeled substrates such as ^{13}C, combined with isotopic labeling measurement by NMR and/or MS provides the underdetermined stoichiometric network with a large amount of additional information (2, 18, 24, 26, 33). Conversion of ^{13}C-labeled substrates in the metabolic network gives distinct, flux-dependent ^{13}C labeling patterns of metabolic products that can be detected by NMR and/or MS. The isotope measurements provide many additional constraints for MFA. Therefore, the problems depicted in Fig. 2 can be solved in most cases by measuring the ^{13}C labeling states of various metabolic products.

3. ^{13}C Metabolic Flux Analysis

The use of ^{13}C isotopic labeling experiments combined with mathematical models and analytical techniques is of increasing importance for various fields of bioscience (18, 24, 26, 34, 35). Among those, MFA utilizing stable isotope tracer techniques is expanding continuously along with increasing interest (2). In particular, the use of ^{13}C labeling is the most prominent for MFA because carbon transfer reactions from substrates to products in a biological network are well-studied and well-defined by the specificity of the enzymes (9, 26). The methods developed for MFA utilize predominantly ^{13}C labeling patterns obtained from biomass constituents such as amino acids from cell protein (33, 36), nucleotides from RNA and DNA (37), or glucose from glycogen (38) formed during growth. Such biological macromolecules are typically not applicable to nongrowing cells, e.g., in production processes of primary or secondary metabolites as well as in immobilized cells, tissue, or whole organisms. As an alternative approach, the labeling of secreted metabolites can be analyzed (39, 40). For instance, Yang et al. (14) demonstrated ^{13}C MFA carried out for the central metabolism of *Corynebacterium glutamicum* solely using carbon dioxide labeling information.

^{13}C MFA estimates immeasurable fluxes from the measurements of ^{13}C labeling states of metabolic products formed by cells using a numerical parameter fitting procedure. There are two factors making the ^{13}C labeling patterns distinct. These are metabolic states and specific labeling patterns of ^{13}C substrates. Hence, the ^{13}C labeling patterns can be modeled as a function of the flux variables.

Typically, determining fluxes from the ^{13}C labeling measurements is computationally expensive due to nonlinearity of the system. Due to the nonlinearity, direct analytical solutions are restricted to models with a few pathways containing less than two branch points (41, 42). For a realistic network, no inverse function of the model is usually available, and thus, the computation of metabolic fluxes from a ^{13}C labeling experiment involves a numerical method as depicted in Fig. 3.

The experiment provides kinetic data such as substrate uptake, product and biomass formation, and ^{13}C labeling data, whereas the simulation creates a synthetic data set corresponding to experimental data in parametrized flux space. By means of numerical optimization, a constrained minimum of independent flux variables ($\boldsymbol{\Theta}$) to an objective function that calculates the weighted sum of squares of differences between measured and simulated data can be found. This is generally referred to as a constrained and weighted nonlinear programming problem, for which the mathematical formulation is:

$$\min_{\boldsymbol{\Theta}\in\Re^m} f(\boldsymbol{\Theta}), \quad \text{where } f(\boldsymbol{\Theta}) = \tfrac{1}{2}(\boldsymbol{\eta} - \mathbf{F}(\boldsymbol{\Theta}))^{\mathrm{T}}\boldsymbol{\Sigma}_{\eta}^{-1}(\boldsymbol{\eta} - \mathbf{F}(\boldsymbol{\Theta})) \\ \text{subject to } \boldsymbol{\nu}_{\text{depend}} = \mathbf{n}_{\text{flux}}(\boldsymbol{\Theta}) \geq \mathbf{0} \tag{17}$$

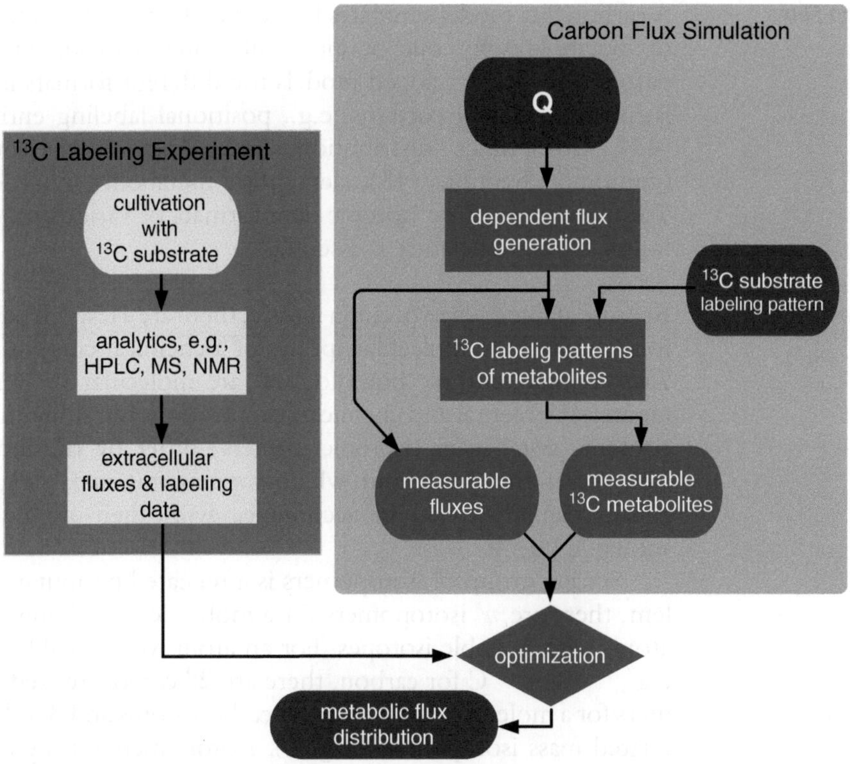

Fig. 3. Flow chart of ^{13}C flux estimation procedure by a carbon flux simulation model and a ^{13}C labeling experiment. For the estimation of Θ, the numerical optimization against measured data of rates and labelings is the typical choice.

Here, $f(\boldsymbol{\Theta})$ denotes the objective function to be minimized, $\boldsymbol{\eta} = (\eta_1, \eta_2, \ldots, \eta_n)^{\mathrm{T}}$ is the measured data set consisting of ^{13}C labeling data extracellular fluxes measured, and $\mathbf{F}(\boldsymbol{\Theta}) = (f_1, f_2, \ldots, f_n)^{\mathrm{T}}$ is the model function corresponding to $\boldsymbol{\eta}$. Further, $\boldsymbol{\Theta} = (\boldsymbol{\Theta}_1, \boldsymbol{\Theta}_2, \ldots, \boldsymbol{\Theta}_m)^{\mathrm{T}}$ is the set of independent variables (design parameter) to be determined by the optimization process, $\boldsymbol{\Sigma}_\eta$ is the measurement covariance matrix, and $\boldsymbol{\nu}_{\mathrm{depend}}$ are the fluxes functionally dependent on $\boldsymbol{\Theta}$ and $n \geq m$. The inverse of $\boldsymbol{\Sigma}_\eta$ acts as a weighting term such that measured values with smaller variances are more weighted during the minimization process and $\mathbf{n}_{\mathrm{flux}}(\boldsymbol{\Theta}) \geq 0$ is the function constraining $\boldsymbol{\Theta}$, namely, the constrained weighted nonlinear least-squares minimization.

Such numerical minimization involves repeated computation of ^{13}C labeling states in a parametrized metabolic flux space using a model that maps carbon atoms or carbon isotope isomers (isotopomer). Moreover, several 100–1,000 nonlinear equations have to be solved to generate simulation data for a realistic central metabolic network (7, 25). Hence, developing a model suited to the simulation is critically important for ^{13}C MFA. Considering this context, we discuss in the following sections how to parametrize a metabolic flux network to get $\boldsymbol{\nu}_{\mathrm{depend}} = \mathbf{n}_{\mathrm{flux}}(\boldsymbol{\Theta})$ and introduce the models developed to simulate ^{13}C labeling states in a parametrized flux space.

3.1. Carbon Flux Network

A carbon flux model simulates flux-dependent ^{13}C labeling patterns of metabolites for one or more substrates with known labeling pattern(s). The developed models use different formats in formulating the labeling patterns, e.g., positional labeling enrichments (43), isotopomer distributions (44), cumulated isotopomer (cumomer) fractions (45), elementary metabolite units (42), etc. To understand those isotopic data formats of various models, the following nomenclature is essential.

3.1.1. Nomenclature

Because stable *isotopes* occur in nature, there are a few different terms for grouping the molecular species of a chemical compound (46). *Isotopologues* (isotopic homologues) are molecular species having identical elemental and chemical compositions but differ in isotopic content. *Isotopomers* (isotopic isomers) differ by the location of isotopes on the compound, whereas *mass isotopomers* are groups of isotopomers classified in accordance with their nominal mass, shown in Fig. 4.

Since a group of isotopomers is a repeated permutation problem, there are n^p isotopomers for a molecule containing p specific atoms with n stable isotopes. For an atom with **2** stable isotopes, e.g., ^{12}C and ^{13}C for carbon, there are $\mathbf{2^3}$ carbon-related isotopomers for a molecule consisting of **3** carbon atoms and **3** + 1 carbon-related mass isotopomers (Fig. 4). Isotopomers can be expressed using binary numbers, e.g., "000," "001," "010," "011," "100," "101," "10," and "111" for the isotopomers in Fig. 4. Note that the digit "0" denotes ^{12}C (nonlabeled as it is the most frequent isotope of carbon) and "1" is ^{13}C (labeled). The use of the binary code both declares the positional labeling patterns and indexes isotopomers when converting it into decimal numbers.

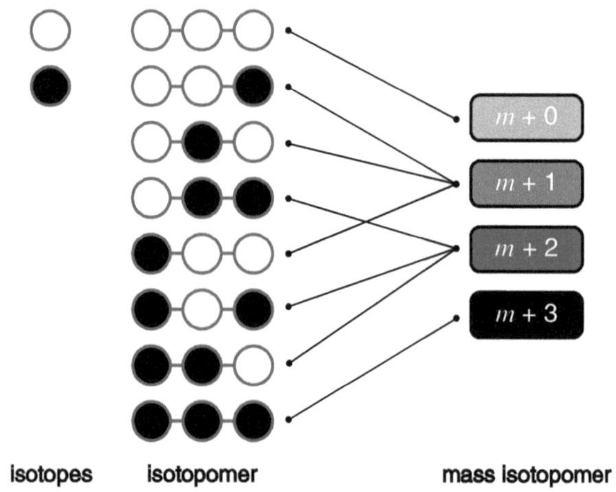

Fig. 4. Isotopes, isotopomers, and mass isotopomers: *white-colored circles* indicate ^{12}C (nonlabeled); *black-colored circles* indicate ^{13}C (labeled). Isotopomers can be transformed into mass isotopomers (see Sect. 3.1.3).

For instance, the above binary numbers are 0, 1, 2,. . ., 7. Thus, the isotopomer of "100" is the fifth (4 + 1) isotopomer of a compound with three carbon atoms. Vice versa, the fourth isotopomer of the compound has the positional labeling pattern of "011" (4 − 1 = 3 into decimal number). Positional carbon isotopomers can be quantified using ^{13}C NMR in terms of ^{13}C multiplet analysis. Complete carbon isotopomers can be analyzed using a combination of ^{1}H NMR and ^{13}C NMR, as described in Chap. 6.

Mass isotopomers of a compound are always measured in mass spectrometers with better than unit mass resolution. Considering naturally occurring stable isotopes of carbon (^{12}C, ^{13}C), oxygen (^{16}O, ^{17}O, ^{18}O), hydrogen (^{1}H, ^{2}H), and nitrogen (^{14}N, ^{15}N), a biologically relevant compound $C_aH_bO_cN_d$ has $a + b + 2c + d + 1$ mass isotopomers and $a + 1$ mass isotopomers for its carbon skeleton. Not all mass isotopomers of a compound can practically be measured, e.g., due to MS detection limits. We denote the mass isotopomers of a compound X by ^{m+i}X, where superscript "m" represents the monoisotopic mass of the compound and "i" the mass addition. For instance, CO_2 has the monoisotopic mass of 44, i.e., $m = 44$ and $i = 0$, when it is composed of one ^{12}C and two ^{16}O. In case either the carbon is ^{13}C or one of the oxygen is ^{17}O, $m = 44$ and $i = 1$ and so forth.

3.1.2. Parametrization of a Stoichiometric System

As depicted in Fig. 3, two key steps of the simulation of a carbon flux network are (1) generation of metabolic flux states that obey stoichiometry and (2) calculation of ^{13}C labeling states of intracellular as well as measurable extracellular metabolites as a function of ^{13}C labeling patterns of substrates and metabolic fluxes. During numerical flux estimation using the ^{13}C labeling measurement data, steps (1) and (2) have to be repeated at each cycle of iterative flux estimation. Therefore, the generation of certain flux states complying with stoichiometry is centrally important for the flux estimation. This can simply be done by parametrizing an underdetermined stoichiometric network (25) by choosing independent and dependent fluxes. The parametrization also provides explicit expressions of fluxes and of analytical partial derivatives, which are useful for numerical computation.

For instance, an underdetermined system with eight fluxes (two measurable and six immeasurable fluxes) and four balances in Fig. 5 can be parametrized either using Gauss–Jordan elimination or supplying additional linear equations specified by the modeler. According to (1), the steady-state material balances for the network in Fig. 5 are given by:

$$\boldsymbol{\nu}_7 + \boldsymbol{\nu}_3 - (\boldsymbol{\nu}_1 + \boldsymbol{\nu}_2) = 0 \quad \text{around metabolite A} \tag{18}$$

$$\boldsymbol{\nu}_2 + \boldsymbol{\nu}_4 - (\boldsymbol{\nu}_3 + \boldsymbol{\nu}_5) = 0 \quad \text{around metabolite B} \tag{19}$$

$$\boldsymbol{\nu}_4 + 2\boldsymbol{\nu}_5 - \boldsymbol{\nu}_6 = 0 \quad \text{around metabolite C} \tag{20}$$

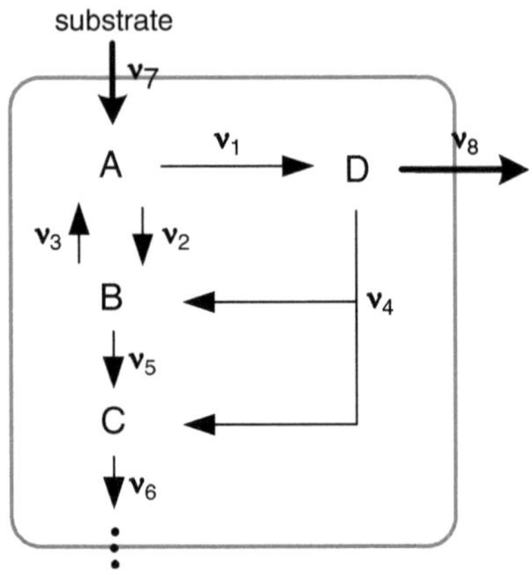

Fig. 5. An example of an underdetermined stoichiometric reaction network: v_7 and v_8 are measurable extracellular fluxes, whereas the intracellular fluxes (v_1, v_2,..., v_6) are immeasurable. Overall balance region is given by the *gray-colored line*.

$$\boldsymbol{v}_1 - (2\boldsymbol{v}_4 + \boldsymbol{v}_8) = 0 \quad \text{around metabolite D} \tag{21}$$

The above linear algebraic system can be rewritten using matrix and vector notation.

$$\mathbf{S}\boldsymbol{v} = \begin{pmatrix} -1 & -1 & 1 & 0 & 0 & 0 & 1 & 0 \\ 0 & 1 & -1 & 1 & -1 & 0 & 0 & 0 \\ 0 & 0 & 0 & 1 & 2 & -1 & 0 & 0 \\ 1 & 0 & 0 & -2 & 0 & 0 & 0 & -1 \end{pmatrix} \boldsymbol{v} = \mathbf{0} \tag{22}$$

Here, $\mathbf{S}$ denotes the stoichiometric matrix with a dimension of 4×8, equaling the Jacobian matrix of the linear system of (18)–(21), $\boldsymbol{v} = (\boldsymbol{v}_1, \boldsymbol{v}_2, \boldsymbol{v}_3, \boldsymbol{v}_4, \boldsymbol{v}_5, \boldsymbol{v}_6, \boldsymbol{v}_7, \boldsymbol{v}_8)^{\mathrm{T}}$, the flux variable vector with a dimension of 8×1 and $\mathbf{0}$ a 4×1 vector whose entries are all zero.

As the flux vector $\boldsymbol{v}$ is arranged such that the immeasurable intracellular fluxes, $\boldsymbol{v}_{\text{intra}} = (\boldsymbol{v}_1, \boldsymbol{v}_2, \boldsymbol{v}_3, \boldsymbol{v}_4, \boldsymbol{v}_5, \boldsymbol{v}_6)^{\mathrm{T}}$, are followed by measurable extracellular fluxes, $\boldsymbol{v}_{\text{extra}} = (\boldsymbol{v}_7, \boldsymbol{v}_8)^{\mathrm{T}}$, $\mathbf{S}$ can correspondingly be partitioned into $\mathbf{S}_{\text{intra}}$ and $\mathbf{S}_{\text{extra}}$. Here, $\mathbf{S}_{\text{intra}}$ equals the matrix consisting of the columns from the first to sixth of $\mathbf{S}$ and the $\mathbf{S}_{\text{extra}}$ are those from the seventh to eighth. Therefore, (22) can alternatively be expressed as:

$$\mathbf{S}_{\text{intra}}\boldsymbol{v}_{\text{intra}} = -\mathbf{S}_{\text{extra}}\boldsymbol{v}_{\text{extra}} \tag{23}$$

In this example, the rank of $\mathbf{S}_{\text{intra}}$ is 4, whereas six unknown intracellular fluxes are present in four linearly independent equations. This means the system is nonredundant (consistent), as the number of equations equals the rank number and is underdetermined with two degrees of freedom. Hence, either two intracellular fluxes have to be chosen as independent or two additional equations that are linearly independent from the material balances have to be supplied by the modeler.

Gauss–Jordan Elimination: Applying the Gauss–Jordan elimination with partial pivoting transforms the matrix **S** into its reduced row echelon form, $\mathbf{S}_{\mathrm{RRE}}$.

$$\mathbf{S}_{\mathrm{RRE}}\boldsymbol{\nu} = \begin{pmatrix} 1 & 0 & 0 & 0 & 0 & 2 & -4 & 3 \\ 0 & 1 & -1 & 0 & 0 & -2 & 3 & -3 \\ 0 & 0 & 0 & 1 & 0 & 1 & -2 & 2 \\ 0 & 0 & 0 & 0 & 1 & -1 & 1 & -1 \end{pmatrix} \boldsymbol{\nu} = \mathbf{0} \tag{24}$$

The first nonzero element that is always 1 in each row of $\mathbf{S}_{\mathrm{RRE}}$ is called "leading 1." If the *i*th column of $\mathbf{S}_{\mathrm{RRE}}$ contains only zeros and one leading 1, then the *i*th flux variable is dependent, otherwise independent. The number of fluxes selected as independent equals the intrinsic degrees of freedom in the stoichiometric network, that is, the difference between the number of variables and the rank of **S**. In this example, the first, second, fourth, and fifth fluxes are dependent, whereas the remaining fluxes are independent. This can simply be visualized by rearranging (24) such that:

$$\mathbf{S}_{\mathrm{RRE}}\boldsymbol{\nu} = \begin{pmatrix} 1 & 0 & 0 & 0 \\ 0 & 1 & 0 & 0 \\ 0 & 0 & 1 & 0 \\ 0 & 0 & 0 & 1 \end{pmatrix} \begin{pmatrix} \boldsymbol{\nu}_1 \\ \boldsymbol{\nu}_2 \\ \boldsymbol{\nu}_4 \\ \boldsymbol{\nu}_5 \end{pmatrix} + \begin{pmatrix} 0 & 2 & -4 & 3 \\ -1 & -2 & 3 & -3 \\ 0 & 1 & -2 & 2 \\ 0 & -1 & 1 & -1 \end{pmatrix} \begin{pmatrix} \boldsymbol{\nu}_3 \\ \boldsymbol{\nu}_6 \\ \boldsymbol{\nu}_7 \\ \boldsymbol{\nu}_8 \end{pmatrix} = \mathbf{0} \tag{25}$$

Since the matrix in the first term is an identity matrix, (25) gives an explicit functional representation between independent and dependent fluxes.

$$\begin{pmatrix} \boldsymbol{\nu}_1 \\ \boldsymbol{\nu}_2 \\ \boldsymbol{\nu}_4 \\ \boldsymbol{\nu}_5 \end{pmatrix} = \begin{pmatrix} 0 & -2 & 4 & -3 \\ 1 & 2 & -3 & 3 \\ 0 & -1 & 2 & -2 \\ 0 & 1 & -1 & 1 \end{pmatrix} \begin{pmatrix} \boldsymbol{\nu}_3 \\ \boldsymbol{\nu}_6 \\ \boldsymbol{\nu}_7 \\ \boldsymbol{\nu}_8 \end{pmatrix} \tag{26}$$

As a result of the parametrization, all possible states of dependent intracellular fluxes, $\boldsymbol{\nu}_{\mathrm{depend}} = (\boldsymbol{\nu}_1, \boldsymbol{\nu}_2, \boldsymbol{\nu}_4, \boldsymbol{\nu}_5)^{\mathrm{T}}$, can be generated by solely varying the independent fluxes, $\boldsymbol{\nu}_{\mathrm{independ}} = (\boldsymbol{\nu}_3, \boldsymbol{\nu}_6, \boldsymbol{\nu}_7, \boldsymbol{\nu}_8)^{\mathrm{T}}$, and this always obeys the stoichiometry of the system. It must be noted that the flux vector must be arranged such that the intracellular fluxes precede the measurable extracellular fluxes, i.e., $\boldsymbol{\nu} = (\boldsymbol{\nu}_{\mathrm{intra}} | \boldsymbol{\nu}_{\mathrm{extra}})$ to render $\boldsymbol{\nu}_{\mathrm{extra}}$ independent. Afterward, by differentiating the linear algebraic system of metabolite balances with respect to $\boldsymbol{\nu}$, one can straightforwardly obtain an appropriate stoichiometric matrix making $\boldsymbol{\nu}_{\mathrm{extra}}$ independent. Otherwise, the measurable fluxes may be selected as dependent.

It is obvious that v_7 and v_8 can be determined from the corresponding extracellular flux measurements. With only the kinetic data, the independent intracellular fluxes v_3 and v_7 would remain unknown. They are estimated from the functional correlation between metabolic flux states and ^{13}C labeling states which can be measured. Once the components of $\boldsymbol{v}_{\text{independ}}$ have been computed, we get all the fluxes as determined by (26).

Additional Equations Specified by the Modeler: The stoichiometric matrix for the intracellular reactions, $\mathbf{S}_{\text{intra}}$, can be augmented by providing additional "flux constraints." This is usually done by manually introducing additional user-defined equations that are linearly independent of stoichiometric balance equations (25), e.g., exchange fluxes, flux partitioning ratios, and/or reversibilities (14, 27, 39, 47–49). The flux partitioning ratios and the exchange fluxes are scaled to [0, 1]-range. This so-called compactification transforms the poorly scaled [0, ∞)-scaled fluxes (e.g., unknown fluxes in $\boldsymbol{v}_{\text{independ}}$) into the [0, 1]-scaled variables, which seems to be advantageous for the numerical computation of fluxes (49). However, these approaches necessitate logical operators to set the net directions of bidirectional reactions (exchange flux) or the direction has to be assumed in advance (reversibility).

Alternatively, one defines flux constraints using the information obtained from the reduced row echelon form (24). As shown by (24) and (25), the independent fluxes can be detected using matrix operation in a single effort. Among these, the extracellular fluxes have the corresponding measurements and do not need to be rescaled. Their true values lie between, for example:

$$-\sigma_{\text{extra},i}\sqrt{\chi^2_{1,\phi}} \leq \boldsymbol{v}^*_{\text{extra},i} \leq +\sigma_{\text{extra},i}\sqrt{\chi^2_{1,\phi}} \tag{27}$$

Here $\boldsymbol{v}^*_{\text{extra},i}$ denotes the true flux value, $\sigma_{\text{extra},i}$ is the measurement error, and $\chi^2_{1,\phi}$ is the inverse of χ^2-cumulative distribution function value at a certain confidence level of ϕ. Hence, the range covers $100 \times \phi$ % of possible experimental observations. As a result, the search space for the extracellular fluxes can be reduced for the optimization process such as (17).

In comparison, the intracellular fluxes selected as independent can be compactified using a simple single rule such that:

$$\varphi_i = \frac{\boldsymbol{v}_i}{\alpha + \boldsymbol{v}_i} \quad \text{with } 0 \leq \boldsymbol{v}_i < \infty \wedge \alpha > 0 \Rightarrow \varphi_i \in [0, 1) \tag{28}$$

The φ_i is the additional flux constraint defined by user and α is a certain real number satisfying $\alpha > 0$. For convenience, we denote φ_i the [0, 1)-flux and α as the parameter scaling constant. Because v_3 and v_6 are independent among the intracellular fluxes, we get two [0, 1)-fluxes for the example network in Fig. 5.

$$\varphi_3 = \frac{\boldsymbol{v}_3}{\alpha + \boldsymbol{v}_3} \tag{29}$$

$$\varphi_6 = \frac{\boldsymbol{v}_6}{\alpha + \boldsymbol{v}_6} \tag{30}$$

The above compactification of fluxes, the [0, 1)-fluxes $\boldsymbol{\varphi}$, is a bijection of the [0, ∞) domain onto a [0, 1) range: if $v_i \to 0$, $\varphi_i \to 0$, and if $v_i \to \infty$, $\varphi_i \to 1$ for a certain parameter scaling constant where $\alpha > 0$. The equations are linear with respect to the fluxes and are linearly independent of each other as well as of the stoichiometric balances (18)–(21).

These [0, 1)-fluxes can potentially elevate the output sensitivity for flux estimation. We define that the output sensitivities of ^{13}C labeling system with respect to fluxes and [0, 1)-fluxes are $\partial \mathbf{x}_{\text{ext}}/\partial \boldsymbol{v}$ and $\partial \mathbf{x}_{\text{ext}}/\partial \boldsymbol{\varphi}$, respectively, where the latter equals $(\partial \mathbf{x}_{\text{ext}}/\partial \boldsymbol{v})\cdot(\partial \boldsymbol{v}/\partial \boldsymbol{\varphi})$ by the chain rule. Differentiating v_i with respect to φ_i results in the following, from (28):

$$\frac{\mathrm{d}\boldsymbol{v}_i}{\mathrm{d}\varphi_i} = \frac{\alpha}{(1-\varphi_i)^2} \tag{31}$$

Obviously, the sensitivity increases by the compactification if $\alpha > (1-\varphi_i)^2$, i.e., $\mathrm{d}v_i/\mathrm{d}\varphi_i > 1$ holds. This is because $\partial \mathbf{x}_{\text{ext}}/\partial \varphi = (\partial \mathbf{x}_{\text{ext}}/\partial \boldsymbol{v}) \cdot (\partial \boldsymbol{v}/\partial \varphi)$. In particular, a higher sensitivity can always be obtained by setting $\alpha \geq 1$ due to the finite values of fluxes, that is, $0 \leq v_i < \infty$ or $0 \leq \varphi_i < 1$. Hence, setting the parameter scaling constant $\alpha \geq 1$ is more reasonable for numerical optimization than $\alpha > 0$.

By introducing the flux constraints, the matrices of (23) are augmented by two additional equations of (29) and (30) such that $\mathbf{S}_{\text{intra.aug}}\boldsymbol{v}_{\text{intra}} = -\mathbf{S}_{\text{extra.aug}}\boldsymbol{\Theta}$, i.e.:

$$\begin{pmatrix} -1 & -1 & 1 & 0 & 0 & 0 \\ 0 & 1 & -1 & 1 & -1 & 0 \\ 0 & 0 & 0 & 1 & 2 & -1 \\ 1 & 0 & 0 & -2 & 0 & 0 \\ 0 & 0 & \varphi_3 - 1 & 0 & 0 & 0 \\ 0 & 0 & 0 & 0 & 0 & \varphi_6 - 1 \end{pmatrix} \cdot \begin{pmatrix} \boldsymbol{v}_1 \\ \boldsymbol{v}_2 \\ \boldsymbol{v}_3 \\ \boldsymbol{v}_4 \\ \boldsymbol{v}_5 \\ \boldsymbol{v}_6 \end{pmatrix}$$
$$= \begin{pmatrix} -1 & 0 & 0 & 0 \\ 0 & 0 & 0 & 0 \\ 0 & 0 & 0 & 0 \\ 0 & 1 & 0 & 0 \\ 0 & 0 & -\alpha & 0 \\ 0 & 0 & 0 & -\alpha \end{pmatrix} \cdot \begin{pmatrix} \boldsymbol{v}_7 \\ \boldsymbol{v}_8 \\ \varphi_3 \\ \varphi_6 \end{pmatrix} \tag{32}$$

Here, $\boldsymbol{\Theta} = (\boldsymbol{v}_7, \boldsymbol{v}_8, \varphi_3, \varphi_6)^{\mathrm{T}}$ is the independent variable (design parameter) to be determined by solving (17), where the [0, 1)-fluxes, φ_3 and φ_6, need to be estimated from ^{13}C labeling measurements. The flux constraints defined in this manner are always linearly independent with the mass balances of (18)–(21). In our example, $\mathbf{S}_{\text{intra.aug}}$ with a dimension of 6×6 has a rank of 6 (full rank) unless both φ_3 and φ_6 are one, which is a priori satisfied as φ_i

is (0, 1)-scaled. Generalized, the matrix $\mathbf{S}_{\text{intra.aug}}$ is always invertible when independent fluxes are rescaled by (28), which gives explicit expressions for the intracellular fluxes.

Due to the occurrence of φ_i in the system matrix ($\mathbf{S}_{\text{intra.aug}}$), explicit expressions for the dependent fluxes are nonlinear with respect to $\mathbf{\Theta}$. By solving (32), we obtain:

$$\boldsymbol{\nu}_{\text{depend}} = \mathbf{n}_{\text{flux}}(\mathbf{\Theta}) \tag{33}$$

Here $\mathbf{n}_{\text{flux}} = (n_{\text{flux},1}, n_{\text{flux},2}, \ldots, n_{\text{flux},6})^{\text{T}}$ denotes the vector with analytical expressions for the dependent fluxes. The expressions can be obtained, e.g., by the symbolic equation-solving packages such as Maple (Maplesoft, Waterloo, ON, Canada) or the Symbolic Math Toolbox of MATLAB (The Mathworks, Natick, MA).

As a result of the parametrization, a certain flux state can be generated with respect to $\mathbf{\Theta}$, which always obeys stoichiometry, and the corresponding ^{13}C labeling states of intra- and extracellular metabolites can be computed for a certain ^{13}C substrate. To exclude physiologically meaningless ranges of the fluxes, $\boldsymbol{\nu} < \mathbf{0}$, the range of the independent variables has to be set as:

$$\Omega_{\text{flux}} = \{\mathbf{\Theta} \in \Re^{\mathbf{dim}\,\mathbf{\Theta}_{\text{free}}} | \mathbf{n}_{\text{flux}}(\mathbf{\Theta}) \geq \mathbf{0}\} \tag{34}$$

The Ω_{flux} denotes the feasible region of fluxes and flux parameters and "**dim**" is the dimension of the corresponding vector. Note that $\mathbf{\Theta}$ is bounded such that $0 \leq \varphi_i < 1$ and $v_{\text{extra},i}$ are as given by (27).

3.1.3. Representations of Isotopic Labeling Pattern

The central key of the carbon flux simulation is the computation of ^{13}C labeling states of metabolites. When a certain flux state is generated by the parametrization (33), one can compute ^{13}C labeling states of metabolites for one or more ^{13}C-labeled substrates. Currently, three methods suited for application to large-scale metabolic networks are widely used. They compute (1) positional labeling enrichments (Fig. 6a) based on carbon atom balances using atom mapping matrices (43) or (2) isotopomer distributions (Fig. 6b) based on carbon isotopomer balances and isotopomer mapping matrices (IMM) (44), (3) using cumomer fractions (Fig. 6c) and cumomer balances (45), respectively. The approaches (1) and (2) utilize numerical methods such as the Gauss–Seidel algorithm or a root-finding algorithm to solve labeling states, whereas (3) allows analytically solving the isotopomer distributions from a cascade of linear equations by linearly transforming the isotopomer space into cumomer space. These approaches utilize mapping matrices describing the mechanisms of carbon atom or isotopomer transitions. A more recent approach developed by Antoniewicz et al. (42) does not rely on such matrices; the so-called "elementary metabolite unit" concept reduces the number of variables involved in carbon flux simulation using a decomposition

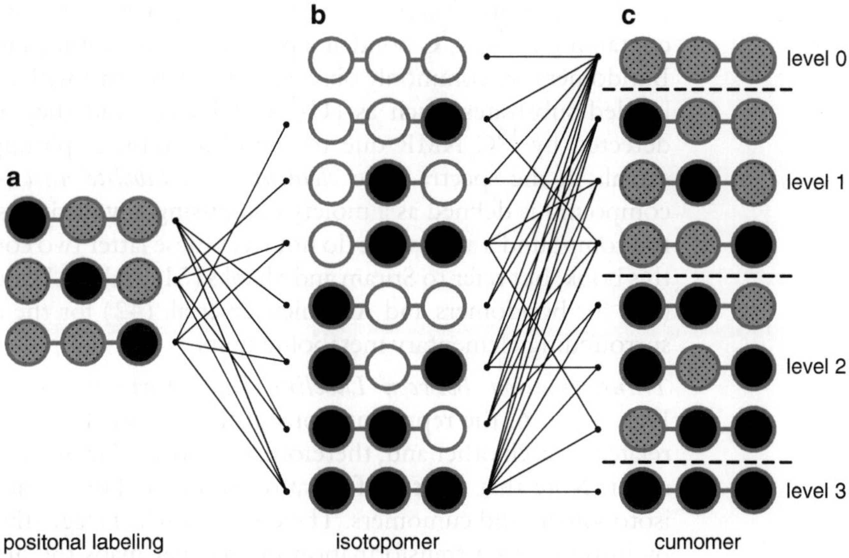

Fig. 6. Different representations of ^{13}C labeling patterns of positional labeling (**a**), isotopomer (**b**), and cumomer (**c**) and relations between the data formats: *white-colored circles* indicate ^{12}C (nonlabeled), *black-colored circles* are ^{13}C (labeled), and *gray-colored circles with dots* can be either ^{12}C or ^{13}C (nonlabeled or labeled).

method and gives same information as isotopomer or cumomer system.

As shown in Fig. 6a, the *positional representation* focuses on a particular carbon atom position of a compound that is labeled. For the molecule with three carbons in our example, it raises three variables representing the fractional labeling enrichment for each position, which can be measured using ^{1}H NMR.

In comparison, *carbon isotopomers* are all possible labeling patterns given by 2^n as explained in Sect. 3.1.1. The isotopomers can be transformed into mass isotopomers by summing the fractions of the isotopomers with the same mass and into the positional format by summing the fractions of the isotopomers labeled at a certain position as well (Fig. 6). Obviously, the isotopomer representation (Fig. 6b) has larger information than the positional representation. However, measuring the entire isotopomers of a compound is still restricted (50).

Cumomers (cumulated isotopomers) are a set of one or more isotopomers whose particular carbon positions are labeled. According to the number of the positional ^{13}C-labels considered, cumomers are grouped into different levels (Fig. 6b). For instance, level 0 indicates that any positions can be ^{12}C or ^{13}C. Level 1 indicates a particular position is ^{13}C but the other is ^{12}C or ^{13}C. Level 2 indicates two certain positions are ^{13}C but the other is ^{12}C or ^{13}C and so forth. The level 1 equals the positional representation. In Sect. 3.1.6, we show that grouping cumomers into different levels is essential for transforming a nonlinear isotopomer system into a linear one.

In addition, *bondomers* (51, 52) are a set of isotopomers containing a ^{13}C–^{13}C bond at a particular place within a molecule. Bondomers are commonly observed in experiments with uniformly labeled substrates, such as [U-$^{13}C_6$]glucose, and they are easily detected by ^{13}C NMR due to the characteristic splitting of the signals in the spectra. The *elementary metabolite unit* (42) of a compound is defined as a moiety comprising any distinct subset of the compound's atoms. We do not treat these latter two concepts in this book, but refer to Sriram and Shanks (51) and van Winden et al. (52) for bondomers and Antoniewicz et al. (42) for the concepts surrounding elementary metabolite units.

Transformation Between Labeling Data Formats: As shown by Figs. 4 and 6, the representations of the ^{13}C labeling patterns are related to each other and, therefore, transformed from one into the other. Note that the transformation is only bidirectional between isotopomers and cumomers. The conversion can elegantly be done by introducing a transformation matrix that maps the linear relations between two different data formats.

The conversion of the carbon isotopomer distribution into the corresponding mass isotopomer distribution (Fig. 4) can be represented as:

$$\mathbf{x}^{\mathrm{mdv}} = \mathbf{T}_{\mathrm{idv}\rightarrow\mathrm{mdv}}\mathbf{x}^{\mathrm{idv}} \stackrel{\mathrm{def}}{=} \begin{pmatrix} {}^{m+0}x \\ {}^{m+1}x \\ {}^{m+2}x \\ {}^{m+4}x \end{pmatrix}$$

$$= \begin{pmatrix} 1 & 0 & 0 & 0 & 0 & 0 & 0 & 0 \\ 0 & 1 & 1 & 0 & 1 & 0 & 0 & 0 \\ 0 & 0 & 0 & 1 & 0 & 1 & 1 & 0 \\ 0 & 0 & 0 & 0 & 0 & 0 & 0 & 1 \end{pmatrix} \begin{pmatrix} x_{000} \\ x_{001} \\ x_{010} \\ x_{011} \\ x_{100} \\ x_{101} \\ x_{110} \\ x_{111} \end{pmatrix} \tag{35}$$

Here $\mathbf{x}^{\mathrm{mdv}} = ({}^{m+0}x, {}^{m+1}x, {}^{m+0}x, {}^{m+0}x)^{\mathrm{T}}$ signifies the mass isotopomer distribution, $\mathbf{x}^{\mathrm{idv}} = (x_{000}, x_{001}, \ldots, x_{111})^{\mathrm{T}}$ is the isotopomer distribution, and $\mathbf{T}_{\mathrm{idv}\rightarrow\mathrm{mdv}}$ is the transformation matrix. The subscripts "000," "001,"..., "111" are the binary codes denoting the specific positional labeling patterns of isotopomers. As the rank of the transformation matrix is 4, the system is underdetermined when carbon isotopomers are calculated from the mass isotopomers, i.e., the conversion from $\mathbf{x}^{\mathrm{mdv}}$ into $\mathbf{x}^{\mathrm{idv}}$ using the pseudoinverse $\mathbf{x}^{\mathrm{idv}} = ({\mathbf{T}_{\mathrm{idv}\rightarrow\mathrm{mdv}}}^{\mathrm{T}}\mathbf{T}_{\mathrm{idv}\rightarrow\mathrm{mdv}})^{-1}{\mathbf{T}_{\mathrm{idv}\rightarrow\mathrm{mdv}}}^{\mathrm{T}}\mathbf{x}^{\mathrm{mdv}}$ is not possible.

Similarly, the positional labeling enrichment can also be obtained from $\mathbf{x}^{\mathrm{idv}}$.

$$\mathbf{x}^{\mathrm{p}} = \mathbf{T}_{\mathrm{idv}\to\mathrm{p}}\mathbf{x}^{\mathrm{idv}} \overset{\mathrm{def}}{=} \begin{pmatrix} x_1 \\ x_2 \\ x_3 \end{pmatrix}$$

$$= \begin{pmatrix} 0 & 0 & 0 & 0 & 1 & 1 & 1 & 1 \\ 0 & 0 & 1 & 1 & 0 & 0 & 1 & 1 \\ 0 & 1 & 0 & 1 & 0 & 1 & 0 & 1 \end{pmatrix} \mathbf{x}^{\mathrm{idv}} \qquad (36)$$

The vector $\mathbf{x}^{\mathrm{p}} = (x_1, x_2, x_3)^{\mathrm{T}}$ denotes the labeling enrichment of each carbon position and $\mathbf{T}_{\mathrm{idv}\to\mathrm{p}}$ is the transformation matrix from $\mathbf{x}^{\mathrm{idv}}$ to $\mathbf{x}^{\mathrm{p}}$, which is also rank-deficient (a singular matrix).

The cumomer fractions are related to its corresponding isotopomer distribution as follows.

$$\mathbf{x}^{\mathrm{cmf}} = \mathbf{T}_{\mathrm{idv}\to\mathrm{cmf}}\mathbf{x}^{\mathrm{idv}} \overset{\mathrm{def}}{=} \begin{pmatrix} x_{xxx} \\ x_{1xx} \\ x_{x1x} \\ x_{xx1} \\ x_{11x} \\ x_{1x1} \\ x_{x11} \\ x_{111} \end{pmatrix}$$

$$= \begin{pmatrix} 1 & 1 & 1 & 1 & 1 & 1 & 1 & 1 \\ 0 & 0 & 0 & 0 & 1 & 1 & 1 & 1 \\ 0 & 0 & 1 & 1 & 0 & 0 & 1 & 1 \\ 0 & 1 & 0 & 1 & 0 & 1 & 0 & 1 \\ 0 & 0 & 0 & 0 & 0 & 0 & 1 & 1 \\ 0 & 0 & 0 & 0 & 0 & 1 & 0 & 1 \\ 0 & 0 & 0 & 1 & 0 & 0 & 0 & 1 \\ 0 & 0 & 0 & 0 & 0 & 0 & 0 & 1 \end{pmatrix} \begin{pmatrix} x_{000} \\ x_{001} \\ x_{010} \\ x_{011} \\ x_{100} \\ x_{101} \\ x_{110} \\ x_{111} \end{pmatrix} \qquad (37)$$

Here $\mathbf{x}^{\mathrm{cmf}} = (x_{xxx}, x_{1xx}, \ldots, x_{111})^{\mathrm{T}}$ denotes the cumomer fractions of a compound, the subscript "1" is the ^{13}C-labeled position, and "x" is the position(s) either labeled or nonlabeled. Because the transformation is done by a square matrix $\mathbf{T}_{\mathrm{idv}\to\mathrm{cmf}}$ whose determinant is nonzero (full-rank), the inverse of $\mathbf{T}_{\mathrm{idv}\to\mathrm{cmf}}$ exist; the formats of $\mathbf{x}^{\mathrm{cmf}}$ and $\mathbf{x}^{\mathrm{idv}}$ are inter-convertible by (37) and $\mathbf{x}^{\mathrm{idv}} = (\mathbf{T}_{\mathrm{idv}\to\mathrm{cmf}})^{-1}\mathbf{x}^{\mathrm{idv}}$. Consequently, we can obtain $\mathbf{x}^{\mathrm{p}}$ or $\mathbf{x}^{\mathrm{mdv}}$ from $\mathbf{x}^{\mathrm{cmf}}$ as well. Thus, the models computing either $\mathbf{x}^{\mathrm{cmf}}$ or $\mathbf{x}^{\mathrm{idv}}$ can be applied to ^{13}C MFA in terms of NMR or MS measurements.

It has to be stated that $\mathbf{x}^{\mathrm{p}}$ and $\mathbf{x}^{\mathrm{mdv}}$ are not transformable into each other. This means MS measurements cannot straightforwardly be applied to a model computing $\mathbf{x}^{\mathrm{p}}$ or that measurements of xmdv and xp cannot be compared directly. In this case one can rely on the so-called "summed fractional labeling (x^{sfl})" (53). From $\mathbf{x}^{\mathrm{p}}$ and $\mathbf{x}^{\mathrm{mdv}}$, x^{sfl} is calculated by:

$$x^{\mathrm{sfl}} = \sum_{i=1}^{n} x_i \quad \text{with}\, \mathbf{x}^{\mathrm{p}} = (x_1, x_2, \ldots, x_n)^{\mathrm{T}} \qquad (38)$$

and

$$x^{\mathrm{sfl}} = \sum_{j=0}^{n} (j \cdot {}^{m+j}x) \quad \text{with } \mathbf{x}^{\mathrm{mdv}} = \left({}^{m+0}x, {}^{m+1}x, \ldots, {}^{m+n}x\right)^{\mathrm{T}} \tag{39}$$

respectively, where n is the number of carbon atoms of a compound.

3.1.4. Carbon Atom Model

The positional carbon transition from a reactant to a product follows a specific mechanism governed by the enzyme that catalyzes the intracellular reaction. As a result, we get the flux-dependent ^{13}C labeling patterns of metabolic products from one or more ^{13}C-labeled substrates. This is the underlying principle of ^{13}C MFA. The intracellular carbon atom fluxes can be modeled by setting up balances for the carbon atoms of each metabolite involved in the metabolic network as given by Zupke and Stephanopoulos (43). This can be most conveniently done by the use of the matrices which map the mechanism of the carbon transition.

Atom Mapping Matrices: An atom mapping matrix (AMM) has a dimension $p \times q$ for a reactant "**rea**" with q and a product "**met**" with p carbons. The (i, j)th element of the matrix is 1 if the ith carbon atom of the product originates from the jth of the reactant; otherwise, it is 0.

$$j\text{th carbon atom}_{\mathrm{rea}} \xrightarrow{\text{enzyme}} i\text{th carbon atom}_{\mathrm{met}} \Rightarrow \mathbf{AMM}_{\mathrm{rea>met}}(i,j) = 1 \tag{40}$$

For instance, pyruvate dehydrogenase releases the first carbon of pyruvate as CO_2, whereas its second and third carbon atom becomes the first and the second of acetyl-CoA, respectively. These positional transitions from pyruvate to acetyl-CoA can be arranged into a 2×3 matrix as follows:

$$\mathbf{AMM}_{\mathrm{pyr>acCoA}} = \begin{pmatrix} 1 & 0 & 0 \\ 0 & 1 & 0 \end{pmatrix} \tag{41}$$

Applying the above AMM, the positional isotopic enrichments of acetyl-CoA, $\mathbf{x}^{\mathrm{p}}_{\mathrm{acCoA}}$, can be calculated from that of pyruvate, $\mathbf{x}^{\mathrm{p}}_{\mathrm{pyr}}$, such that $\mathbf{x}^{\mathrm{p}}_{\mathrm{acCoA}} = \mathbf{AMM}_{\mathrm{pyr>acCoA}} \cdot \mathbf{x}^{\mathrm{p}}_{\mathrm{pyr}}$.

Stationary Carbon Atom Balances: For a large-scale problem where only the positional isotopic enrichment vectors (PIV) of input substrates $\mathbf{x}^{\mathrm{p}}_{\mathrm{inp},j}$ are known, those of other metabolites can be determined by solving an equation system of the carbon atom balances. Assuming the stationary or quasi-stationary state of an intracellular metabolite **met** with n carbon atoms evolving from p different reactions and reacting to q different metabolites, a carbon atom balance at an isotopic stationary state can be set up as follows:

$$\sum_{i=1}^{p} \left(\boldsymbol{\nu}_{\mathrm{in},i} s_i \mathbf{AMM}_{\mathrm{rea>met}} \mathbf{x}^{\mathrm{p}}_{\mathrm{rea},i}\right) - \mathbf{x}^{\mathrm{p}}_{\mathrm{met}} \sum_{j=1}^{q} \left(\boldsymbol{\nu}_{\mathrm{out},j} s_j\right) = 0 \tag{42}$$

Here, $\mathbf{x}^{\mathrm{p}}_{\mathrm{rea},i}$ are the PIVs of incoming reactants into the pool of **met**, $\mathbf{x}^{\mathrm{p}}_{\mathrm{met}}$ are the PIV of the **met** pool equaling the outgoing positional isotopic enrichments, v_{in} are the incoming fluxes, v_{out} are the outgoing fluxes, and s are the stoichiometric coefficients. Each entry of a PIV represents the fractional isotopic enrichment of the corresponding carbon position and is constrained such that:

$$\mathbf{x}^{\mathrm{p}}_{i} = \{\mathbf{x}^{\mathrm{p}}_{i} \in \Re^{n_{\mathrm{C}}} | \forall k : 0 \leq \mathbf{x}^{\mathrm{p}}_{i}(k) \leq 1\} \tag{43}$$

Here, n_{C} denotes the number of carbon atoms in the skeleton of a metabolite and k is the index from 1 to n_{C}. For a network with n metabolites, a linear system $\mathbf{F}(\mathbf{x}^{\mathrm{p}})$ containing n balances of (42) with n PIVs can be constructed.

$$\mathbf{F}(\mathbf{x}^{\mathrm{p}}) = \begin{pmatrix} \mathbf{f}_1(\mathbf{x}^{\mathrm{p}}_1, \mathbf{x}^{\mathrm{p}}_2, \ldots, \mathbf{x}^{\mathrm{p}}_n) \\ \mathbf{f}_2(\mathbf{x}^{\mathrm{p}}_1, \mathbf{x}^{\mathrm{p}}_2, \ldots, \mathbf{x}^{\mathrm{p}}_n) \\ \vdots \\ \mathbf{f}_n(\mathbf{x}^{\mathrm{p}}_1, \mathbf{x}^{\mathrm{p}}_2, \ldots, \mathbf{x}^{\mathrm{p}}_n) \end{pmatrix} = \mathbf{A}\mathbf{x}^{\mathrm{p}} + \mathbf{B}\mathbf{x}^{\mathrm{p}}_{\mathrm{inp}} = \mathbf{0} \tag{44}$$

The $\mathbf{f}_i$ is the carbon atom balance equation set up around n metabolites, $\mathbf{x}^{\mathrm{p}}$ is the set of all unknown n variables, i.e., $\mathbf{x}^{\mathrm{p}} = (\mathbf{x}^{\mathrm{p}}_1, \mathbf{x}^{\mathrm{p}}_2, \ldots \mathbf{x}^{\mathrm{p}}_n)^{\mathrm{T}}$, and $\mathbf{x}^{\mathrm{p}}_{\mathrm{inp}}$ is the set of m input substrates with known PIV, i.e., $\mathbf{x}^{\mathrm{p}}_{\mathrm{inp}} = (\mathbf{x}^{\mathrm{p}}_{\mathrm{inp},1}, \mathbf{x}^{\mathrm{p}}_{\mathrm{inp},2}, \ldots, \mathbf{x}^{\mathrm{p}}_{\mathrm{inp},n})^{\mathrm{T}}$. The system $\mathbf{F}(\mathbf{x}^{\mathrm{p}}) = \mathbf{0}$ is a linear problem that can be formulated as $\mathbf{A}\mathbf{x}^{\mathrm{p}} + \mathbf{B}\mathbf{x}^{\mathrm{p}}_{\mathrm{inp}} = \mathbf{0}$. The matrix $\mathbf{A}$ equals the partial derivatives of $\partial\mathbf{F}/\partial\mathbf{x}^{\mathrm{p}}$ and $\mathbf{B}$ those of $\partial\mathbf{F}/\partial\mathbf{x}^{\mathrm{p}}_{\mathrm{inp}}$. Because there are as many scalar variables as the sum of n_{C} of each n metabolite, $\mathbf{A}$ is a square matrix. If $\mathbf{A}$ is nonsingular and thus invertible, we get $\mathbf{x}^{\mathrm{p}}$ at a certain flux state by solving $-\mathbf{A}^{-1}\mathbf{B}\mathbf{x}^{\mathrm{p}}_{\mathrm{inp}}$. Alternatively, an indirect method can be applied instead of the matrix inversion, e.g., the Gauss–Seidel method (54).

Example: Suppose the carbon atom transitions between the metabolites A, B, C, D, and the substrate (S) in the example metabolic network (Fig. 5) as given in Fig. 7.

For the enzyme reactions involved in the network, the following AMMs can be formulated: $\mathbf{AMM}_{\mathrm{S>A}} = \mathbf{AMM}_{\mathrm{A>B}} = \mathbf{AMM}_{\mathrm{B>A}} = (1,0,0;0,1,0;0,0,1)$, $\mathbf{AMM}_{\mathrm{A>D}} = (0,1,0;0,0,1)$, $\mathbf{AMM}_{\mathrm{B>C}} = ½((0,1,0)+(0,0,1))$, $\mathbf{AMM}_{\mathrm{D_1>B}} = (0,0;0,0;1,0)$, $\mathbf{AMM}_{\mathrm{D_2>B}} = (0,1;1,0;0,0)$, $\mathbf{AMM}_{\mathrm{D_1>C}} = (0,1)$, and $\mathbf{AMM}_{\mathrm{D_2>C}} = (0,0)$. Here, the factor is ½ for $\mathbf{AMM}_{\mathrm{B>C}}$ because C can be formed either from the first or the third carbon of B. The conversion of D into B as well as into B and C is a bimolecular reaction: 2D → B and 2D → B + C. We define D_1 (dotted red line) and D_2 (dotted red line) to distinguish two different carbon transition mechanisms from D to B or C as shown by the above AMMs. This is also convenient later when modeling the carbon isotopomer network.

As given by (42), stationary carbon atom balances can be set up around metabolites in the network using the AMMs defined above.

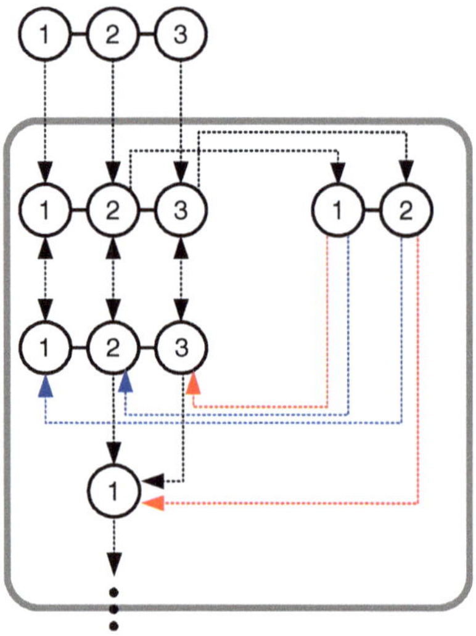

Fig. 7. Carbon atom transitions in the example network shown in Fig. 5. The *digits* in the circles indicate the positions of the carbon atom. The first carbon of metabolite A and B is released out of the system when converted into D and C, respectively.

$$
\begin{aligned}
&(\boldsymbol{\nu}_1+\boldsymbol{\nu}_2)\mathbf{x}_{\mathrm{A}}^{\mathrm{P}}-(\boldsymbol{\nu}_3\mathbf{AMM}_{\mathrm{B>A}}\mathbf{x}_{\mathrm{B}}^{\mathrm{P}}+\boldsymbol{\nu}_7\mathbf{AMM}_{\mathrm{S>A}}\mathbf{x}_{\mathrm{S}}^{\mathrm{P}})=\mathbf{0}\\
&(\boldsymbol{\nu}_3+\boldsymbol{\nu}_5)\mathbf{x}_{\mathrm{B}}^{\mathrm{P}}-(\boldsymbol{\nu}_2\mathbf{AMM}_{\mathrm{A>B}}\mathbf{x}_{\mathrm{A}}^{\mathrm{P}}+\boldsymbol{\nu}_4\mathbf{AMM}_{\mathrm{D_1>B}}\mathbf{x}_{\mathrm{D}}^{\mathrm{P}}+\boldsymbol{\nu}_4\mathbf{AMM}_{\mathrm{D_2>B}}\mathbf{x}_{\mathrm{D}}^{\mathrm{P}})=\mathbf{0}\\
&\boldsymbol{\nu}_6\mathbf{x}_{\mathrm{C}}^{\mathrm{P}}-(\boldsymbol{\nu}_4\mathbf{AMM}_{\mathrm{D_1>C}}\mathbf{x}_{\mathrm{D}}^{\mathrm{P}}+\boldsymbol{\nu}_4\mathbf{AMM}_{\mathrm{D_2>C}}\mathbf{x}_{\mathrm{D}}^{\mathrm{P}}+2\boldsymbol{\nu}_5\mathbf{AMM}_{\mathrm{B>C}}\mathbf{x}_{\mathrm{B}}^{\mathrm{P}})=\mathbf{0}\\
&(2\boldsymbol{\nu}_4+\boldsymbol{\nu}_8)\mathbf{x}_{\mathrm{D}}^{\mathrm{P}}-\boldsymbol{\nu}_1\mathbf{AMM}_{\mathrm{A>D}}\mathbf{x}_{\mathrm{A}}^{\mathrm{P}}=\mathbf{0}
\end{aligned}
\tag{45}
$$

The above linear system consisting of four vector-valued equations represents the nine balance equations for all nine carbon atoms involved in the network. It is clear that the use of AMMs facilitates formulating balances for a large system.

1. *Direct Method by Matrix Inversion*: The above system can be rewritten in terms of matrix-vector notation such that:

$$
\begin{pmatrix}
(\boldsymbol{\nu}_1+\boldsymbol{\nu}_2)\mathbf{I}_{3\times3} & -\boldsymbol{\nu}_3\mathbf{AMM}_{\mathrm{B>A}} & \mathbf{0}_{3\times1} & \mathbf{0}_{3\times2}\\
-\boldsymbol{\nu}_2\mathbf{AMM}_{\mathrm{A>B}} & (\boldsymbol{\nu}_3+\boldsymbol{\nu}_5)\mathbf{I}_{3\times3} & \mathbf{0}_{3\times1} & -\boldsymbol{\nu}_4(\mathbf{AMM}_{\mathrm{D_1>B}}+\mathbf{AMM}_{\mathrm{D_2>B}})\\
\mathbf{0}_{1\times3} & 2\boldsymbol{\nu}_5\mathbf{AMM}_{\mathrm{B>C}} & \boldsymbol{\nu}_6\mathbf{I}_{1\times1} & -\boldsymbol{\nu}_4(\mathbf{AMM}_{\mathrm{D_1>C}}+\mathbf{AMM}_{\mathrm{D_2>C}})\\
-\boldsymbol{\nu}_1\mathbf{AMM}_{\mathrm{A>D}} & \mathbf{0}_{2\times3} & \mathbf{0}_{2\times1} & (2\boldsymbol{\nu}_4+\boldsymbol{\nu}_8)\mathbf{I}_{2\times2}
\end{pmatrix}
\mathbf{x}^{\mathrm{P}}+
\begin{pmatrix}
\boldsymbol{\nu}_7\mathbf{AMM}_{\mathrm{S>A}}\\
\mathbf{0}_{3\times3}\\
\mathbf{0}_{1\times3}\\
\mathbf{0}_{2\times3}
\end{pmatrix}
\mathbf{x}_{\mathrm{inp}}^{\mathrm{P}}=\mathbf{0}
\tag{46}
$$

The first matrix equals $\partial\mathbf{F}/\partial\mathbf{x}^{\mathrm{P}}$, the second equals $\partial\mathbf{F}/\partial\mathbf{x}_{\mathrm{inp}}^{\mathrm{P}}$ where $\mathbf{x}^{\mathrm{P}}=(\mathbf{x}_{\mathrm{A}}^{\mathrm{P}},\mathbf{x}_{\mathrm{B}}^{\mathrm{P}},\mathbf{x}_{\mathrm{C}}^{\mathrm{P}},\mathbf{x}_{\mathrm{D}}^{\mathrm{P}})$ and $\mathbf{x}_{\mathrm{inp}}^{\mathrm{P}}=\mathbf{x}_{\mathrm{S}}^{\mathrm{P}}$. $\mathbf{I}_{n\times m}$ denotes an identity matrix with a dimension of $n\times m$ and $\mathbf{0}_{n\times m}$ is an empty matrix with a dimension of $n\times m$. The matrix $\partial\mathbf{F}/\partial\mathbf{x}^{\mathrm{P}}$

is diagonal dominant, i.e., the absolute value of each diagonal element is greater than or equal to the sum of the absolute values of the other elements in its row. Obviously, the sum of outgoing fluxes (diagonal element) cannot be smaller than the sum of incoming fluxes (elements in the corresponding row), given by (1). In addition, the sum of a row or an AMM cannot be greater than 1 as defined in (40). Thus, the diagonal dominance always holds true and is sufficient for matrix invertiblity (a noninvertible matrix cannot be diagonal dominant). In this regard, the matrix $\partial \mathbf{F}/\partial \mathbf{x}^{\mathrm{P}}$ is always invertible unless disconnections occur in the network. (A network is disconnected when one or more intracellular fluxes are zero, which results in zero elements in the diagonal.) Finally, computing $-(\partial \mathbf{F}/\partial \mathbf{x}^{\mathrm{P}})^{-1}(\partial \mathbf{F}/\partial \mathbf{x}^{\mathrm{P}}_{\mathrm{inp}})\mathbf{x}^{\mathrm{P}}_{\mathrm{inp}}$ results in the flux-dependent $\mathbf{x}^{\mathrm{P}}$ values for one or more ^{13}C inputs defined in $\mathbf{x}^{\mathrm{P}}_{\mathrm{inp}}$.

2. *Gauss–Seidel Algorithm*: Alternatively, a linear problem $\mathbf{b} - \mathbf{A} \cdot \mathbf{x} = \mathbf{0}$ can also be solved iteratively. The system matrix $\mathbf{A}$ can be decomposed into three matrices, i.e., a diagonal ($\mathbf{I}$), a lower triangular ($\mathbf{L}$), and an upper triangular matrix ($\mathbf{U}$), which results in $\mathbf{b} - (\mathbf{I} + \mathbf{L} + \mathbf{U}) \cdot \mathbf{x} = \mathbf{0}$. Subsequently, we obtain an equation of:

$$\mathbf{x} = \mathbf{b} - (\mathbf{Lx} + \mathbf{Ux}) \tag{47}$$

The above equation can be solved iteratively by redefining the problem as:

$$\mathbf{x}_{k+1} = \mathbf{b} - (\mathbf{L}\mathbf{x}_{k+1} + \mathbf{U}\mathbf{x}_k) \tag{48}$$

Its sufficient condition for convergence is the matrix norm of:

$$||-(\mathbf{I} + \mathbf{L})^{-1}\mathbf{U}|| \leq 1 \tag{49}$$

Initiating an iteration loop with an arbitrary set of variables, e.g., $\mathbf{x}_k = \mathbf{x}_0$, the next iterate $\mathbf{x}_{k+1}$ can be updated from the current iterate $\mathbf{x}_k$ because $\mathbf{x}_{k+1}$ appears only in the diagonal and the lower triangular matrix (Fig. 8). By repeating the iterative process, $\mathbf{x}$ will converge to its solution, which equals the minimum of $||\mathbf{d}_x||^2 = (\mathbf{x}_k - \mathbf{x}_{k+1})^{\mathrm{T}} \cdot (\mathbf{x}_k - \mathbf{x}_{k+1})$. To apply the algorithm, the carbon atom balances have to be formulated such as (48). Here, the key of modeling is how to define the kth and (k + 1)th variables.

As depicted in Fig. 8, each of the diagonal variables for which the corresponding balance is set up are placed as the (k + 1)th variables at the left-hand side. At the right-hand side of the ith equation, a variable is the kth if its balance equation appears later than the index i (upper triangular variables); otherwise, we use the (k + 1)th variable (lower triangular variables). Finally, we get a proper formulation whose variables in the diagonal and the lower triangular matrix can be updated from

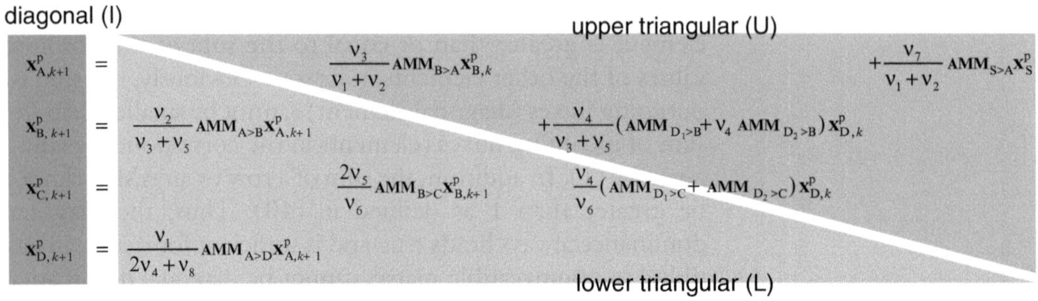

Fig. 8. An example of decomposing the carbon atom balances of (8.45) in two/three parts suited to the Gauss–Seidel algorithm.

those of the upper triangular matrix. As a consequence, the flux-dependent $\mathbf{x}^{\mathrm{P}}$ values can be computed for known ^{13}C input of $\mathbf{x}^{\mathrm{P}}_{\mathrm{inp}}$ by iteration.

In practice, the achievable minimum of $||\mathbf{d}_x||^2$ does not usually equal zero due to finite precision of numerical computation. Thus, an appropriate termination criterion is required to prevent unnecessary iteration cycles with negligible decrease in $||\mathbf{d}_x||^2$. For instance, one can set the termination criterion such that $||\mathbf{d}_x||^2 \leq$ a small number, e.g., the floating-point relative accuracy.

3.1.5. Carbon Isotopomer Model

For a molecule with n_{C} carbon atoms, there are $2^{n_{\mathrm{C}}}$ stable carbon isotopomers resulting from k-subset (repeatable variations; $k = n_{\mathrm{C}}$) of stable carbon isotopes of ^{12}C and ^{13}C. Due to the positional carbon atom transitions of intracellular reactions, the distributions of carbon isotopomers are also characteristic for flux states. Therefore, these distributions can also be used as additional information to perform MFA when the metabolic network is underdetermined.

As shown in Sect. 3.1.4, each enzyme reaction of a carbon atom network involves q reactant carbon atoms to be mapped into p product carbon atoms, whereas 2^q reactant isotopomers are converted into 2^p product isotopomers in a carbon isotopomer network. Therefore, large numbers of balance equations occur in a carbon isotopomer model and it would be cumbersome to set up all balances individually. Analogous to the carbon atom model, mapping matrices can be used to group all isotopomer reactions involved in an enzyme reaction, which simplifies the balancing problems.

Isotopomer Mapping Matrices: These so-called IMMs can be constructed using AMMs and possible labeling patterns of isotopomers as proposed by Schmidt et al. (44). As explained in Sect. 3.1.1, one can express the isotopomer labeling patterns (ILPs) of a compound using 0 and 1 representing ^{12}C and ^{13}C carbon, respectively. For example, the ith ILP is obtained by converting the decimal number "$i - 1$" into binary digits. In case the number of digits n_{bin} is smaller than the number of carbon atoms n_C, additional $n_C - n_{bin}$ zeros have to be prefixed to the binary digits. For instance, the fourth ILP gives binary digits of "11" and for a compound with six carbons, four zeros have to be prefixed to the digits, i.e., "000011." The digits denote that the fifth and the sixth carbon of the fourth isotopomer are ^{13}C atoms (indicated by digit "1"), whereas the other positions are ^{12}C atoms (indicated by digit "0"). In this manner, all possible 2^{n_C} ILPs of a compound can be digitized.

Composing a matrix (**IPL**) whose each row is the particular binary digit, e.g., (0, 0, 0, 0, 1, 1), and multiplying this with the corresponding AMM gives the labeling pattern of the isotopomer produced from the reactant isotopomer. Subsequently, the resulting vector can be converted into its decimal number n_{dec}, which is the index of the product isotopomer when i is obtained, i.e., $i = n_{dec} - 1$. When repeating the procedure for all possible isotopomers of the reactant, it can be declared which isotopomers of the product originate from which isotopomers of the reactant. Using the indices, the reactant–product relations of isotopomer reactions can be mapped using a matrix. For a monomolecular reaction **rea** → **met**, the (i, j)th element of an IMM is 1 if the ith ILP of **met** originates from the jth of **rea**; otherwise, it is 0.

$$\mathbf{AMM}_{\text{rea>met}}(j\text{th row of }\mathbf{ILP}_{\text{rea}})^{\mathrm{T}} = (i\text{th row of }\mathbf{ILP}_{\text{met}})^{\mathrm{T}} \Rightarrow \mathbf{IMM}_{\text{rea>met}}(i,j) = 1 \quad (50)$$

When more than one mole of product is produced from one mole of reactant, as in the reaction from B to C in Fig. 7, we need to consider each carbon transition mechanism separately. For the above example, we first get an IMM using (0 1 0) and the other using (0 0 1). We obtain $\mathbf{IMM}_{B > C}$ by summing the two IMMs and dividing by two.

For a bimolecular reaction **rea1** + **rea2** → **met**, we get two separate matrices $\mathbf{IMM}_{\text{rea1 > met}}$ and $\mathbf{IMM}_{\text{rea2 > met}}$. Hereto, all possible combinations of two reactant isotopomers have to be taken into account. The matrices can be obtained using a double-nested loop operation. For instance, $\mathbf{IMM}_{\text{rea1 > met}}$ can be obtained by the following loop operation:

Initialize the first loop with $k = 1$.

Repeat operation from 1 to 4.

1. Get vector 1 by multiplying $\mathbf{AMM}_{\text{rea1 > met}}$ with the transpose of the kth row of $\mathbf{ILP}_{\text{rea1}}$.
2. Initialize the second loop with $j = 1$.

   Repeat operation from (a) to (f).

   (a) Get vector 2 by multiplying $\mathbf{AMM}_{\text{rea2 > met}}$ with the transpose of the jth row of $\mathbf{ILP}_{\text{rea2}}$.

   (b) Add vector 1 and vector 2 to get vector 3.
   (c) Get index $\boldsymbol{i}$ by converting the binary digits consisting of the elements in vector 3 into a decimal number.
   (d) Set ($\boldsymbol{i}$ − 1, k)th element of $\mathbf{IMM}_{\mathrm{rea1>met}}$ as 1.
   (e) Increase j by one.
   (f) Stop operation from (a) to (e) if j reaches 2^q.
3. Increase k by one.
4. Stop operation from 1 to 3 if k reaches 2^p.

Here, p is the number of carbon atoms of **rea1** and q that of **rea2**.

Stationary Carbon Isotopomer Balances: Assuming the stationary or quasi-stationary state of an intracellular metabolite **met** with n_C carbon atoms evolving from p different reactions and reacting to q different metabolites, a stationary isotopomer balance equation can be set up as follows:

$$\sum_{i=1}^{p}\left(\boldsymbol{\nu}_{\mathrm{in},i}s_i\mathbf{x}_{\mathrm{met},i}^{\mathrm{idv}^*}\right)-\mathbf{x}_{\mathrm{met}}^{\mathrm{idv}}\sum_{j=1}^{q}\left(\boldsymbol{\nu}_{\mathrm{out},j}s_j\right)=0 \tag{51}$$

Here, $\mathbf{x}_{\mathrm{met}}^{\mathrm{idv}^*}$ denotes the isotopomer distribution vector (IDV) of an incoming metabolite into the pool of **met** and $\mathbf{x}_{\mathrm{met}}^{\mathrm{idv}}$ is the IDV of the pool, equaling the outgoing isotopomer distribution. An IDV is constrained such that:

$$\mathbf{x}_i^{\mathrm{idv}}=\{\mathbf{x}_i^{\mathrm{idv}}\in\Re^{2^{n_C}}\,|\sum_{k=1}^{2^{n_C}}\mathbf{x}_i^{\mathrm{idv}}(k)=1\wedge\forall k:0\le\mathbf{x}_i^{\mathrm{idv}}(k)\le 1\} \tag{52}$$

The n_C denotes the number of carbon atoms in the skeleton of a metabolite and k is the index of each IDV element of **met**.

To calculate $\mathbf{x}_{\mathrm{met}}^{\mathrm{idv}*}$, both isotopomer distribution of reactants $\mathbf{x}_{\mathrm{rea}}^{\mathrm{idv}}$ and the corresponding IMM are required. For a monomolecular reaction (**rea** → **met**), we get:

$$\mathbf{x}_{\mathrm{met}}^{\mathrm{idv}*}=\mathbf{IMM}_{\mathrm{rea>met}}\cdot\mathbf{x}_{\mathrm{rea}}^{\mathrm{idv}} \tag{53}$$

For a bimolecular reaction (**rea1** + **rea2** → **met**), we get:

$$\mathbf{x}_{\mathrm{met}}^{\mathrm{idv}*}=\left(\mathbf{IMM}_{\mathrm{rea1>met}}\cdot\mathbf{x}_{\mathrm{rea1}}^{\mathrm{idv}}\right)\otimes\left(\mathbf{IMM}_{\mathrm{rea2>met}}\cdot\mathbf{x}_{\mathrm{rea2}}^{\mathrm{idv}}\right) \tag{54}$$

The **rea** denotes a reactant molecule in a monomolecular reaction, **rea1** and **rea2** are the reactant pair in a bimolecular reaction, $\mathbf{IMM}_{\mathrm{rea>met}}$ is the isotopomer mapping matrix for an isotopomer reaction from **rea** to **met**, and ⊗ is the element-wise multiplication of two vectors. For a network with n metabolites, a nonlinear system $\mathbf{F}(\mathbf{x}^{\mathrm{idv}})$ containing n balances of (51) with n vector-valued variables (IDVs) is constructed.

$$\mathbf{F}(\mathbf{x}^{\mathrm{idv}}) = \begin{pmatrix} \mathbf{f}_1(\mathbf{x}_1^{\mathrm{idv}}, \mathbf{x}_2^{\mathrm{idv}}, \ldots, \mathbf{x}_n^{\mathrm{idv}}) \\ \mathbf{f}_2(\mathbf{x}_1^{\mathrm{idv}}, \mathbf{x}_2^{\mathrm{idv}}, \ldots, \mathbf{x}_n^{\mathrm{idv}}) \\ \vdots \\ \mathbf{f}_n(\mathbf{x}_1^{\mathrm{idv}}, \mathbf{x}_2^{\mathrm{idv}}, \ldots, \mathbf{x}_n^{\mathrm{idv}}) \end{pmatrix} = 0 \tag{55}$$

Here, **f** is an isotopomer balance equation that is nonlinear due to the element-wise multiplication, **F** is the equation system containing n variables and n equations, $\mathbf{x}^{\mathrm{idv}}$ is the set of all unknown n IDVs, and $\mathbf{x}^{\mathrm{idv}} = (\mathbf{x}_1^{\mathrm{idv}}, \mathbf{x}_2^{\mathrm{idv}}, \ldots, \mathbf{x}_n^{\mathrm{idv}})^{\mathrm{T}}$.

For the example network in Fig. 7, the following balances can be set up:

$$\begin{aligned}
&(\boldsymbol{\nu}_1 + \boldsymbol{\nu}_2)\mathbf{x}_{\mathrm{A}}^{\mathrm{idv}} - (\boldsymbol{\nu}_3 \mathbf{IMM}_{\mathrm{B>A}}\mathbf{x}_{\mathrm{B}}^{\mathrm{idv}} + \boldsymbol{\nu}_7 \mathbf{IMM}_{\mathrm{S>A}}\mathbf{x}_{\mathrm{S}}^{\mathrm{idv}}) = \mathbf{0} \\
&(\boldsymbol{\nu}_3 + \boldsymbol{\nu}_5)\mathbf{x}_{\mathrm{B}}^{\mathrm{idv}} - (\boldsymbol{\nu}_2 \mathbf{IMM}_{\mathrm{A>B}}\mathbf{x}_{\mathrm{A}}^{\mathrm{idv}} + \boldsymbol{\nu}_4 (\mathbf{IMM}_{\mathrm{D_1>B}}\mathbf{x}_{\mathrm{D}}^{\mathrm{idv}}) \otimes (\mathbf{IMM}_{\mathrm{D_2>B}}\mathbf{x}_{\mathrm{D}}^{\mathrm{idv}})) = \mathbf{0} \\
&\boldsymbol{\nu}_6 \mathbf{x}_{\mathrm{C}}^{\mathrm{idv}} - ((\boldsymbol{\nu}_4 \mathbf{IMM}_{\mathrm{D_1>C}}\mathbf{x}_{\mathrm{D}}^{\mathrm{idv}}) \otimes (\mathbf{IMM}_{\mathrm{D_2>C}}\mathbf{x}_{\mathrm{D}}^{\mathrm{idv}}) + 2\boldsymbol{\nu}_5 \mathbf{IMM}_{\mathrm{B>C}}\mathbf{x}_{\mathrm{B}}^{\mathrm{idv}}) = \mathbf{0} \\
&(2\boldsymbol{\nu}_4 + \boldsymbol{\nu}_8)\mathbf{x}_{\mathrm{D}}^{\mathrm{idv}} - \boldsymbol{\nu}_1 \mathbf{IMM}_{\mathrm{A>D}}\mathbf{x}_{\mathrm{A}}^{\mathrm{idv}} = \mathbf{0}
\end{aligned} \tag{56}$$

The above 4 vector equations imply 22 variables for the isotopomers of 4 metabolites. To solve flux- and ^{13}C-input ($\mathbf{x}_{\mathrm{S}}^{\mathrm{idv}}$)-dependent isotopomer distributions, a numerical method is required because we have a nonlinear problem. Hereto, methods such as relaxation techniques (44) or certain root-finding algorithm (55) can be employed.

Root Finding for a System of Nonlinear Equations: In many applications we need to find values of the variables in a model satisfying a number of given relations. In particular, when these relations take the form of n equalities for n variables such as (55), the problem is termed as root finding, i.e., finding **x** that satisfy:

$$\mathbf{F}(\mathbf{x}) = \mathbf{0} \tag{57}$$

The **F**: $\mathcal{R}^n \rightarrow \mathcal{R}^n$ is a vector function. This root finding is typically involved in solving a nonlinear system. There are various methods apropos of the root finding as exemplified in Nocedal and Wright (19) and Press (56). Among those, we treat two approaches here, which can be applied for solving (55) or the example (56).

1. *Newton Method*: Using the Taylor's first-order approximation around the current iterate $\mathbf{x}_k$ (in the neighborhood of $\mathbf{x}_k$), the vector function $\mathbf{F}(\mathbf{x}_k)$ can be expanded about the point $\mathbf{x}_{k+1} = \mathbf{x}_k + \mathbf{d}_x$ such that:

$$\mathbf{F}(\mathbf{x}_k + \mathbf{d}_x) = \mathbf{F}(\mathbf{x}_{k+1}) = \mathbf{F}(\mathbf{x}_k) + \mathbf{J}(\mathbf{x}_k)\mathbf{d}_x \tag{58}$$

Here $\mathbf{x} = (x_1, x_2, \ldots, x_n)^{\mathrm{T}}$, $\mathbf{F} = (f_1, f_2, \ldots, f_n)^{\mathrm{T}}$, $\mathbf{d}_x$ is the so-called Newton step, and the matrix $\mathbf{J}(\mathbf{x}_{\mathrm{k}})$ denotes the Jacobian matrix that are the partial derivatives of $\mathbf{F}(\mathbf{x})$ evaluated at $\mathbf{x}_k$. By setting $\mathbf{F}(\mathbf{x}_k + \mathbf{d}_x) = 0$, we obtain a set of linear equations for the next iterate $\mathbf{x}_{k+1}$ that move $\mathbf{F}(\mathbf{x})$ closer to zero, namely:

$$\mathbf{x}_{k+1} = \mathbf{x}_k - \mathbf{J}(\mathbf{x}_k)^{-1}\mathbf{F}(\mathbf{x}_k) \quad \text{or} \quad \mathbf{d}_x = -\mathbf{J}(\mathbf{x}_k)^{-1}\mathbf{F}(\mathbf{x}_k) \tag{59}$$

The process updating $\mathbf{x}_{k+1}$ from $\mathbf{x}_k$ by computing $\mathbf{d}_x$ is iterated to convergence. Once either changes in functions or variables reach machine accuracy, the process can be stopped (56).

2. *Trust Region Method*: The Newton method cannot be guaranteed to converge to a solution set of $\mathbf{F}(\mathbf{x}^*) = \mathbf{0}$ unless they are started close to that solution (19). The method can be made more robust by defining a merit function, e.g., the sum of squares formulation defined as:

$$f(\mathbf{x}) = \frac{1}{2} \parallel \mathbf{F}(\mathbf{x}) \parallel_2^2 = \frac{1}{2}\mathbf{F}(\mathbf{x})^{\mathrm{T}}\mathbf{F}(\mathbf{x}) \tag{60}$$

Here $f(\mathbf{x})$: $\mathcal{R}^n \to \mathcal{R}$. By iteratively minimizing the merit function $f(\mathbf{x})$ until either (1) the function value reaches machine accuracy or (2) no more changes in the function values are detected, a local minimizer $\mathbf{x}^*$ of (60) can be obtained. Any root of $\mathbf{F}$ clearly renders $f(\mathbf{x})$ to become 0, and since $f(\mathbf{x}) \geq 0$ for all $\mathbf{x}$, each root is at least a local minimizer of f. At the same time, this means the local minimizers are not necessarily roots of $\mathbf{F}$. However, any local minimizer $\mathbf{x}^*$ must be a stationary point according to the first-order necessary optimality condition, i.e.:

$$\nabla f(\mathbf{x}^*) = \mathbf{J}(\mathbf{x}^*)^{\mathrm{T}}\mathbf{F}(\mathbf{x}^*) = 0 \tag{61}$$

The $\nabla f = (\partial f/\partial \mathbf{x})^{\mathrm{T}}$ is the gradient. The local minimizers that are not roots of $\mathbf{F}$ satisfy an interesting property; such a nonroot local minimizer giving $\mathbf{F}(\mathbf{x}^*) \neq 0$ is obtainable only if $\mathbf{J}(\mathbf{x}^*)$ is singular. Hence, the singularity of $\mathbf{J}(\mathbf{x}^*)$ must be checked at the termination of the optimization using (60) to ensure the root.

The trust-region (TR) method (57) improves robustness when starting far from the solution. Instead of minimizing (60), the TR method minimizes a different merit function, which reasonably reflects the behavior of (60) in a neighborhood around the current iterate, i.e., the sum of squares using Taylor's first-order approximation of $\mathbf{F}$ (Gauss–Newton linearization of $\mathbf{F}$):

$$q(\mathbf{d}_x) = \frac{1}{2} \parallel \mathbf{F}_k(\mathbf{x}_k) + \mathbf{J}_k(\mathbf{x}_k)\mathbf{d}_x \parallel^2 \tag{62}$$

Here $\mathbf{J}_k$ is the Jacobian matrix evaluated at the kth iterate $\mathbf{x}_k$. The trial step $\mathbf{d}_x$ is generated by minimizing the so-called TR subproblem (62), i.e.:

$$\min_{\mathbf{d}_x} q(\mathbf{d}_x), \quad \text{subject to } \mathbf{d}_x{}^{\mathrm{T}}\mathbf{d}_x \leq \Delta_k \tag{63}$$

where Δ_k is the radius of the TR. The gradient of $q(\mathbf{d}_x)$ with respect to $\mathbf{d}_x$, that is, $\nabla q(\mathbf{d}_x) = \mathbf{J}^{\mathrm{T}}(\mathbf{J}\mathbf{d}_x + \mathbf{F}) = 0$ at any solution

$\mathbf{d}^{GN}$ of the TR subproblem (63) occurs similarly to (61). Thus, it gives:

$$\mathbf{J}_k{}^{T}\mathbf{J}_k\mathbf{d}^{GN} = -\mathbf{J}_k{}^{T}\mathbf{F}_k \tag{64}$$

This so-called Gauss–Newton step $\mathbf{d}^{GN}$ can simply be calculated by solving the above linear problem. The current point is updated to be $\mathbf{x}_k + \mathbf{d}_x$ if the sum of squares function $f(\mathbf{x}_k + \mathbf{d}_x) < f(\mathbf{x}_k)$; otherwise, the current point remains unchanged and the radius of the $n\Delta_k$ is shrunk and the computation of $\mathbf{d}_x$ is repeated.

Jacobian Matrix of the Carbon Isotopomer System: As shown by (59) and (64), the key of the iterative root-finding is computing the Jacobian matrix. The Jacobian matrix for the system of isotopomer balances $\mathbf{F}(\mathbf{x}^{idv})$ in (55) usually has a high dimension and a large number of partial derivatives are involved. For instance, the small network in Fig. 7 has a dimension of 22 × 22 and involves 484 partial derivatives. For a realistic metabolic network, it would be a very expensive process to compute the matrix numerically using finite differencing approximation. Additionally, due to the nonlinearity of the equation system, the numerical differentiation can suffer from inaccuracy and errors. Hence, the analytically calculated Jacobian matrix of the equation system is preferable for improving accuracy and rapidity of convergence. Since $\mathbf{F}(\mathbf{x}^{idv})$ is a square system, its Jacobian matrix $\mathbf{J}$ becomes accordingly square. The (i, j)th element of $\mathbf{J}$ can be defined as:

$$\mathbf{J}(i,j) = \frac{\partial \mathbf{f}_i(\mathbf{x}^{idv})}{\partial \mathbf{x}_j^{idv}} \tag{65}$$

Here $\mathbf{f}_i$ is a certain isotopomer balance (51) belonging to $\mathbf{F}(\mathbf{x}^{idv})$ with $\mathbf{F} = (\mathbf{f}_1, \mathbf{f}_2, \ldots, \mathbf{f}_n)^T$ containing n vector-valued balance equations and variables of $\mathbf{x}^{idv} = (\mathbf{x}_1^{idv}, \mathbf{x}_2^{idv}, \ldots, \mathbf{x}_n^{idv})^T$ with i and $j = 1, 2, \ldots, n$. Because $\mathbf{x}_j^{idv}$ is a vector, the (i, j)th element $\partial \mathbf{f}_i / \partial \mathbf{x}_j^{idv}$ is a matrix. As each $\mathbf{f}_i$ is a vector function containing matrices (IMMs) and the vector variable $\mathbf{x}_j^{idv}$, it is laborious to analytically calculate the Jacobian matrix directly from the equation system $\mathbf{F}(\mathbf{x}^{idv})$. Therefore, instead of writing up all single scalar equations that are the components of $\mathbf{f}_i$, a stepwise procedure was chosen to simplify the derivation of the Jacobian. The calculation of the Jacobian matrix proceeds in three steps (55). (1) A symbolic Jacobian is created whose elements are the symbolic partial derivatives $\partial \mathbf{f}_i / \partial \mathbf{x}_j^{idv}$, where the *symbolic Jacobian* has a dimension of $n \times n$. (2) Subsequently, the resulting elements of the symbolic Jacobian are compiled into executable commands, constituting an *executable Jacobian*, according to groups of derivatives given below. (3) By evaluating the executable Jacobian, it is expanded to the *full Jacobian* with a dimension of $\mathbf{dim}\ \mathbf{x}^{idv} \times \mathbf{dim}\ \mathbf{x}^{idv}$.

1. *Groups of Partial Derivatives*: Since all isotopomer balance equations are based on (51), all possible derivatives in the first step (1) can be classified into three groups. First, for all balances where a particular compound and, correspondingly, all its isotopomers are not taking part, the partial derivatives are zero (*group 1*). Second, all partial derivatives with respect to those compounds, for which the balance was set up, are essentially the product of the stoichiometric coefficient and the sum of all fluxes leaving that pool, $\boldsymbol{\Sigma}\,(v_{\text{out}}s)$ (*group 2*). This corresponds to the partial derivative of (51) with respect to $\mathbf{x}_{\text{met}}$. The last group of elements is corresponding to the partial derivatives of (51) with respect to the incoming IDV of reactants, $\mathbf{x}_{\text{rea}}$ (monomolecular reaction) or $\mathbf{x}_{\text{rea1}}$ and $\mathbf{x}_{\text{rea2}}$ (bimolecular reaction). This group includes elements $v_{\text{in}}s\mathbf{IMM}_{\text{rea}>\text{met}}$, $\boldsymbol{v}_{\text{in}}s\{(\mathbf{IMM}_{\text{rea1}>\text{met}}\mathbf{x}_{\text{rea1}}) \otimes \mathbf{IMM}_{\text{rea2}>\text{met}}\}$, and $\boldsymbol{v}_{\text{in}}s\{\mathbf{IMM}_{\text{rea1}>\text{met}} \otimes (\mathbf{IMM}_{\text{rea2}>\text{met}}\mathbf{x}_{\text{rea2}})\}$ (*group 3*).

   In the second step (2), the groups of all the (i, j)th elements of the symbolic Jacobian are identified and coded as the matrix commands using the rules given in the following section. Hence, a submatrix of the full Jacobian can be determined in the third step (3) by evaluating each command code, which is the (i, j)th element of the executable Jacobian.

2. *Compilation of Partial Derivatives*: Since the variables in (51) are vectors, each element of the symbolic Jacobian, $\partial \mathbf{f}_i/\partial \mathbf{x}_j^{\text{idv}}$, is a matrix. We define, for convenience, an element of the symbolic Jacobian as a submatrix and its (k, l)th element as $\partial f_k/\partial x_l$ with x_l denoting the subvariable which is the lth element of $\mathbf{x}_j^{\text{idv}} = (x_1, x_2, \ldots, x_q)^{\text{T}}$ and f_k as the subfunction which is the kth element of $\mathbf{f}_i = (f_1, f_2, \ldots, f_p)^{\text{T}}$. The full Jacobian for the equation system can be obtained by vertically and horizontally concatenating the submatrices. For $k = 1, 2, \ldots, p$ and $l = 1, 2, \ldots, q$, the (i, j)th element of the symbolic Jacobian can be a square or a nonsquare matrix with a dimension of $p \times q$.

$$\frac{\partial \mathbf{f}_i}{\partial \mathbf{x}_j^{\text{idv}}} = \begin{pmatrix} \dfrac{\partial f_1}{\partial x_1} & ,\ldots, & \dfrac{\partial f_1}{\partial x_q} \\ \vdots & \ddots & \vdots \\ \dfrac{\partial f_p}{\partial x_1} & ,\ldots, & \dfrac{\partial f_p}{\partial x_q} \end{pmatrix} \qquad (66)$$

   Consequently, for the p subbalance regions of the ith $\mathbf{f}$, $\boldsymbol{\psi}_{\text{met}} = \psi_{\text{met},1}, \psi_{\text{met},2}, \ldots, \psi_{\text{met},p}$, which are set up for p subvariables for the ith $\mathbf{x}_{\text{met}}^{\text{idv}} = \{\mathbf{x}_{\text{met}}^{\text{idv}} \in \Re^{\mathbf{dim\,f}} | \mathbf{x}_{\text{met}}^{\text{idv}} = (x_{\text{met},1}, x_{\text{met},2}, \ldots, x_{\text{met},p})^{\text{T}}\}$, there are p subbalance equations for the ith $\mathbf{f} = (f_1, f_2, \ldots, f_p)^{\text{T}}$ to be differentiated with respect to q subvariables of each $\mathbf{x}^{\text{idv}}$ to replace a row of (65) into a set of the submatrices. The entire size of the full Jacobian, which is a square matrix, becomes:

$$\left[\sum_{i=1}^{n} p_i, \sum_{j=1}^{n} q_j\right] \quad \text{where} \sum_{i=1}^{n} p_i = \sum_{i=1}^{n} q_j \tag{67}$$

Here n is the number of equations and variables in the equation system $\mathbf{F}(\mathbf{x}^{\mathrm{idv}})$, p_i is the number of subbalance regions of the ith balance equation $\mathbf{f}_i$, and q_j is the number of subvariables of the jth variable $\mathbf{x}_j^{\mathrm{idv}}$ with $i = 1, 2, \ldots, n$ and $i = j$. The derivatives are compiled by evaluating the executable Jacobian.

If the (i, j)th element of the symbolic Jacobian is identified as zero (group 1), i.e., none of the lth subvariables of $\mathbf{x}_j^{\mathrm{idv}}$ are present in all the kth subbalance equations of $\mathbf{f}_i$, then the corresponding (i, j)th command of the executable Jacobian is a zero matrix of dimension $p \times q$ (*rule 1*). Differentiating all the kth subbalance equations, f_p, of $\mathbf{f}_i$ with respect to all the lth subvariables $x_{\mathrm{met},l}$ of $\mathbf{x}_{\mathrm{met}}^{\mathrm{idv}}$ for which the kth subbalance region $\psi_{\mathrm{met},k}$ is set up ($i = j$ and $p = q$) results in the coefficient of the subvariable at the index $(k, l; k = l)$ and zeros at $(k, l; k \neq l)$ in the submatrix. Therefore, the diagonal element of the executable matrix is a multiplication of the coefficient, $\mathbf{\Sigma}(v_{\mathrm{out}}s)$, and a $p \times p$ identity matrix (*rule 2*). For a monomolecular reaction, the coefficient of the lth subvariable of $\mathbf{x}_{\mathrm{rea},j}^{\mathrm{idv}}$ in the kth subbalance equation is the multiplication of $v_{\mathrm{in}}s$ with the (k, l)th element of the $\mathbf{IMM}_{\mathrm{rea}>\mathrm{met}}$. Hence, the $p \times p$ submatrix is identical to the (i, j)th element of the symbolic Jacobian (*rule 3*$_m$). The element-wise multiplication of two vectors $\mathbf{a}$ and $\mathbf{b}$ is identical to the multiplication of a diagonal matrix of a vector with the other vector, i.e., diag($\mathbf{a}$)$\mathbf{b}$ or diag($\mathbf{b}$)$\mathbf{a}$. Subsequently, for a bimolecular isotopomer reaction from $\mathbf{x}_{\mathrm{rea1},j1,[q1\times 1]}$ and $\mathbf{x}_{\mathrm{rea2},j2,[q2\times 1]}$ to $\mathbf{x}_{\mathrm{met},i,[p\times 1]}$, the bimolecular formula (54) can be rewritten as:

$$\mathbf{x}_{\mathrm{met},i,[p\times 1]}^{\mathrm{idv}*} = \{\mathrm{diag}(\mathbf{IMM}_{\mathrm{rea1}>\mathrm{met},[p\times q_1]}\mathbf{x}_{\mathrm{rea1},j_1,[q_1\times 1]}^{\mathrm{idv}})_{[p\times p]} \\ \mathbf{IMM}_{\mathrm{rea2}>\mathrm{met},[p\times q_2]}\}\mathbf{x}_{\mathrm{rea2},j_2,[q_2\times 1]}^{\mathrm{idv}} \tag{68}$$

or

$$\mathbf{x}_{\mathrm{met},i,[p\times 1]}^{\mathrm{idv}*} = \{\mathrm{diag}(\mathbf{IMM}_{\mathrm{rea2}>\mathrm{met},[p\times q_2]}\mathbf{x}_{\mathrm{rea2},j_2,[q_2\times 1]}^{\mathrm{idv}})_{[p\times p]} \\ \mathbf{IMM}_{\mathrm{rea1}>\mathrm{met},[p\times q_1]}\}\mathbf{x}_{\mathrm{rea1},j_1,[q_1\times 1]}^{\mathrm{idv}} \tag{69}$$

Here $[a \times b]$ denotes the dimension of a matrix or a vector. Hence, the partial derivatives of the group 3 becomes:

$$\frac{\partial \mathbf{f}_i}{\partial \mathbf{x}_{\mathrm{rea1},j_1,[q_1\times 1]}^{\mathrm{idv}}} = \boldsymbol{v}_{\mathrm{in}}s\{\mathrm{diag}(\mathbf{IMM}_{\mathrm{rea2}>\mathrm{met},[p\times q_2]}\mathbf{x}_{\mathrm{rea2},j_2,[q_2\times 1]}^{\mathrm{idv}})_{[p\times p]} \\ \mathbf{IMM}_{\mathrm{rea1}>\mathrm{met},[p\times q_1]}\} \tag{70}$$

and

$$\frac{\partial \mathbf{f}_i}{\partial \mathbf{x}^{\mathrm{idv}}_{\mathrm{rea2},j_2,[q_2\times 1]}} = \boldsymbol{\nu}_{\mathrm{in}} s\{\mathrm{diag}(\mathbf{IMM}_{\mathrm{rea1>met},[p\times q_1]}\mathbf{x}^{\mathrm{idv}}_{\mathrm{rea1},j_1,[q_1\times 1]})_{[p\times p]} \mathbf{IMM}_{\mathrm{rea2>met},[p\times q_2]}\} \tag{71}$$

For both cases, differentiating the kth subbalance equation of $\mathbf{f}_i$ with respect to the qth subvariable of $\mathbf{x}_j^{\mathrm{idv}}$ results in the (p, q) th element of the matrix $\boldsymbol{\nu}_{\mathrm{in}} s\,\mathrm{diag}(\mathbf{IMMx}_j^{\mathrm{idv}})\mathbf{IMM}$. Therefore, a command which compiles a $p \times q_1$ matrix, $\boldsymbol{\nu}_{\mathrm{in}} s\,\mathrm{diag}(\mathbf{IMM}\,\mathbf{x}_{j1}^{\mathrm{idv}})\mathbf{IMM}$, and a $p \times q_2$ matrix, $\boldsymbol{\nu}_{\mathrm{in}} s\,\mathrm{diag}(\mathbf{IMMx}_{j2}^{\mathrm{idv}})\mathbf{IMM}$, becomes the submatrix representing the (i, j_1)th and (i, j_2)th elements of the executable Jacobian, respectively (*rule* 3_b). Note that differentiating $(\mathbf{Ax})\otimes(\mathbf{Bx})$ with respect to a single variable $\mathbf{x}$ gives $\mathrm{diag}(\mathbf{Ax})\mathbf{B} + \mathrm{diag}(\mathbf{Bx})\mathbf{A}$.

In practice, the symbolic Jacobian of the isotopomer balance equation system can be acquired by using a symbolic computation package, which results in an $n \times n$ matrix. Subsequently, using string reading and writing techniques, the analytical expressions in the symbolic Jacobian matrix are rewritten, e.g., using certain matrix commands based on the above rules 1, 2, 3_m, and 3_b. Accordingly, an element of the $n \times n$ Jacobian becomes an executable single command line that designates whether an element of the executable Jacobian has a zero matrix, identity matrix, or a diagonal matrix. The dimensions of those matrices are directly identified by the known dimension of the variables (p, q, q_1, q_2). Once evaluated, the complete Jacobian with a dimension of (67) is obtained by concatenating all submatrices.

The analytical Jacobian matrix of the example system (56) is:

$$\mathbf{J} = \begin{pmatrix} (v_1+v_2)\mathbf{I}_{8\times 8} & -v_3\mathbf{IMM}_{\mathrm{B>A}} & \mathbf{0}_{8\times 2} & \mathbf{0}_{8\times 4} \\ -v_2\mathbf{IMM}_{\mathrm{A>B}} & (v_3+v_5)\mathbf{I}_{8\times 8} & \mathbf{0}_{8\times 2} & -v_4\mathrm{diag}(\mathbf{IMM}_{\mathrm{D_1>B}}\mathbf{x}_{\mathrm{D}}^{\mathrm{idv}})\mathbf{IMM}_{\mathrm{D_2>B}} - v_4\mathrm{diag}(\mathbf{IMM}_{\mathrm{D_2>B}}\mathbf{x}_{\mathrm{D}}^{\mathrm{idv}})\mathbf{IMM}_{\mathrm{D_1>B}} \\ \mathbf{0}_{2\times 8} & 2v_5\mathbf{IMM}_{\mathrm{B>C}} & v_6\mathbf{I}_{2\times 2} & -v_4\mathrm{diag}(\mathbf{IMM}_{\mathrm{D_1>C}}\mathbf{x}_{\mathrm{D}}^{\mathrm{idv}})\mathbf{IMM}_{\mathrm{D_2>C}} - v_4\mathrm{diag}(\mathbf{IMM}_{\mathrm{D_2>C}}\mathbf{x}_{\mathrm{D}}^{\mathrm{idv}})\mathbf{IMM}_{\mathrm{D_1>C}} \\ -v_1\mathbf{IMM}_{\mathrm{A>D}} & \mathbf{0}_{4\times 8} & \mathbf{0}_{4\times 2} & (2v_4+v_8)\mathbf{I}_{4\times 4} \end{pmatrix} \tag{72}$$

Using the Jacobian matrix and a certain root-finding algorithm, we can now compute $\mathbf{x}^{\mathrm{idv}}$ values that result in $\mathbf{F}(\mathbf{x}^{\mathrm{idv}}) = \mathbf{0}$, where each $\mathbf{x}_j^{\mathrm{idv}}$ is constrained by (52). Its computational implementation is discussed in Yang et al. (55) in detail.

3.1.6. Cumomer Model

The cumomer-based model developed by Wiechert et al. (45) provides explicit solutions for the carbon isotopomer system. This is done by transforming the bilinear isotopomer system into a cascade of linear systems. As a result, it allows a stable computation of flux-dependent isotopomer distributions, whereas the above root-finding algorithm can suffer from instability, e.g., when net flux values approach zero (**J** becomes singular).

Generation of Cumomer Labeling Pattern (CLP): As shown in Fig. 6 and (37), the arrangement of cumomers differs from that of isotopomers. They are arranged by weight equaling the number of the specific labeling positions indicated by ones in $\mathbf{x}^{\mathrm{cmf}}$ in (37). The cumomers that belong to a particular level have the same weight but different labeling patterns. The CLPs at a certain level can be generated as follows.

1. Symbolize *x*.
2. Set level as *k*.
3. Create a matrix whose rows consist of all possible combinations of the all elements of $\mathbf{a} = (1, 2, \ldots, n_{\mathrm{C}})^{\mathrm{T}}$ taken *k* at a time.
4. Get dimension of A, which is $a \times b$.
5. Create a matrix $\mathbf{CLP}_k$ with a dimension of $a \times n_{\mathrm{C}}$ whose elements are all *x*.
6. Initialize a loop with $i = 1$.

   Repeat

1. Replace the *i*th row and any *j*th column of $\mathbf{CLP}_k$ by 1, where *j* is every element in the *i*th row of **A**.
2. Stop if *i* reaches *a*.

Here, "*x*" is a symbol to create expressions such as *xxx*, 1*xx*, 11*x*, etc., where "1" denotes the ^{13}C-labeled position(s) and "*x*" can be either ^{12}C or ^{13}C. The operation in line 3 can be obtained by the command nchoosek(**a**, *k*) in MATLAB. $\mathbf{CLP}_k$ is the matrix of what row equals the vector notation of the *k*th level CLP such as $(1, x, x)$ instead of "1*xx*." For instance, we get $\mathbf{A} = (1, 2; 1, 3; 2, 3)$ for the second level of a compound with three carbons, where $\mathbf{a} = (1, 2, 3)$ and $k = 2$. Hence, we have three different cumomers in the second level ($a = 3$). The elements in each row of A denote the particular labeling positions of the corresponding cumomer. Accordingly, we have the cumomers of "11*x*," "1*x*1," and "*x*11" for the second level. The fifth line gives a 3×3 matrix whose elements are *x*. Subsequently, the loop substitutes "*x*" by "1" from the *i*th to *a*th row of $\mathbf{CLP}_k$ using the information contained in **A**. In this manner we get all CLPs from level 1 to n_{C}, where CLP of level 0 equals "*xxx*." The cumomer fractions of a metabolite, $\mathbf{x}^{\mathrm{cmf}}$, are constrained such that:

$$\mathbf{x}_i^{\mathrm{cmf}} = \{\mathbf{x}_i^{\mathrm{cmf}} \in \Re^{2^{n_{\mathrm{C}}}} | \mathbf{x}_i^{\mathrm{cmf}}(1) = 1 \land \forall j : 0 \leq \mathbf{x}_i^{\mathrm{cmf}}(j) \leq 1\} \quad (73)$$

The index $j = 1, 2, 3, \ldots, 2^{n_{\mathrm{C}}}$. Note that $\mathbf{x}_i^{\mathrm{cmf}}$ includes all cumomer fractions from the 0th to the n_{C}th level.

Cumomer Mapping Matrices: The mapping matrices can be generated from AMMs using the similar manner applied to isotopomers. The difference is mainly that one has to take the so-called weight preservation rule (45) into account. A cumomer reaction is restricted for the cumomers with the same weight, that is, cumomers of the *k*th level can be formed either from the *k*th level cumomers or from the cumomers of the *i*th and *j*th levels with $0<i \wedge j<k$ and $i + j = k$. In particular, the latter is applicable to bimolecular reactions. For a reaction **rea** → **met** at the *k*th cumomer level, the (p, q)th element of a mapping matrix $\mathbf{P}_{k,\mathrm{rea}>\mathrm{met}}$ is 1 if the *p*th cumomer of **met** originates from the *q*th of **rea**; otherwise, it is 0.

$$\mathbf{AMM}_{\mathrm{rea}>\mathrm{met}}(q\text{th row of } \mathbf{CLP}_{k,\mathrm{rea}})^{\mathrm{T}} = (p\text{th row of } \mathbf{CLP}_{k,\mathrm{met}})^{\mathrm{T}} \Rightarrow \mathbf{P}_{k,\mathrm{rea}>\mathrm{met}}(p, q) = 1 \quad (74)$$

Note that $\mathbf{P}_{k,\mathrm{rea}>\mathrm{met}}$ maps the reactant and product cumomers of the *k*th level. Consequently, a bimolecular reaction **rea1** + **rea2** → **met** gives two independent mapping matrices of $\mathbf{P}_{k,\mathrm{rea1}>\mathrm{met}}$ and $\mathbf{P}_{k,\mathrm{rea2}>\mathrm{met}}$ as shown below in (76) (the *k*th level cumomers of **met** are determined by those of either **rea1** or **rea2**).

For a bimolecular reaction from the *i*th and *j*th level to the *k*th with $0<i \wedge j<k$ and $i + j = k$ (weight preservation), the mapping matrices $\mathbf{Q}_{ki,\mathrm{rea1}>\mathrm{met}}$ and $\mathbf{Q}_{kj,\mathrm{rea2}>\mathrm{met}}$ are required that are dependent on each other, which involves element-wise multiplication in (77). In this case, the *k*th level cumomers of **met** are determined by both the *i*th and *j*th level of **rea1** and **rea2**, respectively. To get $\mathbf{Q}_{ki,\mathrm{rea1}>\mathrm{met}}$ and $\mathbf{Q}_{kj,\mathrm{rea2}>\mathrm{met}}$, a double-nested loop operation is required to consider all possible combinations of **rea1** and **rea2** as demonstrated in Sect. 3.1.5 for isotopomers.

Stationary Cumomer Balances and its Explicit Solutions: As shown in Fig. 6c, the cumomers of a compound are grouped according to the level. Thus, balances have to be set up for each *k*th subnetwork, which results in the cascade of linear equation systems. Accordingly, the cumomer balances are set up for the cumomer fractions of ${}^{k}\mathbf{x}_{\mathrm{met}}^{\mathrm{cmf}}$ belonging to the *k*th subnetwork. The balances can be formulated analogously to those of isotopomers. Assuming the stationary or quasi-stationary state of an intracellular metabolite **met**, which evolves from *p* different reactions and reacts to *q* different metabolites, a stationary cumomer balance equation can be set up for the *k*th subnetwork as follows:

$$\sum_{n=1}^{p} (\boldsymbol{\nu}_{\mathrm{in},n} s_n \, {}^{k}\mathbf{x}_{\mathrm{met},n}^{\mathrm{cmf}*}) - {}^{k}\mathbf{x}_{\mathrm{met}}^{\mathrm{cmf}} \sum_{m=1}^{q} (\boldsymbol{\nu}_{\mathrm{out},m} s_m) = 0 \quad (75)$$

Here, ${}^{k}\mathbf{x}_{\mathrm{met}}^{\mathrm{cmf}*}$ denotes the cumomer fractions coming into the pool of **met** and ${}^{k}\mathbf{x}_{\mathrm{met}}^{\mathrm{cmf}}$ are the outgoing cumomer fractions. In the *k*th subnetwork, the variables ${}^{k}\mathbf{x}_{\mathrm{met}}^{\mathrm{cmf}}$ for which the balances are set up are cumomer fractions of the *k*th level, whereas ${}^{k}\mathbf{x}_{\mathrm{met}}^{\mathrm{cmf}*}$ can be cumomer fractions of the level equal to or lower than the *k*th.

Similarly to the carbon isotopomer or carbon atom models, the incoming cumomer fractions into the kth subnetwork, ${}^{k}\mathbf{x}_{\mathrm{met}}^{\mathrm{cmf}*}$, are calculated using mapping matrices ($\mathbf{P}_k$, $\mathbf{Q}_{ki}$) containing zeros and ones. Depending on the subnetworks to which reactants belong, these matrices map cumomer reactions in terms of the weight preservation rule. The cumomer reactions between the metabolites with the level are mapped such that:

$$
{}^{k}\mathbf{x}_{\mathrm{met}}^{\mathrm{cmf}*} = \mathbf{P}_{k,\mathrm{rea}>\mathrm{met}}\,{}^{k}\mathbf{x}_{\mathrm{rea}}^{\mathrm{cmf}} \quad \text{and} \quad {}^{k}\mathbf{x}_{\mathrm{met}}^{\mathrm{cmf}*} = \mathbf{P}_{k,\mathrm{rea1}>\mathrm{met}}\,{}^{k}\mathbf{x}_{\mathrm{rea1}}^{\mathrm{cmf}} + \mathbf{P}_{k,\mathrm{rea2}>\mathrm{met}}\,{}^{k}\mathbf{x}_{\mathrm{rea2}}^{\mathrm{cmf}} \quad (76)
$$

These are set up for a monomolecular (**rea** → **met**) and a bimolecular (**rea1** + **rea2** → **met**) cumomer reaction, respectively. Furthermore, the cumomers in the kth subnetwork can originate from a bimolecular reaction of two metabolites balanced in the ith and jth subnetwork on a lower level than the kth, respectively. In this case, ${}^{k}\mathbf{x}_{\mathrm{met}}^{\mathrm{cmf}*}$ can be calculated using the corresponding mapping matrices $\mathbf{Q}_{ki}$ and $\mathbf{Q}_{kj}$ as follows:

$$
{}^{k}\mathbf{x}_{\mathrm{met}}^{\mathrm{cmf}*} = (\mathbf{Q}_{ki,\mathrm{rea1}>\mathrm{met}} \cdot {}^{i}\mathbf{x}_{\mathrm{rea1}}^{\mathrm{cmf}}) \otimes (\mathbf{Q}_{kj,\mathrm{rea2}>\mathrm{met}} \cdot {}^{j}\mathbf{x}_{\mathrm{rea2}}^{\mathrm{cmf}}) \quad (77)
$$

Note that $k = i + j$ with $0<i \wedge j<k$ according to the weight preservation rule, and $\otimes$ denotes the element-wise multiplication of two vectors. Because the variables ${}^{i}\mathbf{x}_{\mathrm{rea1}}^{\mathrm{cmf}}$ and ${}^{j}\mathbf{x}_{\mathrm{rea2}}^{\mathrm{cmf}}$ in the bilinear term (77) are solved in the corresponding lower ith and jth subnetwork, respectively, the kth subnetwork is linear with respect to all kth variables by (75) and (76). Due to this, the cumomer system as a cascade system is linear and can be directly solved from the lowest (first) to the highest level, e.g., using matrix inversion.

The cumomer balances can be separately set up for the intracellular ($\mathbf{F}_{\mathrm{int}}$) and measurable extracellular metabolites ($\mathbf{F}_{\mathrm{ext}}$) such that:

$$
\begin{aligned}
&{}^{1}\mathbf{F}_{\mathrm{int}}({}^{1}\mathbf{x}_{\mathrm{int}}^{\mathrm{cmf}}, {}^{1}\mathbf{x}_{\mathrm{inp}}^{\mathrm{cmf}}) = \mathbf{0}\\
&{}^{2}\mathbf{F}_{\mathrm{int}}({}^{1}\mathbf{x}_{\mathrm{int}}^{\mathrm{cmf}}, {}^{2}\mathbf{x}_{\mathrm{int}}^{\mathrm{cmf}}, {}^{1}\mathbf{x}_{\mathrm{inp}}^{\mathrm{cmf}}, {}^{2}\mathbf{x}_{\mathrm{inp}}^{\mathrm{cmf}}) = \mathbf{0}\\
&\vdots\\
&{}^{n}\mathbf{F}_{\mathrm{int}}({}^{1}\mathbf{x}_{\mathrm{int}}^{\mathrm{cmf}}, {}^{2}\mathbf{x}_{\mathrm{int}}^{\mathrm{cmf}}, \ldots, {}^{n}\mathbf{x}_{\mathrm{int}}^{\mathrm{cmf}}, {}^{1}\mathbf{x}_{\mathrm{inp}}^{\mathrm{cmf}}, {}^{2}\mathbf{x}_{\mathrm{inp}}^{\mathrm{cmf}}, \ldots, {}^{n}\mathbf{x}_{\mathrm{inp}}^{\mathrm{cmf}}) = \mathbf{0} \quad (78)
\end{aligned}
$$

and

$$
\begin{aligned}
&{}^{1}\mathbf{F}_{\mathrm{ext}}({}^{1}\mathbf{x}_{\mathrm{ext}}^{\mathrm{cmf}}, {}^{1}\mathbf{x}_{\mathrm{int}}^{\mathrm{cmf}}) = \mathbf{0}\\
&{}^{2}\mathbf{F}_{\mathrm{ext}}({}^{2}\mathbf{x}_{\mathrm{ext}}^{\mathrm{cmf}}, {}^{1}\mathbf{x}_{\mathrm{int}}^{\mathrm{cmf}}, {}^{2}\mathbf{x}_{\mathrm{int}}^{\mathrm{cmf}}) = \mathbf{0}\\
&\vdots\\
&{}^{m}\mathbf{F}_{\mathrm{ext}}({}^{m}\mathbf{x}_{\mathrm{ext}}^{\mathrm{cmf}}, {}^{1}\mathbf{x}_{\mathrm{int}}^{\mathrm{cmf}}, {}^{2}\mathbf{x}_{\mathrm{int}}^{\mathrm{cmf}}, \ldots, {}^{m}\mathbf{x}_{\mathrm{int}}^{\mathrm{cmf}}) = \mathbf{0} \quad (79)
\end{aligned}
$$

Here, the vectors ${}^{k}\mathbf{x}_{\text{int}}^{\text{cmf}} = ({}^{k}\mathbf{x}_{\text{int},1}^{\text{cmf}}, {}^{k}\mathbf{x}_{\text{int},2}^{\text{cmf}}, \ldots)^{\text{T}}$, ${}^{k}\mathbf{x}_{\text{inp}}^{\text{cmf}} = ({}^{k}\mathbf{x}_{\text{inp},1}^{\text{cmf}}, {}^{k}\mathbf{x}_{\text{inp},2}^{\text{cmf}}, \ldots)^{\text{T}}$, and ${}^{k}\mathbf{x}_{\text{ext}}^{\text{cmf}} = ({}^{k}\mathbf{x}_{\text{ext},1}^{\text{cmf}}, {}^{k}\mathbf{x}_{\text{ext},2}^{\text{cmf}}, \ldots)^{\text{T}}$ include the cumomer fractions of intracellular metabolites, input substrates, and measurable extracellular metabolites involved in the *k*th subnetwork, respectively. ${}^{k}\mathbf{F}_{\text{int}}$ is a square linear equation system with respect to ${}^{k}\mathbf{x}_{\text{int}}^{\text{cmf}}$ and ${}^{k}\mathbf{F}_{\text{ext}}$ is with respect to ${}^{k}\mathbf{x}_{\text{ext}}^{\text{cmf}}$. Moreover, all $\mathbf{x}_{\text{int}}^{\text{cmf}}$ whose level is lower than *k* are solved in advance. Therefore, ${}^{k}\mathbf{x}_{\text{int}}^{\text{cmf}}$ can be obtained by solving the cascade of ${}^{1}\mathbf{F}_{\text{int}}$ to ${}^{n}\mathbf{F}_{\text{int}}$ of (78), ultimately giving ${}^{k}\mathbf{x}_{\text{ext}}^{\text{cmf}}$.

To get explicit solutions of cumomer balance equation systems, (78) and (79) have to be transformed into matrix formulation, i.e., $\mathbf{Ax} = \mathbf{0}$. Due to the element-wise multiplication (77) for the bimolecular reactions from a lower to a higher subnetwork, the following rule must be taken into account. A matrix vector equation system $\mathbf{Ax}_1 - (\mathbf{Bx}_2 + \mathbf{Cx}_3 \otimes \mathbf{Dx}_4) = \mathbf{0}$ can be rewritten as $(\mathbf{A}, \mathbf{B}, \tfrac{1}{2}\,\text{diag}(\mathbf{Dx}_4)\mathbf{C}, \tfrac{1}{2}\,\text{diag}(\mathbf{Cx}_3)\mathbf{D})\mathbf{x} = \mathbf{0}$, where $\mathbf{A}$, $\mathbf{B}$, $\mathbf{C}$, and $\mathbf{D}$ are matrices and $\mathbf{x} = (\mathbf{x}_1, \mathbf{x}_2, \mathbf{x}_3, \mathbf{x}_4)^{\text{T}}$. Accordingly, the *k*th cumomer balances ${}^{k}\mathbf{F}_{\text{int}}$ and ${}^{k}\mathbf{F}_{\text{ext}}$ can be formulated such that:

$$\left(\frac{\partial^{k}\mathbf{F}_{\text{int}}}{\partial^{k}\mathbf{x}_{\text{int}}^{\text{cmf}}}, \frac{\partial^{k}\mathbf{F}_{\text{int}}}{\partial^{k}\mathbf{x}_{\text{inp}}^{\text{cmf}}}, \frac{1}{2}\frac{\partial^{k}\mathbf{F}_{\text{int}}}{\partial^{1}\mathbf{x}_{\text{inp}}^{\text{cmf}}}, \ldots, \frac{1}{2}\frac{\partial^{k}\mathbf{F}_{\text{int}}}{\partial^{k-1}\mathbf{x}_{\text{inp}}^{\text{cmf}}}, \frac{1}{2}\frac{\partial^{k}\mathbf{F}_{\text{int}}}{\partial^{1}\mathbf{x}_{\text{int}}^{\text{cmf}}}, \ldots, \frac{1}{2}\frac{\partial^{k}\mathbf{F}_{\text{int}}}{\partial^{k-1}\mathbf{x}_{\text{int}}^{\text{cmf}}}\right){}^{k}\mathbf{x}_1 = 0 \tag{80}$$

$$\left(\frac{\partial^{k}\mathbf{F}_{\text{ext}}}{\partial^{k}\mathbf{x}_{\text{ext}}^{\text{cmf}}}, \frac{\partial^{k}\mathbf{F}_{\text{ext}}}{\partial^{k}\mathbf{x}_{\text{int}}^{\text{cmf}}}, \frac{1}{2}\frac{\partial^{k}\mathbf{F}_{\text{ext}}}{\partial^{1}\mathbf{x}_{\text{int}}^{\text{cmf}}}, \ldots, \frac{1}{2}\frac{\partial^{k}\mathbf{F}_{\text{ext}}}{\partial^{k-1}\mathbf{x}_{\text{int}}^{\text{cmf}}}\right){}^{k}\mathbf{x}_2 = 0 \tag{81}$$

Here the vector ${}^{k}\mathbf{x}_1 = ({}^{k}\mathbf{x}_{\text{int}}^{\text{cmf}} | {}^{k}\mathbf{x}_{\text{inp}}^{\text{cmf}} | {}^{1}\mathbf{x}_{\text{int}}^{\text{cmf}}, {}^{2}\mathbf{x}_{\text{int}}^{\text{cmf}}, \ldots, {}^{k-1}\mathbf{x}_{\text{int}}^{\text{cmf}} | {}^{1}\mathbf{x}_{\text{inp}}^{\text{cmf}}, {}^{2}\mathbf{x}_{\text{inp}}^{\text{cmf}}, \ldots {}^{k-1}\mathbf{x}_{\text{inp}}^{\text{cmf}})^{\text{T}}$ and the vector ${}^{k}\mathbf{x}_2 = ({}^{k}\mathbf{x}_{\text{ext}}^{\text{cmf}} | {}^{k}\mathbf{x}_{\text{int}}^{\text{cmf}} | {}^{1}\mathbf{x}_{\text{int}}^{\text{cmf}}, {}^{2}\mathbf{x}_{\text{int}}^{\text{cmf}}, \ldots, {}^{k-1}\mathbf{x}_{\text{int}}^{\text{cmf}})^{\text{T}}$. Now, solving (80) and (81) for ${}^{k}\mathbf{x}_{\text{int}}^{\text{cmf}}$ and ${}^{k}\mathbf{x}_{\text{ext}}^{\text{cmf}}$ results in the following explicit solutions for ${}^{k}\mathbf{F}_{\text{int}}$ and ${}^{k}\mathbf{F}_{\text{ext}}$, respectively.

$${}^{k}\mathbf{x}_{\text{int}}^{\text{cmf}} = -\left(\frac{\partial^{k}\mathbf{F}_{\text{int}}}{\partial^{k}\mathbf{x}_{\text{int}}^{\text{cmf}}}\right)^{-1}\left\{\frac{\partial^{k}\mathbf{F}_{\text{int}}}{\partial^{k}\mathbf{x}_{\text{inp}}^{\text{cmf}}}{}^{k}\mathbf{x}_{\text{inp}}^{\text{cmf}} + \frac{1}{2}\sum_{i=1}^{k-1}\left(\frac{\partial^{k}\mathbf{F}_{\text{int}}}{\partial^{i}\mathbf{x}_{\text{inp}}^{\text{cmf}}}{}^{i}\mathbf{x}_{\text{inp}}^{\text{cmf}}\right) + \frac{1}{2}\sum_{j=1}^{k-1}\left(\frac{\partial^{k}\mathbf{F}_{\text{int}}}{\partial^{i}\mathbf{x}_{\text{int}}^{\text{cmf}}}{}^{i}\mathbf{x}_{\text{int}}^{\text{cmf}}\right)\right\} \tag{82}$$

$${}^{k}\mathbf{x}_{\text{ext}}^{\text{cmf}} = -\left(\frac{\partial^{k}\mathbf{F}_{\text{ext}}}{\partial^{k}\mathbf{x}_{\text{ext}}^{\text{cmf}}}\right)^{-1}\left\{\frac{\partial^{k}\mathbf{F}_{\text{ext}}}{\partial^{k}\mathbf{x}_{\text{int}}^{\text{cmf}}}{}^{k}\mathbf{x}_{\text{int}}^{\text{cmf}} + \frac{1}{2}\sum_{j=1}^{k-1}\left(\frac{\partial^{k}\mathbf{F}_{\text{ext}}}{\partial^{j}\mathbf{x}_{\text{int}}^{\text{cmf}}}{}^{j}\mathbf{x}_{\text{int}}^{\text{cmf}}\right)\right\} \tag{83}$$

Note that all the *k*th as well as *i*th $\mathbf{x}_{\text{inp}}^{\text{cmf}}$ values are known (input substrates) and all the *j*th $\mathbf{x}_{\text{int}}^{\text{cmf}}$ ($j < k$) are obtained from the corresponding subnetworks lower than the *k*th in advance (cascade equations system). Therefore, (82) as well as (83) are linear systems. The ${}^k\mathbf{x}_{\text{int}}^{\text{cmf}}$ obtained from (82) is further utilized to get ${}^k\mathbf{x}_{\text{ext}}^{\text{cmf}}$ as specified by (83). The ${}^k\mathbf{x}_{\text{ext}}^{\text{cmf}}$ can further be converted into isotopomer distributions and mass isotopomer distributions using a transformation matrix such as (37).

Example: For the example network in Fig. 7, the largest number of carbon atoms given for a compound is three. Hence, we get a cascade of the following three equation systems.

$$\begin{aligned}
\text{Level 1:}\quad & (\boldsymbol{\nu}_1+\boldsymbol{\nu}_2){}^1\mathbf{x}_{\text{A}}^{\text{cmf}} - (\boldsymbol{\nu}_3\mathbf{P}_{1,\text{B>A}}{}^1\mathbf{x}_{\text{B}}^{\text{cmf}} + \boldsymbol{\nu}_7\mathbf{P}_{1,\text{S>A}}{}^1\mathbf{x}_{\text{S}}^{\text{cmf}}) = \mathbf{0}\\
& (\boldsymbol{\nu}_3+\boldsymbol{\nu}_5){}^1\mathbf{x}_{\text{B}}^{\text{cmf}} - (\boldsymbol{\nu}_2\mathbf{P}_{1,\text{A>B}}{}^1\mathbf{x}_{\text{A}}^{\text{cmf}} + \boldsymbol{\nu}_4\mathbf{P}_{1,\text{D}_1\text{>B}}{}^1\mathbf{x}_{\text{D}}^{\text{cmf}}\\
& \qquad +\boldsymbol{\nu}_4\mathbf{P}_{1,\text{D}_2\text{>B}}{}^1\mathbf{x}_{\text{D}}^{\text{cmf}}) = \mathbf{0}\\
& \boldsymbol{\nu}_6{}^1\mathbf{x}_{\text{C}}^{\text{cmf}} - (\boldsymbol{\nu}_4\mathbf{P}_{1,\text{D}_1\text{>C}}{}^1\mathbf{x}_{\text{D}}^{\text{cmf}} + \boldsymbol{\nu}_4\mathbf{P}_{1,\text{D}_2\text{>C}}{}^1\mathbf{x}_{\text{D}}^{\text{cmf}}\\
& \qquad +2\boldsymbol{\nu}_5\mathbf{P}_{1,\text{B>C}}{}^1\mathbf{x}_{\text{B}}^{\text{cmf}}) = \mathbf{0}\\
& (2\boldsymbol{\nu}_4+\boldsymbol{\nu}_8){}^1\mathbf{x}_{\text{D}}^{\text{cmf}} - \boldsymbol{\nu}_1\mathbf{P}_{1,\text{A>D}}{}^1\mathbf{x}_{\text{A}}^{\text{cmf}} = \mathbf{0}\\
\text{Level 2:}\quad & (\boldsymbol{\nu}_1+\boldsymbol{\nu}_2){}^2\mathbf{x}_{\text{A}}^{\text{cmf}} - (\boldsymbol{\nu}_3\mathbf{P}_{2,\text{B>A}}{}^2\mathbf{x}_{\text{B}}^{\text{cmf}} + \boldsymbol{\nu}_7\mathbf{P}_{2,\text{S>A}}{}^2\mathbf{x}_{\text{S}}^{\text{cmf}}) = \mathbf{0}\\
& (\boldsymbol{\nu}_3+\boldsymbol{\nu}_5){}^2\mathbf{x}_{\text{B}}^{\text{cmf}} - (\boldsymbol{\nu}_2\mathbf{P}_{2,\text{A>B}}{}^2\mathbf{x}_{\text{A}}^{\text{cmf}} + \boldsymbol{\nu}_4\mathbf{P}_{1,\text{D}_2\text{>B}}{}^2\mathbf{x}_{\text{D}}^{\text{cmf}})\\
& \qquad -\boldsymbol{\nu}_4(\mathbf{Q}_{21,\text{D}_1\text{>B}}{}^1\mathbf{x}_{\text{D}}^{\text{cmf}}) \otimes (\mathbf{Q}_{21,\text{D}_2\text{>B}}{}^1\mathbf{x}_{\text{D}}^{\text{cmf}}) = \mathbf{0}\\
& (2\boldsymbol{\nu}_4+\boldsymbol{\nu}_8){}^2\mathbf{x}_{\text{D}}^{\text{cmf}} - \boldsymbol{\nu}_1\mathbf{P}_{1,\text{A>D}}{}^2\mathbf{x}_{\text{A}}^{\text{cmf}} = \mathbf{0}\\
\text{Level 3:}\quad & (\boldsymbol{\nu}_1+\boldsymbol{\nu}_2){}^3\mathbf{x}_{\text{A}}^{\text{cmf}} - (\boldsymbol{\nu}_3\mathbf{P}_{3,\text{B>A}}{}^3\mathbf{x}_{\text{B}}^{\text{cmf}} + \boldsymbol{\nu}_7\mathbf{P}_{3,\text{S>A}}{}^3\mathbf{x}_{\text{S}}^{\text{cmf}}) = \mathbf{0}\\
& (\boldsymbol{\nu}_3+\boldsymbol{\nu}_5){}^3\mathbf{x}_{\text{B}}^{\text{cmf}} - \boldsymbol{\nu}_2\mathbf{P}_{3,\text{A>B}}{}^3\mathbf{x}_{\text{A}}^{\text{cmf}} - \boldsymbol{\nu}_4(\mathbf{Q}_{31,\text{D}_1\text{>B}}{}^1\mathbf{x}_{\text{D}}^{\text{cmf}})\\
& \qquad \otimes(\mathbf{Q}_{32,\text{D}_2\text{>B}}{}^2\mathbf{x}_{\text{D}}^{\text{cmf}}) = \mathbf{0}
\end{aligned}$$

The system of level 1 is identical to the carbon atom model (45), which is a linear system. Solving level 1 by (82) gives the flux-dependent ${}^1\mathbf{x}^{\text{cmf}}$ values for the input labeling given by ${}^1\mathbf{x}_{\text{S}}^{\text{cmf}}$. This provides the values for the variables involved in the bilinear term in the system of level 2. Due to this, the equation system of level 2 becomes linear. The same happens for the system of level 3 when level 2 has been solved. Additionally, it has to be stated that the reaction from D to B by the mechanism of $\mathbf{AMM}_{\text{D}_1\text{>B}} = (0,0;0,0;1,0)$ gives $\mathbf{P}_{2,\text{D}_1\text{>B}} = \mathbf{0}$ and $\mathbf{Q}_{32,\text{D}_1\text{>B}} = \mathbf{0}$. Therefore, the term "$\boldsymbol{\nu}_4\mathbf{P}_{2,\text{D}_1\text{>B}}{}^2\mathbf{x}_{\text{D}}^{\text{cmf}}$" and "$\boldsymbol{\nu}_4(\mathbf{Q}_{32,\text{D}_1\text{>B}}{}^2\mathbf{x}_{\text{D}}^{\text{cmf}}) \otimes (\mathbf{Q}_{31,\text{D}_2\text{>B}}{}^1\mathbf{x}_{\text{D}}^{\text{cmf}})$" are omitted in the second equation of level 2 and level 3, respectively.

3.2. Numerical Flux Estimation

In Sect. 3.1, we discussed how to parametrize the stoichiometric balance systems and how to model carbon labeling system. In terms of the parametrized stoichiometric network, that is:

$$\boldsymbol{\nu}_{\text{depend}} = \mathbf{n}_{\text{flux}}(\boldsymbol{\Theta}) \qquad (84)$$

One can generate any flux states that obey stoichiometry by varying independent variables $\boldsymbol{\Theta} = (\varphi_1, \varphi_2, \ldots, \boldsymbol{\nu}_{\text{ext1}}, \boldsymbol{\nu}_{\text{ext2}}, \ldots)^{\text{T}}$ as shown in Fig. 3. Subsequently, using a carbon flux model:

$$\mathbf{F}(\mathbf{x}, \boldsymbol{\nu}(\boldsymbol{\Theta}), \mathbf{x}_{\text{inp}}) = \mathbf{0} \qquad (85)$$

The flux-dependent labeling state of intra- as well as extracellular metabolites, $\mathbf{x} = (\mathbf{x}_{\text{int}}, \mathbf{x}_{\text{ext}})^{\text{T}}$, can be computed for one or more ^{13}C-labeled substrates ($\mathbf{x}_{\text{inp}}$). Here, $\boldsymbol{\nu}$ comprises all dependent ($\boldsymbol{\nu}_{\text{depend}}$) and independent fluxes (extracellular fluxes: $\boldsymbol{\nu}_{\text{ext}}$).

As shown, both the metabolic state ($\boldsymbol{\nu}$) and the labeling state ($\mathbf{x}$) are functionally dependent on the design parameter $\boldsymbol{\Theta}$. This means $\boldsymbol{\Theta}$ can be determined once extracellular fluxes and the labeling state of metabolites corresponding to $\boldsymbol{\nu}_{\text{ext}}$ and $\mathbf{x}_{\text{ext}}$, respectively, have been acquired from a tracer experiment using one or more selected ^{13}C labeled substrates. According to this relationship, the following model function $\boldsymbol{\Phi}(\boldsymbol{\Theta})$ can be formulated.

$$\Phi(\boldsymbol{\Theta}) = \begin{pmatrix} \boldsymbol{\nu}_{\text{ext}} = \mathbf{T}_{\text{flux}}\boldsymbol{\Theta} \\ \mathbf{x}_{\text{ext}} = \mathbf{T}_{\text{labeling}}\mathbf{x} \end{pmatrix} \tag{86}$$

Here, $\mathbf{T}_{\text{flux}}$ is a matrix consisting of ones and zeros that maps $\boldsymbol{\nu}_{\text{ext}}$ and $\boldsymbol{\Theta}$, and $\mathbf{T}_{\text{labeling}}$ maps $\mathbf{x}_{\text{ext}}$ and $\mathbf{x} = (\mathbf{x}_{\text{int}}, \mathbf{x}_{\text{ext}})^{\text{T}}$. As shown by (81) and (83), $\mathbf{x}_{\text{ext}}$ can also be derived by solving an implicit function. Because the inverse function of $\boldsymbol{\Phi}(\boldsymbol{\Theta})$ is typically not available, $\boldsymbol{\Theta}$ has to be estimated numerically. This can be done by formulating a nonlinear regression model.

3.2.1. Nonlinear Regression Model

A nonlinear regression model $\boldsymbol{\eta} = \Phi(\boldsymbol{\Theta}) + \boldsymbol{\varepsilon}$ can be termed as a covariance-weighted nonlinear least-squares minimization problem given by:

$$\min_{\boldsymbol{\Theta}\in\Omega} f(\boldsymbol{\Theta}), \quad \text{subject to } \mathbf{n}_{\text{flux}}(\boldsymbol{\Theta}) \geq \mathbf{0}$$
$$\text{where } f(\boldsymbol{\Theta}) = \tfrac{1}{2}(\boldsymbol{\eta} - \Phi(\boldsymbol{\Theta}))^{\text{T}}\boldsymbol{\Sigma}_{\eta}^{-1}(\boldsymbol{\eta} - \Phi(\boldsymbol{\Theta})) \tag{87}$$

Here $f(\boldsymbol{\Theta})$ denotes the objective function to be minimized with respect to the design parameters $\boldsymbol{\Theta}$. The measured data set $\boldsymbol{\eta} = (\eta_1, \eta_2, \ldots, \eta_n)^{\text{T}}$ corresponds to the model function $\boldsymbol{\Phi}(\boldsymbol{\Theta})$ defined for $\boldsymbol{\nu}_{\text{ext}}$ and $\mathbf{x}_{\text{ext}}$ in (86). The error $\boldsymbol{\varepsilon}$ associated with $\boldsymbol{\eta}$ is typically assumed to have a normal distribution such that $\boldsymbol{\varepsilon} \in N(0, \boldsymbol{\Sigma}_{\eta})$, where $\boldsymbol{\Sigma}_{\eta}$ is the covariance matrix of measurements. The inverse of $\boldsymbol{\Sigma}_{\eta}$ acts as a weighting term such that measured values with smaller variances are more weighted during the minimization process.

The problem (87) is solved by nonlinear optimization methods. For ^{13}C MFA, the applied algorithms are mainly gradient-based local optimizations such as sequential quadratic programming (14, 28, 58) or gradient-free global optimization (41, 47, 59) such as evolutionary programming, simulated annealing, or genetic algorithms. Also, a hybrid technique of global-local optimization has been applied (60). Those algorithms are described in detail elsewhere (19, 56, 61). The stochastic global optimization methods can be inefficient due to the time required obtaining the solution in high dimensional parameter spaces (62, 63). In comparison, the gradient-based local optimizations have a much higher convergence speed, but the solution quality heavily depends on starting points (19, 63). Furthermore, only the convex minimization problem ensures reaching the global optimum, whereas the convexity of general nonlinear problems with nonlinear constraints is nontrivial to determine in practice (64). Thus, one may obtain solutions that are not necessarily global and that might vary depending on starting points.

When a gradient-based optimization method is applied, the model's Jacobian matrix $\mathbf{J} = \partial\mathbf{\Phi}/\partial\mathbf{\Theta}$ is required to compute the gradient ∇f of the objective function, the transpose of the first partial derivatives of $f(\mathbf{\Theta})$ with respect to $\mathbf{\Theta}$, i.e.,

$$\nabla f(\mathbf{\Theta}) = \frac{\partial\Phi}{\partial\mathbf{\Theta}}^{\mathrm{T}} \mathbf{\Sigma}_{\eta}^{-1}(\Phi(\mathbf{\Theta}) - \boldsymbol{\eta}) \tag{88}$$

and to linearly approximate the model function. The linear approximation of $\mathbf{\Phi}$ in the neighborhood of the current iterate $\mathbf{\Theta}_k$ yields:

$$\nabla f(\mathbf{\Theta}_k) = \mathbf{J}(\mathbf{\Theta}_k)^{\mathrm{T}}\mathbf{\Sigma}_{\eta}^{-1}(\Phi(\mathbf{\Theta}_k) + \mathbf{J}(\mathbf{\Theta}_k)\Delta\mathbf{\Theta}_k - \boldsymbol{\eta}) \tag{89}$$

Here $\mathbf{J}(\mathbf{\Theta}_k)$ is $\partial\mathbf{\Phi}/\partial\mathbf{\Theta}$ evaluated at $\mathbf{\Theta}_k$. As shown by (61), the basic idea of solving (87) is that we seek a certain minimizer satisfying the first-order necessary optimality condition, that is, $\nabla f = \mathbf{0}$. The solution of the above linearization obtained by solving $\nabla f = \mathbf{0}$ for $\Delta\mathbf{\Theta}_k$ is:

$$\Delta\mathbf{\Theta}_k = (\mathbf{J}(\mathbf{\Theta}_k)^{\mathrm{T}}\mathbf{\Sigma}_{\eta}^{-1}\mathbf{J}(\mathbf{\Theta}_k))^{-1}\mathbf{J}(\mathbf{\Theta}_k)^{\mathrm{T}}\mathbf{\Sigma}_{\eta}^{-1}(\boldsymbol{\eta} - \mathbf{F}(\mathbf{\Theta}_k)) \tag{90}$$

This is used to get a new estimate of the optimum, that is, $\mathbf{\Theta}_{k+1} = \mathbf{\Theta}_k + \Delta\mathbf{\Theta}_k$. The whole process is repeated until we get both ∇f and $\Delta\mathbf{\Theta}$ to approach zero or a small value defined by the modeler (termination criteria). Hence, obtaining the model's Jacobian matrix $\mathbf{J}$, i.e., the partial derivatives of the model function $\mathbf{\Phi}$ with respect to $\mathbf{\Theta}$, are essential. Moreover, the Jacobian matrix is necessitated to design ^{13}C tracer experiments, which be shown in Sect. 3.3.

When $\mathbf{J}$ is available, the Hessian matrix ($\mathbf{H}$), i.e., the second derivative of $f(\mathbf{\Theta})$, can also be computed. It specifies the curvature of the search surface and provides a quadratic representation of it in its vicinity. Using this information, the convergence can be accelerated. The numerical calculation of $\mathbf{H}$ involves a large amount of computation. Therefore, it is advantageous to provide the Hessian analytically. For the nonlinear problem (87), $\mathbf{H}$ can be obtained by linearization (19, 56), i.e.:

$$\mathbf{H} = \frac{\partial(\nabla f)}{\partial\mathbf{\Theta}} \approx \frac{\partial\Phi}{\partial\mathbf{\Theta}}^{\mathrm{T}} \mathbf{\Sigma}_{\eta}^{-1} \frac{\partial\Phi}{\partial\mathbf{\Theta}} \tag{91}$$

In practice, the constrained nonlinear minimization problem (87) is formulated as the Lagrangian function, a linear combination of the objective function and the constraints. The frequently applied algorithm associated with the Lagrangian method is the sequential quadratic programming, of which details are described elsewhere (19, 65).

3.2.2. Key Partial Derivatives

To get the model's Jacobian matrix, the measured extracellular fluxes $\boldsymbol{\nu}_{\text{ext}}$ and labeling data $\mathbf{x}_{\text{ext}}$ have to be differentiated with respect to $\boldsymbol{\Theta}$. The Jacobian matrix for (86) equals:

$$\frac{\partial \Phi}{\partial \boldsymbol{\Theta}} = \begin{pmatrix} \frac{\partial \boldsymbol{\nu}_{\text{ext}}}{\partial \boldsymbol{\Theta}} & \mathbf{0} \\ \mathbf{0} & \frac{\partial \mathbf{x}_{\text{ext}}}{\partial \boldsymbol{\Theta}} \end{pmatrix} = \begin{pmatrix} \mathbf{T}_{\text{flux}} & \mathbf{0} \\ \mathbf{0} & \mathbf{T}_{\text{labeling}} \frac{\partial \mathbf{x}}{\partial \boldsymbol{\Theta}} \end{pmatrix} \tag{92}$$

$\mathbf{T}_{\text{flux}}$ and $\mathbf{T}_{\text{labeling}}$ are simple matrices containing zeros and ones, e.g., $\mathbf{T}_{\text{flux}} = (0,\ 0,\ 1,\ 0;\ 0,\ 0,\ 0,\ 1)$ if $\boldsymbol{\Theta} = (\varphi_1, \varphi_2, \boldsymbol{\nu}_{\text{ext1}}, \boldsymbol{\nu}_{\text{ext2}})^{\text{T}}$, where ν_{ext1}, ν_{ext2} are the measurable extracellular fluxes. In contrast, the equation system consisting of carbon atom and isotopomer balances such as (44) and (55), respectively, is the implicit function of the labeling $\mathbf{x}$ and flux state $\boldsymbol{\nu} = (\boldsymbol{\nu}_{\text{depend}}, \boldsymbol{\nu}_{\text{ext}})$ with ν being the function of $\boldsymbol{\Theta}$ by (84) and $\mathbf{T}_{\text{flux}}\boldsymbol{\Theta}$ as shown by (85). For a certain constant input labeling of $\mathbf{x}_{\text{inp}}$, we get the key partial derivatives $\partial \mathrm{x}/\partial \Theta$ by differentiating the implicit function $\mathrm{F}(\mathbf{x}, \boldsymbol{\nu}(\boldsymbol{\Theta})) = \mathbf{0}$ and by applying the chain rule.

$$\begin{aligned} \frac{\partial \mathbf{x}}{\partial \boldsymbol{\Theta}} &= -\left(\frac{\partial \mathbf{F}}{\partial \mathbf{x}}\right)^{-1} \left(\frac{\partial \mathbf{F}}{\partial \boldsymbol{\nu}} \frac{\partial \boldsymbol{\nu}}{\partial \boldsymbol{\Theta}}\right) \\ &= -\left(\frac{\partial \mathbf{F}}{\partial \mathbf{x}}\right)^{-1} \left(\frac{\partial \mathbf{F}}{\partial \boldsymbol{\nu}_{\text{depend}}} \frac{\partial \boldsymbol{\nu}_{\text{depend}}}{\partial \boldsymbol{\Theta}} + \frac{\partial \mathbf{F}}{\partial \boldsymbol{\nu}_{\text{ext}}} \frac{\partial \boldsymbol{\nu}_{\text{ext}}}{\partial \boldsymbol{\Theta}}\right) \end{aligned} \tag{93}$$

We explained how to get $\partial \mathbf{F}/\partial \mathbf{x}$ for carbon isotopomer systems in Sect. 3.1.5. The partial derivatives $\partial \boldsymbol{\nu}_{\text{depend}}/\partial \boldsymbol{\Theta}$ can be obtained by differentiating with respect to $\boldsymbol{\Theta}$, and $\partial \boldsymbol{\nu}_{\text{ext}}/\partial \boldsymbol{\Theta}$ is simply $\mathbf{T}_{\text{flux}}$.

The partial derivatives of cumomer fractions with respect to $\boldsymbol{\Theta}$ are obtained by differentiating each kth level $\mathbf{F}_{\text{ext}}$ that is an implicit function of ${}^{k}\mathbf{x}_{\text{ext}}^{\text{cmf}}, {}^{1}\mathbf{x}_{\text{int}}^{\text{cmf}}, \ldots, {}^{k-1}\mathbf{x}_{\text{int}}^{\text{cmf}}, {}^{k}\mathbf{x}_{\text{int}}^{\text{cmf}}$, and $\boldsymbol{\nu}$, i.e.:

$$\begin{aligned} \frac{\partial^k \mathbf{x}_{\text{ext}}^{\text{cmf}}}{\partial \boldsymbol{\Theta}} = -\left(\frac{\partial^k \mathbf{F}_{\text{ext}}}{\partial^k \mathbf{x}_{\text{ext}}^{\text{cmf}}}\right)^{-1} &\left\{ \frac{\partial^k \mathbf{F}_{\text{ext}}}{\partial^k \mathbf{x}_{\text{int}}^{\text{cmf}}} \frac{\partial^k \mathbf{x}_{\text{int}}^{\text{cmf}}}{\partial \boldsymbol{\Theta}} + \frac{1}{2} \sum_{j=1}^{k-1} \left(\frac{\partial^k \mathbf{F}_{\text{ext}}}{\partial^j \mathbf{x}_{\text{int}}^{\text{cmf}}} \frac{\partial^j \mathbf{x}_{\text{ext}}^{\text{cmf}}}{\partial \boldsymbol{\Theta}}\right) \right. \\ &\left. + \frac{\partial^k \mathbf{F}_{\text{ext}}}{\partial \boldsymbol{\nu}} \frac{\partial \boldsymbol{\nu}}{\partial \boldsymbol{\Theta}} \right\} \end{aligned} \tag{94}$$

The partial derivatives of ${}^k\mathbf{x}_{\text{int}}^{\text{cmf}}$ with respect to $\boldsymbol{\Theta}$ are:

$$\frac{\partial^k \mathbf{x}_{\text{int}}^{\text{cmf}}}{\partial \boldsymbol{\Theta}} = -\left(\frac{\partial^k \mathbf{F}_{\text{int}}}{\partial^k \mathbf{x}_{\text{int}}^{\text{cmf}}}\right)^{-1} \cdot \left\{ \frac{1}{2} \sum_{j=1}^{k-1} \left(\frac{\partial^k \mathbf{F}_{\text{int}}}{\partial^j \mathbf{x}_{\text{int}}^{\text{cmf}}} \cdot \frac{\partial^j \mathbf{x}_{\text{int}}^{\text{cmf}}}{\partial \boldsymbol{\Theta}} \right) + \frac{\partial^k \mathbf{F}_{\text{int}}}{\partial \boldsymbol{v}} \cdot \frac{\partial \boldsymbol{v}}{\partial \boldsymbol{\Theta}} \right\} \quad (95)$$

By vertically concatenating resulting matrices, we get:

$$\frac{\partial \mathbf{x}_{\text{ext}}^{\text{cmf}}}{\partial \boldsymbol{\Theta}} = \left(\frac{\partial^1 \mathbf{x}_{\text{ext}}^{\text{cmf}}}{\partial \boldsymbol{\Theta}}; \ \frac{\partial^2 \mathbf{x}_{\text{ext}}^{\text{cmf}}}{\partial \boldsymbol{\Theta}} \ ; \ldots ; \ \frac{\partial^k \mathbf{x}_{\text{ext}}^{\text{cmf}}}{\partial \boldsymbol{\Theta}} \right) \quad (96)$$

As shown in Sect. 3.1.3, x can be transformed to be suited to measurements using the transformation matrices of $\mathbf{T}_{\text{idv} \rightarrow \text{mdv}}$, $\mathbf{T}_{\text{idv} \rightarrow \text{p}}$ or $\mathbf{T}_{\text{cmf} \rightarrow \text{idv}}$. For instance, when carbon isotopomers are transformed into mass isotopomers $\partial \mathbf{x}_{\text{ext}}/\partial \boldsymbol{\Theta} = \mathbf{T}_{\text{idv} \rightarrow \text{mdv}} \mathbf{T}_{\text{labeling}} \partial \mathbf{x}/\partial \boldsymbol{\Theta}$, and when cumomer fractions are transformed into mass isotopomer distributions, $\partial \mathbf{x}_{\text{ext}}/\partial \boldsymbol{\Theta} = \mathbf{T}_{\text{idv} \rightarrow \text{mdv}} \mathbf{T}_{\text{cmf} \rightarrow \text{idv}} \partial \mathbf{x}_{\text{ext}}^{\text{cmf}}/\partial \boldsymbol{\Theta}$.

In terms of the model's Jacobian matrix, we can provide the nonlinear problem (87) with the gradient (88) analytically and also obtain optimal designs of ^{13}C tracer experiments as well as statistical qualities of flux estimates.

3.3. Designing ^{13}C Tracer Experiments

When the model $\boldsymbol{\Phi}$ has been set up and its Jacobian matrix is available, computer-aided designs can be carried out to optimize experimental conditions based on a particular optimality criterion. There are various forms of optimality criteria used to select the points for a design. One popular criterion is the *D*-optimality, which seeks to maximize the determinant (**det**) of the information matrix of the model. The determinant is important because the inverse of $\mathbf{A}$ exists only if $\mathbf{det}(\mathbf{A}) \neq 0$. Numerically, smaller determinant results in larger inaccuracy for calculating the inverse of $\mathbf{A}$. The *D*-optimality criterion is a well-established method for multilevel experimental design concerning a regression model and is useful when accuracy of the parameters themselves is the primary concern (66).

As given by (90), solving the problem (87) requires inversion of a matrix $\mathbf{J}(\boldsymbol{\Theta})\boldsymbol{\Sigma}_{\eta}^{-1}\mathbf{J}(\boldsymbol{\Theta})$, which is the inverse of the covariance of the design parameter ($\boldsymbol{\Sigma}_{\Theta}$). Clearly, the experimental design maximizing the determinant of this matrix will give the most accurate numerical estimation of $\boldsymbol{\Theta}$. The inverse of $\boldsymbol{\Sigma}_{\Theta}$ is named Fisher's information matrix, i.e., $\boldsymbol{\Sigma}_{\Theta}{}^{-1} = \text{Fish}(\boldsymbol{\Theta})$. Maximizing the determinant of Fish($\boldsymbol{\Theta}$) is an identical process to minimizing its reciprocal value. Thus, the so-called *D*-value, the reciprocal of **det**(Fish ($\boldsymbol{\Theta}$)), is used to quantitate optimality of a design and is defined as:

$$D = \frac{1}{\mathbf{det}(\text{Fish}(\boldsymbol{\Theta}))} = \frac{1}{\mathbf{det}(\mathbf{J}(\boldsymbol{\Theta})^{\text{T}} \cdot \boldsymbol{\Sigma}_{\eta}^{-1} \cdot \mathbf{J}(\boldsymbol{\Theta}))} \quad (97)$$

The *D*-value gives the generalized variance of the estimates, i.e., the squared volumes of the confidence ellipsoids for a specified model. As the Jacobian matrix of the model is involved in the calculation of the *D*-value, the *D*-optimality is model-dependent.

The use of the *D*-optimality criterion to design ^{13}C tracer experiments has been introduced by Mollney et al. (67) and has proven useful for the identification of informative tracer substrates. To identify the optimal design, *D*-values have to be numerically minimized with respect to input tracer substrate to identify which ^{13}C-labeled tracer substrate is the optimal choice for determining the design parameter $\boldsymbol{\Theta}$ from an experiment. Yang et al. (68) suggested that one may implement a parallel set of tracer experiments using differently ^{13}C-labeled substrates to increase information content when measurable output metabolites are limited.

In case a previous experimental design is available, the quality of information expected from the new design can be evaluated by referencing it to the previous design. To this end, the relative information index $\boldsymbol{I}$ can be applied (59, 67, 68).

$$\boldsymbol{I} = \left(\frac{D_{\mathrm{REF}}(\mathbf{x}_{\mathrm{inp1}})}{D_{\mathrm{ND}}(\mathbf{x}_{\mathrm{inp2}})} \right)^{(1/(2N_{\mathrm{free}}))} \tag{98}$$

Here D_{REF} denotes the *D*-value of the reference design, D_{ND} is that of the new design, and N_{free} is the number of the independent variables in the model. The larger the relative information index resulting from an experimental design, the more information can be predicted with respect to the input labeling pattern used for the reference experiment.

3.4. Statistical Analysis

Once a system's characteristics have been estimated by solving the nonlinear problem (87), it is also important to determine statistical qualities of the results. There are two different approaches. One of them is the Monte Carlo simulation (MCS), which is useful for nondifferentiable models. However, the method is time-consuming for computation because a few hundred parameter estimation steps have to be performed repeatedly. The alternative method is the regression analysis. Its implementation can be mathematically complex for a nonlinear model with high dimensionality due to the requirement of analytical partial derivatives in vector space, but the computation time can be reduced.

3.4.1. Monte Carlo Method

The MCS methods refer to any simulations or computational experiments involving the use of random numbers (69). By performing statistical sampling experiments on a computer, the MCS provides, e.g., statistical characteristics of design parameters involved in the nonlinear least-squares minimization problems. Hereto, the procedure of the MCS can be outlined as follows.

1. Determine the pseudopopulation representing the true population of interest.
2. Generate a set of random numbers from the pseudopopulation.
3. Perform parameter estimation using the random numbers.
4. Repeat steps 2 and 3 for N trials and store N parameter estimates.
5. Evaluate statistical properties of the resulting pseudopopulations of design parameters.

The pseudopopulations of the measurement data $\boldsymbol{\eta}$ are determined from its corresponding measurement errors. Hereto, a measurement model can be generalized such that:

$$\boldsymbol{\eta} = \Phi(\boldsymbol{\Theta}) + \boldsymbol{\varepsilon} \tag{99}$$

The measurement error vector $\boldsymbol{\varepsilon}$ is typically assumed to be normally distributed with expectation vector $\mathbf{0}$ and its covariance matrix such that $\boldsymbol{\varepsilon} \in N(\mathbf{0}, \boldsymbol{\Sigma}_\eta)$. Accordingly, a random data set $\boldsymbol{\eta}_{\mathrm{RND}}$ can be generated using the statistic of $\boldsymbol{\eta}$. By repeatedly generating $\boldsymbol{\eta}_{\mathrm{RND}}$ and performing parameter estimation steps with an objective of ½ $||\boldsymbol{\eta}_{\mathrm{RND}} - \boldsymbol{\Phi}(\boldsymbol{\Theta})||^2$ weighted by the covariance $\boldsymbol{\Sigma}_\eta$, we get the statistical behavior of parameter estimates. For MCS, the number of trials N should be at least 50 when estimating the standard error of a statistic (70).

The MCS method is useful when (1) model is nondifferentiable, (2) its Jacobian matrix is ill-conditioned, or (3) it requires some constants k with uncertainties, e.g., a nonlinear model such as $\boldsymbol{\Phi}(\boldsymbol{\Theta}, k)$.

3.4.2. Nonlinear Regression Analysis

A least-squares problem is called regression analysis in statistics. The implementation of a nonlinear regression model begins with model linearization based on first-order Taylor's expansion. Due to this, the local behavior of the nonlinear model is linearly approximated. Assuming the parameter estimate is close to its true value, the nonlinear regression model (99) can be approximated in the neighborhood of the estimate (66). Assuming the parameter estimate $\boldsymbol{\Theta}^*$ is not biased and normally distributed such as $N(\boldsymbol{\Theta}^*, \boldsymbol{\Sigma}_\Theta)$, its covariance matrix results in (20):

$$\boldsymbol{\Sigma}_\Theta = (\mathbf{J}(\boldsymbol{\Theta}^*)^{\mathrm{T}} \cdot \boldsymbol{\Sigma}_\eta^{-1} \cdot \mathbf{J}(\boldsymbol{\Theta}^*))^{-1} \tag{100}$$

The main diagonal elements in $\boldsymbol{\Sigma}_\Theta$ equal the variances of $\boldsymbol{\Theta}^*$, i.e., $\boldsymbol{\sigma}^2 = \mathbf{diag}(\boldsymbol{\Sigma}_\Theta)$. Further, intracellular fluxes are functionally related to $\boldsymbol{\Theta}$ by (84). Thus, the covariance matrix given for the fluxes ($\boldsymbol{\Sigma}_{\mathrm{flux}}$) can be obtained according to the Gaussian error propagation.

$$\boldsymbol{\Sigma}_{\mathrm{flux}} = \frac{\partial \boldsymbol{v}_{\mathrm{depend}}}{\partial \boldsymbol{\Theta}}(\boldsymbol{\Theta}^*) \cdot \boldsymbol{\Sigma}_\Theta \cdot \frac{\partial \boldsymbol{v}_{\mathrm{depend}}}{\partial \boldsymbol{\Theta}}(\boldsymbol{\Theta}^*)^{\mathrm{T}} \tag{101}$$

From this, one can calculate the confidence intervals of each flux at a significant level of α.

$$[\boldsymbol{\nu}_i - \Delta, \boldsymbol{\nu}_i + \Delta] \quad \text{with}\, \Delta^2 = \chi_1^2(1-\alpha)\cdot\sigma_i^2 \tag{102}$$

If there is redundancy for the parameter estimation, this can be used for a hypothesis test to verify whether the data can be described by the model. This can be performed by using the following χ^2-test.

$$\| \boldsymbol{\eta} - \Phi(\boldsymbol{\Theta}^*) \|_{\boldsymbol{\Sigma}_\eta}^2 \leq \chi^2_{\dim\, \boldsymbol{\eta} - \dim\, \boldsymbol{\Theta}}(1-\alpha) \tag{103}$$

Glossary

Cumomers (cumulated isotopomers)	A set of one or more isotopomers whose particular carbon positions are labeled
Gradient	A vector field whose components are the partial derivatives of a scalar function f
Hessian matrix	The square matrix of second-order partial derivatives of a function
Isotopologues (isotopic homologues)	Molecular species having identical elemental and chemical compositions but differ in isotopic content
Isotopomers (isotopic isomers)	Molecular species that differ by the location of isotopes on a compound
Jacobian matrix	The matrix of all first-order partial derivatives of a vector-valued function
Least-squares minimization	Numerical estimation of regression parameters by minimizing the sum of the squared residuals resulting from the difference between the model-predicted and measured values
Mass isotopomers	Groups of isotopomers classified in accordance with their nominal mass
Metabolic flux	The rate at which material is processed through a metabolic pathway defined in a metabolic network
Metabolic flux analysis	Quantification of metabolic fluxes in a metabolic network
Nonlinear programming	A numerical process of solving a system containing nonlinear nature
Null space of a matrix A	The set of all vectors $\mathbf{x}$ for which $\mathbf{Ax} = \mathbf{0}$. The null space of a matrix with n columns is a linear subspace of n-dimensional Euclidean space
Parametrization	A process writing a function so that all the variables depend on the same variable (parameter)

Rank of a matrix	Maximal number of linearly independent rows (columns) in a matrix
Reduced row echelon form	A matrix obtained using Gauss–Jordan elimination with partial pivoting of its parent matrix

References

1. Stephanopoulos G, Aristidou AA, Nielsen JH. Metabolic engineering: principles and methodologies. San Diego, CA: Academic Press; 1998.
2. Stephanopoulos G. Metabolic fluxes and metabolic engineering. Metab Eng. 1999;1(1): 1–11.
3. Bailey JE. Reflections on the scope and the future of metabolic engineering and its connections to functional genomics and drug discovery. Metab Eng. 2001;3(2):111–4.
4. Brunengraber H, Kelleher JK, Des Rosiers C. Applications of mass isotopomer analysis to nutrition research. Annu Rev Nutr. 1997;17: 559–96.
5. Hellerstein MK. In vivo measurement of fluxes through metabolic pathways: the missing link in functional genomics and pharmaceutical research. Annu Rev Nutr. 2003;23:379–402.
6. Stephanopoulos G. Metabolic engineering. Biotechnol Bioeng. 1998;58(2–3):119–20.
7. Arauzo-Bravo MJ, Shimizu K. Estimation of bidirectional metabolic fluxes from MS and NMR data using positional representations. Genome Inform Ser Workshop Genome Inform. 2001;12:63–72.
8. Klamt S, Schuster S, Gilles ED. Calculability analysis in underdetermined metabolic networks illustrated by a model of the central metabolism in purple nonsulfur bacteria. Biotechnol Bioeng. 2002;77(7):734–51.
9. Wiechert W. Modeling and simulation: tools for metabolic engineering. J Biotechnol. 2002; 94 (1):37–63.
10. Matsuda F, Morino K, Miyashita M, Miyagawa H. Metabolic flux analysis of the phenylpropanoid pathway in wound-healing potato tuber tissue using stable isotope-labeled tracer and LC-MS spectroscopy. Plant Cell Physiol. 2003;44(5):510–7.
11. Yang C, Hua Q, Shimizu K. Metabolic flux analysis in *Synechocystis* using isotope distribution from ^{13}C-labeled glucose. Metab Eng. 2002;4(3):202–16.
12. Forbes NS, Meadows AL, Clark DS, Blanch HW. Estradiol stimulates the biosynthetic pathways of breast cancer cells: detection by metabolic flux analysis. Metab Eng. 2006;8 (6):639–52.
13. Puccetti C, Aureli T, Manetti C, Conti F. ^{13}C-NMR isotopomer distribution analysis: a method for measuring metabolic fluxes in condensation biosynthesis. NMR Biomed. 2002; 15(6):404–15.
14. Yang TH, Wittmann C, Heinzle E. Respirometric ^{13}C flux analysis—part II: in vivo flux estimation of lysine-producing *Corynebacterium glutamicum*. Metab Eng. 2006;8 (5):432–46.
15. Vo TD, Palsson BO. Isotopomer analysis of myocardial substrate metabolism: a systems biology approach. Biotechnol Bioeng. 2006;95(5):972–83.
16. Ratcliffe RG, Shachar-Hill Y. Measuring multiple fluxes through plant metabolic networks. Plant J. 2006;45(4):490–511.
17. Wiechert W, Noh K. From stationary to instationary metabolic flux analysis. Adv Biochem Eng Biotechnol. 2005;92:145–72.
18. Wiechert W. ^{13}C metabolic flux analysis. Metab Eng. 2001;3(3):195–206.
19. Nocedal J, Wright SJ. Numerical optimization. New York, NY: Springer; 1999.
20. Arnold SF. Mathematical statistics. Englewood Cliffs, NJ: Prentice-Hall; 1990.
21. Vallino JJ, Stephanopoulos G. Metabolic flux distributions in *Corynebacterium glutamicum* during growth and lysine overproduction [reprinted from Biotechnol Bioeng 1993;41: 633–46]. Biotechnol Bioeng. 2000;67(6): 872–85.
22. Varma A, Palsson BO. Stoichiometric flux balance models quantitatively predict growth and metabolic by-product secretion in wild-type *Escherichia coli* W3110. Appl Environ Microbiol. 1994;60(10):3724–31.
23. van der Heijden RT, Heijnen JJ, Hellinga C, Romein B, Luyben KC. Linear constraint relations in biochemical reaction systems: I. Classification of the calculability and the balanceability of conversion rates. Biotechnol Bioeng. 1994;43:3–10.
24. Nielsen J. Metabolic engineering. Appl Microbiol Biotechnol. 2001;55(3):263–83.

25. Wiechert W, Mollney M, Petersen S, de Graaf AA. A universal framework for ^{13}C metabolic flux analysis. Metab Eng. 2001;3(3):265–83.
26. Wittmann C. Metabolic flux analysis using mass spectrometry. Adv Biochem Eng Biotechnol. 2002;74:39–64.
27. Marx A, de Graaf AA, Wiechert W, Eggeling L, Sahm H. Determination of the fluxes in the central metabolism of *Corynebacterium glutamicum* by nuclear magnetic resonance spectroscopy combined with metabolite balancing. Biotechnol Bioeng. 1996;49(2):111029.
28. Wittmann C, Heinzle E. Genealogy profiling through strain improvement by using metabolic network analysis: metabolic flux genealogy of several generations of lysine-producing *Corynebacteria*. Appl Environ Microbiol. 2002;68(12):5843–59.
29. Pfeiffer T, Schuster S, Bonhoeffer S. Cooperation and competition in the evolution of ATP-producing pathways. Science. 2001;292(5516): 504–7.
30. Varma A, Palsson BO. Metabolic capabilities of *Escherichia coli*: I. Synthesis of biosynthetic precursors and cofactors. J Theor Biol. 1993;165 (4):477–502.
31. Edwards JS, Palsson BO. Systems properties of the *Haemophilus influenzae* Rd metabolic genotype. J Biol Chem. 1999;274(25): 17410–6.
32. Bonarius HP, Timmerarends B, de Gooijer CD, Tramper J. Metabolite-balancing techniques vs. ^{13}C tracer experiments to determine metabolic fluxes in hybridoma cells. Biotechnol Bioeng. 1998;58(2–3):258–62.
33. Dauner M, Sauer U. GC-MS analysis of amino acids rapidly provides rich information for isotopomer balancing. Biotechnol Prog. 2000;16 (4):642–9.
34. Stephanopoulos G, Alper H, Moxley J. Exploiting biological complexity for strain improvement through systems biology. Nat Biotechnol. 2004;22(10):1261–7.
35. Sauer U. High-throughput phenomics: experimental methods for mapping fluxomes. Curr Opin Biotechnol. 2004;15(1):58–63.
36. Christensen B, Nielsen J. Isotopomer analysis using GC-MS. Metab Eng. 1999;1(4):282–90.
37. Macallan DC, Fullerton CA, Neese RA, Haddock K, Park SS, Hellerstein MK. Measurement of cell proliferation by labeling of DNA with stable isotope-labeled glucose: studies in vitro, in animals, and in humans. Proc Natl Acad Sci U S A. 1998;95(2):708–13.
38. Shulman RG, Rothman DL. ^{13}C NMR of intermediary metabolism: implications for systemic physiology. Annu Rev Physiol. 2001;63: 15–48.
39. Wittmann C, Heinzle E. Application of MALDI-TOF MS to lysine-producing *Corynebacterium glutamicum*: a novel approach for metabolic flux analysis. Eur J Biochem. 2001;268(8):2441–55.
40. Bonarius HP, Ozemre A, Timmerarends B, et al. Metabolic-flux analysis of continuously cultured hybridoma cells using $^{13}CO_2$ mass spectrometry in combination with ^{13}C-lactate nuclear magnetic resonance spectroscopy and metabolite balancing. Biotechnol Bioeng. 2001;74(6):528–38.
41. Forbes NS, Clark DS, Blanch HW. Using isotopomer path tracing to quantify metabolic fluxes in pathway models containing reversible reactions. Biotechnol Bioeng. 2001;74(3): 196–211.
42. Antoniewicz MR, Kelleher JK, Stephanopoulos G. Elementary metabolite units (EMU): a novel framework for modeling isotopic distributions. Metab Eng. 2007;9(1):68–86.
43. Zupke C, Stephanopoulos G. Modeling of isotope distributions and intracellular fluxes in metabolic networks using atom mapping matrixes. Biotechnol Prog. 1994;10(5): 489–98.
44. Schmidt K, Carlsen M, Nielsen J, Villadsen J. Modeling isotopomer distributions in biochemical networks using isotopomer mapping matrixes. Biotechnol Bioeng. 1997;55(6): 831–40.
45. Wiechert W, Mollney M, Isermann N, Wurzel M, de Graaf AA. Bidirectional reaction steps in metabolic networks: III. Explicit solution and analysis of isotopomer labeling systems. Biotechnol Bioeng. 1999;66(2):69–85.
46. Hellerstein MK, Neese RA. Mass isotopomer distribution analysis at eight years: theoretical, analytic, and experimental considerations. Am J Physiol. 1999;276(6 pt 1):E1146–70.
47. Dauner M, Bailey JE, Sauer U. Metabolic flux analysis with a comprehensive isotopomer model in *Bacillus subtilis*. Biotechnol Bioeng. 2001;76(2):144–56.
48. Follstad BD, Stephanopoulos G. Effect of reversible reactions on isotope label redistribution—analysis of the pentose phosphate pathway. Eur J Biochem. 1998;252(3):360–71.
49. Wiechert W, de Graaf A. Bidirectional reaction steps in metabolic networks: I. Modeling and simulation of carbon isotope labeling experiments. Biotechnol Bioeng. 1997;55(1):102–17.
50. de Graaf AA, Mahle M, Mollney M, Wiechert W, Stahmann P, Sahm H. Determination of full ^{13}C isotopomer distributions for metabolic flux analysis using heteronuclear spin echo difference NMR spectroscopy. J Biotechnol. 2000; 77(1):25–35.

51. Sriram G, Shanks JV. Improvements in metabolic flux analysis using carbon bond labeling experiments: bondomer balancing and Boolean function mapping. Metab Eng. 2004;6(2): 116–32.
52. van Winden WA, Heijnen JJ, Verheijen PJ. Cumulative bondomers: a new concept in flux analysis from 2D [^{13}C,^{1}H] COSY NMR data. Biotechnol Bioeng. 2002;80(7):731–45.
53. Christensen B, Christiansen T, Gombert AK, Thykaer J, Nielsen J. Simple and robust method for estimation of the split between the oxidative pentose phosphate pathway and the Embden-Meyerhof-Parnas pathway in microorganisms. Biotechnol Bioeng. 2001;74 (6):517–23.
54. Kreyszig E. Advanced engineering mathematics. 7th ed. New York, NY: Wiley; 1993.
55. Yang TH, Wittmann C, Heinzle EE. Metabolic network simulation using logical loop algorithm and Jacobian matrix. Metab Eng. 2004; 6(4):256–67.
56. Press WH. Numerical recipes in C: the art of scientific computing. 2nd ed. Cambridge, UK: Cambridge University Press; 1992.
57. Conn AR, Gould NIM, Toint PL. Trust-region methods. Philadelphia, PA: Society for Industrial and Applied Mathematics; 2000.
58. Wiechert W, Siefke C, de Graaf A, Marx A. Bidirectional reaction steps in metabolic networks: II. Flux estimation and statistical analysis. Biotechnol Bioeng. 1997;55(1):118–35.
59. Arauzo-Bravo MJ, Shimizu K. An improved method for statistical analysis of metabolic flux analysis using isotopomer mapping matrices with analytical expressions. J Biotechnol. 2003;105(1–2):117–33.
60. Zhao J, Shimizu K. Metabolic flux analysis of *Escherichia coli* K12 grown on ^{13}C-labeled acetate and glucose using GC-MS and powerful flux calculation method. J Biotechnol. 2003; 101(2):101–17.
61. Floudas CA, Pardalos PM. Recent advances in global optimization. Princeton, NJ: Princeton University Press; 1992.
62. Schmidt K, Nielsen J, Villadsen J. Quantitative analysis of metabolic fluxes in *Escherichia coli*, using two-dimensional NMR spectroscopy and complete isotopomer models. J Biotechnol. 1999;71(1–3):175–89.
63. Mendes P, Kell D. Non-linear optimization of biochemical pathways: applications to metabolic engineering and parameter estimation. Bioinformatics. 1998;14(10):869–83.
64. Nash SG, Sofer A. Linear and nonlinear programming. New York, NY: McGraw-Hill; 1996.
65. Schittowski K. NLQPL: a FORTRAN-subroutine solving constrained nonlinear programming problems. Ann Oper Res. 1985;5: 485–500.
66. Massart DL. Handbook of chemometrics and qualimetrics. Amsterdam, The Netherlands: Elsevier; 1997.
67. Mollney M, Wiechert W, Kownatzki D, de Graaf AA. Bidirectional reaction steps in metabolic networks: IV. Optimal design of isotopomer labeling experiments. Biotechnol Bioeng. 1999;66(2):86–103.
68. Yang TH, Heinzle E, Wittmann C. Theoretical aspects of ^{13}C metabolic flux analysis with sole quantification of carbon dioxide labeling. Comput Biol Chem. 2005;29(2):121–33.
69. Martinez WL, Martinez AR. Computational statistics handbook with MATLAB. Boca Raton, FL: Chapman & Hall/CRC; 2002.
70. Efron B, Tibshirani R. An introduction to the bootstrap. New York, NY: Chapman & Hall; 1993.

Chapter 9

Introduction to Metabolic Control Analysis (MCA)

Maliackal Poulo Joy, Timothy C. Elston, Andrew N. Lane, Jeffrey M. Macdonald, and Marta Cascante

Abstract

Metabolic Control Analysis (MCA) provides a conceptual framework for understanding the control of fluxes though metabolic pathways at the molecular level. It further provides a theoretical underpinning for an experimental approach to determining metabolic control. In this chapter, the basic principles of MCA are introduced, and the kinds of applications that are accessible to this approach. The relationship to flux analysis and measurement of metabolic fluxes is outlined.

Key words: Metabolic control analysis, Flux control, Elasticity

1. Introduction

In the preceding chapters, methods of determining the concentrations of metabolites and obtaining flux information by analysis of isotopomers have been presented. However, the number of metabolites that can be determined with sufficient accuracy and precision, and the time dependence of their changes, remains comparatively limited, and as such a complete description of the entire system at the atomic level is underdetermined. Even with this limitation, it is possible to make use of existing knowledge about biochemical pathways and networks to address general questions about flux control at a systems level. There are several approaches to this complex problem, as described in Chaps. 8, 10, and 11. A comparatively simple approach that is commonly used is Metabolic Control Analysis (MCA). In this chapter, we present the basic theoretical background to this approach.

To understand why some enzymes have a strong influence on cell physiology and how they control cell growth and transformation, two main theoretical frameworks have been developed

Teresa Whei-Mei Fan et al. (eds.), *The Handbook of Metabolomics*, Methods in Pharmacology and Toxicology, DOI 10.1007/978-1-61779-618-0_9,

during the last 3 decades, the Biochemical Systems Theory (BST) developed by Savageau (1–4) and the MCA (5, 6). These theories have been developed largely independently of each other, and although they use different nomenclatures, they both provide a formalism for a quantitative description of substrate flux in response to changes in various system parameters in complex enzyme systems (7–10). In this chapter, we use the MCA formalism. MCA and metabolic profiling are closely related fields because carbon flow changes are the combined results of changes in enzyme activity, substrate availability, and redistribution.

If one assumes that, under appropriate conditions, the metabolic network is in a steady state, then the properties of pathways can be described simply in terms of the component enzymes and metabolites. How these steady state fluxes and metabolite concentrations are influenced by enzyme properties or other parameters in the system can be understood using a mathematical technique called MCA (6, 11). MCA helps us to predict the metabolic effects of perturbations on the system and tell us how metabolic system properties are controlled and shared among different enzymes in the pathway. An important conclusion of MCA is that control may be distributed over the entire system, rather than there being a single rate-limiting step. MCA provides a framework for quantifying the degree of flux control exerted by any given enzyme in a pathway. This has important ramifications for targeting enzymes for inhibition in a therapeutic context, as well as for understanding the influence of xenobiotics on entire metabolic pathways, and is therefore a valuable tool for designing approaches for modulating metabolic activity for therapeutics, as well as for understanding the response of organisms to environmental toxicants.

First, we introduce some basic concepts that relate thermodynamics to kinetics in a cellular context.

1.1. Thermodynamics and Kinetics

A live cell is thermodynamically an open system for example that maintains a nonequilibrium state. The same is true for tissues and an entire organism, but at a different level. For a biological system, this all requires very careful choice of standard states, and exactly what constitutes the system.

The Gibbs free energy (constant pressure) defines the state of a system in relative to equilibrium. The chemical potential, μ is the partial molar free energy (i.e., normalized to the molar concentration). The actual value of the free energy G depends on the conditions, including the concentrations of all species present in the system. Thus it is necessary to define the free energy difference between two states, such as a chemical reaction, under a defined set of conditions that represent a reference state. In biochemistry, this is often taken to be pH 7, 310 K, and 100 mM ionic strength and the activity of water = 1 for 55.5 M (12). The free energy change under these conditions is the standard Gibbs energy, ΔG^0, which is related to the equilibrium constant K by

$$\Delta G^0 = -\mathrm{RTln}\, K = \Delta H^0 - T\Delta S^0 \tag{1}$$

Where ΔH is the change in enthalpy, which is effectively heat (and is what is measured in a calorimeter). $T\Delta S$ is the entropic term, which in very crude terms relates to a change in the order or number of degrees of freedom in the reaction.

If ΔH is not zero, then K is dependent on temperature. K may also depend on ionic strength, water activity, pressure, and a wide variety of other variables.

By definition, at equilibrium, there is no net flux, i.e., the rates in the forward and reverse directions are identically equal. This standard free energy is rarely if ever realized in real systems. The important value is the available free energy ΔG, which defines the departure from equilibrium. The equilibrium constant is equal to the ratio of the chemical activities of the products and reactants, namely:

$$K = \Pi{<}a_{\mathrm{p}}{>}/\Pi{<}a_{\mathrm{s}}{>} \tag{2}$$

where $<a_{\mathrm{p}}>$ and $<a_{\mathrm{s}}>$ are the activities of the products and reactants at equilibrium respectively.

Activities are generally cast in the form $a = \gamma c$ where c is the concentration and γ is the activity coefficient in concentration terms. Under ideal conditions, or at the defined standard state, γ is unity, so under these conditions the activity is equal to the concentration. Unfortunately, the interior of cells is not close to the biochemical standard state, as different compartments may have quite different pH values, and the concentration of protein approaches 200 mg/mL, i.e., far from thermodynamic ideality. If the activity of water at 55.5 M is set to 1, then a is around 0.7 for cellular water. Furthermore, in addition to compartmentation making cells inhomogeneous, even individual compartments are irregular solutions (cf. membrane surfaces and various fibers or filaments). These conditions can certainly influence the activity coefficients markedly (13).

The equilibrium constant is expressed as an activity ratio. For a system not at equilibrium, a similar activity ratio can be calculated, i.e., $\Gamma = a_{\mathrm{p}}/a_{\mathrm{s}}$, which is simply the experimental value of the ratio of the activities (concentrations) at a particular time or sample.

The free energy associated with this ratio is then $\Delta G = -\mathrm{RTln}$ $(a_{\mathrm{p}}/a_{\mathrm{s}})$, and thus the deviation from equilibrium can be written as:

$$\Delta G - \Delta G^0 = -\mathrm{RTln}\ \Gamma/K \tag{3}$$

This equation simply indicates the direction of the spontaneous reaction depending on the departure of the activity ratio from that at equilibrium. If $\Gamma/K < 1$ the reaction proceeds toward P, whereas if

$\Gamma/K > 1$, it goes from P to S. As this is a path-independent process, it matters not whether the individual reactions are catalyzed or not, as a catalyst (e.g., an enzyme) does not influence ΔG, only the rate at which equilibrium is attained. The corollary to this statement is that an enzyme does not influence the direction of a reaction.

It is common in biochemical systems for the available free energy to favor the reaction in the "wrong" direction. Anabolic reactions fall into this category, as they are thermodynamically uphill. To drive a reaction against its thermodynamic driving force requires a net input of energy. This is achieved by coupling to another reaction or set of reactions that is thermodynamically more favorable such as the hydrolysis of ATP to ADP, inorganic phosphate and a proton. This reaction is biochemically favorable in a live cell because the ratio of ATP to ADP and Pi is maintained high compared with the equilibrium constant, at the expense of an input of energy in the form of glucose some of which is recovered from the of oxidation to CO_2. In a dead cell, this reaction lies far to the right.

Thus for the reaction A⇔B where $K_1 = b/a$ lies very much in the direction A, then A can be converted to B by coupling to the reaction:

$$\mathrm{ATP} + \mathrm{H_2O} \Leftrightarrow \mathrm{ADP} + \mathrm{Pi} \ + \mathrm{H}^+ : \mathrm{K_2}$$

The free energies of these reactions are

$$\Delta G_1 = \Delta G_1^0 - \mathrm{RTln}\, b/a$$

$$\Delta G_2 = \Delta G_2^0 - \mathrm{RTln(adp.pi.h^+/atp)} \approx -7\ \mathrm{kcal/mol}\ (\mathrm{at\,pH}\ 7)$$

Suppose that $\Delta G_1^0 = -\Delta G_2^0$, and favors A over B ca. 10^5-fold at equilibrium. Under these conditions, the coupled equilibrium would be $K_1K_2 = 1$ thus making the ratio $b/a = 1$ instead of 10^{-5}. This assumes that all the standard free energy is available, i.e., starting from ATP and A in their standard states. The actual free energy available depends on the ratio of the concentrations to the equilibrium values. For example, if the ratio atp/adp.pi were maintained at 5 mM^{-1} (e.g., 2 mM ATP, 0.1 mM ADP and 4 mM Pi), the available free energy is −6 kcal/mol, then the ratio of b/a would be 0.2.

The net flux of a reaction *does* depend on the degree of departure from equilibrium.

1.2. A Simple Example: Linear pathway

Consider an unbranched pathway from S to P,

$$\mathrm{S} \Leftrightarrow \mathrm{B} \Leftrightarrow \mathrm{C} \Leftrightarrow \mathrm{D} \Leftrightarrow \mathrm{P}$$

$$\mathrm{E1} \quad \mathrm{E2} \quad \mathrm{E3} \quad \mathrm{E4} \tag{4}$$

The flux from substrate S to product P depends on the concentrations of the metabolites S and P, the concentrations of the enzymes E_1–E_4, their intrinsic catalytic power (e.g., k_{cat}/K_m) and the overall equilibrium constant, $K_{eq} = p_{eq}/s_{eq}$. Here, we use lower case letters to denote the concentrations of upper case species, e.g., e is the concentration of E. At the steady state, the rate at each step is the same. At chemical equilibrium, the flux J is by definition zero, which occurs when the product/substrate ratio is equal to the equilibrium ratio. The disequilibrium ratio Γ is defined as the ratio $(p/s)/K_{eq}$, which is unity at equilibrium. The critical parameter thermodynamically is then the departure from equilibrium $(1-\Gamma)$. The net flux is maintained by a continued input of substrate, e.g., from the exterior of the cell. If the disequilibrium ratio is much less than 1, then the flux J is maximal in the forward direction (S to P), whereas if $\Gamma > 1$, the flux is in the reverse direction (i.e., P to S). The steady state flux for an enzyme-catalyzed reaction can be written in terms of the free (uncomplexed) concentrations for enzyme (e) and substrates (s) and the disequilibrium ratio as (14):

$$J = (k_{cat}/K_m)e.s(1 - \Gamma) \qquad (5)$$

In some pathways, e.g., glycolysis, most of the metabolites are present at concentration below both their K_m values (15), and also the active site concentrations (16, 17), in which case, the free enzyme concentration is close to the total enzyme concentration, and the enzyme is far from saturation.

For a simple scheme as in (4), the flux can be written as

$$J = f(k_i).s.(1 - \Gamma) \qquad (6)$$

Where $f(k_i)$ is a function of the enzyme activities e_i,

In the linear scheme (4), the net flux at steady state is the same at each step, i.e., J(S–B) = J(B–C) etc. Using the formalism of (5), in terms of free enzyme and substrate concentration, the flux from S to P can be written:

$$J(S - P) = k_1k_2k_3k_4s(1 - p/s/K_{eq})/[k_{-1}k_{-2}(k_{-3} + k_4) + k_3k_4(k_{-1} + k_2)] \qquad (7)$$

where $k_i = (k_{cat}/K_m)_ie_i$ The same enzyme catalyzes a given step in both the forward and reverse directions, and therefore $k_1 = (k_{cat}/K_m)_{1i}e_1$ and $k_{-1} = (k_{cat}/K_m)_{-1}e_i$, etc.

Hence, (7) predicts that the flux at constant $s(1-\Gamma)$ is essentially hyperbolic in each enzyme concentration, e_i (Fig. 1a). As the activity of any one enzyme is increased from a very low value to a very high value, the flux J will increase hyperbolically to a maximum rate that is determined by the activities of all the other enzymes in the pathway. In the limit that the activity of one enzyme is very low, then it would become the rate-limiting

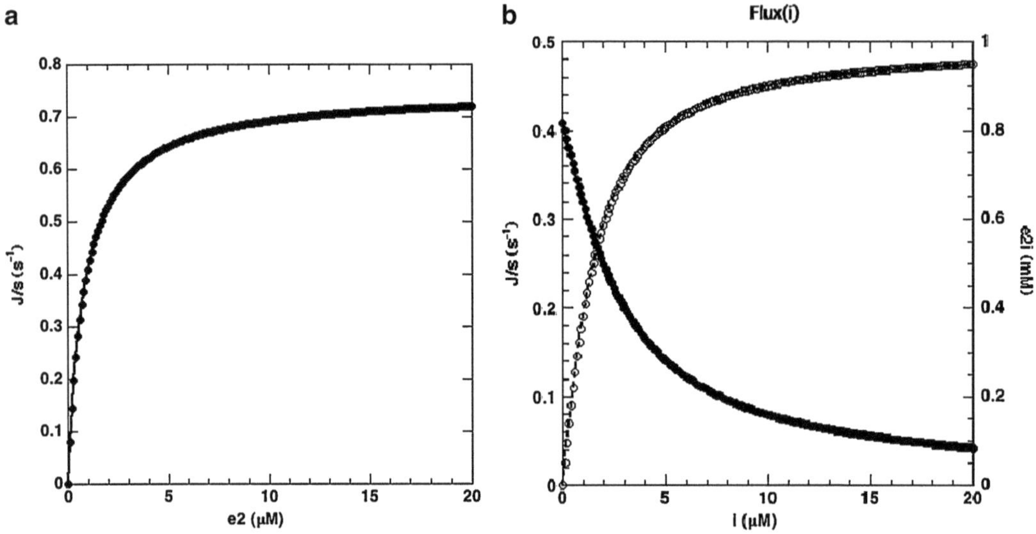

Fig. 1. Dependence of net flux on enzyme concentration and inhibitor concentration for a simple pathway. The linear pathway in scheme 1 was used with the following parameters. All forward rate constants k_1, k_2, k_3, $k_4 = k_{cat,i}/K_{m,i}$ were set to 1 $\mu M^{-1}\ s^{-1}$, and all enzyme concentrations except E2 were set to 1 μM. All reverse rate constants were set to 1 $\mu M^{-1}\ s^{-1}$ except for E1 which was 0.1 $\mu M^{-1}\ s^{-1}$. The term $1-\Gamma$ was set to 0.9, i.e., strong forward flux. Dependence of *J*/*s* on the concentration of E2. (**b**) Dependence of the flux on the concentration of a competitive inhibitor I binding to E2 with a dissociation constant of 1 μM. The left ordinate shows the flux, the right ordinate the concentration of EI complex. All other parameters as in (**a**).

component, whereas once it becomes in large excess over the capacities of the other enzymes, it exerts no further influence on the flux and hence has no control over the flux. From Fig. 1a, we can see that under the condition where the enzyme activities are balanced ($(k_{cat}/K_m)e = 1$ μM for all the enzymes and $1 - \Gamma = 0.9$) the maximum increase in the flux obtainable from increasing the concentration of an enzyme (e2) is of the order twofold. In contrast, if a particular enzyme is inhibited, for example by adding a competitive inhibitor of one enzyme, the flux can be made to decrease ultimately to zero (Fig. 1b). However, for abundant enzymes, such as those found in glycolysis, the concentration of the inhibitor needed to effect a substantial decrease in flux can be very high. For 1 μM enzyme, and a modest affinity of inhibitor of 1 μM, even a 20-fold excess of the inhibitor, sufficient to reduce the free enzyme concentration to 5%, the flux decreased to 10% in this example. As discussed by Fell (6), the shape of this curve depends strongly on the conditions and the intrinsic control coefficient of the enzyme to be inhibited.

Such considerations do not take into account changes in concentration of intermediates that arise due to changes in activity of a particular enzyme (but see below). The question then is how to assess the degree of flux control over the net pathway flux; this is the goal of MCA, which provides a means to estimate the quantitative contribution to flux control for each enzyme in a pathway, and the response to changes in concentrations of intermediates.

2. Metabolic Control Analysis as a Tool to Identify Control Steps

MCA provides a quantitative description of substrate flux in response to changes in system parameters of complex enzyme systems. Medical applications of the approach include identifying candidate enzymes in pathways suitable as targets for cancer therapy (7) (and Chap. 10). MCA complements current studies of genomics and proteomics, providing a link between biochemistry and functional genomics that relates the expression of genes and gene products to cellular biochemical and physiological events. Thus, it is an important tool for the study of genotype–phenotype correlations. It allows genes to be ranked according to their importance in controlling and regulating cellular metabolic networks. We can expect that MCA will have an increasing impact on the choice of targets for intervention in drug discovery.

Therefore, MCA characterizes system behavior and identifies crucial steps in metabolic pathway regulation. Such information is necessary for predicting critical enzymatic target sites for genetic, chemical, or metabolic intervention (through gene therapy, small-molecule drugs, or dietary treatments) and to identify key points of intervention in metabolic pathways linked to cancer.

An important puzzle in drug discovery is how to identify key targets in disease pathways. Differential expression of genes between diseased and healthy tissue is commonly taken as an indication of the specific targets of disease pathways. Such an approach ignores the obvious fact that the robust metabolic network of feedback loops and regulatory mechanisms within cells has evolved to maintain homeostasis and to withstand a variety of genetic and environmental insults. The interlinking of disease pathways through such a metabolic network increases the difficulty of identifying therapeutic targets using information from gene expression analysis. On the other hand, MCA approaches the problem of drug targeting by examining the contribution of individual components within a metabolic network, providing a theoretical framework for describing metabolic/signaling/genetic systems of any complexity.

MCA is concerned with understanding the effects of changes in the parameters such as enzyme concentrations, temperature, pH, etc., on the metabolic system quantities such as flux or metabolite concentrations (6, 11). Thus, it provides a framework for estimating the sensitivity of a metabolic network function to system parameters. Sensitivity of metabolic flux and concentrations on the enzyme activities or other parameters are characterized by control coefficients.

It has been observed that the flux control coefficients in many metabolic pathways are similar for several steps along the pathways (18), that is, the control does not reside in any single enzyme. Furthermore, certainly for central pathways like glycolysis, the maximum possible rate as expressed by V_{max} of individual enzymes may exceed the flux by an order of magnitude or more (19, 20) in some tissues. This implies that the flux capacity is not maximal under many operating conditions. To materially affect the flux through such a balanced pathway, in principle any one of the enzymes can be a target for an inhibitor, which would have to reduce the activity of the enzyme by a high fraction, and indeed maintain that level of inhibition in the face of continued enzyme synthesis and turnover. However, in high flux cases, the V_{max} values may be comparable to the actual fluxes in vivo (20).This underlines the importance of considering the actual tissue and its physiological function.

MCA was introduced to biochemical systems in the 1970s by Kacser and Burns (21, 22) and Heinrich and Rapaport (23–25). MCA involves calculating the control coefficients, and here, we list some of them and relationships among them.

3. Flux and Concentration Control Coefficients

In contrast to the conventional belief that there is only one enzyme determining the flux through a pathway, it is quite clear that due to the complex network of metabolic systems, activities of several enzymes control the flux or rate of a particular reaction. Hence, it is necessary to identify the contributions of each enzyme on the flux of a reaction, as they can be very different. This control is quantified by Flux Control Coefficients (FCC). Consider the steady state flux, v_j of a reaction in a metabolic pathway to be J and let e_i be the concentration of an enzyme in the reaction pathway. The ratio of the fractional change of flux to the fractional change in the concentration of the enzyme is defined as the Flux Control Coefficient, C^J_{Ei}

$$C^J_{\mathrm{Ei}} = (e_i/J)\partial J/\partial e_i = \partial \ln(J)/\partial \ln e_i \qquad (8)$$

The FCC can be considered as the fractional change in flux for a small relative change in enzyme concentration.

Figure 2 is a plot of the flux control coefficient. As expected from Fig. 1, in a linear metabolic chain where all the enzymes obey Michaelis–Menten kinetics, the flux control coefficient changes for a high value at low enzyme concentration, and approaches zero once the concentration of enzyme i exceeds the capacity of the remaining enzymes in the pathway. Interestingly, enzymes with sigmoidal kinetics can maintain or even gain control with an

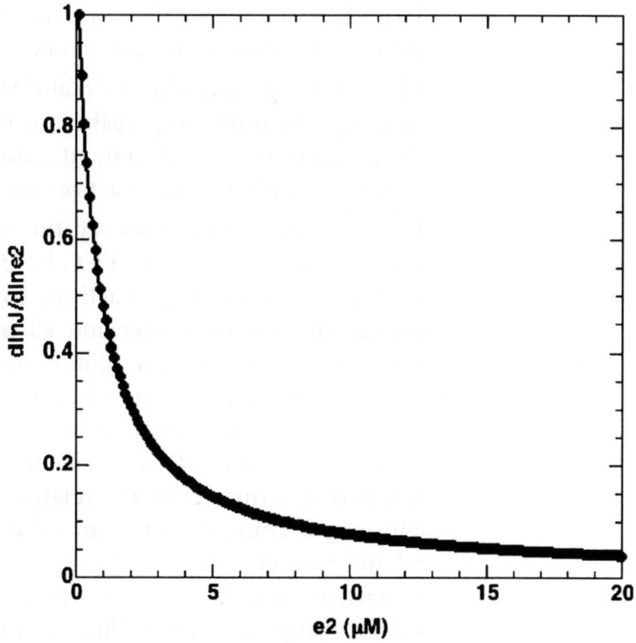

Fig. 2. Flux control coefficient. The control coefficient for enzyme 2 in scheme 1 was calculated from the slope of the *J/s* curve in Fig. 1, multiplied by the ratio *e2/J*, according to (5) in the text.

increase in enzyme activity or concentration. This has been described as "paradoxical control" and it has been experimentally demonstrated that hepatic glucokinase, which has a very high flux control coefficient and displays sigmoidal behavior within the hepatocyte in situ as a result of interaction with a regulatory protein, displays sustained or increased control over an extended range of enzyme concentrations when the regulatory protein is overexpressed (26, 27). It should be noted that the existence of sustained or increased control of a step in a metabolic pathway could be important in biotechnology as activation of an enzyme that displays this property would have similar effects on the flux over a wide range of enzyme activities.

Furthermore, since the control coefficients are the fractional changes in flux for fractional changes in activity, the maximum values of C must be unity, assuming reactions that are linear in enzyme activity. This further implies that the sum of the control coefficients cannot exceed unity, which can be expressed as the summation theorem, namely

$$\sum_{i=1} C^{J}_{\mathrm{Ei}} \qquad (9)$$

This immediately shows that under balanced conditions, all of the flux coefficients are similar, and therefore must be of the order

$1/n$ where n is the number of steps. Thus, in an n-step pathway, the control of each enzyme can be said to be large if the actual value of C^J_{Ei} is much greater than $1/n$ and vice versa. If one enzyme has a large C^J_{Ei}, then it is responsible for most of the flux control under the conditions of measurement, and the remaining enzymes contribute a much smaller fraction to the control (i.e., collectively, $1 - C^J_{\mathrm{Ei}}$). In a linear pathway the maximum FCC value is unity and for that case all other FCC have to be zero. This corresponds to a true rate limiting reaction. In reality a few of the control coefficients will be higher and all others will be essentially zero. Those enzymes that have high control coefficients can be considered as the most important ones controlling the particular flux. For example, in the scheme given by (4), the control coefficients for the balanced case will be 0.25, which implies that the relative change in flux is only a quarter of the relative change in enzyme activity. In contrast, a control coefficient of 0.75 in this instance implies a relative flux change of 0.75 times the relative change in enzyme activity, and for the remaining three enzymes, the control is at most a 25% change in relative flux per unit change in relative enzyme activity, and on average only 8% for those three enzymes. Thus, if C^J_{E2} is 0.75, and C^J_{E1}, C^J_{E3} and C^J_{E4} are 0.083 each, then the relative flux control is nine times as much for E2 as the other three enzymes.

However, changes in the activity of an enzyme in the pathway are likely also to change the concentration of metabolites. The effect of this is characterized using the concentration control coefficient (CCC), $C^{\mathrm{S}}_{\mathrm{Ei}}$. Analogously to FCC, it is defined as the ratio of the fractional change of concentration of substrate to the fractional change in the concentration of the enzyme.

$$C^{\mathrm{S}}_{\mathrm{Ei}} = (e_i/s_j)\partial s_j/\partial e_i = \partial \ln(s_j)/\partial \ln e_i \tag{10}$$

A change in the activity of enzyme i may change the concentrations of the substrate and products of that reaction. But because these are then substrates and product of the sequential neighbors in the reaction network, (cf. scheme 4) this may alter the flux and balances of intermediates throughout the pathway. The net result is that a depletion of intermediate i is compensated for any depletion of connected intermediates, such that the sum of all of the concentration control coefficient is zero, as expressed by:

$$\sum C^{\mathrm{S}}_{\mathrm{Ei}} = 0 \tag{11}$$

Summation theorems clearly indicate the "whole system" nature of metabolic activity. Since the control coefficients with respect to different enzymes of a flux or a metabolite concentration obey these equalities, they are constrained and one can deduce the most important enzymes that control the activity. In general several enzymes of the pathway share the control of flux and concentrations. In all these analyses, we assume that the changes in the activities of enzymes are infinitesimal and the system has dynamic and structural stability, meaning that the steady states are retained under small perturbations and in the case of parameter perturbations, the resulting steady states are close enough to the unperturbed case. Moreover, we always consider only the case where the activity of an enzyme is proportional to its concentration. Cases where enzymes interact to form complexes in which the properties of the individual components are changed need additional attention (28), such as where substrate channeling occurs or at certain branch points (29). A generalization of MCA that addresses these complications has been presented (10, 30, 31).

An attractive feature of MCA is that it does not require all system components to be characterized a priori (6, 32). Moreover, control coefficients can be estimated for different components of the network and for pertinent environmental factors. The control coefficients give a first approximation of which proteins or pathways may exert more control on the system properties to be modified. Targeting the steps with higher control coefficients on relevant system properties, such as tumor growth or obesity, could be a good strategy to design effective therapeutic agents (7). In the case of the pentose phosphate pathway, which is enhanced in tumor cells, an in vivo tumor growth control coefficient of 0.9 was measured in mice with Ehrlich's ascites tumor for transketolase (33), while for glucose-6-phosphate dehydrogenase a control coefficient of 0.41 was computed (34) and these enzymes are ranked as new promising anticancer drug targets (27, 35). These control coefficients indicate that these two enzymes are important for the tumor cell progression and therefore could be good candidates for a combined multiple-hit anticancer therapy (36). The expanded understanding of crucial proliferative processes provided by MCA and metabolic profiling make it clear that target metabolic enzymes for new anticancer therapies have to be those that are demonstrated to have high control coefficients (see below) to limit substrate flow for nucleic acid ribose synthesis. This is, of course, also a crucial criterion in drug development efforts in which the efficacy of potential antiproliferative drugs is determined by metabolic screening.

As an inhibitor of a specific enzyme is titrated in, the activity of that enzyme will decrease, i.e., its FCC will increase; at some point it will become the rate-limiting step in the pathways, implying a redistribution of all other control coefficients, and also the concentrations of intermediates within the pathways. This in itself could have serious metabolic consequences, even if the enzyme is not completely inhibited. It is generally difficult to achieve 100% inhibition because of protein turnover, limited affinity and dose/delivery. Clearly it is desirable to target an enzyme that has a high

FCC (say>0.8) than one with a low FCC (<0.2), as in the former case, a substantial decrease in flux will be achieved for relatively small degree of inhibition of the enzyme, whereas for the latter case, a much higher effective dose of inhibitor would be needed, and this will cause a larger redistribution of intermediates, as shown below.

Specific examples of applications of MCA are presented in the Chaps 10 and 11.

4. Elasticity Coefficients

The effect of changing the metabolite concentration on the rate of a reaction, v_i, is quantified by elasticity coefficients. Since the concentration of products also can affect the rate, one can calculate the elasticity coefficient not only with respect to substrates but also with respect to products. Instead of considering the enzyme concentration as a parameter, one can consider any other parameter which affects the metabolic activity to calculate this coefficient. In those cases it is called the π-elasticity and the former is called ε-elasticity.

$$\varepsilon_{\mathrm{S}}^{\mathrm{V}} = (s_i/v_j)\partial v_j/\partial s_i = \partial \ln(v_j)/\partial \ln s_i \quad \varepsilon - \text{elasticities} \tag{12a}$$

$$p_{\mathrm{S}}^{\mathrm{V}} = (p_i/v_j)\partial v_j/\partial p_i = \partial \ln(v_j)/\partial \ln p_i \quad \pi - \text{elasticities} \tag{12b}$$

For a Michaelis–Menten enzyme,

$$\varepsilon_{\mathrm{S}}^{\mathrm{v}} = K_{\mathrm{m}}/(s + K_{\mathrm{m}}) \tag{12c}$$

$\varepsilon_{\mathrm{s}}^{\mathrm{v}}$ approaches unity at low substrate concentrations, and zero at saturating concentrations. Indeed, any reaction rate curve that shows a saturation behavior has these properties, though the steepness of the slope of ε in the neighborhood of the substrate concentration that gives half maximal velocity varies according to the degree of cooperativity for example, as shown in Fig. 3. The elasticity, or the response of the flux through reaction j to the concentration of substrate is much steeper for a cooperative enzyme than for an enzyme obeying Michaelis–Menten kinetics.

4.1. Connectivity Theorems

Elasticity is a local quantity in the sense that it is independent of changes in other parts of the pathway. However the system level properties become manifest when we take into consideration the relations between FCC, CCC, and elasticity coefficients. The connectivity theorems describe this interconnectedness of a biochemical pathway.

The connectivity theorem for FCC is:

$$\sum C_{\mathrm{Ei}}^{J} \varepsilon_{\mathrm{s}}^{v_i} = 0 \tag{13a}$$

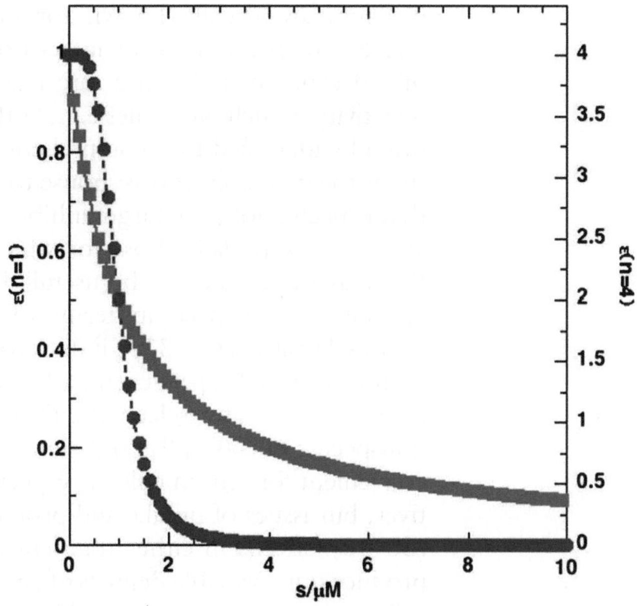

Fig. 3. Elasticity coefficients. Elasticity coefficients were calculated for the Michaelis–Menten model (*filled circles*) and for the Hill model with $n = 4$ (*filled squares*). The K_m and $K_{0.5}$ values were 1 μM in each simulation. Left ordinate $n = 1$, right ordinate $n = 4$.

and for each pair of metabolites of the system S_j and S_k the connectivity theorem for CCC is:

$$\sum C^{S_j}_{E_i\,ij}\varepsilon^{v_i}_{S_k} = -\delta_{jk} \quad \text{where } \delta_{jk} = 0 \text{ if } j \neq k \text{ and } \delta_{jk} = 1 \text{ if } j = k \tag{13b}$$

These relationships are very powerful in terms of constraints on metabolic networks, and the relationship between global fluxes and the properties of individual enzymes. One can use these relations to calculate some of the unknown coefficients using a few known ones. For example, consider enzymes 2 and 3 for scheme 4, which catalyze the interconversion of B to C and C to D, respectively. The relevant FCC are C^J_{E2} and C^J_{E3} and the elasticities are ε^{v2}_{B} and ε^{v3}_{C}. If C is shared only by these two enzymes (no branching or feedback inhibition involving B or C), then from (10), $C^J_{B}\varepsilon^{v2}_{B} = -C^J_{E3}\varepsilon^{v3}_{C}$, i.e., there are only three independent parameters. In an extended pathway, the number of such equations can be used to solve explicitly for all of the control coefficients if the elasticities are known (6).

Direct measurement of FCC and CCC can done by perturbing the enzyme activity using specific inhibitors, siRNA and antisense oligonucleotides, titration with purified enzymes, or by genetic modification to over express enzymes or even groups of enzymes. Although affinities of small molecule inhibitors for the target enzymes are usually known for purified systems in vitro, the effective does required for intact cells or tissues has to be determined experimentally, and care taken to account for the limited selectivity of such molecules e.g., "off target" effects. The latter can often by identified by a comprehensive metabolite profiling analysis, as the metabolic flux response to an inhibitor may deviate from that expected for pure target inhibition. Off target effects of drugs are legion, especially those for which the affinity is only modest. Whereas these may still be useful clinically (multiple targets may actually be beneficial in terms of cell killing and suppressing acquired resistance—(37)), it does complicate the analysis of effects on flux thorough a particular pathways. The siRNA approach offers in principle greater selectivity, though care has to be taken over nonspecific effects (38), and similarly for antisense. The latter is convenient for cells in culture, especially using morpholino derivatives, but issues of uptake and protein binding must be addressed (38–40). siRNA in either transient or stable transfected cells can produce quite variable degrees of enzyme activity depending on the cell type and mode of delivery. However, under the best conditions, >90% suppression can be achieved. For the purposes of MCA or flux analysis, the stable transfection approach is preferred, because it is possible to select the transected cell population, and further place the expression of the siRNA under the control of an inducible promoter, such as the Tet repressor/doxycycline (41, 42), thereby providing control over the timing of the knockdown. It is essential always to determine not only the degree of knockdown of the specific message (such as by qRTPCR) but also the enzyme level (e.g., by Western), and indeed ultimately by the specific activity of the enzyme in the cell population. The disadvantage of the mRNA manipulation is that it can be difficult to control the level of knockdown; MCA analysis is in its initial derivation couched in terms of infinitesimal changes in activity. This limitation has in part been overcome as in recent years control coefficients for large changes have been defined and summation theorems, in terms of enzyme concentrations as well as expressions to calculate these control coefficients in terms of the elasticity coefficients for large changes have been derived (43, 44).

As discussed above, the control coefficients must themselves change as the activity of an enzyme is deceased for a high excess over the pathways flux capacity to becoming essentially a rate-limiting enzyme. Upregulation of enzyme activity is complementary, and similar arguments apply. These considerations are nicely exemplified by MCA of respiring mitochondria. The control coefficients of different steps vary greatly according to the availability of substrates, glycolytic enzyme capacity and the proton leakage pathways. Thus, in the transition from state 4 to state 3, the control coefficient for the proton leak decreases from around 0.9 in state 3 to <0.1 in state 4, whereas the ATP turnover reactions increase from zero in state 3, reach a maximum of about 0.75 at 50% maximal respiration rates, and then decline. The slack is largely taken up by increasing succinate utilization in the state 3 to state 4 transition (45).

Indirect measurements involve first finding elasticity coefficients and then using connectivity theorems to evaluate the control coefficients. This involves a kinetic model, and hence, kinetic constants are needed. Whereas a pathway model is likely to be available because of extensive literature biochemistry and now the large number of sequenced genomes (albeit many incompletely annotated), estimation of appropriate kinetic constants is not straightforward. Even where the catalytic constants and K_m values for all substrates have been measured in vitro, these can differ substantially from the relevant values in vivo, particularly where there are multiple allosteric effectors, whose concentrations may not be well determined in vivo. However, one can use approximate kinetic descriptions such as lin-log kinetics (46, 47) to model biochemical pathways where there is no need for the explicit knowledge of kinetic parameters.

4.2. How Much Perturbation Can Be Tolerated Experimentally?

The foregoing presents a formalism for analyzing the control of flux through pathways. In practical terms, this requires making measurements of carefully perturbed systems. As Figs. 1–3 show, the control coefficients are themselves in general concentration dependent. However, such considerations suggest practical rules of thumb as to the size of the perturbation that can be used experimentally, such that the various equations apply. Experimentally, one will generally measure typically $\Delta J/\Delta p$ (where p is some experimentally perturbed parameter) at a small number of points. In the limit of a high value of C, i.e., when the enzyme exerts most of the control, then the control coefficient for that enzyme has the maximum dependence on the enzyme concentration, and small perturbations are needed to define it (Fig. 2). In contrast, at sufficiently high values of a particular enzyme activity, the flux is insensitive to its concentration, and relatively large perturbations are both necessary to measure a change in flux at all, and introduce relatively little error. However, small control coefficients are of lesser interest.

5. Conclusions

MCA is a relatively simple formalism for assessing the distribution of control within metabolic pathways, and provides a framework for designing appropriate experiments. Its major achievements are to show that flux control is in general distributed and that control and regulation should be considered as different things. For example, feedback regulation, so common in bacteria, leads to a decrease in the flux control coefficient of the feedback regulated enzyme, exactly the opposite of general expectation. It does, however, serve to stabilize metabolic concentrations (i.e., homeostasis), which is not only the hallmark of well-performing systems but also a desirable trait (6).

6. Resources and Further Reading

http://bip.cnrs-mrs.fr/bip10/mcafaq.htm
http://dbkgroup.org/mca_home.htm
http://www.copasi.org/tiki-index.php (48)

Glossary

Disequilibrium ratio	Deviation of a reaction from equilibrium as expressed by the ratio of the actual reactants to the values they have at equilibrium, under the prevailing conditions $\Gamma = (p/s)/K\text{eq}$. This is related to the available free energy difference for driving a reaction: $\Delta G = \Delta G^0 - \text{RTln}\,\Gamma$
Elasticity	Is a property of an enzyme and determines how the flux through a particular step depends on the substrate concentration: $\partial \ln v_i / \partial \ln s_i$
Flux	Net rate of a reaction or of a pathway. Flux is the difference between the forward rate and the reverse rate, $J = v_f - v_r$
Flux Control	The extent to which flux is determined and is a system property. If J is the net flux, the control is determined by the sensitivity of the net flux to changes in activity at individual steps
Flux Control Coefficient (FCC)	Fractional change in flux due to a fractional change in enzyme activity a: $\text{FCC} = \partial \ln J / \partial \ln a$
Hill equation	Proteins that interact with multiple substrates or ligands, such as hemoglobin, may show cooperativity between binging sites. The Hill equation represents an all or none cooperative binding equation of the form $F = s^n/(K + s^n)$ where n is the Hill coefficient. A value $n > 1$ implies positive cooperativity, and $n < 1$ is negative cooperativity. N is always less than the number of binding

	sites. Cf. Monod–Wyman–Changeux and Koshland–Nemethy–Filmer models (15)
k_{cat}, K_m	In the Michaelis–Menten mechanism, k_{cat} is the turnover number for an enzyme and represents the apparent first order rate constant for the breakdown of ES complexes. K_m is operationally the concentration of substrate at which the reaction velocity is half its maximum possible, as determined by $V_{max} = k_{cat}$.[enzyme]. k_{cat}/K_m is the apparent second order rate constant or substrate-enzyme complex formation and determines the specificity of the enzyme for its substrate (15)
Rate	Speed of a reaction. For a Michaelis–Menten reaction, the initial rate is $v_i = V_{max}.s/(K_m + s)$
Regulation	In MCA, control and regulation are distinct properties. Control is defined through the coefficients such as FCC. In contrast, regulation refers to the maintenance of homeostasis (i.e., resistance change), and a regulated enzyme is one that performs this task. Such an enzyme does not have to have a high FCC
Response	How flux changes with respect to a local parameter p such as an effector $Ri = \partial \ln J/\partial \ln pi$

References

1. Savageau MA, Voit EO, Irvine DH. Biochemical systems-theory and metabolic control-theory.1. fundamental similarities and differences. Math Biosci. 1987;86(2):127–45.
2. Savageau MA, Voit EO, Irvine DH. Biochemical systems-theory and metabolic control-theory. 2. the role of summation and connectivity relationships. Math Biosci. 1987;86(2):147–69.
3. Savageau MA. Design of molecular control mechanisms and demand for gene-expression. Proc Natl Acad Sci USA. 1977;74(12):5647–51.
4. Voit EO. Computational analysis of biochemical systems: a practical guide for biochemists & molecular biologists. Cambridge, UK: Cambridge University Press; 2000.
5. Fell DA. Metabolic control analysis—a survey of its theoretical and experimental development. Biochem J. 1992;286:313–30.
6. Fell D. Understanding the control of metabolism. In: Snell K, editor. Frontiers in metabolism. London: Portland Press; 1997.
7. Cascante M, Boros LG, Comin-Anduix B, de Atauri P, Centelles JJ, Lee PWN. Metabolic control analysis in drug discovery and disease. Nat Biotechnol. 2002;20(3):243–9.
8. Cornishbowden A. Metabolic control-theory and biochemical systems-theory—different objectives, different assumptions, different results. J Theor Biol. 1989;136(4):365–77.
9. Cascante M, Franco R, Canela EI. Use of implicit methods from general sensitivity theory to develop a systematic-approach to metabolic control.1. unbranched pathways. Math Biosci. 1989;94(2):271–88.
10. Cascante M, Franco R, Canela EI. Use of implicit methods from general sensitivity theory to develop a systematic-approach to metabolic control.2. complex-systems. Math Biosci. 1989;94(2):289–309.
11. Heinrich R, Schuster S. The regulation of cellular systems. New York: Chapman & Hall; 1996.

12. Nicholls DG, Ferguson SJ. Bioenergetics3. San Diego: Academic Press; 2001.
13. Hall D, Minton AP. Macromolecular crowding: qualitative and semiquantitative successes, quantitative challenges. Biochim Biophys Acta-Proteins and Proteomics. 2003;1649 (2):127–39.
14. Roberts JKM, Lane AN, Clark RA, Nieman RH. Relationships between the rate of synthesis of ATP and the concentrations of reactants and products of ATP hydrolysis in maize roottips, determined by P-31 nuclear magnetic-resonance. Arch Biochem Biophys. 1985;240 (2):712–22.
15. Fersht A. Structure and mechansim in protein science. Structure and mechansim in protein science. New York: W.H. Freeman & Co; 1999.
16. Albe KR, Butler MH, Wright BE. Cellular concentrations of enzymes and their substrates. J Theor Biol. 1990;143(2):163–95.
17. Srivastava DK, Bernhard SA. Enzyme enzyme interactions and the regulation of metabolic reaction pathways. Curr Top Cell Regul. 1986;28:1–68.
18. Werle M, Jahn L, Kreuzer J, Hofele J, Elsasser A, Ackermann C, Katus HA, Vogt AM. Metabolic control analysis of the Warburg-effect in proliferating vascular smooth muscle cells. J Biomed Sci. 2005;12(5):827–34.
19. Marin-Hernandez A, Rodriguez-Enriquez S, Vital-Gonzalez PA, Flores-Rodriguez FL, Macias-Silva M, Sosa-Garrocho M, Moreno-Sanchez R. Determining and understanding the control of glycolysis in fast-growth tumor cells—flux control by an over-expressed but strongly product-inhibited hexokinase. FEBS J. 2006;273(9):1975–88.
20. Suarez RK, Staples JF, Lighton JRB, West TG. Relationships between enzymatic flux capacities and metabolic flux rates: Nonequilibrium reactions in muscle glycolysis. Proc Natl Acad Sci USA. 1997;94(13):7065–9.
21. Kacser H, Burns J. The control of flux. Symp Soc Exp Biol. 1973;27:65–104.
22. Kacser H, Burns J, Fell D. The control of flux. Biochem Soc Trans. 1995;1923:1341–66.
23. Heinrich R, Rapoport TA. Linear steady-state treatment of enzymatic chains—general properties, control and effector strength. Eur J Biochem. 1974;42(1):89–95.
24. Heinrich R, Rapoport TA. Linear steady-state treatment of enzymatic chains—critique of crossover theorem and a general procedure to identify interaction sites with an effector. Eur J Biochem. 1974;42(1):97–105.
25. Rapoport TA, Heinrich R, Jacobasc G, Rapoport S. Linear steady-state treatment of enzymatic chains—mathematical-model of glycolysis of human erythrocytes. Eur J Biochem. 1974;42(1):107–20.
26. Kholodenko BN, Brown GC. Paradoxical control properties of enzymes within pathways: Can activation cause an enzyme to have increased control? Biochem J. 1996;314:753–60.
27. de Atauri P, Acerenza L, Kholodenko BN, de la Iglesia N, Guinovart JJ, Agius L, Cascante M. Occurrence of paradoxical or sustained control by an enzyme when overexpressed: necessary conditions and experimental evidence with regard to hepatic glucokinase. Biochem J. 2001;355:787–93.
28. Kacser H, Sauro HM, Acerenza L. Enzyme-enzyme interazctions and control analysis.1. the case of nonadditivity—monomer-oligomer associations. Eur J Biochem. 1990;187 (3):481–91.
29. Kohdolenko BN, Lyubarev AE, Kurganov BI. Control of the metabolic flux in a system with high enzyme concentrations and moiety-conserved cycles. Eur J Biochem. 1992;210:147–53.
30. Kholodenko BN, Cascante M, Westerhoff HV. Control-theory of metabolic channeling. Mol Cell Biochem. 1995;143(2):151–68.
31. Kholodenko BN, Westerhoff HV, Puigjaner J, Cascante M. Control in channeled pathways—a matrix-method calculating the enzyme control coefficients. Biophys Chem. 1995;53 (3):247–58.
32. Cornish-Bowden A, Cárdenas ML. Technological and medical implications of metabolic control analysis. Dordrecht: Kluwer; 2000.
33. Comin-Anduix B, Boren J, Martinez S, Moro C, Centelles JJ, Trebukhina R, Petushok N, Lee WNP, Boros LG, Cascante M. The effect of thiamine supplementation on tumour proliferation—a metabolic control analysis study. Eur J Biochem. 2001;268(15):4177–82.
34. Boren J, Montoya AR, de Atauri P, Comin-Anduix B, Cortes A, Centelles JJ, Frederiks WM, Van Noorden CJF, Cascante M. Metabolic control analysis aimed at the ribose synthesis pathways of tumor cells: a new strategy for antitumor drug development. Mol Biol Rep. 2002;29(1–2):7–12.
35. Bowden AC. Metabolic control analysis in biotechnology and medicine. Nat Biotechnol. 1999;17(7):641–3.
36. Ramos-Montoya A, Lee WNP, Bassilian S, Lim S, Trebukhina RV, Kazhyna MV, Ciudad CJ, Noe V, Centelles JJ, Cascante M. Pentose phosphate cycle oxidative and nonoxidative balance: a new vulnerable target for

overcoming drug resistance in cancer. Int J Cancer. 2006;119(12):2733–41.

37. Weinberg RA. The Biology of Cancer. Garland Science: New York; 2007.

38. Summerton JE. Morpholino, siRNA, and S-DNA compared: impact of structure and mechanism of action on off-target effects and sequence specificity. Curr Top Med Chem. 2007;7(7):651–60.

39. Robu ME, Larson JD, Nasevicius A, Beiraghi S, Brenner C, Farber SA, Ekker SC. p53 activation by knockdown technologies. PLoS Genet. 2007;3(5):787–801.

40. Du LT, Pollard JM, Gatti RA. Correction of prototypic ATM splicing mutations and aberrant ATM function with antisense morpholino oligonucleotides. Proc Natl Acad Sci USA. 2007;104(14):6007–12.

41. Liu YM, Borchert GL, Donald SP, Surazynski A, Hu CA, Weydert CJ, Oberley LW, Phang JM. MnSOD inhibits proline oxidase-induced apoptosis in colorectal cancer cells. Carcinogenesis. 2005;26(8):1335–42.

42. Monroe DG, Getz BJ, Johnsen SA, Riggs BL, Khosla S, Spelsberg TC. Estrogen receptor isoform-specific regulation of endogenous gene expression in human osteoblastic cell lines expressing either ER alpha or ER beta. J Cell Biochem. 2003;90(2):315–26.

43. Acerenza L. Design of large metabolic responses. Constraints and sensitivity analysis. J Theor Biol. 2000;207(2):265–82.

44. Acerenza L, Ortega F. Metabolic control analysis for large changes: extension to variable elasticity coefficients. Iee Proceedings Systems Biology Syst Biol (Stevenage). 2006;153(5):323–6.

45. Nicholls DG, Ferguson SJ, The chemiosmotic proton circuit. In: Bioenergetics3. San Diego: Academic Press; 2001

46. Hatzimanikatis V, Bailey JE. Effects of spatiotemporal variations on metabolic control: approximate analysis using (log)linear kinetic models. Biotechnol Bioeng. 1997;54(2):91–104.

47. Wu L, Wang WM, van Winden WA, van Gulik WM, Heijnen JJ. A new framework for the estimation of control parameters in metabolic pathways using lin-log kinetics. Eur J Biochem. 2004;271(16):3348–59.

48. Hoops S, Sahle S, Gauges R, Lee C, Pahle J, Simus N, Singhal M, Xu L, Mendes P, Kummer U. COPASI—a complex pathway simulator. Bioinformatics. 2006;22:3067–74.

Chapter 10

Application of Tracer-Based Metabolomics and Flux Analysis in Targeted Cancer Drug Design

Marta Cascante, Vitaly Selivanov, and Antonio Ramos-Montoya

Abstract

Metabolic profiling using stable-isotope tracer technology enables the measurement of substrate redistribution within major metabolic pathways in living cells. This technique has demonstrated that transformed human cells present acute metabolic shifts and that some anticancer drugs induce their effects by forcing the reversion of these metabolic changes. This chapter introduces the application of tracer-based metabolomics and flux analysis in the design of new anticancer therapies, and discusses differential metabolic adaptations of cancer cells that can be new complementary targets in the design of rational combinational treatments in chemotherapy.

Key words: Metabolic Control Analysis, Cancer Therapy, Metabolic Profiling

Abbreviations

e4p	Erythrose-4-phosphate
f6p	Fructose-6-phosphate
g3p	Glyceraldehyde-3-phosphate
MS	Mass spectrometry
NMR	Nuclear magnetic resonance
PPP	Pentose phosphate pathway
r5p	Ribose-5-phosphate
s7p	Sedoheptulose-7-phosphate
TA	Transaldolase
TK	Transketolase
xu5p	Xylulose-5-phosphate

Teresa Whei-Mei Fan et al. (eds.), *The Handbook of Metabolomics*, Methods in Pharmacology and Toxicology, DOI 10.1007/978-1-61779-618-0_10, © Springer Science+Business Media New York 2012

1. Introduction

Metabolites as the end products of cellular regulatory processes ultimately reflect the response of biological systems to genetic or environmental intervention. Metabolite profiling consists of the identification of the specific metabolic profile that characterizes a given sample, i.e., the set of all the metabolites detected by analyzing a sample using appropriate analytical techniques (1, 2). Metabolomics complements genomics and proteomics, which characterize a more static state of the cell, while the global dynamic study of cellular metabolism is exclusively provided by flux analysis. Therefore, development of metabolomics is urgent and vital for Systems Biology application to Biomedicine and Biotechnology. Actually, approaching the cell as a complex system has long been an established principle in metabolic engineering (3, 4) and, by making possible the detection of new drug targets in biochemical networks for therapeutic use, this should improve the process of validating drug targets and finally increase the rate of pharmaceutical innovation. The most critical challenges are to identify the commonly elusive controlling enzymatic steps that strongly affect metabolic substrate flux and thus operate as adequate targets of further genetic, chemical, or metabolic interventions.

Analysis of the central metabolic processes and their regulation in normal and cancer cells allows obtaining information, which complements that from genomics and proteomics, and to identify the best drug targets for intervention at pharmacologic or genetic levels. This knowledge will also serve for prevention of diseases or early treatment avoiding extensive use of drugs (5, 6). The behavior of metabolic networks in mammalian cells, as indicated by the flow of substrates, is defined by interconnected elements of the cell function regulation, it is complex, and it is governed at each level by different mechanisms (7, 8). Signaling events lead to related metabolic reactions, which in turn modify other metabolic functions or gene expression, thus forming a biological system of complex regulatory mechanisms (8, 9). Metabolic profiling supplies essential information beyond the achieve of signal transduction and genetic studies, showing whether the adjustments in carbon flow, i.e., pentose cycle metabolism, that are crucial for fast cell proliferation are taking place. Additionally, the use of metabolic profiling to both identify important targets and fully determine if a candidate anticancer drug in fact induces a growth-limiting effect makes molecular profiling a precious new tool in the efficient development of effective mechanism-based antitumor drugs. The fact that although molecular genetic studies can anticipate changes in metabolism, they cannot entirely explain if metabolic network enzymes with strong control properties are active and their substrates abundantly present demonstrates the necessity for metabolic profiling using stable isotope-labeled substrates.

Drug discovery today puts serious emphasis on discovering new anticancer products that work by interfering with cell growth by targeting specific signal transduction pathways or genes. The use of metabolic profiles in the drug discovery process facilitates the determination of the important enzymatic steps that control carbon flow into proliferation-related macromolecules. It is possible, using metabolic profiling, to identify new targets for anticancer compounds that selectively disrupt the unique metabolic network adaptation of cancer cells (10–12). There still are potential targets to be explored, with the notion that a combined approach of studying signaling, genetic, and metabolic events on the same bench will enable to better define the metabolic adaptations crucial for cancer cell growth and death. Using such an approach, a much larger set of anticancer compounds could be screened according to their signaling properties and metabolic profiles during the industrial drug development process (12–14).

1.1. Differential Metabolic Adaptation of Cancer Cells Can Be New Complementary Targets in the Design of Rational Combinational Therapies in Chemotherapy

The latest molecular studies have demonstrated that quite a few of the multiple genetic alterations that cause tumor development directly affect cellular energy metabolism through the glucose metabolic network (15–18). Particularly, it has been demonstrated that most tumors produce high levels of lactate and fructose 1,6-bisphosphate and have high rates of aerobic glycolysis, with correspondingly high rates of biosynthesis of both lipids and nucleic acids (9). This collection of metabolic adaptations of cancer cells is vital for their capability for uncontrolled proliferation in a hypoxic tumor environment and confers a strong robustness to cancer cells for the development of drug resistance. Nevertheless, the sharing of precursor substrates and cofactors of other interconnecting pathways, which make cancer cells vulnerable to perturbation of the network, restrict these adaptive mechanisms. Such restrictions imply the existence of rare points of fragility, which could become logical new drug targets. Consequently, it has been suggested that strategies designed to prevent metabolic network adaptation essential for cancer cell proliferation would be particularly efficacious in the treatment of cancer drug resistance (8, 9, 19–21).

Conceiving a combination drug therapy to prevent drug resistance is not an easy duty. The interconnected network of alternative pathways can be rearranged by the cancer cells to overcome the effects of drug inhibition of a single pathway (22, 23). Besides, there is convincing evidence showing that many of the intracellular metabolic networks are robust and that major changes in their outputs may not occur in spite of dramatic changes in a single component of the network (24, 25). One of the main changes in tumor cell metabolic network happens at a proteomic level, by changing the isoenzymatic pattern of important glucose central metabolism enzymes, like the pyruvate kinase, hexokinase, or transketolase (26–29). An isoenzyme is an enzyme that takes part in the same reaction, but presents a different structure and has a different response towards metabolites. The expression of an isoenzyme could give some advantageous metabolic characteristics to the tumor cell, but at the same time researchers might use this difference between the tumor cell and its normal counterpart as a new target in anticancer therapy. The situation of pyruvate kinase is very descriptive (26). This enzyme presents four different isoforms: L-PK, predominant in gluconeogenic tissues like liver or kidney; R-PK, predominant in erythrocytes; M1-PK, predominant in tissues with high glycolysis and high energy production, as muscle and brain; and M2-PK, predominant in lung and high nucleogenic tissues, as it is the case of proliferant cells, embryonic cells, stem cells, and tumoral cells. M2-PK presents a feature which is precious to the tumoral cell: it can alternate between a dimeric form, which seems to be generated by the direct interaction of M2-PK with several oncoproteins and presents lower affinity towards phosphoenolpyruvate, thus provoking an accumulation of glycolytic intermediates that derive to nucleic acid, phospholipid, and aminoacid synthesis; and a tetrameric form, which favors the conversion of glucose to pyruvate with the generation of energy. Tumoral cells appear to be able to modify this dimeric/tetrameric conformation according to their necessities of energy and cell division. Moreover, recently Stetak et al. (30) showed that the tumor marker M2-PK plays a general role in caspase-independent cell death of tumor cells and thereby defines this glycolytic enzyme as a novel target for cancer therapy development.

Changes of glucose metabolic fluxes distribution also appear to be decisive for the tumor cell as well as the changes in the isoenzyme expression. In previous studies, it has been exposed that metabolic adaptation of tumor metabolism contains an enhancement of pentose phosphate cycle fluxes and a specific balance between oxidative and nonoxidative branches to maintain the high proliferative rates (31, 32). It has been hypothesized that this balance between oxidative and nonoxidative branches of the pentose phosphate cycle is indispensable to maintain the metabolic efficiency of the cancer cell for growth and proliferation (11, 33, 34). Ramos-Montoya et al. (11) validated this hypothesis by showing that the perturbation of this balance using a multiple-hit drug strategy results in metabolic inefficiency and cell death.

2. Metabolic Control Analysis as a Tool to Identify Control Steps and Potential Drug Targets

To comprehend why some enzymes have a strong influence on cell physiology and how they control cell growth and transformation, the two main theoretical frameworks have been the Biochemical Systems Theory (BST) developed by Savageau (35), Voit (36) and Metabolic Control Analysis (MCA) (8, 37). These theories have been developed almost independently of each other during the past decades, and although they use different nomenclatures, they are equivalent in providing a quantitative description of substrate flux in response to changes in various system parameters in complex enzyme systems (38, 39). MCA and metabolic profiling are, in fact, closely related fields since carbon flow changes are the combined results of enzyme activity changes and substrate availability and redistribution. The control exerted over substrate flux or any systemic parameter (e.g., cell proliferation) can be quantitatively described in MCA as a control coefficient for each and every enzyme in a metabolic network (and see Ch. 9). As an example, pentose phosphate pathway (PPP) enzymes have been characterized in terms of their flux control coefficients in different mammalian cells, including tumor cells. The growth control coefficients of glucose-6-phosphate dehydrogenase and transketolase in the Ehrlich's tumor model have been shown to be high (33), becoming new promising targets for anticancer drugs (20). The extended comprehension of essential proliferative processes provided by MCA and metabolic profiling makes it obvious that target metabolic enzymes for new anticancer therapies have to be those that are demonstrated to have high control coefficients to limit substrate flow for nucleic acid ribose synthesis. This is, certainly, also a fundamental condition in drug development efforts in which metabolic screening is necessary to determine the efficacy of potential antiproliferative drugs.

As described in the Chap. 9, MCA provides a quantitative description of substrate flux in response to changes in system parameters of complex enzyme systems.

How to identify key targets in disease pathways becomes a significant puzzle in drug discovery. Differential expression of genes between diseased and healthy tissue is usually taken as a sign of the specific targets of disease pathways. Such an approach pays no attention to the obvious fact that the robust metabolic network of feedback loops and regulatory mechanisms within cells has evolved to maintain homeostasis and to withstand a variety of genetic and environmental unexpected changes. The interlinking of disease pathways through such a metabolic network increases the complexity of identifying therapeutic targets using information from gene expression analysis. In contrast, MCA approaches the problem of drug targeting by exploring the contribution of individual components within a metabolic network, providing a theoretical framework for describing metabolic/signaling/genetic systems of any complexity. An attractive feature of MCA is that it does not require all system components to be characterized a priori (37, 40). Furthermore, control coefficients can be estimated for different components of the network and for pertinent environmental factors. The control coefficients provide a first approximation of which proteins or pathways may exert more control on the system properties to be modified. Targeting the steps with higher control coefficients on relevant system properties, such as tumor growth or obesity, could be a good strategy to design an effective therapeutic agent (8). In the case of the PPP, which is enhanced in tumor cells, an in vivo tumor growth control coefficient of 0.9 was measured in mice with Ehrlich's ascites tumor for transketolase (33), while for glucose-6-phosphate dehydrogenase a control coefficient of 0.41 was computed (41). These control coefficients indicate that these two enzymes are central for the tumor cell progression and consequently could be good candidates for a combined multiple-hit anticancer therapy (11). The analysis and comparison of control coefficient profile between tumor cells and their normal counterpart allow the identification of differences in metabolic adaptation that can be exploited to identify selective drug targets against cancer with lower side effects.

3. Metabolic and Fluxomic Profiling of Tumor Cells

The measurement of substrate redistribution within major metabolic pathways in living cells is enabled by metabolic profiling using stable-isotope tracer technology. This technique has demonstrated that transformed human cells present acute metabolic shifts and that some anticancer drugs induce their effects by forcing the reversion of these metabolic changes. By enlightening tumor-specific metabolic shifts in tumor cells, metabolic profiling enables drug developers to identify the metabolic steps that control cell proliferation, therefore helping the identification of new anticancer targets and the screening of lead compounds for antiproliferative metabolic effects. The metabolic profile of a given cell represents the integrated end-point of many growth-modifying signaling events against the background of the cell's genetic makeup. As a result, metabolic profiling is the simultaneous assessment of substrate flux within and among major metabolic pathways of macromolecule synthesis and energy production under various physiological conditions, growth phases, and substrate environments (13). It can seriously support the industrial drug discovery process by revealing metabolic adaptive changes that occur as a consequence of gene expression and changes in microenvironment, and is, consequently, complementary to genetic profiling. Getting metabolic profiles can both characterize the efficacy of new antiproliferative drugs and provide a screening tool for drug development. Then, the changes in substrate carbon flow and redistribution among various metabolic pathways observed in the transformed proliferating-cell phenotypes observed in cancer can be used throughout metabolic profiling to identify decisive enzymes and their substrate analogues to make easy drug development.

The use of mass spectrometry (MS) and glucose molecules labeled with stable (nonradiating) isotope (^{13}C) can reveal the distribution of labeled carbons in various intermediates during de novo macromolecule synthesis in cancer cells. Metabolic profiling is designed to expose detailed substrate-flow modifications in response to pathological processes or new antitumor therapies. Here we discuss the specific application of [1,2-$^{13}C_2$]-glucose in metabolic profiling. The changing pattern of distribution of ^{13}C from [1,2-$^{13}C_2$]-glucose in intracellular metabolic intermediates gives a measure of carbon flow towards the PPP, glycolysis, direct glucose oxidation, the tricarboxylic acid (TCA) cycle, and fatty acid synthesis, simultaneously. Metabolic profiling reveals specific flux changes in lactate, glutamate, nucleic acid ribose, and palmitate during oncogenesis and during antiproliferative treatments. As a result, it shows major changes in glucose use for macromolecule synthesis in cancer, information that can also be used for drug target development. The stable-isotope tracers generate a vast number of metabolite forms that differ according to the number and position of labeled isotopes in the carbon skeleton (isotopomers) and such a big variety makes the analysis of isotopomer data highly complex. In contrast, this diversity of forms does provide adequate information to address cell operation in vivo (42). Metabolic networks of living cells produce the complicated redistribution of carbon skeleton atoms of substrates. When these substrates are artificially labeled by stable isotopes (such as ^{13}C) at specific positions, the reorganization of carbon skeleton becomes measurable and its quantification provides insight to the respective metabolic reactions. Interconnection of several isotope-exchange reactions generates in each metabolite a variety of forms, which differ by the number and positions of ^{13}C isotopes (^{13}C isotopomers). A given set of metabolic fluxes generates a specific distribution of isotopomer fractions, and as a result, the isotopomer distribution indicates the underlying set of fluxes.

The study of metabolic profiles in response to cell-transforming agents or cancer growth-controlling compounds by means of stable isotopes in cancer cell cultures or in vivo can expose how the growth signaling and metabolic processes are connected and to what extent metabolic pathway flux influences cell growth.

Successful anticancer therapeutics is expected to limit carbon flow towards nucleic acid synthesis and shift glucose toward oxidation. These changes can easily be shown by metabolic profiling, making it an excellent tool for screening potential new drugs to treat cancer. Isotopomer distribution in different metabolic pools shows different distributions between codon 12 mutant KRAS (K12)-transformed cells and codon 13 mutant KRAS (K13)-transformed cells. It reveals that K12 cells display greatly increased glycolysis with only a slight increase in activity along pathways that produce nucleic acid and lipid synthesis precursors in the oxidative branch of the PPP and via pyruvate dehydrogenase flux. In contrast, K13 mutants present a modest increase in anaerobic glycolysis associated with a large increase in oxidative PPP activity and pyruvate dehydrogenase flux. The distinctive differences in metabolic profiles of K12 and K13 codon mutated cells point out that a strong correlation exists between the flow of glucose carbons towards either increased anaerobic glycolysis, and resistance to apoptosis (K12), or increased macromolecule synthesis, rapid proliferation, and increased sensitivity to apoptosis (17). These differences indicate PPP regulatory enzymes as good targets to inhibit K13 cells proliferation, as well as the proliferation of other types of tumor cells which hold similar metabolic adaptations.

The metabolic network of cancer cells confers adaptive mechanisms against many chemotherapeutic agents, but also presents serious constraints, which make cells vulnerable to perturbation of the network due to drug therapy. Combination therapies based on targeting the nucleic acid synthesis metabolic network at multiple points have exposed that cancer cells overcome single hit strategies through different metabolic network adaptations making obvious the robustness of cancer cell metabolism. In a biological network, the inhibition of one pathway may result in the adaptive use of alternative pathways compensating for the effects of the drug and leaving the net substrate flux unaffected. On the contrary, when inhibitory agents are used in combination, the inhibition of cell growth can be either simply additive or synergistic, depending on the relationships and mechanisms within the pathways targeted. The full knowledge of the entire network of nucleic acid biosynthesis pathways and the complex interactions among its regulatory mechanisms eagerly suggests a new approach to the rational design of chemotherapeutic agents: targeting multiple sites of the network (11). The analysis of cancer metabolic adaptations using this approach has also identified the maintenance of pentose phosphate cycle oxidative and nonoxidative balance to be critical for cancer cell survival and vulnerable to chemotherapeutic intervention (11). This delicate balance is essential to maintain proliferation in cancer cells and is a vulnerable target within the cancer metabolic network for potential novel therapies in overcoming drug resistance, as the inhibition of cell proliferation becomes stronger as the imbalance of pentose phosphate cycle in favor of the oxidative branch caused by different drug combinations gets stronger.

This novel principle for rational drug discovery and cancer therapy design, developed in the last years from the integrative biology point of view, is an exciting departure from the current, more limited thinking in cancer chemotherapy. Chemotherapy designed to target metabolic pathways is innovative and potentially more effective than those designed by gene-targeting or protein-targeting to reach for desired effects. As an example, drug combinations resulting in a more dramatic imbalance between oxidative/nonoxidative PPPs are efficient to inhibit tumor cell growth and therefore the targeting of the pentose phosphate metabolic network flux balance can be a new strategy for novel cancer therapies to overcome drug resistance. Additionally, the understanding of metabolic constraints within the cancer metabolic network presents new insight into vulnerability of the metabolic network to disturbance at key spots and new strategies in the design of cancer therapy to control the robustness of cancer cell metabolic adaptations. However, the above-described isotopomer distribution analysis, although it indicates the most active metabolic pathways, is qualitative and too approximate, while quantitative results are needed to be applied in cancer therapy. A quantitative description of metabolic flux adaptation needs simulation of the isotopomer distribution data in a model, which integrates capacity to calculate dynamics for each isotopomer concentration and to account for enzyme kinetic mechanisms.

4. Quantitative Metabolic Flux Analysis

The comprehensive analysis of mass isotopomer data obtained by MS or NMR demands that all possible individual isotopomers are computed. This requires solving 2^n equations for a substance consisted of n carbons. In this way even for the model description of all isotopomers formation in glycolysis and PPP, the algorithm must construct the equations automatically, since it is practically impossible to write such a huge number of equations by hand. Schmidt et al. (43) developed a simulation algorithm for the computation of all possible isotopomers. This algorithm of isotopomer mapping matrices evolved from the earlier approach of atom mapping matrices (44, 45), allowed to construct and solve automatically hundreds of equations that describe all isotopomers transformation according to the specific reaction mechanisms. This method made it possible to simulate all isotopomers steady-state distribution for the given set of metabolic fluxes, while the best fit to the experimental distribution pointed to the set compatible with the measured distribution. However, the presence of large exchange fluxes caused severe instability of numerical solution or convergence problems, which restricted the application of this method. Wiechert et al. (46) found an elegant way to overcome the problem of instability by reformulating isotopomer balance equations into cumomer balance equations. The term cumomer (from cumulative isotopomers) designates a sum of isotopomers with fixed positions of label (a 1-cumomer fraction is a sum of the positional enrichments). Such reformulation of the equations in terms of cumomers simplified the task and made possible to obtain the solution in one step based on matrix calculus. The equations formulated in terms of cumomer fractions can be solved explicitly as a cascade of linear systems, evaluating the cumomer fractions one by one starting from the 0-cumomer fraction. Then the cumomer fractions can be transformed back into isotopomer fractions.

This method was well elaborated (46–49) including the development of a computer program based on the cumomer-balance method, which performs the complete isotopomer analysis and finds the flux profile by experimental isotopomer distribution fitting (46) (see also Chap. 8).

However, there are at least three reasons to develop one more approach to isotopomer analysis. First, although the above-described algorithm overcomes the problem of instability of iterative numerical solution, it is restricted by stationary flux analysis thus leaving without any examination the available time course of label distribution, which could be more informative than steady-state analysis. Second, all the above approaches to the computation of isotopomer transformations consider fluxes as independent variables. This was noted as an advantage of the method because such an analysis did not need any assumptions regarding the biochemical basics of considered fluxes (46). However, if the amount of isotopomer information is insufficient, additional data are necessary for the unambiguous evaluation of flux profile. In this case, the known kinetic characteristics of analyzed enzyme reactions and results of classical kinetic modeling could provide such additional necessary information. Third, even if the analysis reveals the fluxes taking them as independent, the fluxes remain disconnected from the detailed mechanisms of the catalysis and regulation considered in kinetics models, thus the biochemical reasons for the observed behavior remain unclear. In this case, the use of kinetic modeling could also solve this problem. Long era of classical biochemistry developed a number of kinetic models of complex systems that use known characteristics of enzyme catalysis and regulation. These parameters could be employed in metabolic flux analysis, providing the necessary additional information. An excellent example is a model of erythrocyte central metabolism (50), which includes kinetic models of all involved enzymes with known regulatory and catalytic mechanisms and kinetic constants, verified by numerous experiments.

On the other hand, the kinetic models of complex systems, analyzing the experimentally observed cellular functions as a result of operation of many regulated processes, include many parameters and therefore, like the flux analysis, also suffer from insufficiency of experimental data. Moreover, the kinetic models normally include characteristics of enzymatic reactions obtained in vitro, and such data cannot always be used for the interpretation of in vivo experiments. The use of in vivo tracer data would animate the old classical district of kinetic studies. In this situation, integration of kinetic modeling with complete isotopomer analysis would provide:

- For kinetic study of in vivo cell operation, the new area of tracer data, which are necessary for understanding the organization and regulation of the processes in living cells and applicability of classical in vitro information
- For metabolic flux analysis, the additional information to restrict the number of acceptable sets of metabolic fluxes by the ones that are compatible not only with a given pattern of isotopomer distribution, but also with the data of previous biochemical studies

5. Algorithms for Integrated Kinetic Model and Isotopomer Distribution Analysis in Metabolic Flux Analysis

The module of the software developed by Selivanov et al. (51–53), which performs simulation of isotopomer dynamics, operates not independently, but as an extension of a kinetic model of an analyzed system. It could be compatible with various kinetic models of central metabolism, so that it accepts the total fluxes and metabolite concentrations predetermined by the kinetic model constituting the first part of the analytic software. Thus, the first step of analysis is the solution of ordinary differential equations (ODEs), which describe the total concentration change as the sum of the production rate of the given metabolite minus the rates of its consumption. The metabolite concentration obtained from the ODEs solution become initial values of nonlabeled isotopomers of internal metabolites in the following step of analysis. Other isotopomers are initially set to 0, except the outside metabolites, which have the initial distribution according to that added experimentally. Fluxes, also obtained from the solution of ODEs, are also used to simulate the respective reactions between the isotopomers.

To connect the ordinary kinetic model execution with isotopomer simulation, a specific interface is necessary. For kinetic models, an enzyme reaction could be described as one net metabolic flux derived based on the reaction kinetic mechanism and expressed as the difference between forward and reverse reactions. This is sufficient because only net fluxes define changes in the calculated total metabolite concentrations. In contrast, for the isotopomer analysis, forward and reverse fluxes make independent contributions into isotope exchange, therefore they should be computed separately. Also there are additional fluxes, which also redistribute the tracer atoms but do not change the total metabolite concentrations. A classical example of a variety of fluxes is the nonoxidative PPP, the most problematic metabolic part related to numerous isotope-exchange reactions catalyzed by transketolase (TK) and transaldolase (TA), described in details by Selivanov et al. (42). One of the reactions of nonoxidative PPP catalyzed by transketolase is:

$$\mathrm{xu5p} + \mathrm{r5p} \leftrightarrow \mathrm{g3p} + \mathrm{s7p} \qquad (1)$$

The catalytic cycle of this reaction consists of a series of reversible elementary steps: binding of donor substrate (xu5p) and formation of a covalent enzyme–substrate complex (E*xu5p); splitting of donor substrate and formation of a covalently bound intermediate (the α-carbanion of α, β-dihydroxyethyl-ThDP, the so-called "active glycolaldehyde") and an aldose (g3p); both are localized in the active site of the enzyme (EG*g3p). This complex dissociates into the complex of the enzyme with active glycolaldehyde (EG) and the first product, free aldose (g3p). These steps could be shown as follows:

$$\mathrm{xu5p} + \mathrm{E} \leftrightarrow \mathrm{E^{*}xu5p} \leftrightarrow \mathrm{EG^{*}g3p} \leftrightarrow \mathrm{EG} + \mathrm{g3p}$$

In the second half-reaction, active glycolaldehyde interacts with the other aldose (r5p) available in the reaction mixture. The new ketose (s7p) is released from the enzyme–substrate complex after passing through the same reaction steps in reverse order.

$$\mathrm{EG} + \mathrm{r5p} \leftrightarrow \mathrm{EG^{*}r5p} \leftrightarrow \mathrm{E^{*}s7p} \leftrightarrow \mathrm{xu5p} + \mathrm{E}$$

Various isotope-exchange fluxes are created in this TK-catalyzed reaction. The first half-reaction, even in the absence of the substrates for the second half-reaction, can catalyze isotope exchange between xu5p and g3p, which in the presence of labeled g3p would result in labeling of xu5p. It can transfer forward and reverse the last *n*-2 atoms of ketose-substrate to the pool of aldose-product (e.g., xu5p ↔ g3p) through the three steps of the first half-reaction. The same isotope exchange could proceed in the second half-reaction between s7p and r5p. The whole cycle could result in the exchange of the first two carbons between s7p and xu5p, delivering the atoms through six steps

$$\mathrm{xu5p} \leftrightarrow \mathrm{E^{*}xu5p} \leftrightarrow \mathrm{EG^{*}g3p} \leftrightarrow \mathrm{EG} \leftrightarrow \mathrm{EG^{*}r5p} \leftrightarrow \mathrm{E^{*}s7p} \leftrightarrow \mathrm{s7p}$$

Thus, the following six fluxes of the carbon skeleton parts could be expressed through the elementary steps of the catalytic mechanism:

$$\text{vxg} : \text{xu5p} \rightarrow \text{g3p}$$

$$\text{vgx} : \text{g3p} \rightarrow \text{xu5p}$$

$$\text{vxs} : \text{xu5p} \rightarrow \text{s7p}$$

$$\text{vsx} : \text{s7p} \rightarrow \text{xu5p}$$

$$\text{vsr} : \text{s7p} \rightarrow \text{r5p}$$

$$\text{vrs} : \text{r5p} \rightarrow \text{s7p}$$

The difference between forward and reverse fluxes is the same for all isotope-exchange reactions and it corresponds to the net flux:

$$\text{vxg} - \text{vgx} = \text{vxs} - \text{vsx} = \text{vrs} - \text{vsr} = \text{vnet}$$

from which it follows that

$$\text{vxg} - \text{vxs} = \text{vgx} - \text{vsx} \quad \text{and} \quad \text{vsr} - \text{vsx} = \text{vrs} - \text{vxs}$$

The whole reaction cycle exchanges carbons between xu5p and s7p expressed by the fluxes vxs and vsx, but also it is accompanied by the exchange inside half-reactions, i.e., between xu5p and g3p, and also between s7p and r5p. The last expressions show that forward and reverse exchanges in the half-reactions are the same. Taking into account equality of the half-reaction exchanges, the four fluxes define the entire isotope exchanges associated with the considered TK reaction:

- Forward flux xu5p $\rightarrow$ s7p (vxs)
- Reverse flux s7p $\rightarrow$ xu5p (vsx)
- Exchange xu5p $\leftrightarrow$ g3p (vxg $-$ vxs)
- Exchange s7p $\leftrightarrow$ r5p (vsr $-$ vsx)

The above fluxes could be expressed through the elementary rates (42). The elementary rates, in turn, could be expressed through the elementary rate constants and substrate and product concentrations using, for instance, King and Altman algorithm (as described e.g., in (54)). Thus, all TK fluxes are considered not as independent but as interrelated through the elementary rate constants, which could be determined in independent experiments as described elsewhere (52). Presence of different substrates in the intracellular volume, which compete for the same enzyme, further complicates the situation. The whole scheme of the TK reactions in the cell includes two more reactions:

$$\text{xu5p} + \text{e4p} \leftrightarrow \text{g3p} + \text{f6p}$$

$$\text{s7p} + \text{e4p} \leftrightarrow \text{r5p} + \text{f6p} \qquad (2)$$

In this situation, the number of isotope-exchange fluxes related to the TK reactions increases, but all of them can be expressed through the elementary rate constants (42). Taking into account that each half-reaction is common for two of the three whole reactions, nine different isotope-exchange fluxes could be associated with them:

$$\text{xu5p} + \text{E} \rightarrow \text{Exu5p} \rightarrow \text{EGg3p} \rightarrow \text{EG} \rightarrow \text{EGrSp} \rightarrow \text{Es7p} \rightarrow \text{E} + \text{s7p}$$

$$\text{xu5p} + \text{E} \leftarrow \text{Exu5p} \leftarrow \text{EGg3p} \leftarrow \text{EG} \leftarrow \text{EGrSp} \leftarrow \text{ES} \leftarrow \text{E} + \text{s7p}$$

$$\text{xu5p} + \text{E} \rightarrow \text{Exu5p} \rightarrow \text{EGg3p} \rightarrow \text{EG} \rightarrow \text{EGe4p} \rightarrow \text{Ef6p} \rightarrow \text{E} + \text{f6p}$$

$$\text{xu5p} + \text{E} \leftarrow \text{Exu5p} \leftarrow \text{EGg3p} \leftarrow \text{EG} \leftarrow \text{EGe4p} \leftarrow \text{Ef6p} \leftarrow \text{E} + \text{f6p}$$

$$\text{s7p} + \text{E} \rightarrow \text{Es7p} \rightarrow \text{EGr5p} \rightarrow \text{EG} \rightarrow \text{EGe4p} \rightarrow \text{Ef6p} \rightarrow \text{E} + \text{f6p}$$

$$\text{s7p} + \text{E} \leftarrow \text{Es7p} \leftarrow \text{EGr5p} \leftarrow \text{EG} \leftarrow \text{EGe4p} \leftarrow \text{Ef6p} \leftarrow \text{E} + \text{f6p}$$

$$\text{xu5p} + \text{E} \leftrightarrow \text{Exu5p} \leftrightarrow \text{EGg3p} \leftrightarrow \text{EG} + \text{g3p}$$

$$\text{f6p} + \text{E} \leftrightarrow \text{Ef6p} \leftrightarrow \text{EGe4p} \leftrightarrow \text{EG} + \text{e4p}$$

$$\text{s7p} + \text{E} \leftrightarrow \text{Es7p} \leftrightarrow \text{EGrSp} \leftrightarrow \text{EG} + \text{r5p}$$

Expressed through the elementary rate constants, such isotope exchange fluxes are evaluated for all the enzymes after the kinetic model execution. The obtained values represent the necessary interface which connects the kinetic model with simulation of isotopomer distribution.

6. Reactions Between Isotopomers

The algorithm passes all the computed isotope-exchange fluxes to the next module, which computes dynamics of all isotopomers produced in the analyzed pathway. For isotopomer designation, we use a binary notation for the ^{13}C and ^{12}C atoms as it is helpful in optimization of references to a specific isotopomer as described in more details elsewhere (42, 51). Since each carbon atom of a molecule can exist in one of the two states, labeled (marked as "1") or unlabeled ("0"), each metabolite in the model can be represented by an array of 2^n of possible isotopomers, where n is the number of carbon atoms in the molecule. Each isotopomer in the model is represented as binary numbers; its digits correspond to the carbon atoms in a molecule (3 digits for trioses, 4 for erythrose, etc.). A "1" or a "0" in certain position in a string signifies that corresponding carbon atom is labeled or unlabeled. For instance, all isotopomers for glyceraldehyde-3-phosphate (g3p) are:

$$000, 001, 010, 011, 100, 101, 110, 111$$

This representation of isotopomers as successive integer numbers is very convenient because the model uses it as references to the respective position in the existing array of concentrations of all isotopomers, different for each metabolite. This ordering of the isotopomers in the array allows optimization of referring the isotopomer products for any isotopomer substrate related to the considered reactions, as it is explained below. For instance, the reaction (xu5p + r5p ↔ s7p + g3p) between arbitrarily chosen isotopomers of xu5p (10011) and r5p (10000) produces the following isotopomers of s7p and g3p:

$$10011(\mathrm{xu5p}) + 10000(\mathrm{r5p}) \leftrightarrow 1010000(\mathrm{s7p}) + 011(\mathrm{g3p}) \quad (3)$$

Then the change of concentrations according to the succession of reaction is calculated. Assuming that all isotopomers have the equal affinity, the rate of reaction between pair of isotopomers is proportional to their concentrations, while the sum of reaction rates for all isotopomers gives the global metabolic flux calculated also at the previous, kinetic, step. If, for instance, Vf is the global forward flux for the TK reaction between xu5p and r5p, the flux for this reaction between isotopomers i and j (Vf_{ij}) would be expressed as follows:

$$\mathrm{Vf}_{ij} = \mathrm{Vf} \times [\mathrm{xu5p}_i] \times [\mathrm{r5p}_j]/([\mathrm{xu5p}_{\mathrm{tot}}] \times [\mathrm{r5p}_{\mathrm{tot}}]) \quad (4)$$

Here, the indices i and j refer to the concentrations of the respective isotopomers and the index "tot" refers to the total concentration of the metabolite, as calculated in the kinetic model. In this way, the first part, ODE solving, is linked to the part that computes the label distribution: the kinetic model calculates global fluxes and concentrations and defines the values (as in the above example $\mathrm{Vf}/([\mathrm{xu5p}_{\mathrm{tot}}] \times [\mathrm{r5p}_{\mathrm{tot}}])$), which are used to get the fluxes in reactions between isotopomers (as in (4)). Given isotopomers are consumed in interactions with other isotopomers in the course of considered reaction, and also in other fluxes created by the same enzyme and in other enzymatic reactions. The program sums all of them to define the derivative for each isotopomer:

$$\mathrm{d}[\mathrm{xu5p}_i]/\mathrm{d}t = -\mathrm{Vf}_{ij} - \Sigma V[\mathrm{xu5p}_i]_{\mathrm{cons}} + \Sigma V[\mathrm{xu5p}_i]_{\mathrm{prod}}$$

$$\mathrm{d}[\mathrm{r5p}_j]/\mathrm{d}t = -\mathrm{Vf}_{ij} - \Sigma V[\mathrm{r5p}_j]_{\mathrm{cons}} + \Sigma V[\mathrm{r5p}_j]_{\mathrm{prod}} \quad (5)$$

Here, the indices cons and prod indicate the other rates of production and consumption of the considered isotopomers in all other isotope-exchange reactions. Software offers a choice of methods for numerical solution of differential equations for isotopomers, usually fourth order Runge–Kutta works well. Consumption of substrates corresponds to the product formation:

$$\mathrm{d}[\mathrm{g3p}_{\mathrm{ra}}]/\mathrm{d}t = \mathrm{Vf}_{ij} - \Sigma V[\mathrm{g3p}_{\mathrm{ra}}]_{\mathrm{cons}} + \Sigma V[\mathrm{g3p}_{\mathrm{ra}}]_{\mathrm{prod}}$$

$$\mathrm{d}[\mathrm{s7p}_{\mathrm{rd}}]/\mathrm{d}t = \mathrm{Vf}_{ij} - \Sigma V[\mathrm{s7p}_{\mathrm{rd}}]_{\mathrm{cons}} + \Sigma V[\mathrm{s7p}_{\mathrm{rd}}]_{\mathrm{prod}} \quad (6)$$

Here ra and rd are the reference numbers of the acceptor ($g3p_{ra}$) and donor ($s7p_{rd}$) produced in the reaction between $xu5p_i$ and $r5p_j$. In the considered above example (3), if i in binary presentation is 10011 and j is 10000, then ra is 011 and rd is 1010000. Analysis of experimental data starts from execution of the kinetic model simulating time course of metabolite concentrations and all isotope-exchange fluxes, which then are used to simulate the corresponding isotopomer distribution. Experimental data fitting finds the flux profile and kinetic parameters compatible with the analyzed data. A combination of kinetic modeling with isotopomer distribution analysis allows combining also the respective experimental data, which can be analyzed. Moreover, our algorithm expands the usual steady-state isotopomer analysis to the nonsteady-state conditions. The following kinds of experimental data could be subjects of fitting:

- Measured rate of production of various metabolites in cell cultures under different conditions of incubation and intracellular concentration of some metabolites
- Total metabolite concentrations
- Distribution of labeled atoms such as ^{13}C isotopes in metabolites (^{13}C isotopomers), when the label was added with some of the substrates

The program performs fitting of the experimental data and statistical analysis of the best-fit as it was described elsewhere (52, 53).

7. An Example: Colon Cancer Cell Line HT29, Transketolase Inhibition

An example of the application of this software could be estimation of glucose metabolism fluxes in HT29 cells that were incubated with D-[1,2-^{13}C]-glucose; the cells were studied in the absence and presence of oxythiamine (OT), an irreversible inhibitor of TK. Since the drug effect is known and the extent of TK inhibition could be measured, here we use this study to demonstrate the capacity of the program to predict the metabolic flux distribution after the controlled distortion of cellular metabolism. The program evaluated the set of metabolic fluxes included in the model, which gave the minimal deviation from the experimentally measured mass isotopomer distribution in r5p from RNA and lactate. It was found that including the detailed kinetic mechanisms of TK and TA reactions in the model strictly restricts the multidimensional area of flux profiles compatible with the experimental data. The necessity to be consistent with the reaction mechanism filters out the ambiguous combinations of parameters.

Restricted by the interdependency of the fluxes via the TK and TA reactions, the program first has found the dilution of newly

Table 1
Simulated metabolic fluxes related with TK and TA catalysis in HT29 cells utilizing 100% D-[1,2-^{13}C]-glucose incubated in the absence (control) or in the presence of oxythiamine (OT)

		Control	OT
TK	xu5p ↔ g3p	2.260	0.582
	xu5p → Sed7P	0.7	0.237
	xu5p → f6p	0.054	0.0386
	s7p → f6p	0.052	0.0337
TA	f6p ↔ g3p	0.047	0.039
	s7p ↔ e4p	0.0033	0.0092
	s7p → f6p	0.0645	0.068
	[r5p], (mM)	0.006	0.0079

In control, the fluxes correspond to the best fit of ^{13}C distribution measured in r5p of RNA. The effect of OT was simulated as 75% reduction of TK activity (for the details see (52))

synthesized r5p by that initially present in RNA. The extent of dilution exactly corresponded to the whole amount of r5p initially present in RNA. This fact shows that RNA r5p is not degraded, but once synthesized ribose-nucleotides are 100% reutilized through subsequent cell division. The fit of experimental data pointed out to the corresponding set of kinetic parameters, i.e., elementary rate constants, V_{max}, K_m of the included enzymatic reactions. If these parameters were determined correctly, the model would predict the experimental pattern that could be measured after an alteration of the metabolic state, of course, if the reason of such alteration is controlled and could be adequately simulated. An example of such controlled alteration could be a treatment of the cells with oxythiamine, which being transformed into oxythiamine diphosphate inhibits transketolase by substituting its natural cofactor thiamine diphosphate. As it was measured, after such treatment TK activity dropped down to 0.25 of its initial levels. Simulation of this TK activity drop keeping all other parameters unchanged gave the isotopomer distribution in r5p and lactate, which was close to that obtained experimentally after TK inhibition (52). Some metabolic fluxes corresponded to the best fit of the isotopomer distribution before OT treatment and after simulated 75% OT inhibition are shown in Table 1. Some of the isotope-exchange fluxes catalyzed by TK decreased almost proportionally to the total TK activity (xu5p ↔ g3p, xu5p → s7p). However, TK inhibition did not change proportionally all the fluxes which it catalyzes, some of them practically did not change, as xu5p → f6p. TK inhibition also changed the fluxes catalyzed by another enzyme, TA. The flux s7p ↔ e4p increased threefold. This is a result of complex interaction between metabolic fluxes through common intermediates and regulators. A decrease of enzyme activity could result in accumulation of substrates, which activate some isotope exchange even if it is catalyzed by this partially inhibited enzyme. Thus, evaluation of flux profile does not always unambiguously point to the reason of its change.

Another interesting result is that TK inhibition, which is accompanied also by inhibition of cell proliferation, in fact did not decrease r5p concentration; in contrary, Table 1 shows that it even increased, thus confirming that the TK-dependent inhibition of proliferation does not depend on TK-dependent r5p synthesis. Probably, TK performs also another role more related with cell proliferation.

8. The Perspective for Analysis of Bioactive Natural Effectors

The above example, where multiple metabolic effect of known TK inhibitor was evaluated, showed the advantage of kinetic model implementation as a part of metabolic flux analysis. Our algorithm can solve also the reverse problem: after adjusting the model for control conditions, it can find the key step in the metabolic pathway affected by the studied factor, which mechanism of action is unknown. This objective could be of great importance for pharmaceutical-related problems. Classical flux analysis, which considers metabolic fluxes as independent variables, would reveal changes in many, if not all, fluxes. In this situation, it would be impossible to understand the primary effect of analyzed factor since it is hidden among secondary consequences. However, a kinetic model, which takes into account metabolite and effector dependency of metabolic fluxes, could reveal that such complete change of metabolic flux profile is induced by just one enzyme activity changed. The kinetic model, which is integrated in data fit algorithm, can help to find, as the above example shows, that the multiple flux perturbation could be induced by a change of one parameter (TK activity in the above example). This is extremely important for drug development in cancer therapy. The characteristic for tumor cells' loss of capacity to differentiate, to control proliferation and to enter in apoptosis in fact could be restored by specific cancer cell treatment using such agents as butyrate, polyphenols from grapes or tea, Edelphosine (55–57). The biochemical mechanism by which these chemicals induce antitumor effects are in general unknown, although registered associated changes in central metabolism (55) could be primary factors inducing restoring of normal, noncancer, cell behavior. Understanding the biochemical mechanism of such restoring of normal cell properties would allow modulating and augmenting the desired characteristics. Analysis and amplification of the action performed by already existed bioactive substances seems to be more efficient than to invent a completely new strategy of therapy. Such analysis assumes that the kinetic model, which is placed in the basis of it, should reveal the key points, which are modified by the drugs and which modification restores the capacity to differentiate or to enter in apoptosis.

In order to have such predictive capacity, the model must adequately describe the kinetic characteristics of enzyme reactions and their regulation in situ. This seems to be a problem, since such characteristics are usually defined in vitro. However, as the above example shows, the initial model constructed using in vitro data could be refined by analysis of isotopomer distribution data obtained in situ in the desired cell line under various control conditions. Then the model, which already accounts for the in situ properties of metabolic network, could be used to reveal the key drug effect.

Integration of kinetic models with isotopomer dynamic simulation software thus essentially advances both parts. Kinetic models initially constructed based on existed in vitro data could be adopted for intracellular condition by the analysis of isotopomer distribution data through the module, which performs respective simulations. This adaptation has also valuable academic significance providing information about specificity of in situ organization of cellular metabolism. On the other hand, isotopomer distribution analysis, which can find the most probable set of fluxes corresponding to analyzed conditions, cannot define the key underlying metabolic changes; only integration with kinetic models can achieve this. The capacity of defining the drug's key metabolic effect, which can be used for cancer therapy, renders our analytical software a promising tool in cancer research and its biomedicine applications.

Acknowledgments

This work was supported by Grants SAF2011-25726 and ISCIII-RTICC (RD06/0020/0046) from the Spanish government and the European Union FEDER funds), the AGAUR-Generalitat de Catalunya (grant 2009SGR1308, 2009 CTP 00026 and Icrea Academia award 2010 granted to M. Cascante), and the European Commission (FP7-ITN) METAFLUX grant agreement n°264780.

References

1. Schlotterbeck G, Ross A, Dieterle F, Senn H. Metabolic profiling technologies for biomarker discovery in biomedicine and drug development. Pharmacogenomics. 2006;7(7):1055–75.
2. Schnackenberg LK, Beger RD. Monitoring the health to disease continuum with global metabolic profiling and systems biology. Pharmacogenomics. 2006;7(7):1077–86.
3. Bailey JE. Reflections on the scope and the future of metabolic engineering and its connections to functional genomics and drug discovery. Metab Eng. 2001;3(2):111–4.
4. Oksman-Caldentey KM, Saito K. Integrating genomics and metabolomics for engineering plant metabolic pathways. Curr Opin Biotechnol. 2005;16(2):174–9.
5. German JB, Hammock BD, Watkins SM. Metabolomics: building on a century of biochemistry to guide human health. Metabolomics. 2005;1(1):3–9.
6. van der Greef J, Hankemeier T, McBurney RN. Metabolomics-based systems biology and personalized medicine: moving towards n = 1 clinical trials? Pharmacogenomics. 2006;7(7):1087–94.
7. Westerhoff HV, Koster JG, Van Workum M, Rudd KE. On the control of gene expression. In: Cornish-Bowden A, editor. Control of metabolic processes. New York, NY: Plenum; 1990. p. 399–412.
8. Cascante M, Boros LG, Comin-Anduix B, de Atauri P, Centelles JJ, Lee PW. Metabolic control analysis in drug discovery and disease. Nat Biotechnol. 2002;20(3):243–9.
9. Dang CV, Semenza GL. Oncogenic alterations of metabolism. Trends Biochem Sci. 1999;24(2):68–72.
10. Pelicano H, Martin DS, Xu RH, Huang P. Glycolysis inhibition for anticancer treatment. Oncogene. 2006;25(34):4633–46.
11. Ramos-Montoya A, Lee W-NP, Bassilian S, Lim S, Trebukhina RV, Kazhyna MV, Ciudad CJ, Noé V, Centelles JJ, Cascante M. Pentose phosphate cycle oxidative and non-oxidative balance: a new vulnerable target for overcoming drug resistance in cancer. Int J Cancer. 2006;119(12):2733–41.
12. Boros LG, Serkova NJ, Cascante MS, Lee W-NP. Use of metabolic pathway flux information in targeted cancer drug design. Drug Discov Today Ther Strat. 2004;1(4):435–43.
13. Boros LG, Cascante M, Paul Lee W-N. Metabolic profiling of cell growth and death in cancer: applications in drug discovery. Drug Discov Today. 2002;7(6):364–72.
14. Schnackenberg LK. Global metabolic profiling and its role in systems biology to advance personalized medicine in the 21st century. Expert Rev Mol Diagn. 2007;7(3):247–59.
15. Mathupala SP, Rempel A, Pedersen PL. Aberrant glycolytic metabolism of cancer cells: a remarkable coordination of genetic, transcriptional, post-translational, and mutational events that lead to a critical role for type II hexokinase. J Bioenerg Biomembr. 1997;29(4):339–43.
16. Vousden KH, Lane DP. p53 in health and disease. Nat Rev Mol Cell Biol. 2007;8(4):275–83.
17. Vizan P, Boros LG, Figueras A, Capella G, Mangues R, Bassilian S, Lim S, Lee WN, Cascante M. K-ras codon-specific mutations produce distinctive metabolic phenotypes in NIH3T3 mice [corrected] fibroblasts. Cancer Res. 2005;65(13):5512–5.
18. Halabe Bucay A. The biological significance of cancer: mitochondria as a cause of cancer and the inhibition of glycolysis with citrate as a cancer treatment. Med Hypotheses. 2007;69(4):826–8.
19. Cascante M, Ortega F, Marti E. New insights into our understanding of the regulation and organization of cell factories. Trends Biotechnol. 2000;18(5):181–2.
20. Bowden AC. Metabolic control analysis in biotechnology and medicine. Nat Biotechnol. 1999;17(7):641–3.
21. Baggetto LG. Biochemical, genetic, and metabolic adaptations of tumor cells that express the typical multidrug-resistance phenotype. Reversion by new therapies. J Bioenerg Biomembr. 1997;29(4):401–13.
22. Bailey JE. Lessons from metabolic engineering for functional genomics and drug discovery. Nat Biotechnol. 1999;17(7):616–8.
23. Huang S. Rational drug discovery: what can we learn from regulatory networks? Drug Discov Today. 2002;7(20 Suppl):S163–9.
24. Kitano H. Cancer as a robust system: implications for anticancer therapy. Nat Rev Cancer. 2004;4(3):227–35.
25. Kitano H. A robustness-based approach to systems-oriented drug design. Nat Rev Drug Discov. 2007;6(3):202–10.
26. Mazurek S, Boschek CB, Hugo F, Eigenbrodt E. Pyruvate kinase type M2 and its role in

tumor growth and spreading. Semin Cancer Biol. 2005;15(4):300–8.

27. Yasuda S, Arii S, Mori A, Isobe N, Yang W, Oe H, Fujimoto A, Yonenaga Y, Sakashita H, Imamura M. Hexokinase II and VEGF expression in liver tumors: correlation with hypoxia-inducible factor 1 alpha and its significance. J Hepatol. 2004;40(1):117–23.
28. Coy JF, Dressler D, Wilde J, Schubert P. Mutations in the transketolase-like gene TKTL1: clinical implications for neurodegenerative diseases, diabetes and cancer. Clin Lab. 2005;51 (5–6):257–73.
29. Langbein S, Zerilli M, Zur Hausen A, Staiger W, Rensch-Boschert K, Lukan N, Popa J, Ternullo MP, Steidler A, Weiss C, Grobholz R, Willeke F, Alken P, Stassi G, Schubert P, Coy JF. Expression of transketolase TKTL1 predicts colon and urothelial cancer patient survival: Warburg effect reinterpreted. Br J Cancer. 2006;94(4):578–85.
30. Stetak A, Veress R, Ovadi J, Csermely P, Keri G, Ullrich A. Nuclear translocation of the tumor marker pyruvate kinase M2 induces programmed cell death. Cancer Res. 2007;67 (4):1602–8.
31. Poulsen HS, Frederiksen P. Glucose-6-phosphate dehydrogenase activity in human breast cancer. Lack of association with oestrogen receptor content. Acta Pathol Microbiol Scand A. 1981;89(4):263–70.
32. Kuo W, Lin J, Tang TK. Human glucose-6-phosphate dehydrogenase (G6PD) gene transforms NIH 3T3 cells and induces tumors in nude mice. Int J Cancer. 2000;85(6):857–64.
33. Comin-Anduix B, Boren J, Martinez S, Moro C, Centelles JJ, Trebukhina R, Petushok N, Lee WN, Boros LG, Cascante M. The effect of thiamine supplementation on tumour proliferation. A metabolic control analysis study. Eur J Biochem. 2001;268(15):4177–82.
34. Boros LG, Puigjaner J, Cascante M, Lee WN, Brandes JL, Bassilian S, Yusuf FI, Williams RD, Muscarella P, Melvin WS, Schirmer WJ. Oxythiamine and dehydroepiandrosterone inhibit the nonoxidative synthesis of ribose and tumor cell proliferation. Cancer Res. 1997;57 (19):4242–8.
35. Savageau MA. Biochemical system analysis: nonlinear systems analysis. Reading, MA: Addison-Wesley; 1976.
36. Voit EO. Computational analysis of biochemical systems: a practical guide for biochemists and molecular biologists. Cambridge, UK: Cambridge University Press; 2000. 544pp.
37. Fell DA. Understanding the control of metabolism. London, UK: Portland Press; 1997. p. 300.
38. Cascante M, Franco R, Canela EI. Use of implicit methods from general sensitivity theory to develop a systematic approach to metabolic control. I. Unbranched pathways. Math Biosci. 1989;94(2):271–88.
39. Cascante M, Franco R, Canela EI. Use of implicit methods from general sensitivity theory to develop a systematic approach to metabolic control. II. Complex systems. Math Biosci. 1989;94(2):289–309.
40. Cornish-Bowden A, Cárdenas ML. Technological and medical implications of metabolic control analysis. Dordrecht, The Netherlands: Kluwer; 2000.
41. Boren J, Ramos-Montoya A, de Atauri P, Comin-Anduix B, Cortes A, Centelles JJ, Frederiks WM, Van Noorden CJ, Cascante M. Metabolic control analysis aimed at the ribose synthesis pathways of tumor cells: a new strategy for antitumor drug development. Mol Biol Rep. 2002;29(1–2):7–12.
42. Selivanov VA, Sukhomlin T, Centelles JJ, Lee PW, Cascante M. Integration of enzyme kinetic models and isotopomer distribution analysis for studies of in situ cell operation. BMC Neurosci. 2006;7 Suppl 1:S7.
43. Schmidt K, Carlsen M, Nielsen J, Villadsen J. Modeling isotopomer distributions in biochemical networks using isotopomer mapping matrices. Biotechnol Bioeng. 1997;55:831–40.
44. Marx A, de Graaf A, Wiechert W, Eggeling L, Sahm H. Determination of the fluxes in the central metabolism of *Corynebacterium glutamicum* by nuclear magnetic resonance spectroscopy combined with metabolic balancing. Biotechnol Bioeng. 1996;49:111–29.
45. Zupke C, Stephanopoulos G. Modeling of isotope distributions and intracellular fluxes in metabolic networks using atom mapping matrices. Biotechnol Prog. 1994;10:489–98.
46. Wiechert W, Mollney M, Isermann N, Wurzel M, de Graaf A. Bidirectional reaction steps in metabolic networks: III. Explicit solution and analysis of isotopomer labeling systems. Biotechnol Bioeng. 1999;66:69–85.
47. Wiechert W, de Graaf A. In vivo stationary flux analysis by 13C labeling experiments. Adv Biochem Eng Biotechnol. 1996;54:109–54.
48. Wiechert W, de Graaf A. Bidirectional reaction steps in metabolic networks: I. Modeling and simulation of carbon isotope labeling experiments. Biotechnol Bioeng. 1997;55:101–17.
49. Wiechert W, Siefke C, de Graaf A, Marx A. Bidirectional reaction steps in metabolic networks: II. Flux estimation and statistical analysis. Biotechnol Bioeng. 1997;55:118–35.

50. Mulquiney P, Kuchel P. Modelling metabolism with mathematica. Boca Raton, FL: CRC Press; 2003.
51. Selivanov VA, Puigjaner J, Sillero A, Centelles JJ, Ramos-Montoya A, Lee PW, Cascante M. An optimized algorithm for flux estimation from isotopomer distribution in glucose metabolites. Bioinformatics. 2004;20(18):3387–97.
52. Selivanov VA, Meshalkina LE, Solovjeva ON, Kuchel PW, Ramos-Montoya A, Kochetov GA, Lee PW, Cascante M. Rapid simulation and analysis of isotopomer distributions using constraints based on enzyme mechanisms: an example from HT29 cancer cells. Bioinformatics. 2005;21(17):3558–64.
53. Selivanov VA, Marin S, Lee PW, Cascante M. Software for dynamic analysis of tracer-based metabolomic data: estimation of metabolic fluxes and their statistical analysis. Bioinformatics. 2006;22(22):2806–12.
54. Cornish-Bowden A. Fundamentals of enzyme kinetics. 3rd ed. London, UK: Portland Press; 2004.
55. Boren J, Lee WN, Bassilian S, Centelles JJ, Lim S, Ahmed S, Boros LG, Cascante M. The stable isotope-based dynamic metabolic profile of butyrate-induced HT29 cell differentiation. J Biol Chem. 2003;278(31): 28395–402.
56. Matito C, Mastorakou F, Centelles JJ, Torres JL, Cascante M. Antiproliferative effect of antioxidant polyphenols from grape in murine Hepa-1c1c7. Eur J Nutr. 2003;42(1):43–9.
57. Mollinedo F, Gajate C, Martin-Santamaria S, Gago F. ET-18-OCH3 (edelfosine): a selective antitumour lipid targeting apoptosis through intracellular activation of Fas/CD95 death receptor. Curr Med Chem. 2004;11(24): 3163–84.

Chapter 11

Noninvasive Fluxomics in Mammals by Nuclear Magnetic Resonance Spectroscopy

Justyna Wolak, Kayvan Rahimi-Keshari, Rex E. Jeffries, Maliackal Poulo Joy, Abigail Todd, Peter Pediatitakis, Brian J. Dewar, Jason H. Winnike, Oleg Favorov, Timothy C. Elston, Lee M. Graves, John Kurhanewicz, Daniel Vigneron, Ekhson Holmuhamedov, and Jeffrey M. Macdonald

Abstract

Metabolism is an interconnecting network of metabolite consumption and creation. Metabolomics has focused on metabolite concentrations in metabolic networks. Fluxomics is also required in the study of metabolism and quantifies the flux of substrate through each reaction step or a series of reaction steps (i.e., metabolic pathway or cycle), and ultimately is required for energy balance equations of the system. The primary noninvasive method of quantifying fluxes in living systems is by in vivo ^{13}C nuclear magnetic resonance (NMR) spectroscopy. The present state of noninvasive in vivo NMR technology allows for just four simultaneous flux measurements of metabolic pathways: gluconeogenesis, glycogen synthesis, glycolysis, and citric acid cycle. Since the liver is the gatekeeper and metabolic center for the animal, in vivo fluxomics of liver is extensively reviewed. Additionally, other organ systems studies are discussed demonstrating interorgan cycles, such as the Cori and Randall cycles. This review discusses the basics of in vivo fluxomics focusing on the general details of the NMR experimental protocol and required hardware/software needed to analyze the data.

Currently, there are two general methods for determining multiple flux rates. The *dynamic* method entails acquiring serial time points, whereas the *static* method is a single measurement in which flux through metabolic pathways is quantified by isotopomer (i.e., isotope isomers) analysis. The flux data are analyzed by mathematical models to calculate the global flux measurement (in silico fluxomics), and create a mass balance of the biosystem. Models are especially useful for inferring various metabolic states of the system, which are affected by drugs, toxicants, or pathology. As with all in silico models, increasing the number of empirically derived concentrations and fluxes into the model greatly increases the accuracy and utility of the model. NMR spectroscopy (NMRS) is inherently insensitive compared to other analytical modalities, limiting the temporal resolution of the dynamic in vivo measurements. To address the NMR sensitivity, several technological advances have been made. First, magnets are now at higher magnetic field strengths. Second, the technique of dynamic nuclear polarization (DNP) of substrates increases the signal for ^{13}C up to five orders of magnitude.

In vivo fluxomics requires a broad knowledge of biochemistry, in vivo NMRS, and metabolic modeling. Therefore, this chapter is intended as a handbook for upper division undergraduate students and graduate students in biochemistry or engineering and relates the basics of electrical and biochemical engineering and animal handling. The chapter is intended for use in an introductory graduate course on NMR-based fluxomics for physical scientist.

Teresa Whei-Mei Fan et al. (eds.), *The Handbook of Metabolomics*, Methods in Pharmacology and Toxicology, DOI 10.1007/978-1-61779-618-0_11,

Key words: Fluxomics, hyperpolarization, in vivo NMR, modeling

1. Introduction

Decoding of the human genome has brought about the need to phenotype a multitude of genotypes. Current methods for gene sequencing (genomics), quantification of mRNA (transcriptomics), and analysis of proteins (proteomics) require the destruction of the biological sample. On the other hand, metabolite analysis (metabolomics) can be done nondestructively using nuclear magnetic resonance (NMR)-based methods. Metabolomics focuses on the identification and quantification of small molecules (<2 kDa), typically at a single time point. However, missing from "-omics"-based analysis is the flux of substrate through a given pathway (fluxomics). Figure 1 shows how flux links all the "-omics." For example, the environment can quickly change a biological system when stress is applied (Fig. 1). For example, newly exercised muscle tissue in the order of 1 min speeds up the rate of glycolysis 100-fold to maintain ATP for the actin-myosin complex (1, 2). The net effect of this action is that the ATP concentration does not drop by more than 40% (3). Genomic differences can also lead to altered phenotypes because mutations may exist that affect the flow of nutrients into and out of the cell. A cell switching from G_0 to G_1 and entering the cell cycle will exhibit a profound change in metabolism in order to make proteins, lipids, and nucleotides required for mitosis (4).

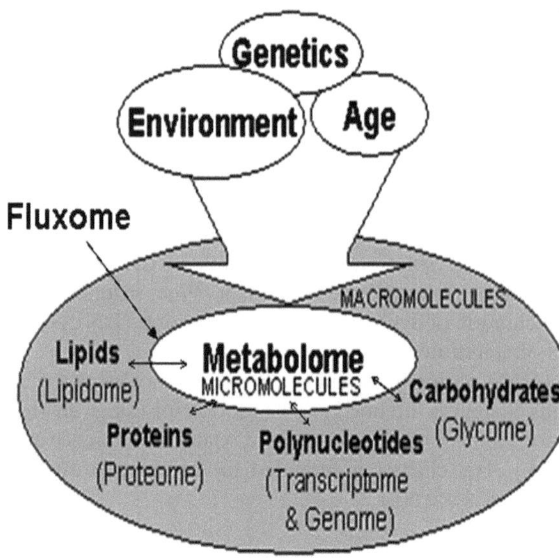

Fig. 1. Metabolomics connects to all the other "-omics" via metabolic turnover with macromolecules.

This is accomplished primarily from the consumption of carbohydrates. During an infection, lymphocytes significantly increase their pyrimidine pool, an order of magnitude, while purines are increased just fourfold (5). During DNA replication, it is essential that the four deoxynucleotides are of roughly equal concentration and not rate-limiting, otherwise a nucleotide substitution can occur causing a mutation. Therefore, cell cycle regulation of nucleotide metabolism is extremely robust (6). Metabolic regulation controls pyrimidine flux and will be discussed in Sect. 2.2.

Fluxomics is the quantification of biochemical reaction rates, or fluxes, in a biological system, while the fluxome is the summation of all fluxes within a biosystem. With current technology, it is not possible to measure all metabolites in vivo, so mathematical models are required to predict the entire fluxome. The commonly used mathematical methods for fluxomics include metabolic flux analysis (MFA) and metabolic control analysis (MCA) discussed in Chaps. 8 and 9, respectively. As an example of MFA, experimentally derived fluxes are used as input for the in silico MFA model, which then generates the fluxome (7, 8). Since technologically it is not yet possible to quantify the fluxome, the flux of measurable metabolites at key pathway junctions or branch points act as surrogate measures of flux through an entire metabolic pathway (9) and the rest is derived in silico (see Chaps. 8 and 9) (10).

The goal of fluxomics is to determine the mass balance within a given biosystem (11, 12). Mass balance is based on the first law of thermodynamics, conservation of mass and energy. Since virtually all reactions for energy generation are known and most experiments are performed in a closed system, a quantitative description of metabolite production and consumption rates can be balanced between the tissue and the environment. When the energy currencies of high-energy phosphagens such as nucleotide triphosphate (NTP) (13) and phosphocreatine (PCr) and redox factors, nicotinamide adenine dinucleotide (NADH), are incorporated, an energy balance is generated that can act as a metabolomic phenotype. For example, at the simplest level of complexity, cells in culture, the metabolites inside the cell (termed the "fingerprint") can be balanced with the media (termed the "footprint") by mass balancing the multitude of coupled reactions thereby generating an energy balance for the system. Dynamic energy and mass budget (DEB) theory and methods were developed in the early 1990s to determine mass balances at multiple levels of complexity: organisms (i.e., a network of organs and tissues), eco-systems (i.e., a network of organisms) (14), and even to assess global warming of the planet (15, 16). In vivo fluxomics can determine the mass balance in a biosystem making it a powerful phenotyping tool. For example, if a malignant tumor is cultured in a dish, the fingerprint will show increased consumption of glucose and glutamine while the footprint will show increased lactate production (glycolytic end product) even under aerobic conditions. This metabolomic phenotype is called the "Warburg effect" (17) and could be given as a mass balance, or less detailed, an energy balance of phosphagens and redox cofactors, in the various compartments (i.e., intra- or intercellular) of the biosystem.

Production and consumption rates of metabolites can be determined by measuring the change in concentrations, or mass, over time using various techniques, including gravimetric, spectroscopic, or chromatographic in the biosystem where the boundary conditions are defined. For example, if the boundary conditions are the borders of a perfused liver, one can calculate the changes in concentration of nutrients or waste products in the perfusate entering and leaving the isolated liver (18, 19). However, in order to determine the contribution from the various metabolic pathways contributing to the nitrogen or carbon "mass balance" in a biosystem, one must use isotope tracers (^{15}N, ^{13}C, ^{14}C, ^{11}C) (20, 21), especially at steady state when concentrations do not change. For example, in the perfused liver example given above, if one were to quantify production and consumption rates inside the perfused liver at steady state, one would use isotopes to obtain rate constants. In vivo NMR spectroscopy (NMRS) has been used to measure flux rates noninvasively in intact animals as well as by high-resolution NMRS of tissue or cell extracts. This review covers all of the types of biochemical fluxes that have been quantified by NMRS with a *focus* on *perfused* and *intact liver and translation to humans.* Although some very elegant in vivo ^{15}N NMR studies were performed to quantify the hepatic urea cycle (22) and transamination (23) reactions using ^{15}N-labeled ammonia, as well as ^{2}H to define hepatic one-carbon metabolism (24), this review will focus on ^{13}C NMR studies.

Flux measurements by ^{13}C NMRS are done by *dynamic* or *static* methods. Examples of these methods at steady state and nonsteady state conditions will be discussed. The concept of time scales is very important in the accurate determination of flux. For a given compound within a biosystem, the time scale of reactions can change due to different compartmentation or *pools* (see Glossary for defining the subtle difference of these two terms). For example, pathways such as glycolysis, the citric acid cycle, and serine formation require temporal resolution on the order of minutes even seconds during a *dynamic* flux measurement in order to obtain accurate flux calculations. In contrast, the primary antioxidant of the body, glutathione, has a turnover of about 10 h and requires a temporal resolution on the order of hours. Total body protein turnover occurs in 3 days (25–27), yet insulin is synthesized in 20 min (28, 29), and some plasma proteins in several hours (30, 31). There are several pools of lipids in a cell with different turnover rates. For example, in brain the turnover of the glycerophospholipids, phosphatidylinositol, phophatidylcholine and phosphatidylethanolamine depends on the attached fatty acids, and for the fatty acid docosohexanoic acid, the half-life 3.9, 22.4, and 57.8 h, respectively (32, 33). This relatively short turnover of phosphatidylinositol reflects its utility in cell signaling. Also, there are different pools within the cell: those undergoing endocytosis forming lysosomes, those being synthesis in the endoplasmic reticulum, and those forming the nuclear and plasma membranes, as well as different pools in the different cell types within the brain (32, 33). These turnover rates depend on the environment (28), genetic disposition and cell cycle (34), and maturational age (21, 35, 36) of a cell. RNA turnover rates have been determined (37) and decrease with age that affects downstream protein translation (36), ultimately affecting mitochondrial function (38). The turnover of RNA (t-RNA, r-RNA, and m-RNA) is also tightly controlled by cell cycle machinery (39). The concept of the various time scales for turnover rates will be demonstrated using a specific example of glycine metabolism in Sect. 3.

Finally, a new technology, dynamic nuclear polarization (DNP), will be reviewed, which increases ^{13}C NMR sensitivity nearly 5 orders of magnitude, making 1 mM metabolites as sensitive as 55.5 M water (111 M protons). DNP ^{13}C spectroscopic imaging is being rapidly translated to the clinic (40). This new technology will be explained in Sect. 6.

2. Background: Fluxomics

2.1. Fluxomics and the Methods Used for Quantification of Flux

The essence of metabolism is captured by the quantification of organic and inorganic substrates defining a mass balance, which is based on the first law of thermodynamics, conservation of energy (see Chap. 3). A comprehensive measurement of mass balance of the biosystem would require measurement of all the concentrations and fluxes depicted in the generalized biochemical scheme shown in Fig. 1 and has never been done for any multicellular species. The primary available chemical potential energy of a biosystem is in the form of ATP and the capacitance stored across mitochondrial membrane (2). Biochemistry texts can be misleading by stating that the driving force of ATP hydrolysis is the high-energy phosphoanhydride bond. The critical thing is that ATP readily couples to other reactions via enzymes, both increasing the speed as well as being able to drive them against their own ΔG. ATP levels can be noninvasively quantified by in vivo ^{31}P NMRS (41). Fluorescence spectroscopy is the most common method used to measure mitochondrial membrane hyperpolarization using fluorescent dyes (42) or the endogenous redox couple $NADH/NAD^+$ (43). It is a relatively unknown fact that NMRS can measure endogenous redox couples, which correlate to the redox potential in the same manner as fluorescent tracers quantify the $NADH/NAD^+$ ratio.

In vivo NMRS is the only method permitting in situ measurements of multiple metabolites simultaneously. Therefore, in vivo NMRS is a powerful noninvasive method for fluxomics. In addition, these methods are easily translated to humans because they employ stable isotopes rather than (unstable) radioactive nuclides, which release ionizing radiation from nuclear decay. Even though doses are within safe ranges of exposure, radioactivity has become stigmatized within the patient population. In fact, the stigma associated with radioactivity prompted dropping the word "nuclear" from NMRS and clinically NMRS is known as magnetic resonance spectroscopy (MRS). By quantifying concentrations by ^{1}H spectroscopic imaging (44) and reaction rates by ^{13}C NMRS (45), production or consumption rates, or net flux rates, can be quantified, permitting determination of the mass balance of a biosystem.

In nuclear imaging, positron-emitters such as the radioactive nuclides, ^{11}C and ^{18}F, are incorporated into nutrients and are extremely useful in the detection and diagnosis of cancer. In particular, the success of positron emission tomography (PET) is due to its ability to detect increased uptake of glucose commonly observed in cancerous tissue. Since children have faster growing tissue than adults, and thereby more susceptible to permanent DNA mutations, it is advised they not be exposed to the positron-emitters used in PET due to radiation exposure. Rather, it is recommended that MRI or ultrasound be used instead (46). The positron-emitting ^{18}F-fluoro-2-deoxy-D-glucose (FDG) is more rapidly taken up in cancer cells, but is not metabolized beyond the hexokinase step due to the absence of the 2-OH group. Furthermore, there is usually a down-regulation of the phosphatase, resulting in a net accumulation of FDG compared with normal tissue. Thus, at most it provides an estimate of glucose transport and not intracellular metabolism. The emitted positrons annihilate electrons in nearby atoms, releasing two gamma rays, in opposite directions. The simultaneously detected gamma ray paths are reconstructed into a three-dimensional image.

PET-CT combination scanners enable a high-resolution X-ray image to register the metabolic PET image to colocalize the signal by dual image modalities for a validated cancer diagnosis (47). In clinical PET systems, the pixel resolution is between 4 and 6.5 mm, while whole body CT can reach a pixel resolution of 0.5 mm with 64 slices. ^{1}H MRI and hyperpolarized ^{13}C MRSI achieve a resolution of less than 0.2 mm with asymmetric voxels in 3 T whole body imagers (48). The advantage of both ^{1}H and hyperpolarized ^{13}C MRSI is the detection of multiple biomarkers enhancing its diagnostic potential (40, 44). However, unlike radioactive tracers in PET scans, which are used at levels of 0.01% thereby creating a true "massless" tracer, in some in vivo ^{13}C NMR experiments the plasma substrate concentrations are an order of magnitude higher during the infusion (45) and therefore cannot be considered a tracer in the true sense of the word (20). Higher field magnets used in animal studies and attention to these steady state issues insure accurate interpretation of the in vivo ^{13}C NMR experimental results.

Dynamic PET imaging in humans is used to obtain rates of glucose uptake in the brain (49). A three-compartment model, which includes the blood–brain barrier, is used for the analysis and is applied to each voxel using a bolus of ^{18}F-FDG (49). However, only a single flux is measured, so fluxomics is not possible with PET. Fluorescence spectroscopy has long been used to obtain rates in isolated cells, but typically pure enzymes or cell preparations are used for enzyme kinetics. Optical imaging is increasingly being used in whole animals and should become useful for determining some rates, but is limited by the ability to detect light due to quenching, especially in deep tissue. Therefore, optical imaging is not as useful in determining kinetics of enzymes, especially in internal organs from intact organisms, as compared to NMR. Also optical methods as well as ultrasound are not amenable to the determination of multiple rates, which is easily accomplished with ^{13}C NMR (50) and will be reviewed in depth in Sect. 6.

2.1.1. Stable Isotopic Labels and ^{13}C NMR Spectroscopy

NMRS generates positional information using stable nonradioactive isotopes such as ^{13}C, ^{15}N, and ^{2}H. Metabolic flux information is encoded in the isotopomers (i.e., isotope isomers or isomers of a chemical composed of varying isotopes $^{13}C/^{12}C$, $^{15}N/^{14}N$, $^{17}O/^{16}O$, etc.) that are generated during metabolism and permits the quantification of "relative" fluxes via isotopomer ratios. Absolute flux is obtained by measuring isotope incorporation rates dynamically (i.e., over time) resulting in a rate constant which when multiplied by concentration results in the absolute flux (see Sect. 2.2). A powerful NMR-observable nuclei in determining metabolic flux is ^{13}C because: (1) it is a naturally abundant tracer (1.1% of all carbons), (2) positional information is generated with superior resolution along the *x*-axis (chemical shift), which is at least fourfold greater than ^{1}H and is far less complex due to inherently fewer coupling partners with superior line widths (see Chap. 3), (3) it has greater sensitivity compared to other common NMR-observable nuclei common in biochemistry, such as ^{15}N, ^{17}O, and (4) compared to in vivo ^{1}H NMRS, it does not require solvent suppression.

What the ^{13}C isotopes provide in metabolic experiments is positional information on isotopomer enrichments. Both the ^{13}C and ^{1}H NMR spectra can aid in determining ^{13}C isotope enrichments, which can vary from 1.1 to 100% (51). Fractional enrichment is defined as the number of molecules with a ^{13}C spin in a given position (label coming from introduced precursor as well as natural abundance), divided by the total number of molecules in the pool. Absolute fractional enrichment is the enrichment above the background natural abundance, which is subtracted from the

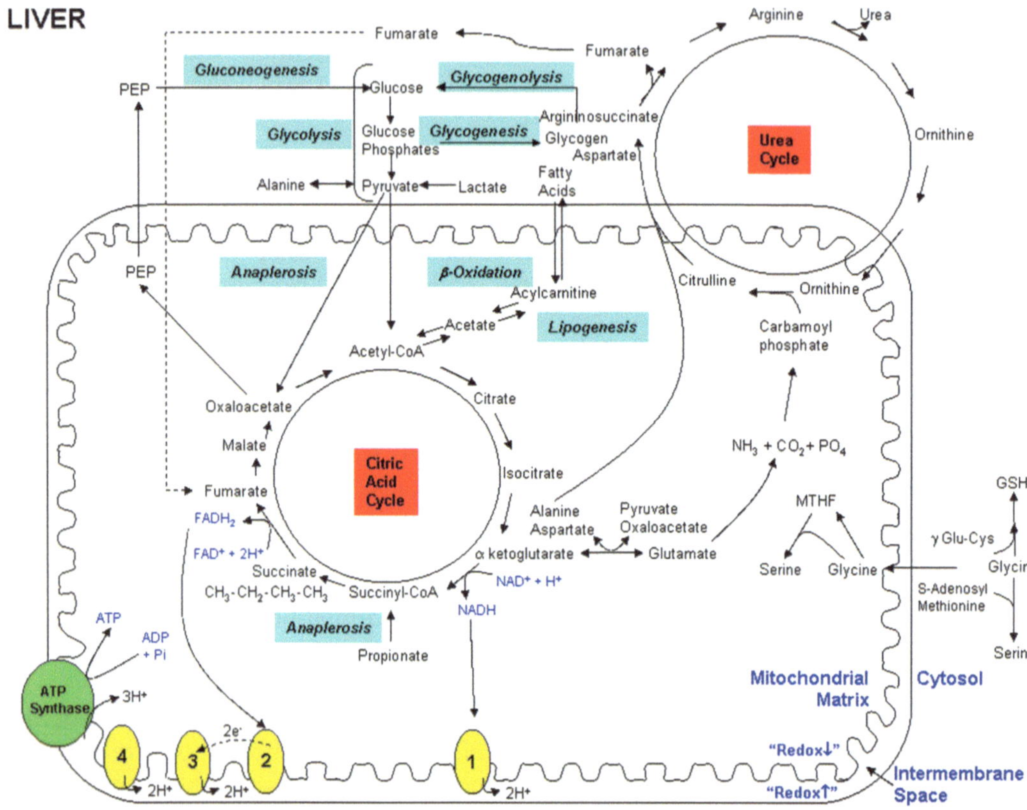

Fig. 2. Biochemical scheme for liver metabolism. The liver is a major organ for nitrogen balance (urea cycle), glucose homeostasis (gluconeogenesis), and lipid homeostasis, including beta-oxidation. Oxidative phosphorylation via the electron transport chain and ATP synthase is shown on the *bottom left*. *PEP* phosphoenolpyruvate; *GSH* glutathione; *MTHF* methyltetrahydrofolate.

total (51); this is solely caused by the metabolism and incorporation of the administered ^{13}C-labeled molecule. Obtaining an absolute fractional enrichment for a particular metabolite therefore allows fluxes to be measured typically via dynamic methods. On the other hand, in order to determine relative flux, isotopomer analysis is executed within a single spectrum. Numerous isotopomers observed within one data set allow for relative ratios to be established between them. Classically, such isotopomer analysis finds applications in static measurements, although dynamic measurements have also been done. NMR methods for determining isotopomer fractional enrichments have been extensively reviewed elsewhere (20, 21, 51, 52). For single time point analysis, flux ratios can only be calculated at isotopic steady state

In vivo ^{13}C NMRS is a powerful technology in metabolic engineering for metabolic flux and control analysis where prokaryotes are used to produce proteins and the majority of the fluxome is experimentally measured (8, 52, 53). In mammals, using 2-^{13}C-glucose multiple net fluxes are quantified for various pathways and can be used to determine metabolic flux through various reaction pathways including gluconeogenesis, glycolysis, Krebs' cycle, and the pentose phosphate pathway (PPP) (54–62). Figure 2 depicts a biochemical schematic of the many biochemical reactions that have been quantified by in vivo NMRS in liver. However, these fluxes for the various reactions depicted in Fig. 2 have not been measured simultaneously by in vivo NMRS. Therefore, fluxomics remains to be performed by this method.

A key reaction in the Krebs cycle is the formation of succinate (Fig. 2), which is a symmetric molecule and ultimately will create multiple glutamate isotopomers that can be used to determine Krebs' flux (54, 63). This is described in Chap. 14 by Fan. Biochemical reactions with high activation energy are accelerated by enzymes, which lower the activation energy. Coupling an energetically unfavorable to a favorable reaction, such as the hydrolysis of ATP, drives biochemical reactions to completion. The coupling is catalyzed by an enzyme or system of enzymes. ATP is made primarily by glycolysis and by oxidative phosphorylation. In glycolysis, ATP is generated from ADP and inorganic phosphate by substrate-level phosphorylation, which utilizes energy released during the oxidation of glucose via the glycolytic reactions. In oxidative phosphorylation, energy from the Krebs cycle is transferred to the respiratory chain by electron shuttles, which creates an electrochemical gradient between the inner and outer leaflet of the inner mitochondrial membrane (Fig. 2). The phosphorylation of ADP is catalyzed by ATP synthase by coupling to the reduction of oxygen to water and this is where most ATP is created in a normal cell (Fig. 2). Moving reducing equivalents (electrons) generated from glycolysis across the mitochondrial membrane depends on shuttles (i.e., malate-aspartate, α-glycerol-phosphate), which require compartmentation of cytosolic and mitochondrial enzyme isozymes for the same reaction. For example, in Fig. 2, two transaminases are shown for the formation of aspartate and alanine from their ketoacids. Therefore, isozymes with similar functions exist in both mitochondrial and cytosolic compartments (114, 170). Figure 2 shows aspartate exiting the mitochondria and entering the urea cycle. Aspartate can also reform oxaloacetate via the cytosolic aspartate transaminase, which in turn is reduced by NADH to malate via malate dehydrogenase and malate reenters the mitochondria shuttling cytosolic reducing equivalents. Measuring redox invasively requires quantifying redox couples in mitochondria and cytosol (64) or use of fluorescence markers (65). Indeed, the action of these shuttles and functional electron transport within the mitochondria are necessary for the continued function of glycolysis in the cytoplasm. In the early 1980s, Robert E. London not only pioneered the use of glutamate and glutamine isotopomers to determine Krebs' flux (54) along with Shulman (63), but also was the first to use ^{13}C-labeled nicotinic acid (essentially vitamin B_3 or niacin) which is incorporated into NADH and ultimately could be used to extrapolate the intracellular redox state from the NADH/NAD^+ ratio (66). NADH is used to drive the electron transport chain and ultimately drives oxidative phosphorylation (Fig. 2). Other redox couples have been used to measure redox state such as lactate-pyruvate, acetoacetate, and β-hydroxybutyrate (67) and oxidized to reduced glutathione (68), which are included in Table 1. In addition, the oxygenation state of myoglobin (69) and hemoglobin (70) has been measured by ^{1}H NMRS. The problem with the NMR measurement of these couples is that they are typically a global measurement and do not distinguish between different compartments, resulting in an averaged overall total cellular ratio affected by the total volume of the various cellular compartments.

2.2. Metabolic Steady and Nonsteady State Conditions: Example of Hepatic Glucose Metabolism

Organisms in their natural environment are in a chronic nonsteady state predictably changing diurnally and unpredictably changing in response to nutritional status and energy demand, which requires substrate fluxes to change by as much several orders of magnitude. A complex metabolic regulatory network controls flux, and this is dominated by a network of signaling pathways in which the enzymes are regulated by interactions with metabolites. This includes covalent modification of kinases via phosphorylation/dephosphorylation, as well as noncovalent ("allosteric") interactions. The latter includes feedback inhibition or activation of key homeostatic enzymes such as PFK-1 (activated by fructose 2,6 bisphosphate, and inhibited by ATP and citrate). In both cases, metabolic regulation is exerted by changes in enzyme activity due to interaction with metabolites.

Although normal metabolism is in nonsteady state most of the time, experimentally, fluxes are best measured at steady state. This is due to the mathematics used, which becomes analytically unmanageable without steady state assumptions. For a linear system, the formal math is rather simple, but the algebra is very tedious. Nonlinearity complicates the treatment of metabolic systems, and regrettably (for modelers), many parts of metabolism are inherently nonlinear. Specifically, the overall enzyme activity will depend on the enzyme, reactant, and product concentrations, but also on allosteric and nonallosteric effectors that may lead to inhibition or activation effects, generally controlled by signaling pathways. This process can be written according to a simple interconversion between reactant and product ratio:

$$\text{Reactants } v_f \Leftrightarrow v_r \text{ Products} \tag{1}$$

where v_f and v_r are the enzyme-catalyzed rates in the forward and reverse direction, respectively.

Table 1
Metabolic investigations of liver

Animal intact isolated tissue extract	Treatment	Metabolic pathway measured	Stable isotopic tracer	Rate/outcome	References
Human	Normal (fed, fasted)	Glycogenesis	Natural abundance	Surface coil; Hepatic glycogen repletion rate of 0.2 mM/min/g of liver (normal hepatic glycogen ~230 mM)	(173)
Human	Normal	Glycogen	Natural abundance	Direct and proton-detected ^{13}C pulse sequences detected glycogen	(174)
Baboon (intact)	Normal (fasted)	Glycogenesis	[1-^{13}C] Glucose	Surface coil; direct (65%)/indirect (35%) glycogenesis	(175)
Human	Normal (fed, fasted)	Glycogenesis Glycogenolysis	[1-^{13}C] Glucose	Under net glycogenesis in humans, glycogen syn. and degradation occur simultaneously; Net glycogenesis is 0.24 μmol/mL of liver per minute in fed state vs. 0.28 in fasted state	(176)
Rabbit (intact, tissue, and extract)	Normal (fed)	Glycogenesis	Natural abundance	Surface coil; Hepatic glycogen levels monitored	(177)
Rabbit (intact and extract)	Normal (fed)	Glycogen	Natural abundance	^{13}C NMR signal of glycogen C-1 100% visible using in vivo and nat. abundance	(98)
Rabbit (extract)	Normal (fasted)	Krebs'	[U-^{13}C] Lactate	Krebs' flow rates; Glutamate labeling by lactate at rate of ~6.0 μmol/kg/min	(178)

(continued)

Table 1 (continued)

Animal intact isolated tissue extract	Treatment	Metabolic pathway measured	Stable isotopic tracer	Rate/outcome	References
Rat (intact and tissue)	Normal (varied diet)	Lipids (triglycerides and phospholipids) Glycogenesis Glycogenolysis Gluconeogenesis	Natural abundance	Surface coil; monitor effects of dietary fat (lipids like triglycerides and phospholipids) and carbohydrate dietary modifications	(179)
Rat (intact and extract)	Normal (fasted)	Ketogenesis Krebs'	[1-^{13}C] Butyrate	Surface coil; Observe ketone body formation via carbonyl spectral region	(180)
Rat (isolated)	Normal (fed)	Krebs'	[2-^{13}C] Acetate	C-4 of glutamate labeled first; monitor glutamine-glutamate futile cycling	(181)
Rat (extract)	Normal (fasted)	Glycogenesis	[1-^{13}C] Glucose	One-third glycogenesis via direct pathway; large amount of glycogen synthesis via another	(62)
Rat (intact and extract)	Normal (fasted, fed)	Krebs' Gluconeogenesis	[3-^{13}C] Alanine	Surface coil; Alanine flows mostly through PC and not PDH	(182)
Rat (extract)	Normal (fasted)	Glycogenesis	[U-^{13}C] Glucose	35% of glycogen synthesized via direct pathway	(183)
Rat (extract)	Normal (fasted)	Krebs' Glycogenesis	[1-^{13}C] Glucose	34% glycogen synthesized directly; Alanine and lactate contribute 55% to glycogen formation	(184)
Rat (extract)	Normal (fasted)	Krebs' Gluconeogenesis	[2-^{13}C] Acetate	7% glucose carbons from Krebs' cycle	(185)
Rat (intact and extract)	Normal (fed, fasted)	Glycolysis Glycogenesis β-Oxidation	[1,2,11,12-$^{13}C_4$] Dodecanedioic acid [1,2-$^{13}C_2$] Glucose [1,6-$^{13}C_2$] Glucose	Apply multilabeled substrates; ^{13}C-^{13}C spin couplings distinguish between endogenous metabolites vs. others	(186)

Rat (intact and extract)	Normal (fasted)	Gluconeogenesis Glycogenesis	[3-^{13}C] Alanine [1-^{13}C] Glucose	Surface coil; 0.075 vs. 0.025 per minute of direct vs. indirect glycogen synthesis	(187)
Rat (intact and tissue)	Normal (fed, fasted)	Glycogenesis Glycogenolysis	Natural abundance [1-^{13}C] Glucose	Surface coil; novel NMR techniques involving gradients allow increased natural abundance detection	(188)
Rabbit (extract) Rat (intact)	Normal (fasted)	Glycogenesis	Natural abundance [1-^{13}C] Glucose	T_1 field dependent while T_2 is not; in vitro and in vivo measurements similar; T_1 (65 ms at 2.1 T, 142 ms at 4.7 T, 300 ms at 8.4 T) T_2 (6 ms at 2.1 T, 9 ms at 4.7 T, 9 ms at 8.4 T)	(189)
Rat (extracts)	Normal (fed)	Fatty acid metabolism	[2-^{13}C] Acetate	Quantitative measurements of exogenous acetate enable acid metabolism monitoring	(190)
Rat (intact)	Normal (fed)	Glycogen	Natural abundance	Surface coil; Adiabatic RF pulses attenuate saturated carbon signals improving glycogen detection	(191)
Rat (extract)	Normal (fasted)	Glycogenesis PPP	[1-^{13}C] Glucose [6-^{13}C] Glucose	29% direct glycogenesis; negligible amount to PPP from infused glucose	(192)
Rat (isolated)	Normal (fasted)	Gluconeogenesis Krebs' PPP	[1,2,3-$^{13}C_3$] Propionate	PPP insignificant; method for determining fractional enrichment of each ^{13}C isotopomer	(193)
Rat (isolated and extract)	Normal (fasted)	Gluconeogenesis Krebs'	[1,2,3-$^{13}C_3$] Propionate	Gluconeogenic flux 1.2 times Krebs' flux (0.37 vs. 0.32 μmol/gww/min)	(116)
Rat (intact and extracts)	Normal (fasted)	Krebs'	[2-^{13}C] Ethanol	Measured Krebs' flux of 0.33 ± 0.09 μmol/g/min	(194)
Rat (intact and extract)	Normal (fed)	Glucose metabolism, ascorbic acid metabolism	[1,2-^{13}C] Glucose [1-^{13}C] Glucose	Turnover rate of hepatic ascorbic acid (vitamin C) in vivo: 1.9 ± 0.4 (nmol/min/g)	(195)

(continued)

Table 1 (continued)

Animal intact isolated tissue extract	Treatment	Metabolic pathway measured	Stable isotopic tracer	Rate/outcome	References
Rat (intact, isolated, and extract)	Normal	Lipogenesis β-Oxidation Lipolysis	[1-^{13}C] Arachidonic acid and [3-^{13}C] γ-linolenic acid	Mobility and turnover of tissue lipids	(196)
Rat (intact and extract)	Normal	Glutathione metabolism	[2-^{13}C] Glycine	GSH fractional isotopic enrichment at rate 0.316 per hour	(45)
Mouse (isolated)	Normal (fasted)	Krebs' Gluconeogenesis	[3-^{13}C] Alanine [2-^{13}C] Ethanol	Krebs' entry when both alanine and ethanol present; alanine enters via carboxylation of pyruvate and ethanol via acetyl-CoA	(80)
Mouse (isolated)	Normal (fasted)	Glycogenesis Glycogenolysis Gluconeogenesis Recycling of triacylglycerols	[2-^{13}C] Glycerol [1,3-^{13}C] Glycerol	Gluconeogenic flux from glycerol followed	(117)
Human	Normal vs. glycogen type IIIA storage disease	Glycogenesis Glycogenolysis	Natural abundance	Surface coil; dietary and exercise effects; glycogen level 2–3 times higher in disease state	(197)
Human	Normal vs. hepatic steatosis	Lipogenesis	Natural abundance	Hepatic triglycerides determination (range of hepatic fat content values for several patients)	(198)
Human	Normal (fed, fasted); insulin and glucagon	Glycogenesis Glycogenolysis Gluconeogenesis	Natural abundance [1-^{13}C] Glucose	Insulin and glucagon influences on glycogenesis and turnover rates (many rates given)	(199)
Human	4 Hypoglucagonemic conditions (fasted); insulin and glucagon	Glycogenesis Glycogenolysis	[1-^{13}C] Glucose	Surface coil; Extensive flux rates in table (e.g., range for net glycogenesis: −0.25 to 0.36 mmol L of liver per minute)	

Rat (intact and extract)	Normal (fed, fasted) vs. phosphorylase kinase deficiency (*gsd/gsd*)	Glycogen	Natural abundance	Surface coil; 3× normal glycogen in *gsd/gsd* strain; NMR can diagnose glycogen storage disease	(200)
Rat (isolated and extract)	Normal (fasted); with and without insulin	Gluconeogenesis Glycogenesis Glycogenolysis Krebs'	[2-^{13}C] Pyruvate [1,2-^{13}C] Ethanol	^{31}P and ^{13}C both recorded glycogen increase at 17 μmol of glucose units/g of liver/h and glucose increased at 17 μmol/g of liver/h	(76)
Rat (isolated and extract)	Normal (fed); glucagon	Glycogenolysis Glycolysis Glycogenesis	Natural abundance [1-^{13}C] Glucose	Glycogen T_1's (0.11–0.24 s) and T_2's (16–31 ms) for in situ and in vitro measurements	(201)
Rat (intact)	Normal (fed, fasted); glucagon	Glycolysis Glycogenesis Glycogenolysis	Natural abundance [1-^{13}C] Glucose	Surface coil; monitor C-1 carbons of glucose to glycogen	(202)
Rat (intact)	Normal (fasted); glucagon and insulin	Glycogenesis Glycogenesis Glycogenolysis	[1-^{13}C] Glucose	Insulin and glucagon effects on glucose; glycogen synthesis increases linearly with glucose concentration	(203)
Rat (intact and extract)	Normal (fasted) vs. diabetic	Ketogenesis Krebs' Gluconeogenesis	[1,3-^{13}C] Butyrate [3-^{13}C] Butyrate [1-^{13}C] Butyrate	Surface coil; Disposal of acetyl-CoA different between fasted/fed rats	(204)
Rat (intact, tissue, and extract)	Normal (fasted) vs. diabetic	Ketogenesis Krebs' Gluconeogenesis	[1,3-^{13}C] Octanoate	Surface coil; Ketone body production control in inner mitochondria space	(205)
Rat (isolated)	Normal (fed, fasted) vs. diabetic; insulin	Gluconeogenesis Krebs'	[3-^{13}C] Alanine [2-^{13}C] Pyruvate	Pyruvate kinase flux = 0.74 of gluconeogenic rate in liver of controls; undetectable in diabetes	(206)
Rat (isolated and extract)	Normal (fed, fasted) vs. diabetic	Krebs' Lipogenesis	[3-^{13}C] Alanine	Flux through Krebs' of PDH vs. PC for control fed (1:1.2), control fasted (1:7.7), diabetic (1:2.6)	(207)
Rat (isolated and extract)	Normal (fasted) vs. diabetic	Gluconeogenesis Krebs'	[3-^{13}C] Alanine [2-^{13}C] Pyruvate	Diabetic gluconeogenesis 2–4-fold greater compared to control	(206)

(continued)

Table 1 (continued)

Animal intact isolated tissue extract	Treatment	Metabolic pathway measured	Stable isotopic tracer	Rate/outcome	References
				(diabetic 52 vs. control 24) units of [μmol(g of liver per wet weight)]/h	
Rat (isolated)	Normal (fasted); insulin	Glycogenolysis Glycogenesis	[1-^{13}C] Glucose [3-^{13}C] Alanine [3-^{13}C] Lactate	Net glycogenesis rate is 0.1–0.15 μmol/g/min	(208)
Rat (intact, tissue, and extract)	Normal (fed, fasted) vs. diabetic	β-Oxidation Krebs' Ketogenesis	[1,12-$^{13}C_2$] or [1,2,11,12-$^{13}C_4$] dodecanedioic acid	Metabolism differences between monocarboxylic acids and dicarboxylic fatty acids	(209)
Rat (isolated)	Normal vs. tumor (fasted)	Gluconeogenesis Glycogenesis	[3-^{13}C] Alanine	Tumor cells show changes in hepatic metabolism of alanine; also decreased glycerol utilization and Krebs' cycle	(210)
Rat (intact)	Normal (fed, fasted); insulin	Glycogenesis Glycogenolysis	[1-^{13}C] Glucose [2-^{13}C] Glucose	Compared fed and fasted; glycogenesis (0.3 μmol/min/g) vs. glycogenolyis (0.045 μmol/min/g) for fasted rats	(211)
Rat (intact and extract)	Normal (fed, fasted); [1,3-^{13}C] ribose	Glycogenesis	[1,2-^{13}C] Glucose	Fed rats: Direct pathway (67%), no indirect detected; Fasted rats: Direct pathway (13%) and some via indirect	(212)
Rat (isolated)	Normal vs. tumor (fasted)	Gluconeogenesis	[3-^{13}C] Alanine	Increases [3-^{13}C] aspartate production and demonstrates increased PC activity in tumors	(213)

Rat (extract)	Normal (fasted); insulin	Gluconeogenesis	[1-^{13}C] Glucose	Hyperglycemia under hyperinsulinemia shows increased hepatic glycogen via direct pathway; glycogenesis rates of 0.16, 0.41, 0.13 μmol glucosyl U g/liver/min under various conditions	(214)
Rat (intact and tissue)	Normal (fed); 2,2-dichloro-1-(2-chlorophenyl)-1-(4-chlorophenyl)-[3-^{13}C]-pronane [^{13}C-DDP]	Xenobiotics	^{13}C-DDP	Surface coil; No metabolites detected; Monitor drug induced intrahepatic changes for 12 days	(215)
Rat (intact and tissue)	Normal (fed); 1-(*o*-chlorophenyl)-1-(*p*-chlorophenyl)-2,2-dichloro-3-^{13}C-proprane	Xenobiotics	^{13}C-DDP	Surface coil; xenobiotic product can be followed noninvasively	(216)
Rat (isolated and extract)	Normal (fasted) vs. triiodothyronine treated, hydroxymalonate	Glycolysis Gluconeogenesis Krebs'	[3-^{13}C] Alanine	Flux through pyruvate kinase + malic enzyme to PC 0.18 ± 0.04 in normal rats vs. 0.44 ± 0.08 in treated; following hydroxymalonate addition, T_3 treated flux decrease to 0.15 ± 0.04	(217)
Rat (intact and extract)	Normal vs. ischemia (fasted)	Krebs' Glycogenesis Gluconeogenesis	[1-^{13}C] Glucose	Glucose and energy metabolism indicates ATP level participates in glycogenesis and gluconeogenesis in liver	(218)
Rat (intact and extract)	Normal vs. endotoxemia (fasted)	Gluconeogenesis Krebs'	[3-^{13}C] Alanine	Endotoxin cause inhibition of gluconeogenesis activity and Krebs' cycle	(219)

(continued)

Table 1 (continued)

Animal intact isolated tissue extract	Treatment	Metabolic pathway measured	Stable isotopic tracer	Rate/outcome	References
Rat (intact and extracts)	Normal pregnancy (ad libitum vs. routine meal feeding) (fed, fasted)	Glycogenesis	[1-^{13}C] Glucose	Meal feeding regimes in pregnant rats have increased glycogenesis as compared to ad libitum diets	(220)
Rat (intact and extract)	Burn vs. sham (fasted)	Gluconeogenesis Krebs'	[U-^{13}C] Lactate	Up-regulation of gluconeogenesis and pyruvate to oxaloacetate at expense of non-Krebs' sources; Increased gluconeogenesis from lactate; Table of fluxes	(221)
Rat (extract)	Burn vs. sham (fasted)	Gluconeogenesis Krebs' cycle	[1,2,3-^{13}C] Propionate	Gluconeogenesis vs. Krebs' not altered by burn; Burn trauma stimulate hepatic anaplerosis	(222)
Rat (intact and isolated)	Normal (fed); insulin and glucose	Glycogenolysis	Natural abundance	Glycogenolysis in control: $-0.53 \pm 0.021\%$/min	(223)
Mouse (isolated and extracts)	Normal vs. malaria (fasted)	Gluconeogenesis Krebs'	[2-^{13}C] Pyruvate	56% reduction of glucose production in malarial animals	(224)
Mouse (isolated)	Normal vs. disease (African trypanosomes)	Krebs'	[3-^{13}C] Alanine	Disease causes no permanent damage to hepatic alanine metabolism	(225)
Mouse (isolated)	Normal vs. leukemia (fasted)	Krebs' Gluconeogenesis Glycolysis	[3-^{13}C] Alanine [1-^{13}C] Glucose	Gluconeogenesis rate lower for leukemia; 34.0 ± 8 vs. 4.0 ± 2 μmol glucose/h/g for control vs. leukemia	(226)

Mouse (isolated and extract)	Normal vs. *Ob/ob* mouse model of obesity and insulin resistance; glucagon	Lipogenesis Gluconeogenesis	[2-^{13}C] Pyruvate	Leptin influence on hepatic metabolism monitored; Gluconeogenesis in control, leptin in vitro, and leptin in vivo over 3 h was, respectively, 0.56, 0.75, and 1.18 μmol/gww/min	(227)
Mouse (intact)	Normal vs. diabetes (fasted)	Glycogenesis Gluconeogenesis	[1-^{13}C] Glucose	Net glycogen synthesis rate 2× higher ADM group vs. control	(228)
Mouse (isolated)	Normal (express human glucagon receptor); glucagon; several antagonists	Glycogenolysis Gluconeogenesis	[3-^{13}C] Pyruvate	Efficacy of glucagon receptor antagonists at different concentrations	(229)

Allosteric and nonallosteric effectors modulate the reaction rates by acting on the enzyme. Rate and flux may be defined by analogy to the two types of electricity, direct current (DC) vs. alternating current (AC). Rate and flux have the same units, which are typically gram or moles per unit time per cell number or weight of tissue—or some other measure of tissue volume such as grams of protein or DNA or cell number. In this model, the net flux, J, is the difference between the two unidirectional rates, i.e.,

$$J = v_f - v_r \tag{2}$$

Net flux is sometimes used to define the total flux through a metabolic pathway, in the same manner as rate is used, as some of the individual fluxes can be in reverse of the net flux direction for the entire metabolic pathway. Also, "flux rate" is often used to define flux. In fact, when performing a kinetic study on an isolated enzyme, generally only the enzyme and substrate are present initially and the "initial velocity," v_0, of product formation is measured in the form of millimoles or milligrams of product per unit time at a given enzyme concentration. This in fact is a rate according to our definition.

The simplest possible mechanism for a single substrate single product reaction as in the above scheme is as follows:

$$\mathrm{K_R} \quad \mathrm{k_2} \quad \mathrm{Kp}$$

$$\mathrm{R + E \Leftrightarrow ER \Leftrightarrow EP \Leftrightarrow E + P} \tag{3}$$

$$\mathrm{k_{-2}}$$

where R, E, and P represent reactant, enzyme, and product, respectively. Under the simplifying assumption that reactants and product very rapidly equilibrate with the enzyme, the initial velocities (rates) in the forward and reverse direction are given by:

$$v_f = \mathrm{d}p/\mathrm{d}t = k_2 e_t r_0/(K_R + r_0) \tag{4a}$$

$$v_r = \mathrm{d}s/\mathrm{d}t = k_{-2} e_t p_0/(K_p + p_0) \tag{4b}$$

where p_0 and r_0 are the initial concentrations of R and P, K_R and K_p are the dissociation constants from the enzyme, k_2 and k_{-2} are the catalytic rate constants, and e_t is the total enzyme concentration. In general, in a cell, the initial rate conditions do not apply. More generally, the flux for the mechanism is given by:

$$J = e_t(k_2 r - k_{-2} K_R p/K_p)/[r + K_R(1 + p/K_p)] \tag{5}$$

k_2, k_{-2}, K_R, and K_P are not all independent; they are related by the overall equilibrium constant for the reaction, which is independent of the enzyme, according to:

$$K_{eq} = (k_2/K_R)/(k_{-2}/K_p) \tag{6}$$

This also embodies the Haldane relationship. The flux J can thus be rewritten as:

$$J = \frac{k_2 e_t r[1 - p/rK_{eq}]}{[r + K_R(1 + p/K_p)]} \quad (7)$$

Effectors can influence the value of K_R, k_2, etc., but not K_{eq}.

Thus, the flux is determined not only by the enzyme properties (k_{cat} and K_m values), but also on the absolute concentrations of the enzyme, reactants, and the deviation or their ratio from the equilibrium value. The thermodynamic disequilibrium component is expressed in the square brackets in the numerator of (7) and this defines the direction of the reaction. Thus, if p/rK_{eq} is equal to unity, there is no net flux (the reaction is at equilibrium), whereas if it is different from unity, the reaction goes in either the forward or the reverse direction.

In the context of an isolated enzyme, at steady state, the rate of production of P is a constant. However, if the substrate is allowed to deplete, then the flux will decrease. Furthermore, the product builds up there will be product inhibition, and eventually the flux will reach zero as equilibrium is approached. In the context of a metabolic pathway, generally homeostatic mechanisms tend to maintain both r and p constant at each step along the pathway, such that at steady state, the flux at each point is the same. Only the end product of the pathway then changes as a function of time. This is described in more detail in Chaps. 1 and 9.

For example, during the short steady state that occurs after a meal, there will be a net production of hepatic glycogen, or during exercise, muscle will produce lactate. In the case of glucose after a meal, the steady state for the organism would be the point where the *rates* of intestinal absorption and hepatic liver formation of glycogen and glucose consumption do not change. In the case of exercise, the steady state could be defined at the point where the rate of lactate production and its secretion into the blood stream and the rate of kidney excretion and hepatic metabolism do not change. As mentioned above, a true steady state is rare for an organism that maintains homeostasis. However, short periods may occur, whereby a pseudosteady state can be assumed. The organism compartmentalizes these reactions in different organs or organelles, whereby one organ has a steady state production of lactate and alanine, for example muscle, and another has a steady state consumption, for example liver. In fact, this transfer of lactate and alanine to liver from muscle and then reformation of glucose and transport of glucose back to the muscle is called the Cori cycle. So, during exercise a steady state can be created even though there is a constant rate of glycogen mobilization from the liver, Cori cycling of lactate, alanine, and glucose, and a net loss of lactate from the kidneys. If the product were to accumulate in one of these organs, this would decrease the rate of product formation according to Eq. (7) and the system would enter a nonsteady state. Organisms have evolved ingenious inter and intracellular compartmentation strategies to achieve metabolic stability, some of which are discussed in Sect. 3.3.

Using stable or radioactive isotopes, one can determine the rate, *k*, from the initial slope of the time course of incorporation or decay of isotopically labeled reactant. A steady state is typically maintained in perfused organs or perfused cell systems, because the concentration of nutrients in media can be maintained relatively constant, which in turn maintains constant intracellular concentrations and thus the flux does not change. The intracellular complement of small molecules is the so-called the metabolomic "fingerprint." In batch mode where the media is changed completely at a given time interval, common in cell culture, the waste products can accumulate in the extracellular media, giving the so-called the metabolomic "footprint" and represents the secreted products or consumed nutrients by the cell (71). However, the nutrients, such as glucose, are typically at sufficiently high concentrations, near the V_{max}, such that the fluxes do not change significantly. Although perfused cells and organs permit a reductionist approach to study metabolomics and fluxomics, ultimately the organism contains all the paracrine and endocrine signaling required for normal metabolism and must be used to obtain the complete scope of the metabolic network.

Metabolic regulation is the sum of the biochemical processes that may increase or decrease substrate flux through the various metabolic pathways and nearly always include cell signaling pathways (allosteric effectors). Besides simply increasing reactants of metabolic pathways, the enzymes can be allosterically or nonallosterically modified, whereby the enzyme is actually covalently modified to change its macromolecular structure or to increase the enzymes activity. A good example of metabolic regulation controlling the response to changes in nutritional status is that of glucose metabolism, in fed and starved states. In order to understand the change in substrate fluxes of metabolic pathways, a detailed analysis of the metabolic regulators must be included, such as, allosteric modification of transporters, signaling proteins (i.e., kinases/phosphatases), and enzymes by covalent modification such as phosphorylation or by noncovalent interactions with small molecules (<1 kDa) such as ATP. Figure 3a is a diagram of the metabolic regulation of signaling proteins and the covalent modification via phosphorylation, thus depicting the effect of hormones, insulin, and glucagon on the small molecule secondary messenger, cyclic adenine mono phosphate (cAMP). Ultimately, these hormones regulate the activity of glycogen synthase (GS) and glycogen phosphorylase (GP) as well as breakdown of triglycerides to free fatty acids (FFA) resulting in the formation of ketone bodies.

Mathematical models are used to plan ^{13}C NMR experiments and to interpret or predict the resulting data (20). The metabolic

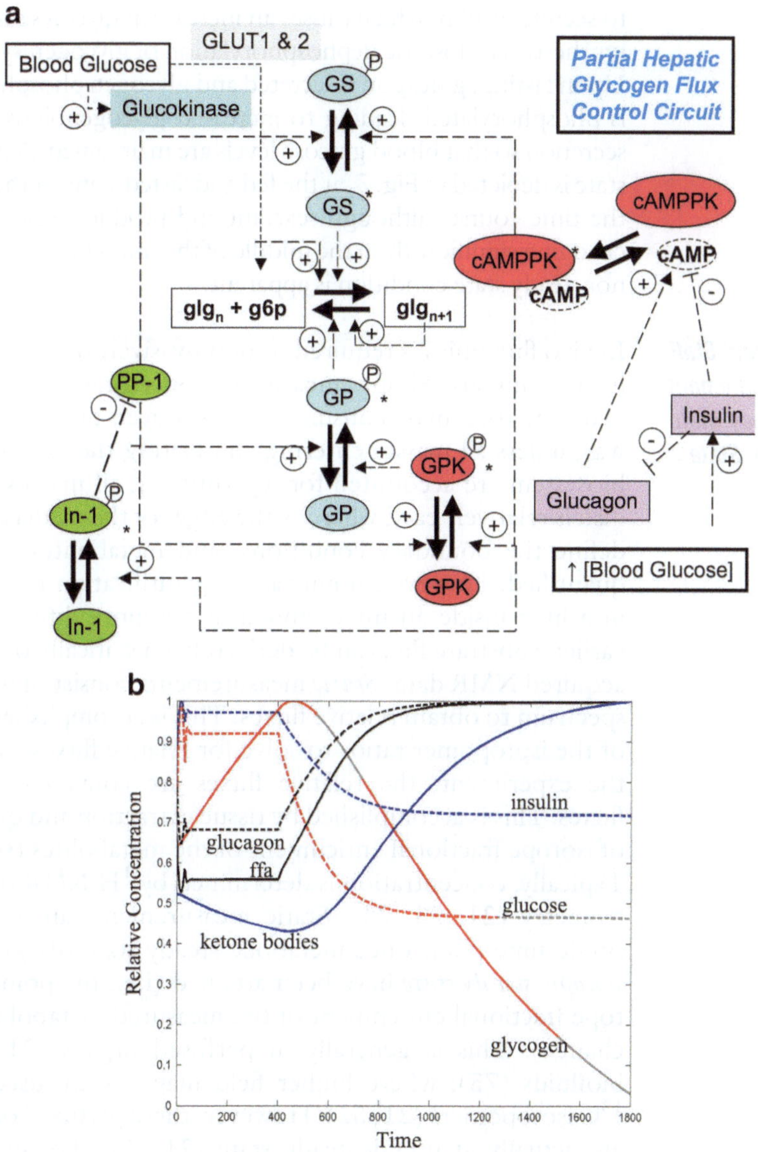

Fig. 3. Metabolic modeling in liver. (**a**) Model of metabolic regulation for glucose and fat metabolism in the fed and fasted states. (**b**) Simulation of hepatic metabolite and hormone concentrations changes over a hypothetical time scale of about 8 h after feeding. *cAMPPK* cAMP protein kinase; *glg* glycogen; *g6p* glucose-6-phosphate; *GLUT 1 and 2* glucose transporters; *ffa* free fatty acids; *GP* glycogen phosphorylase; *GPK* GP kinase; *GS* glycogen synthetase; *In-1* inhibitor protein 1; *PP-1* protein phosphatase 1. Adapted from Todd (72).

regulatory scheme can be translated to a Matlab™ program to predict metabolite levels that can help interpret experimental fluxomic data. Figure 3b is a simulation of hepatic carbohydrate and fat concentration after a meal demonstrating the positive and negative feedback of hormones (i.e., endocrine signals), insulin and glucagon, in response to changes in glucose concentration in blood (72). After a meal, the plasma glucose concentration increases causing the pancreas to secrete insulin, which causes an increase in glycolysis and glycogen synthesis via allosteric dephosphorylation of glycogen synthase (GS). Upon fasting, glucagon is secreted and glycogen phosphorylase (GP) is phosphorylated, leading to increased glycogenolysis and glucose secretion so that blood glucose levels are maintained. A pseudosteady state is depicted in Fig. 3, at the fed and fasted states at the two ends of the time course, although reactant and product concentrations are changing significantly in the middle of the time course, where clearly a nonsteady state condition is apparent.

2.3. Dynamic and Static ^{13}C NMR Measurement of Flux at Steady State and Nonsteady State

In vivo fluxomics is required to noninvasively obtain mass balance in live animals. Simply measuring concentration will underestimate the total mass consumed or produced by a metabolic pathway, unless all masses entering and exiting the boundaries of the biosystem are accounted for. Quantifying all masses in a culture dish is relatively easy, whereby the edges of the media and cell mass define the boundary conditions, and metabolites are invasively quantified. However, noninvasive quantification of mass balance in a liver inside an intact animal is far more difficult. As stated earlier, substrate flux can be derived from statically or dynamically acquired NMR data. *Static* measurements consist of using a single spectrum to obtain relative fluxes. This is accomplished by analysis of the isotopomer ratios to solve for relative fluxes. At the end of the experiment, the relative fluxes are converted to absolute fluxes. This is accomplished by tissue extraction and quantification of isotope fractional enrichment of the metabolites (see Chap. 2). Typically, concentration is determined by ^{1}H NMR or mass spectrometry (21, 73, 74). Static measurements are obtained at a single time point once metabolic steady state ($dC/dT = 0$) and *isotopic steady state* have been attained (i.e., the point where isotope fractional enrichment of the measured metabolites does not change). This is generally in perfused organs (21) or human biofluids (75), where higher field magnets are used to resolve ^{13}C isotopomers (21, 52). However, these perfused organ models are actually at pseudosteady state (21, 76). For example, with perfused Langendorf preparations, the excised heart is taken from a condition of being bathed in a rich mixture of plasma nutrients, to a saline solution composed of a single or mixture of several nutrients. Under these conditions, the tissue relies on more on endogenous substrates (21) that are not typical of normal metabolism. Sometimes blood is used (76, 77). However, although these organs are relatively short-lived, the kinetics are rapid compared to the initial equilibrium phase of the study and are in a pseudosteady state by the time the ^{13}C studies begin (21, 78). Comparing to metabolism of whole organisms always has caveats. Mammalian animal studies are always tainted by the need for anesthesia. In short, one must always consider the limitations of the model as it relates to steady state conditions that are of physiological relevance.

Dynamic measurements of fluxes obtain multiple spectra using dynamic in vivo NMRS to measure isotope enrichment of nutrients (41, 79). This can require several hours of noninvasive monitoring of the biosystem (45). As discussed above, these studies are typically performed under pseudosteady state conditions, so concentrations do not change ($dC/dT = 0$). In contrast, at *isotopic nonsteady state* (i.e., isotope fractional enrichment of the measured metabolites is changing), the time course of isotopic incorporation can be analyzed to derive the rates of the desired metabolic reaction(s). Most *metabolic nonsteady state* NMR fluxomic studies (i.e., concentration changes during kinetic measurement) have been performed dynamically in perfused organs where substrates are controlled and have focused on substrate utilization and citric acid (aka Krebs or TCA) cycle flux (21). Dynamic NMR flux studies using intact organism have used two-state models where fluxes are measured once the new metabolome representing a pathology, nutritional status, or drug/toxicant exposure has reached a new metabolic steady state. Since both flux and concentrations are changing during nonsteady state conditions, one must obtain dynamic measurements of both concentration by ^{1}H NMRS and the corresponding ^{13}C NMR spectra in order to derive the changing flux in response to the changing reactant/product concentrations. This is very complex (Chap. 8). Therefore, two-state models are preferred.

2.3.1. In Vivo ^{13}C NMR Studies in Intact Mammals and Perfused Organs

In vivo ^{13}C NMRS of liver was the first organ studied by this method (80). Very soon after brain, heart, kidney, skeletal muscle, and other tissues were studied using this approach (52). Liver is the central metabolic organ for the entire organism. However, liver produces the poorest NMR spectral conditions because of movement, magnetic susceptibility issues, and short T_2 values, all of which compromise signal-to-noise ratio (SNR) and resolution. Abdominal motion of liver in vivo has been overcome by use of ex vivo perfusion, but this eliminates organ interactions present at the organismal level. The liver is the best organ to monitor for system effects on the metabolome or fluxome, because the liver is the central organ responsible for detoxification, synthesis, storage, and energy generation, and thus the hub through which all organs interact metabolically. The application of in vivo ^{13}C NMR methodology in whole animals has measured all major metabolic pathways including the Citric acid cycle, gluconeogenesis, glycolysis, β-oxidation, glycogenesis, lipogenesis, protein synthesis, nucleotide metabolism, even signaling, and fluxes simultaneously (see Table 1).

Table 1 illustrates the current state of in vivo ^{13}C liver studies in mammals. Not mentioned are other NMR active nuclei such as ^{2}H (81) and ^{31}P (82), which have been utilized in conjunction with ^{13}C tracers to gather metabolism data. The information in Table 1 reveals the widespread and ongoing developments in the field. These studies started with monitoring natural abundance ^{13}C in intact animals and progressed to perfusion and infusion of ^{13}C-labeled nutrients in perfused liver and intact animals, respectively. Presently, only a few fluxes have been quantified simultaneously in the same organism with five metabolic pathways using *static* method in human biofluids (i.e., gluconeogenesis, glycogen synthesis, glycolysis, Krebs', and PPP) (75) and eight metabolites using the *dynamic* method in brain from intact rat (83, 84). Applications in the areas of diabetes, obesity, burns, leukemia, and tumors are just a few examples where these efforts have been successfully applied to liver (Table 1).

Although intact brain and perfused heart are perhaps the most published organs for in vivo ^{13}C NMRS, we have focused on thoroughly reviewing the liver literature. For reviews of in vivo ^{13}C NMR of brain (85, 86) and heart (21, 87–89), refer to the indicated literature. Table 1 presents a comprehensive review of mammalian liver in vivo ^{13}C NMR literature. Four categories of animal sample preparation are examined as indicated in the first column including "non-invasive" intact (whole animal), isolated (excised, perfused liver), tissue (excised pieces of liver tissue), and extracts ("invasive" sample preparation). Advantages and disadvantages accompany each study choice, with typically lower signal-to-noise data in whole animal studies collecting in situ data or increased resolution in isolated liver ex vivo experiments performed under certain assumptions. It is typically necessary to end each ^{13}C time course study with an extraction of the tissue to validate the noninvasive in vivo measurements.

The chronological table is divided into two groups according to treatment type. The first group encompasses normal states and is immediately followed by disease or chemical treatment conditions. Each group is arranged from the largest to the smallest mammals with the most abundant studies exploiting both intact and isolated rat livers.

Within the first normal class, subjects are either fed or fasted and various metabolic pathways are measured using stable isotopic tracers. Typical pathways studied are gluconeogenesis, glycolysis, glycogenesis, glycogenolysis, Krebs' (tricarboxylic or citric acid) cycle, and ketogenesis. Selected references analyze β-oxidation, fatty acid metabolism, and PPP, or simply demonstrate glycogen detection and no flux is measured. Employing appropriate "metabolic" tracers such as 1-^{13}C-glucose or 2-^{13}C-acetate among others and in all the cases not a "massless" tracer as can be assumed with radioactive isotope studies, the authors determine suitable pulse sequences and hardware choices to monitor percentages and flow rates of particular pathways.

The second group of studies primarily focuses on diabetes and the effects of insulin and glucagon on metabolism while also addressing glycogen storage disease, tumors, ischemia, burn

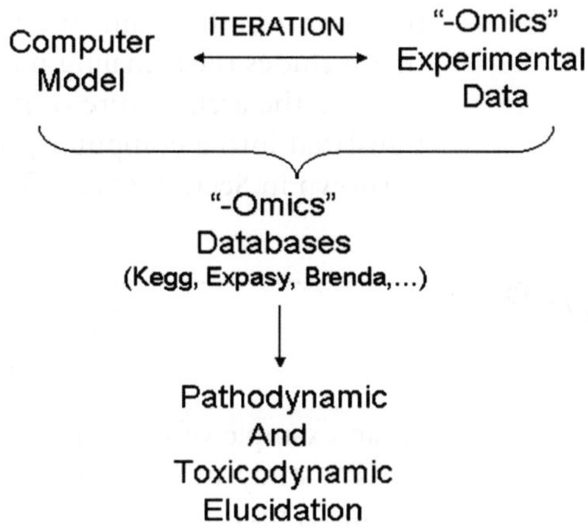

Fig. 4. Pathodynamic and toxicodynamic algorithm.

injuries, and malaria. Similar isotopic tracers as in the normal experiments are utilized with multiple tracers such as 3-^{13}C-alanine and 2-^{13}C-pyruvate in single studies becoming prominent. Turnover rates, T_1 and T_2 measurements, and drug xenobiotics are monitored in the previously mentioned metabolic pathways.

2.3.2. In Silico Mass Balance Models and Algorithm for Toxicodynamics and Pathodynamics

In general, the global analysis accrued by the "-omics" experiments can be arrayed with computational analysis and metabolic databases, to elucidate etiologies of disease and toxicity by defining the cascade of pathological or toxic events. Figure 4 is the "-omics" toxicodynamic or pathodynamic algorithm incorporating the global analysis of all the "-omics" methodologies in an iterative manner with mathematical modeling with the goal of identifying the upstream and downstream toxic or pathological events that define the etiology of toxicity or pathology. Similar to macromolecular structure determination algorithms, empirical data impose constraints on the computer calculations macromolecular structure (90). However, unlike the structure determination algorithm, the "-omics" algorithm has significant dynamic events that occur at a different time scale, a period of seconds to years rather than picoseconds, depending on acute or chronic aspects of the study. To first create these models from scratch, one must perform metabolic reconstruction using metabolic pathway databases, such as KEGG, which can be queried to list the metabolic connections to a substrate, thereby generating your network (91). Next, the boundary conditions of the biosystem must be defined. For example, in a perfused liver system, one can consider the liver "well-stirred" (i.e., homogeneous), and have a three-compartment model defining the boundary conditions: the perfusate, the hepatocytes, and the mitochondria within the hepatocytes. In dynamic PET imaging of the brain, (described in Sect. 1), a three-compartment model was used to define the boundary conditions such as the blood–brain barrier, the plasma in the brain, and the brain cells (49). Finally, a network that includes the signaling molecules as well as the micromolecules creating the architecture of the mathematical model is derived and translated into a computer program permitting input and output, as shown in Sect. 2.2 (Fig. 3).

3. Examples of ^{13}C NMR Studies

3.1. Dynamic Measurements

As an example of the dynamic NMR measurement, an in vivo ^{13}C NMRS study of liver from anesthetized rats infused with 2-^{13}C-glycine is used in order to illustrate the various parts of the experiment. The steady state study was performed by (45) and the non-steady state study was performed as part of Dr. Macdonald's doctoral work in Dr. T.L. James laboratory (92). Although dated, these studies illustrate the multiple hurdles one must consider in performing dynamic in vivo ^{13}C NMR studies.

3.1.1. Steady State, Dynamic Measurements from In Vivo ^{13}C NMR Spectral Time Course Datasets

Figure 5 shows in vivo ^{13}C NMR spectra of liver from intact rat obtained using an implanted surface coil localized to the liver (45) prior (Fig. 5b) and 4 h after (Fig. 5a) 2-^{13}C-glycine infusion (4.4 mM/kg/h), and the high resolution ^{13}C NMR analysis of the perchloric acid extract of the liver (Fig. 5c) corresponding the 4 h time point (Fig. 5a) (figure taken from (92)). Note the superior spectral

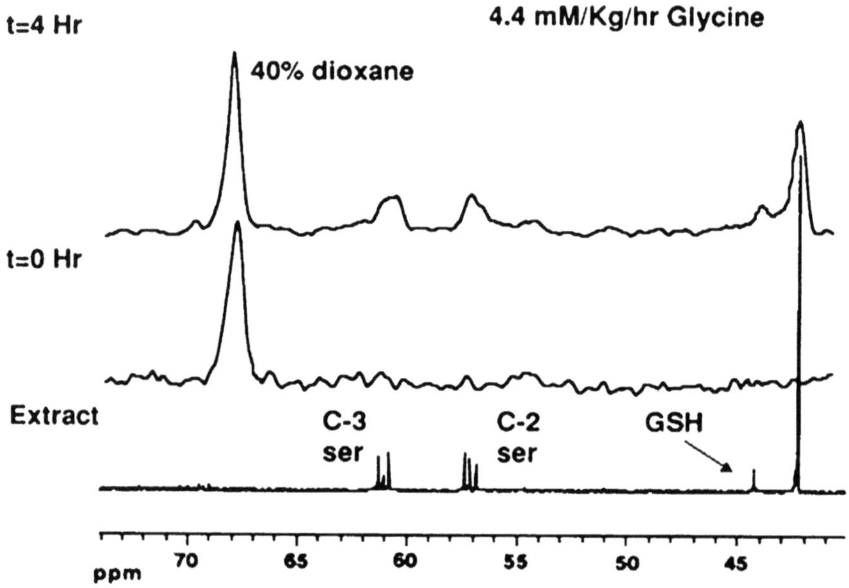

Fig. 5. ^{13}C NMR spectroscopy of rat liver. In vivo ^{13}C NMR spectra (*top*, *middle*) and the high resolution ^{13}C NMR spectrum of the perchloric acid extract (*bottom*) from an anesthetized rat infused with 2-^{13}C-glycine. Modified from (92). *Gly* glycine; *GSH* glutathione; *C-2 ser* C2 carbon of serine; *C3 ser* C3 carbon of serine.

resolution of the perchloric acid extract, demonstrating the effect of iron and motion in decreasing the in vivo T_2 and the T_2^* values (see Chap. 6, for causes of inhomogeneity associated with T_2^*). One notes the increase of four sets of peaks [C2 ser (2-^{13}C-serine), C3 ser (3-^{13}C-serine), GSH ([2-^{13}C-glycyl]glutathione), and Gly (2-^{13}C-glycine)], with a fifth peak 40% dioxane which is present in vivo but not in the perchloric acid extract. This section will explain the analysis of the peaks representing GSH, Gly, and 40% dioxane. Section 3 describes the analysis of the triplet of C2-Ser and C3-Ser in the perchloric acid extract (Fig. 5c). Clearly, the relatively large amount of glycine infused in conjunction with relatively similar kinetics as that of glycine resulting in poor temporal resolution means serine is not at metabolic steady state. Although plasma glycine concentration was not determined, a quick estimation of 4.4 mM/kg/h or about 1.1 mM/h for these 250 g rats infusing into about a 10 mL blood volume would result in 110 mM if it were not metabolized or excreted by the kidneys. The blood concentration of glycine is about 0.3 mM (93). The caveats for why glutathione is at a pseudosteady state are described below and are very important to understand: (1) the glycine is at the V_{max} of glutathione synthetase, and (2) the temporal resolution is sufficient to derive the rate.

3.1.2. Peak Area Determination from Dynamic In Vivo ^{13}C NMR Spectra

The 40% dioxane peak (Fig. 5a, b) is an external standard and that is why it is not present in the perchloric acid extract (Fig. 5c). The external standard is used for quality control and quantification. For example, if experimental conditions suddenly degrade the spectral quality due to pulses affected by detuning of the circuit or uncharacteristic tissue movement, the standard will also be affected, and it is assumed in the same manner as the in vivo peaks of interest. In some cases, an internal standard such as choline *N*-methyl carbons resonances at 54.6 ppm can be used as a reference or calibrant (94); however, an external standard is most commonly used. Typically, a magnetic glass capillary or sphere is placed between the tissue of interest and the NMR probe (45). Magnetic susceptibility effects (see Chap. 6) are still present even with proper placement and container shape, especially for surface coil liver analysis, so the chemical shift difference from pure dioxane can be as much as 0.3 ppm in error, e.g., 68.7 vs. 69.0 ppm.

The peak areas of glutathione and glycine were compared to the dioxane peak area resulting in a peak area ratio that is plotted with respect to time. The temporal resolution of this study was 10 min, and it is important to have sufficient temporal resolution in order to obtain at least four points defining the curve, preferably eight points or more, especially if there is more than one rate that requires derivation. For the peaks representing C-3 ser and C-2 ser, this temporal resolution would need to be at least 3 min in order to analyze the rapid kinetics of serine formation. Also, as mentioned above, serine is not at steady state and would belong in the

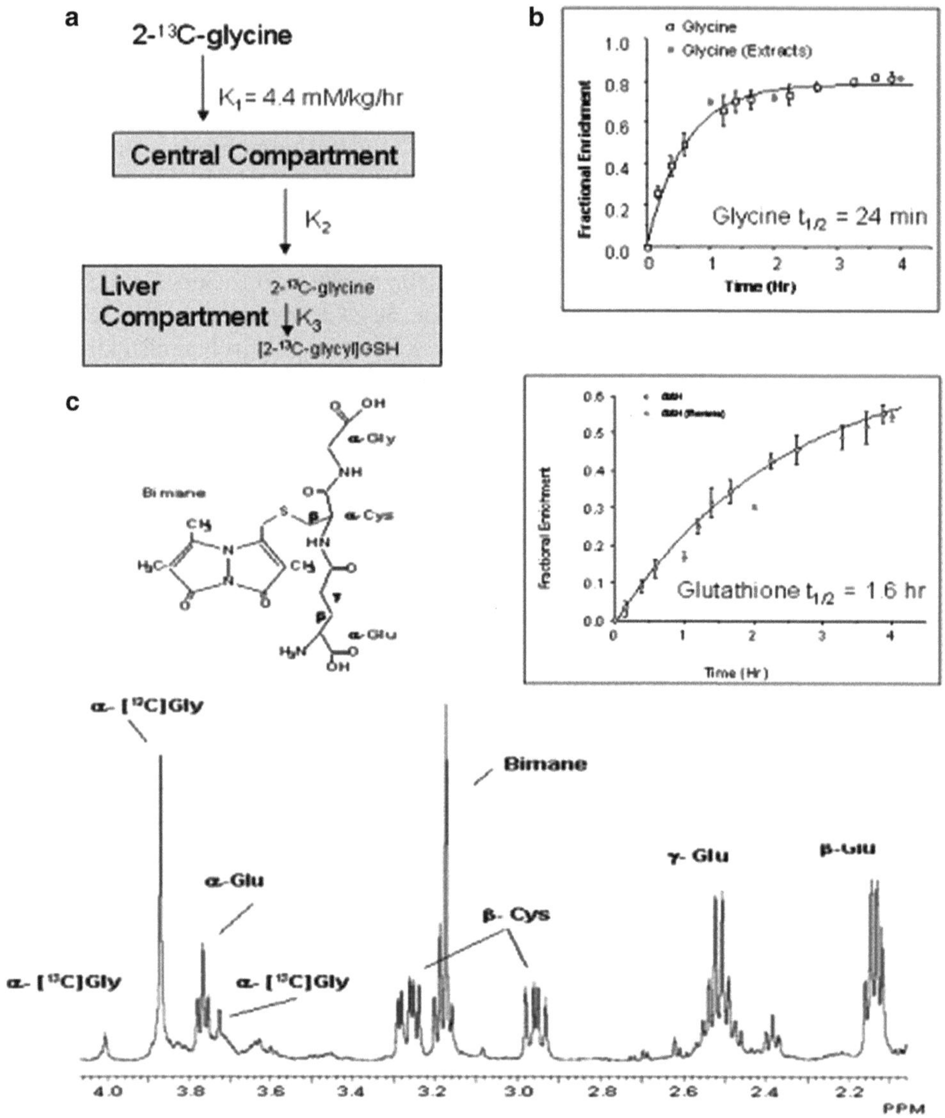

Fig. 6. Compartment Model. (**a**) Definition of kinetic parameters. (**b**)Time courses of ^{13}C enrichment in glycine and glutathione with fits defined by the model in (**a**). (**c**) Structure of bimane and proton spectrum showing fractional enrichments. From ref. (45).

following section on nonsteady state kinetics. Various commercial vendors specialize in software for NMR analysis, and the NMR processing software packages are available, (LCModel, ACD), and some have free downloadable 1D processing versions online (MestreC, Acorn NMR, Swan, NMR Pipe). MacFid (Tecmag Inc., Houston, TX) was used on a MacIntosh computer to fit the peaks in the study shown in Figs. 5 and 6.

The area of the various peaks appearing in a series of in vivo ^{13}C NMR spectra recorded over a period of time can be *integrated* or determined with a least squares fitting algorithms, known as peak fitting or *deconvolution*. *Deconvolution* is used when there are overlapping peaks that are not baseline resolved. Deconvolution is a peak fitting procedure in which a Gaussian or Lorentzian (or commonly a combination of the two) peak shapes plus, in some cases, a baseline function is iteratively fitted to the experimental spectrum using a least squares criterion for example. The peak areas are recovered from the best fit. *Integration* is a point-by-point summation of area. Integration can be done by linearly interpolating the point (trapezoid rule) or polynomial interpolation (Simpson's rule), but both have systematic errors associated with baseline offset or distortion. Correct zero-filling to properly define the shape, peak phasing, baseline correction, and suitable data acquisition parameters are key features in obtaining proper integrals. Due to incomplete baseline separation of the glycine and glutathione peaks, peak fitting, or deconvolution, was used to obtain peak areas in this study (45). Figure 6b shows plots of peak area ratios of glycine-to-dioxane and glutathione-to-dioxane after conversion ^{13}C fractional enrichment.

Single Component Curve Fitting

The in vivo ^{13}C peak intensities obtained as a function of time are fit to the appropriate rate equations to solve for kinetic rate constants using standard mathematical-based software programs, such as, Excel™, Mathematica™, and Matlab™. First, one creates a metabolic model for the biological system. This is done by compartmental analysis whereby the external and internal boundaries of the system are defined. Compartmental analysis is a routine data analysis methodology used in biomedical engineering (95) pharmacokinetics and many other disciplines. Using the example of 2-^{13}C-glycine infusion in rats, we first defined the compartments in Fig. 6a (45, 92). This describes a very simple model in which constant glycine infusion into the central compartment (the blood) is relatively rapid for glycine (~60 min) and is defined by the volume of distribution. The volume of distribution is a pharmacokinetic term described as the volume by which the infused glycine will equilibrate and fill the various compartmental of a biosystem. Essentially, this is the time needed for the central compartment (blood) to reach steady state concentrations with all the organs of the body. It takes some time to fill these compartment(s) and that is defined by the glycine time course shown in Fig. 6b with a half-life of 24 min. It takes five half-lives to reach steady state (45). Once inside the hepatocytes, glycine is metabolized by cytosolic glutathione synthetase to yield the tripeptide glutathione. Glutathione is an antioxidant needed to protect the cell. It has a relatively long half-life (i.e., turnover in order of tens of hours). After being made in the cytosol, glutathione is transported into the mitochondria. Since import into mitochondria is rapid compared to glutathione synthesis in the cytosol, its mitochondrial glutathione was not detected in the time course from the in vivo ^{13}C NMRS (45). Another potential reason mitochondrial glutathione was not detected is that it became NMR-invisible upon import. In the mitochondria, glutathione may noncovalently bind to macromolecules, rendering it NMR-invisible. From the results, we are unable to exclude this possibility (see below) (45). Figure 6b shows the time courses of glycine (top) and glutathione (bottom) from which the kinetic parameter, half-life, was derived. Both glycine and glutathione were fit using a least squares algorithm to the one-compartment model (i.e., monoexponential) to derive the rate constant (k) according to:

$$y = A(1 - e^{-kx}) \tag{8}$$

Since glutathione did not reach a similar fractional enrichment as glycine, it is obvious that the reactions have not reached steady state. The fact that glycine isotopic equilibration was not at steady state until 60 min after start of infusion would affect the kinetic analysis of glutathione if the kinetics were on similar time scales and (8) would need to be modified to subtract the glycine curve representing volume of distribution phase. However, because the half-life of glycine was 24 min and that of glutathione was 1.6 h, it was possible to neglect the rapid glycine exponential when deriving the glutathione kinetic equations. Another potential problem in determining accurate turnover rates is the time course of the observations. Ideally, one should acquire data for five half-lives to obtain the most accurate measure of kinetic parameters. However, this would have been 8 h and the rats could not tolerate 8 h with the surgery they had undergone (45). The physiological perturbation would have had more effects on accurate physiological glutathione kinetic determination than truncating the time course. This study was run for nearly three half-lives and this is sufficient to estimate the turnover rate. However, any time course followed for less than three half-lives should have some proportional error associated with the rate derivation. However, a single exponential can be rather well determined by a small number of very precise measurements.

Although the infused 2-^{13}C-glycine was fit with a one-compartment model, in fact, there is a second component to the curve, and the curve is composed of two rate constants of vastly different rate time scales. The first occurs within 2 h as discussed above—the time it takes glycine to distribute throughout the body to fill the volume of distribution. This extremely fast rate was not detected with this 10 min temporal resolution, the uptake of glycine from the blood to the hepatocytes. The second component takes 3 days to reach equilibrium and is the protein pool becoming labeled and is the reason only 80% of glycine is labeled after 4 h of infusion (25). Therefore, as long as rates are resolved with sufficient temporal resolution so that the peak fitting algorithms can separate out the various resonances, multiple rates can be determined from a single dynamic ^{13}C NMR time course. In short, glycine kinetics reflect the volume of distribution plus whole body protein turnover, whereas the glutathione label represents de novo synthesis.

In the time course (Fig. 6b), the *y*-axis represents the absolute fractional enrichment rather than relative fractional enrichment. To obtain absolute fractional enrichment, a tissue extract of metabolites was made using the previously described perchloric acid extraction method and a high-resolution NMR spectra was obtained and metabolite concentrations were determined. The in vivo time point was calibrated to this value. Figure 6c is a high-resolution ^{1}H NMR spectrum of the tissue extract. The extract was treated with bromobimane, which reacts with free sulfhydryl groups including that of the reduced form of glutathione. Last, the extract was passed over a C18 cartridge to eliminate coresonating biochemicals within the liver extract. The [2-^{13}Cglycyl]glutathione satellite peak areas in the ^{1}H-spectra in Fig. 6c are represented by the [2-^{13}Cglycyl]glutathione peak areas plus [2-^{12}Cglycyl]glutathione peak area. These peak areas are summed up to determine the fractional enrichment. This method of fractional enrichment determination is considered the "gold standard" in NMRS (20, 21, 51, 52). The fractional enrichment obtained at the end of the experiment is then assigned to the peak area ratio of the final in vivo time point and the previous peak area ratios are calibrated to this value to generate the graphs shown in Fig. 6b.

There are several other factors that must be considered that could affect the accurate measurement of turnover rate. In addition to exchange kinetics vs. de novo synthesis that can affect the turnover rate of metabolites (96), factors such as differential saturation of peaks and NMR visibility may alter results as well. To correct for saturation effects (see Chap. 6), saturation factors should be determined (45). The visibility of a metabolite by NMR depends on its SNR and detection limit. Most metabolites interact with macromolecules (see Fig. 1), e.g., the metabolic enzymes, membranes, and polynucleotides, so this is a common recurring problem in metabolite analysis. The bound fraction metabolites are typically broadened (and may also be shifted along the *x*-axis, or chemical shift represented by δ) below the detection limits. Owing to the slow tumbling rate of the protein, R_2 is shortened and peaks broaden (see Chap. 6). NMR detects predominantly the free metabolites. Thus, the total concentration can in some instances be substantially larger than what is actually observed by NMR, and the bound fraction varies from metabolite to metabolite. This raises the issue of how to deal with metabolic fluxes at all if most is bound and NMR-invisible. A classic example of this was the controversy over glycogen (97, 98) ATP (99, 100) and polyamine (101). One solution is to cast all of the appropriate equations in terms of free concentrations when analyzing NMR datasets, rather than total concentrations. However, in vivo NMR visibility should always be determined when possible.

NMR visibility is typically determined by comparing peak area ratio in vivo to the same peak ratios in the extract. Obviously, it is important to know the NMR visibility of one of these metabolites represented by the peak ratio in order to obtain an accurate measure of the peak of interest. Glutathione, for example, binds to the protein compartment in cells creating a mixed disulfide pool (bound fraction) or coordinates with iron or other macromolecules, which broadens the in vivo NMR peak to the point of becoming invisible (see Chap. 6) (45). Macromolecular binding or chelation with paramagnetic ions resulting in NMR invisibility can often be misinterpreted as being a normal condition of the biosystem. However, it could be the nonphysiological conditions of the biosystem causing the protein binding. For example, glutathione rapidly forms mixed-disulfides when cells experience stress conditions. In an early study, Nicholson et al. (102) concluded that glutathione was not ^{1}H NMR-visible due to protein binding in packed hepatocyte suspensions-administered acetaminophen. In fact, they were likely correct and the glutathione was bound, but this was due to the highly hypoxic environments of the packed hepatocytes, which release iron from ferritin pools and ultimately increase the bound fraction and cell death. Later, in perfused MCF-7 cells (103) and intact liver (45), glutathione was ^{13}C NMR-visible. Even the superior R_2 values of ^{13}C (e.g., roughly the width in Hz at half peak height in the spectrum shown in the top spectrum in Fig. 5) compared to ^{1}H nuclei could account for this lack of NMR visibility. Therefore, it is very important to investigate the physiological relevance of the biosystem before blaming NMR visibility. At the back-end of the in vivo NMR experiment, the extraction procedure is very important and can lead to macromolecular binding and loss of micromolecules/metabolites (see Chap. 2). In fact, perchloric acid extraction generates peroxyl radicals from the heavy iron load and increases the bound fraction of glutathione. This made the results from the experiment shown in Fig. 5 to be noninterpretable regarding glutathione NMR-visibility (45).

This effect of line broadening or shortening R_2 values is best illustrated with the endogenous chelator, citrate, and binding to divalent cations such as manganese. In fact, these cations are often added to extracts to shorten R_1 values, so spectra can be obtained more rapidly (104). Depending on the binding constant, the binding of cations can affect the chemical shift, and this phenomenon has been used to determine intracellular magnesium and calcium ions concentrations using endogenous and exogenous chelators such as ATP and FBAPTA, respectively (41, 105). The use of chelators and their relaxation mechanism are used as contrast agents in MRI. Desferrioxime, sold as Desferal™, is used to bind endogenous iron and secreted into the biliary tree from the liver and is an imaging contrast agent, decreasing R_1 values (106). For a physical description of mechanisms of relaxation, the reader is referred to Chap. 6.

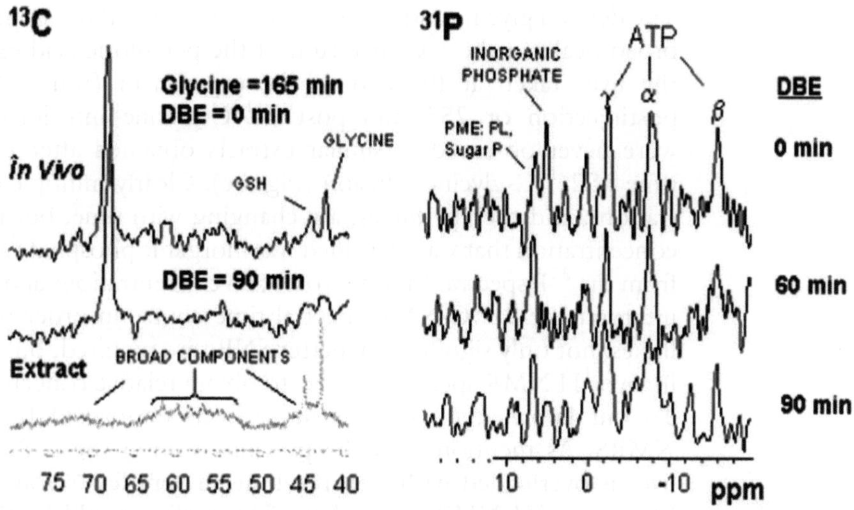

Fig. 7. The time course of in vivo ^{13}C and ^{31}P NMR spectra of liver from intact rats infused with 2-^{13}C-glycine. The glycine was infused for 165 min and followed by administration of half the LD_{50} dose of dibromoethane. Note very little change to the ^{31}P spectra, yet significant changes in the ^{13}C spectra. Adapted from ref. (92).

Finally, there is always the potential of unanticipated physiological perturbation during in vivo experiments as a result of the continual fight for improved NMR spectral quality at the cost of maintaining normal physiology. Often in the process of setting up a biological NMR experiment, experimental parameters may skew results. Parameters affected include hypoxia (e.g., decreasing perfusion of organs, or increasing anesthesia to animals to decrease motion effects), or increase in stress hormones such as adrenalin or IL-6 (e.g., surgical implantation of the NMR surface probe to increase sensitivity). These perturbations will cause rate changes to compensate for the stress and binding effects—both of which will taint in vivo fluxomics data.

3.2. Nonsteady State, Dynamic Measurements from In Vivo ^{13}C NMR Spectral Time Course Data

An example of nonsteady state, dynamic measurement of flux by in vivo ^{13}C NMRS is the administration of dibromoethane during glycine infusion using the same rat model as previously described (45), except 1.1 mM/kg/h infusion was used instead 4.4 mM/kg/h (92), thus the smaller glycine and serine peak areas. Figure 7 shows the results from interleaved in vivo $^{31}P/^{13}C$ NMRS, a method first described by experiments by Cohen (76) using perfused liver. After 165 min intravenous infusion of 1.1 mM/kg/h of 2-^{13}C-glycine ($^{13}C = 0$ min, left; $^{31}P = 0$ min, right), a LD_{50} of the carcinogen dibromoethane dissolved in corn oil was administered by intraperitoneal injection and serial 10 min acquisition $^{31}P/^{13}C$ spectra were obtained during the first 90 min postinjection. While the spectra are very noisy, it is clear that there was little change in the inorganic phosphate and ATP peaks in the ^{31}P spectra, while there is a greater change in the ^{13}C spectrum.

The defined glycine and glutathione peaks redistribute to unknown broad peaks in the ^{13}C spectrum of the perchloric acid extract of the liver taken at the end of the experiment (time = 90 min postinjection or 255 min post 2-^{13}C-glycine infusion), which were never observed in similar extracts obtained after the same time of 2-^{13}C-glycine infusion (Fig. 5c). Clearly multiple concentrations, and thereby fluxes, are changing with time, but the only concentration that was identified was inorganic phosphate and ATP from the ^{31}P spectra. In order to obtain concentrations and thereby interpret the 2-^{13}C NMR spectral time course in order to derive fluxes, not only significantly better SNRs are required, but also the in vivo ^{1}H NMR spectra in order to obtain relative concentrations. To our knowledge, this has never been performed by in vivo NMRS. As mentioned in the previous section (Sect. 3.3.1), rat liver is overloaded with iron resulting in very few resolved peaks by in vivo ^{1}H NMRS, and these first studies would be the most feasible in brain, which delivers some of the spectral quality of any tissue.

3.3. Steady State, Static Measurement of Isotopomer Ratios and Compartmentation

Isotopomers are identical molecules with ^{13}C in different locations. In some metabolic pathways, a single carbon label in a substrate can be incorporated into multiple positions of a downstream metabolite depending on enzymes. Examples showing how such isotopomers can be generated are described in a previous chapter (see Chap. 6) and in Sect. 2.1.1. ^{13}C NMRS has the advantage over other analytical methods, such as mass spectrometry, in analyzing isotopomers because positional information is inherently present in the NMR spectra, and the ^{13}C-^{13}C coupling patterns resolve the various isotopomers. Although MS/MS and analysis of fragmentation patterns can also obtain positional isotope information (see Chap. 4), it is destructive and is not "non-invasive"—the topic of this chapter. The best example of how isotopic scrambling can occur involves the production of succinate in the Krebs' cycle (Fig. 2). Isotopomer analysis can be used to determine the Krebs' flux and anaplerosis by analyzing the glutamate molecule and location of ^{13}C labels (54, 107).

3.3.1. Quantifying Tissue Compartmentation from ^{13}C NMR Spectra

In conjunction with isotopomer analysis, NMR can determine metabolic compartmentalization not only noninvasively in vivo, but the positional isotopomers obtained directly by a single 1D or 2D high-resolution NMR spectrum from tissue extracts (see Chap. 2). The data can be confirmed by MS/MS analysis (see Chap. 4). Metabolism in glia and neurons is encoded with isotopomer information, precluding the need for microdissection of these tissues. These isotopomers contain a "memory" of the metabolic processes or relative fluxes occurring in the various compartments. Compartmentation of neurotransmitters in the various type of cell of the brain is extremely important for proper functioning of the central nervous system;

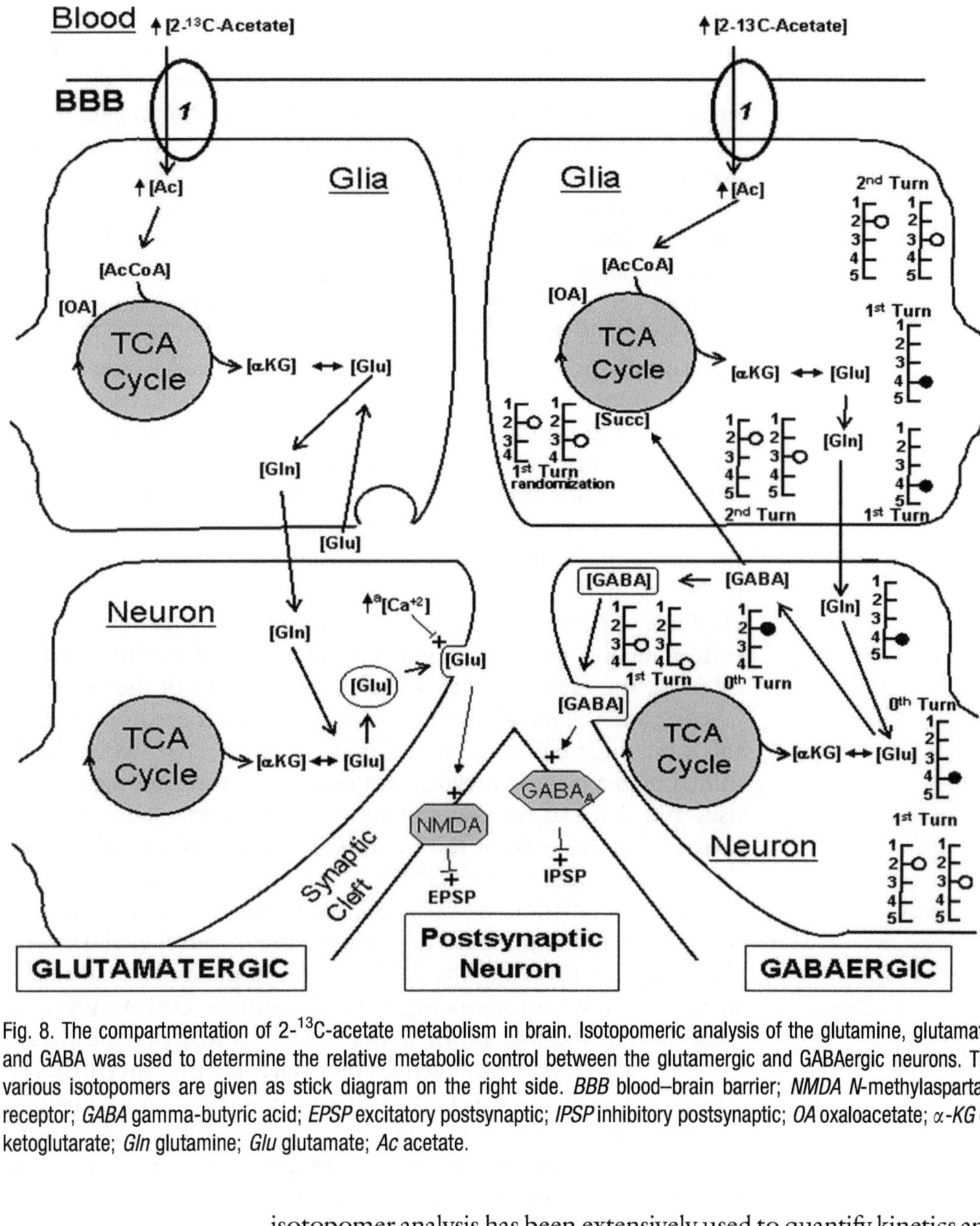

Fig. 8. The compartmentation of 2-^{13}C-acetate metabolism in brain. Isotopomeric analysis of the glutamine, glutamate, and GABA was used to determine the relative metabolic control between the glutamergic and GABAergic neurons. The various isotopomers are given as stick diagram on the right side. *BBB* blood–brain barrier; *NMDA N*-methylaspartate receptor; *GABA* gamma-butyric acid; *EPSP* excitatory postsynaptic; *IPSP* inhibitory postsynaptic; *OA* oxaloacetate; *α-KG* α-ketoglutarate; *Gln* glutamine; *Glu* glutamate; *Ac* acetate.

isotopomer analysis has been extensively used to quantify kinetics and compartmentation (108, 109). The best example of this is the use of glutamine/glutamate cycling in the brain using 2-^{13}C-acetate (110–112). Figure 8 is a diagram of the tissue compartmentation of acetate metabolism in the brain, demonstrating the use of in vivo ^{13}C NMR to map metabolism. The key to quantifying Krebs' flux is the molecular randomization of the ^{13}C-label at the formation of the symmetrical molecule, succinate (Fig. 8). Succinate is a symmetrical compound and the carbons at the 2 and 3 positions are chemically equivalent. If 2-^{13}C-acetate is metabolized by astrocytes, then α-ketoglutarate is labeled at the three position; there is an equal chance of this label being incorporated into the two and three positions of succinate (Fig. 8). That is, what should become the C3 of succinate due to symmetry is the same as the C2 of succinate. As the four-carbon molecule continues through the Krebs' cycle, it becomes nonsymmetric at malate forming 1:1 ratio of 2-^{13}C-oxaloacetate to 3-^{13}C-oxaloacetate on the first turn of the Krebs' cycle (Fig. 8). On the second turn of the Krebs' cycle, α-ketoglutarate is equally labeled at the two and three positions (Fig. 8).

The key to determining metabolic compartmentation in the brain is the fact that 2-^{13}C-acetate is metabolized to glutamine only in glial cells, and then the glutamine is transported to the neuron (Fig. 8). Once inside the neuron, the glutamine is metabolized to glutamate and incorporated into vesicles, which in turn are secreted into the synaptic cleft once activated. In addition to glutamatergic neurons, GABAergic neurons also form GABA from astrocytic formation of glutamine. Any difference in relative abundance of the isotopomers dynamically or at steady state is due to metabolic processes in the different compartments, and therefore one can elucidate on metabolic demand and control by comparing the isotopomers between glutamine, glutamate, and GABA. That is, by using the metabolic "trick" of the scrambling of the succinate labeling and the metabolic memory encoded by the isotopomers of the these three biochemical, not only can the Krebs' flux be determined in glia (i.e., astrocytes) and neurons, but so can the relative uses and demand for the glutamine substrate for neurochemical activity. For example, if the C2-to-C3 isotope ratio of glutamine differs from glutamate or GABA, then one can make conclusions regarding regulation of metabolic coupling between these two tissue types under different conditions (113). Hassel et al. showed that in the steady state, the C3/C4 ratio in glutamine and glutamate (and the corresponding C3/C2 ratio in GABA) gives an indication of the fraction of carbon skeletons that exit the Krebs' cycle on each turn (113). Further, they state that the comparison of this ratio in GABA (C3/C2) to that in glutamate and glutamine (C3/C4) allows an assessment of the fraction of GABA derived from glutamine carbon skeletons vs. skeletons from the glutamate pool that have traversed the neuronal Krebs' cycle.

3.3.2. Quantifying Cellular Compartmentation from ^{13}C NMR Spectra

Figure 9 is a schematic representation of the two different compartments of the cell where the various serine isotopomers are formed, the cytosol and the mitochondria. To the right is a portion of a representative ^{13}C NMR spectrum of PCA extract of rat infused for 3 h with 2-^{13}C-glycine, demonstrating the various peaks corresponding to the three isotopomers. The methyl donor depends on substrate (114), but glycine is a major methyl donor in the mammalian mitochondria (115). The cytosolic methylating

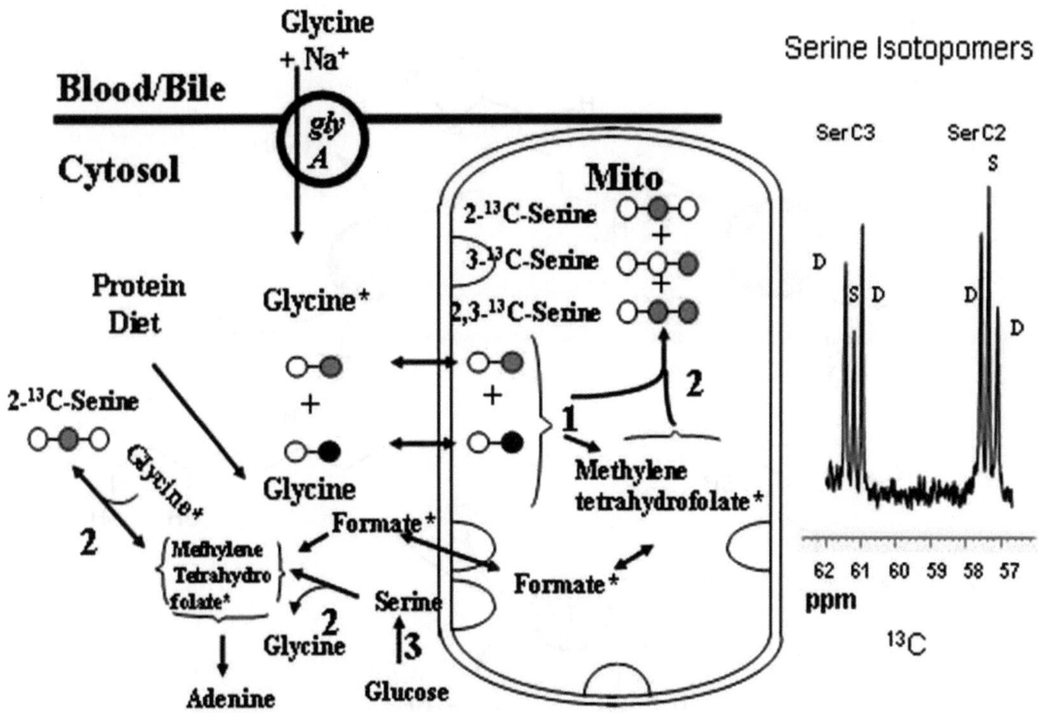

Fig. 9. Compartmentation of serine synthesis and the use of isotopomeric analysis and ^{13}C MRS to determine compartmentation biochemistry and monitor mitochondrial function.

agent, *S*-adenosylmethionine, was unlabeled in this study of anesthetized Sprague-Dawly rat (92), therefore the peak pattern at the C2 and C3 of serine should be the same; however, the singlet C2 peak representing 2-^{13}C-serine isotopomer is larger than the singlet C3 peak, representing the 3-^{13}C-serine isotopomer. The additional C2 singlet represents 20% of the total serine C2 and C3 peak area, and therefore 20 and 80% was formed in the cytosol and mitochondria, respectively (92).

Specifically, the mitochondrial matrix and the cytosol require exchange of metabolites across two mitochondrial membranes: inner and the outer. The difference in glycine metabolism in mitochondria and cytosol provides the approach to quantitatively monitor the activity of these pathways in hepatocytes from profiling of individual serine isotopomers in cellular extracts. Mitochondrial compartment contains four enzymes of the so-called *G*lycine *C*leavage *S*ystem (GCS). Four reactions facilitate decarboxylation and deamination glycine resulting in generation and transfer of CH_2 group of glycine to *T*etra*H*ydroxy*F*olate (THF), a cofactor of mitochondrial *S*erine *H*ydroxy*M*ethyl *T*ransferase (*m*SHMT), thus forming methylene-THF (Fig. 10). At next step, this methyl group from CH_2-THF transferred on another molecule of glycine,

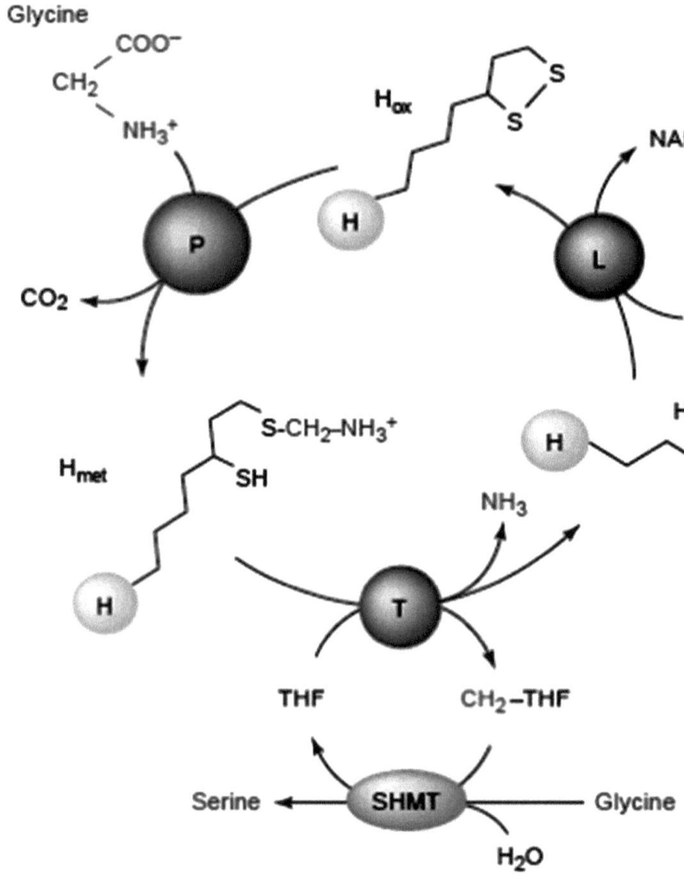

Fig. 10. Glycine cleavage system of mitochondria. P-glycine decarboxylase, T-deaminase, L-reductase, *SHMT Serine HydroxyMethyl Transferase*; *THF TetraHydroxyFolate*, CH_2-THF-methylated THF, H-pyridoxal phosphate: H_{red}, H_{ox}, and H_{met} oxidized, reduced, and methylated forms, respectively.

thus forming the molecule of serine (Fig. 10). This reaction is highly irreversible and this determines unidirectional flow of substrates in mitochondrial GCS from glycine to serine. The carbon atom of methyl group derived from glycine molecule comes from β-position (2C) and incorporated into serine as γ-carbon (3C). The absence of such system in the cytosol results in synthesis of different serine isotopomers by cytosolic SHMT from methyl groups generated using the sources different from glycine (115).

3.4. Multiple Pathway Analysis for Fluxomics

There are a few in vivo ^{13}C NMR studies measuring multiple metabolic fluxes. Jones et al. elegantly demonstrate the feasibility of relating glucose and glutamate ^{13}C-NMR multiplets to corresponding metabolic pathways of gluconeogenesis and pyruvate recycling (116). The study focuses on glucose and glutamate for several reasons with the main goals centering on human applications. Noninvasive collection of urine from human subjects is clinically advantageous and preferred over blood tissue biopsy by patients. The logic behind choosing uniformly [1,2,3-$^{13}C_3$] labeled propionate as a tracer as opposed to a single-labeled carbon is that it manifests multiplets for glucose and glutamate as opposed to singlets, resulting in additional biochemical information; also, utilizing propionate simplified quantification because it enters the Krebs cycle via a single irreversible anaplerotic pathway as opposed to multiple entries for other substrates like alanine or lactate.

The observed isotopomers derived from [1,2,3-$^{13}C_3$] propionate of glucose and glutamate combined with simple mathematical equations of the metabolic model involved was the strategy for obtaining fluxes in this work. A comparison between isolated perfused livers and livers from intact animals showed little difference in the rates (116). Accordingly, gluconeogenesis and pyruvate recycling is easily and reliably measured in a ^{13}C spectrum of blood after an oral dose of [1,2,3-$^{13}C_3$] propionate, without unknown metabolites crowding the multiplets.

4. In Vivo NMR Experimental Considerations

Some tissues have innate biological characteristics resulting in superior NMR spectra (i.e., sharper peaks resulting in better resolution and SNR) as compared to others. It is for this reason that the majority of in vivo multinuclear NMR studies have been on brain and the fewest on internal organs, particularly liver, kidney, spleen, lungs, and intestine, even though the very first ^{13}C NMR studies were on liver (117). Poor NMR spectral quality of these organs is due to high ferromagnetic load, motion, or having air–water interface. To reduce the problem of motion and iron in the blood and enhance sensitivity by the use of higher field magnets with superior NMR probes, the majority of NMR studies on internal organs have used excised tissues that can be perfused in a high-resolution NMR spectrometer (117).

4.1. Animal Handling and NMR Hardware

Animals can be anesthetized with pentobarbital of some other general anesthetic, but a volatile anesthetic such as 3% isoflurane/ nitrous oxide/oxygen and maintained with about 2% isoflurane/oxygen is preferred. Anesthetics, especially general anesthetics, decrease body temperature and animals must be placed on a heating pad to maintain body temperature during the NMR experiment. Animals typically undergo a survival surgical procedure to implant a catheter into the jugular, femoral, or tail vein through which stable-isotope-labeled amino acids can be infused. Although the label can be administered via intraperitoneal injection or gavage, the kinetics is nonsteady state and complex. The animals are anesthetized during the cannulation procedure and kept warm on a warming pad.

The chronic jugular vein cannulation procedure (118) is the most effective and common. An incision across the right side of the neck will reveal the right jugular vein which will be cannulated with polyurethane tubing. The catheter is subcutaneously routed to the back and exteriorized between the shoulder blades. The animal is fitted with a jacket/harness to hold the infusion line in place. The surgical procedure takes a trained surgeon about 20 min to complete. The catheterized animal wakes up from the anesthesia and can be free to move about its cage as the infusion line is attached to a swing arm allowing unhindered mobility. The animal recovers for a day to make sure the surgery does not affect metabolism, as alpha and beta adrenergic hormones (fight or flight hormones) are released during surgery and corticosteroid during the healing process. Once healed, the infusion line is used to deliver stable-isotope-labeled amino acids for periods up to 24 h or more.

4.2. Hardware

Besides the NMR console and magnet, the hardware for in vivo ^{13}C NMRS consists of the NMR probe and the perfusion loop for excised liver and animal infusion and monitoring system for intact animals. High-resolution probes cost in the range of \$20,000–50,000, whereas in vivo surface coils range from \$5,000 to \$10,000 and can be easily constructed with minimal experience beyond a novice education in radiofrequency engineering (119). For animal studies, knowledge of building one's own NMR probe construction is essential due to the fact that one may need to change coil geometries based on the region of interest. Perfused organ studies use a volume coil wherein the entire liver is contained within the NMR coil, and the NMR probe is designed for vertical bore magnets. For animals, typically surface coils are used to localize to the tissue of interest, and typically the NMR probe is designed for a horizontal bore magnet for rats or larger. A drawing of a perfused liver in a volume coil is shown in Fig. 11a with the various components of the perfusion loop (76). It is very important to place a bubble trap just before the media line enters the bore of the vertical bore magnet from the top. Bubbles can get trapped inside the liver and destroy spectral quality due to enormous magnetic susceptibility effects caused by the air–water interface. A picture of a surface coil used for rat studies is drawn in Fig. 11b. The surface coil is localized to liver by implanting or placing it on the right side of the rat over liver (45). Implantation of surface coils was first reported in 1986 (120), and many sophisticated surface coils such as phase-arrays (121, 122), as well as RF coils for microscopy (123) have since been developed. The reader is directed to reviews for in-depth description of RF coil design, theory, and construction (123, 124).

For the direct detection of ^{13}C, various NMR radiofrequency (RF) NMR probes designs have been used for receiving ^{13}C signal and decoupling the ^{1}H signal *d*: (1) two dual surface coils

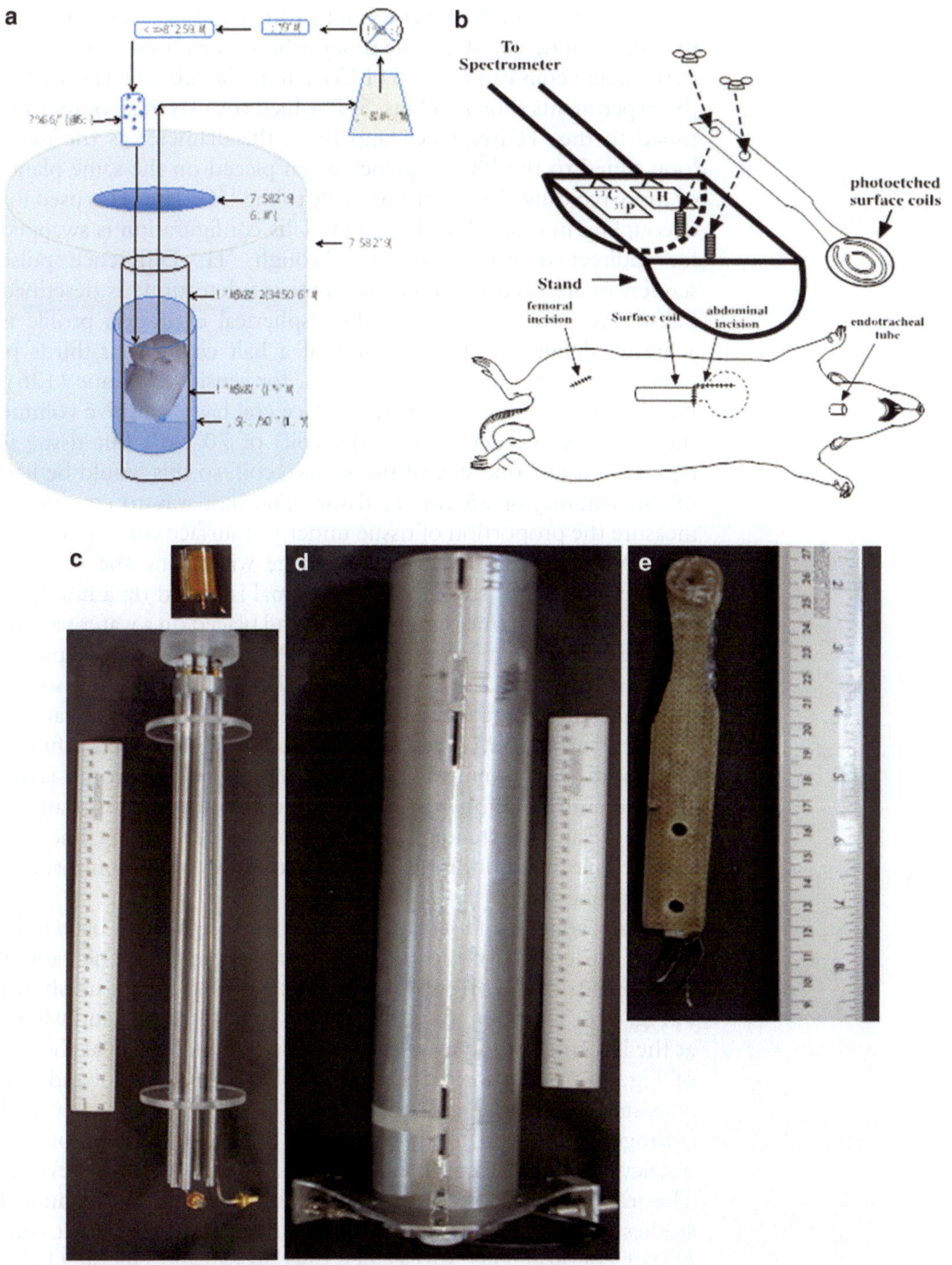

Fig. 11. NMR probes. Examples of the volume (**a**, **c**), and surface (**b**, **e**) NMR probes. The housing (**d**) is necessary to shield from RF noise. Schematic (**b**) was modified from ref. (45), from Macdonald.

in-plane (45) or orthogonal to one another (125), (2) surface coil receive/volume coil decouple designs have been used (85), or (3) two volume coils can be used (125). An implanted coil was used in the experiments shown in Figs. 5–7, which consists of an outer loop tuned to the ^{1}H frequency, and twice the diameter as the inner loop tuned to the ^{13}C frequency when placed on the same plane, or more typically placed orthogonally to the ^{13}C. The ^{1}H is used for decoupling in direct ^{13}C detection. This configuration is swapped for indirect detection of ^{13}C through ^{1}H. Difference pulse sequences are used for direct and indirect detection, as described below. As a rule of thumb, a hemispherical excitation profile is achieved defined by the function of a half circle, four-thirds pi multiplied by radius cubed ($4\pi r^3/3$), for sensitive volume (126). For example, a 6.5 cm diameter surface coil has a sensitive volume (i.e., the volume detected by the coil) of 70 cm^3, but tissue is typically on just one side of the surface coil, so this would be half of this volume, or 35 cm^3 of tissue. The best way to empirically measure the proportion of tissue under the surface coil is to obtain a ^{1}H MRI and the limits of the image will define the sensitive volume (126). The sternum of the animal is placed on a nonmagnetic transducer to measure heart rate and placed on a water bath or heating pad for temperature control. An infusion line is typically used for chronic infusion of the ^{13}C-labeled substrate, and sometimes anesthesia. Preferably, volatile anesthesia is used. The rat and attached surface NMR probe, warm pad, anesthesia and infusion lines, and heart monitoring transducer are contained on a stand and the entire assembly is inserted into the magnet. As many as five lines can be extending from the magnet, including lines for volatile anesthesia, infusion, warm water, heart rate monitor, and NMR probe (45).

Many volume and surface NMR probe designs have been published, but consist of the same primary components. The various components of a NMR probe for vertical bore magnets are shown in Fig. 11c. The volume coil sits at the top of the probe and will be at the isocenter of the magnet during operation. Shown at the top of Fig. 11c is a photoetched Helmholtz coil. A broadband coil consists of an inner coil tuned to ^{13}C Larmor frequency and orthogonally placed to an outer coil tuned to ^{1}H Larmor frequency; an indirect coil configuration has this design in reverse. The implanted surface coil used in the in vivo ^{13}C NMR animal studies of 2-^{13}C-glycine metabolism is shown in Fig. 11e. It consists of a photo-etched surface described in Fan and Higashi (127), which is attached to leads and glued to a fiberglass support coated with polyethylene spray to insulate the circuit. As mentioned above, long leads can cause spurious resonances and so twisting leads can eliminate any large loops that could create an undesired resonating inductor in the circuit. However, in this case, since the NMR surface coil was implanted, the leads needed to be long enough to attach to a circuit outside the animal. More recent studies do not implant the surface and the length of the leads is minimized and localization is achieved using the gradients (125).

4.3. Statistical Analysis of Flux Data

Data obtained in flux experiments can undergo statistical analyses using standard techniques such as Student's t-test or ANOVA, depending on the experimental design. The simplest type of statistical problem is when only one experimental measure, such as metabolite concentration or its flux, is collected in a number of experiments under two different naturally occurring or experimentally induced conditions. In Table 1, the fluxes were minimal and Student's t-test was sufficient for use. However, as the datasets get large and multiple fluxes are compared, ANOVA and other multivariate statistical analyses will need to be applied.

5. Mathematical Models: Metabolic Flux Balance (MFA) and Metabolic Control Analysis (MCA)

5.1. Metabolic Flux Balance Analysis and Metabolic Control Analysis

Mathematical modeling and computational analysis in conjunction with experimental studies can enhance the understanding of metabolic systems greatly (128). Due to various experimental limitations in finding all the metabolic fluxes, to construct a fluxome of a complex metabolic system is very difficult if not impossible. Modeling biological data can be predictive given less, little, or no empirical data or, using empirical NMR-derived fluxomic data using known metabolic pathways is defined as "discrete" models. Using the stoichiometric properties of reactions involved, one can calculate unknown fluxes in metabolic systems, knowing a few of the fluxes by using experimental methods such as ^{13}C NMR. One can use metabolic flux balance analysis (FBA) for this purpose (129, 130). In FBA, one is interested in calculating the intracellular steady state fluxes using a stoichiometric model and applying mass balances around those fluxes. Steady state is assumed to occur in the time scales involved in such experiments, in most biological systems (131). Measured fluxes usually are the uptake rates of substrates and secretion rates of metabolites. MFA assumes reaction stoichiometry, but there is no need to know the kinetic properties of any enzymes involved. How these steady state fluxes and metabolite concentrations are influenced by enzyme properties or other parameters in the system can be understood using a mathematical technique called MCA (131, 132). MCA helps us to predict the metabolic effects of perturbations on the system and tells us how metabolic system properties are controlled and shared among different enzymes in the pathway. One important aspect of biochemical systems is that the control is distributed over the entire system.

5.2. Flux Balance Analysis

One can write the rate equations for metabolic concentrations using simple mass balance; the rate of change of a metabolite at a specific time is equal to the net difference of incoming fluxes and outgoing fluxes (131). Consider a metabolic network with m metabolites and r reactions. We can write the rate of change of the metabolite concentration as:

$$\frac{\mathrm{d}x_i}{\mathrm{d}t} = \sum_{j=1}^{n} S_{ij} v_j, \quad i = 1, \ldots, m \quad \text{and} \quad j = 1, \ldots, r \tag{9}$$

Here x_i is the concentration of the ith metabolite, S_{ij} is the ijth element of the stoichiometric matrix, and v_j is the flux through reaction j. In matrix form, we can write it as:

$$\frac{\mathrm{d}x}{\mathrm{d}t} = Sv \tag{10}$$

Here, the rate v is a function of metabolite concentrations x, kinetic parameters p, and time $t : v = v(x, p, t)$. v is in general a nonlinear function. At steady state, $\mathrm{d}x/\mathrm{d}t = 0$, and hence $Sv = 0$.

If we know a few steady state fluxes, we can write the above equation as a sum of two parts, containing the k known fluxes, v_k, and the u unknown fluxes v_u.

$$S_\mathrm{u} v_\mathrm{u} = -S_\mathrm{k} v_\mathrm{k} \equiv -b \tag{11}$$

Therefore, the unknown fluxes are given by: $v_\mathrm{u} = -S_\mathrm{u}^{-1} b$

When S_u is a square matrix and all the rows are linearly independent, one can calculate the inverse of S_u, S_u^{-1}. Using that one can easily calculate the unknown fluxes by Gaussian elimination.

However, in most of the real situations, S_u is not a square matrix and there will be linear dependencies between different rows. In general, number of reactions r will be more than the number of metabolites, m. Here are some of the different situations that can arise.

- When the rank of S_u is less than u, the system is underdetermined. In such cases, one can use constraints based on biological reasoning and try to find the unknown fluxes using linear optimization and other methods.
- When rank of S_u is equal to u, it is a determined system.
- When rank of $S_\mathrm{u} < m$, we have a redundant system. In such cases, one can still use the above equation to find the unknown fluxes using the generalized inverse of S_u. Generalized inverse provides a least square solution to this overdetermined system. In such systems, some of the rows are linearly dependent and give rise to redundancies. These redundancies can be utilized to estimate errors in the flux values.
- When rank of $S_\mathrm{u} = u = m$, S_u is a square matrix and one can use simple linear algebra, as mentioned above to find the unknown fluxes.

5.3. Metabolic Control Analysis

MCA deals with understanding the effects of changes in the parameters such as enzyme concentrations, temperature, pH, etc., on the metabolic system quantities such as flux or metabolite concentrations (131, 132). Basically, it deals with estimating the sensitivity of a metabolic network function to system parameters. Sensitivity of metabolic flux and concentrations on the enzyme activities or other parameters are characterized by control coefficients.

MCA was introduced to biochemical systems in the 1970s by Kacser and Burns (133) and Heinrich and Rapoport (134, 135). The theory of MCA is given in Chap. 9. Below is an example of MCA using results obtained using in vivo ^{13}C NMR spectral data.

5.4. Example of an MCA NMR Experiment

Jucker et al. (136) used MCA to calculate the distributed control of insulin-stimulated skeletal muscle glucose disposal in awake rats. Due to the limitations of NMR experiments, a top-down approach to MCA where the control is defined over a few metabolic components each consisting of a number of enzymes was used, instead of a bottom-up approach where all the individual components are separately measured. Control of glucose disposal was considered to be distributed between (1) glucose transport through insulin-stimulated GLUT-4 and phosphorylation via hexokinase; (2) glycogen synthesis consisting of phosphoglucomutase, UDP-glucose pyrophosphorylase, and glycogen synthesis enzymes; and (3) glycolysis consisting of numerous enzymes including phosphofructokinase and pyruvate kinase in skeletal muscle.

Using the summation theorem, connectivity theorem, and branch point theorem (132, 137) involving the fluxes of glycolysis, glycogen synthesis, and glucose disposal, and elasticity coefficients with respect to G-6-P concentrations, they calculated the three flux control coefficients. Most of the control of glucose disposal during hyperinsulinemia was determined to be at the glucose transport/phosphorylation step (0.55 ± 0.10) and the rest distributed between glycogen synthesis (0.30 ± 0.06) and glycolysis (0.15 ± 0.02).

For this calculation, three separate hyperinsulinemic infusion protocols were used:

1. Protocol 1: Euglycemic (~6 mM)-hyperinsulinemic (10 mU/kg/min)
2. Protocol 2: Hyperglycemic (~11 mM)-hyperinsulinemic (10 mU/kg/min) clamp with somatostatin
3. Protocol 3: Euglycemic (~6 mM)-hyperinsulinemic (10 mU/kg/min)-lipid/heparin clamp

In this study, [1-^{13}C]glucose was administered in all these protocols for a 3-h period, during which its incorporation into [1-^{13}C]-glycogen, [3-^{13}C]-lactate, and [3-^{13}C]-alanine was determined in the hindlimb of awake rats via ^{13}C-NMR. Glucose-6-phosphate was measured using in vivo ^{31}P-NMR. The three different protocols differentially modulate both the fluxes and intramuscular glucose-6-phosphate (G-6-P) concentrations so that they could calculate the elasticities. Blood samples were taken at different time points to measure the plasma glucose and lactate concentrations. Glycogen synthesis rates were calculated using the individual time point glycogen concentrations. Using the label incorporation into lactate and alanine, the glycolytic flux was calculated. ADP, ADP, Mg^{2+}, pH, and Pi were measured using in vivo ^{31}P-NMR and were constant, in all the three protocols. Such a large number of measurements are essential because the system comprises several intersecting pathways. It is difficult to obtain accurate flux measurements under these conditions, especially with singe time point analyses. Furthermore, the influence of branch points makes the MCA analysis more complex, though rigorous matrix approaches have been developed (see Chap. 9). A key to all MCA models is the assumptions of the summation theorem. In many cases, where multiple experimental treatments are applied, this is false and calculated fluxes may be incorrect. Nevertheless, the study indicates that glycolysis itself contributes little control over the utilization of glucose under insulin stimulation.

5.5. Software for the Analysis of Metabolic Systems

There are several software packages available to do metabolic FBA and MCA. Many of them have both the capabilities and can be used to model and to simulate biochemical systems also. Here we mention a few of them, which are free for academic use.

1. FluxAnalyzer (http://www.mpi-magdeburg.mpg.de/projects/fluxanalyzer) (138): FluxAnalyzer is a Matlab package for integrated pathway and flux analysis with graphical user interface. This can be used for different types of stoichiometric network analysis including FBA.
2. MetaFluxNet (http://mbel.kaist.ac.kr/mfn) (9): MetaFluxNet is a software package for quantitatively and interactively analyzing metabolic fluxes.
3. COPASI (http://www.copasi.org) (139): COPASI is a software application for simulation and analysis of biochemical networks. Functionality of COPASI includes MFA and MCA along with several other biochemical modeling and analysis tools, with a graphical user interface.

6. Novel Technology for Fluxomics: Dynamic Nuclear Polarization

It is well known that ^{13}C NMRS (as well as other nuclei) has been limited in its ability to characterize metabolic states due to its low sensitivity. This low sensitivity is a result of the low natural abundance of ^{13}C (1.1%) in addition to the low gyromagnetic ratio of carbon (6.728284×10^{7} rad/T s). These characteristics reduce the overall sensitivity of ^{13}C nearly four orders of magnitude in comparison to ^{1}H NMR (6,400 fold without NOE or INEPT, 1,600 fold if include INEPT—cf. Chap. 6) and even more impressively for ^{15}N (up to 270,000 fold). Traditionally, the low nuclear polarization and low abundance were compensated by high concentrations of sample as well as the introduction of ^{13}C-enriched substrates. Depending on the nucleus, these direct detection methods require hours to days to record spectra with sufficient signal-to-noise for analysis.

With this difficulty in mind, a number of techniques have been proposed to increase the polarization of nuclear spins to overcome their low gyromagnetic ratios. In addition to enrichment, indirect detection methods have been widely practiced, but these require a convenient scalar coupled proton (cf. Chap. 6). Newer methods that provide a much greater sensitivity enhancement have recently been developed. These methods of hyperpolarization include: *para*-hydrogen-induced polarization (PHIP) (140), optical pumping (141), and DNP (142, 143). Each of these methods has the potential to generate 100% nonthermal polarization of the chosen ½ spin nucleus. PHIP, also known as PASADENA (144, 145) and ALTADENA (146), relies on the introduction of a *para*-hydrogen substrate through catalytic hydrogenation (146). Though this method has been shown to be successful (147), it is only applicable to reactions involving substrates with double and triple bonds. Optical pumping utilizes circularly polarized laser light and has been successfully applied to the hyperpolarization of ^{3}He and ^{129}Xe (141). This method is restricted to a subset of the noble gases and has limited application to the study of metabolism. The final method, DNP, is based on the polarization of nuclear spins in an amorphous solid state at ~1 K through coupling of the nuclear spins and unpaired electrons via an organic-free radical. Recent advances in the field of low temperature physics, electronic paramagnetic resonance (EPR), and NMR have provided for the adaptation of the DNP technique, described as early as the 1950s (148), to metabolically appreciable systems (149–151). Due to its applicability, the purpose of this section is to describe this emerging technique of hyperpolarization and its application to the investigation of metabolic systems.

6.1. DNP Physics: The Solid State Effect and Hyperpolarization

Conceptually, what we consider DNP is an extension of what has been previously described as the "solid state effect" (148). In the early 1950s, Overhauser postulated that an NMR signal could be increased as a result of the interaction between a nucleus and the electrons of a metal (152). This principle was later applied to nonmetals by Abragam (153), and in 1974 (154), demonstrated

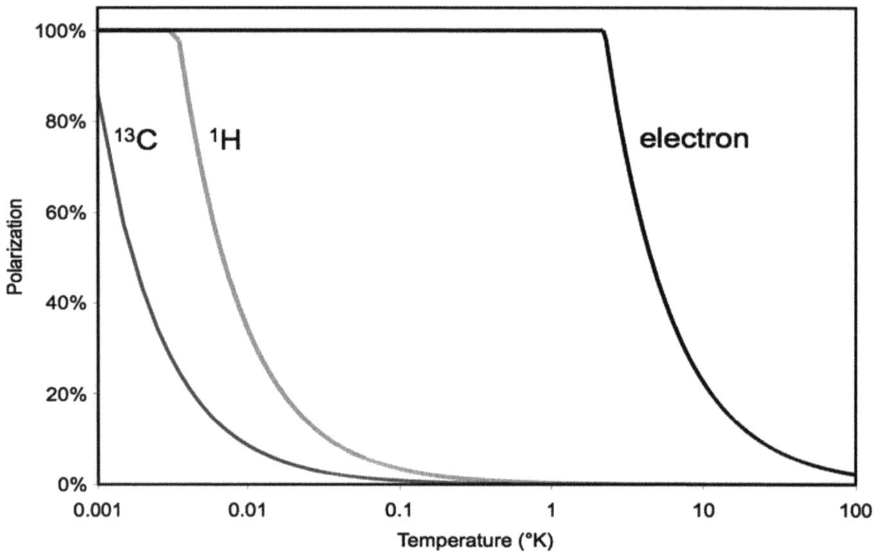

Fig. 12. Fraction polarization for different spins. Plot of the percent polarization as a function of time for each indicated spin. These were calculated using (12) at a magnetic field strength of 3.35 T.

that through thermal contact between nuclear and electronic spins, DNP can be produced (154).

To investigate the underlying physics of the solid state effect, first consider a set of nuclear spins I embedded in a solid containing a small percentage of paramagnetic impurities with spins S. These spins are of ½ and have Larmor frequencies ω_I and ω_S. For a given spin, the spin density where all magnetization is along the z-axis corresponds to the equilibrium among states governed by the Boltzmann distribution. A spin $I = \frac{1}{2}$ can be characterized by two states $|\alpha\rangle$ and $|\beta\rangle$. The probability of finding a spin in each of the states is then proportional to (12):

$$P_\alpha \propto e^{(-E_\alpha/kT)} \approx 1 - \frac{E_\alpha}{kT}, \quad E_\alpha = \frac{-\hbar\gamma_I B_0}{2} \tag{12a}$$

$$P_\beta \propto e^{(-E_\beta/kT)} \approx 1 - \frac{E_\beta}{kT}, \quad E_\beta = \frac{\hbar\gamma_I B_0}{2} \tag{12b}$$

The overall spin polarization of this system is the population difference between the $|\alpha\rangle$ and $|\beta\rangle$ states. This population difference or percent polarization is demonstrated in Fig. 12 for electron, proton, and carbon spins with respect to temperature.

At low temperatures (on the order of 1 K) in a strong magnetic field, the electron polarization is near unity while other nuclei are not, yielding a distribution of uniformly oriented spins S and disoriented spins I (Fig. 13). These spins I and S are coupled through dipolar interactions and this permits the simultaneous reversal of these spins in the same direction (producing two "up" spins) or opposite directions (producing one spin "up" and one spin "down") if the spins

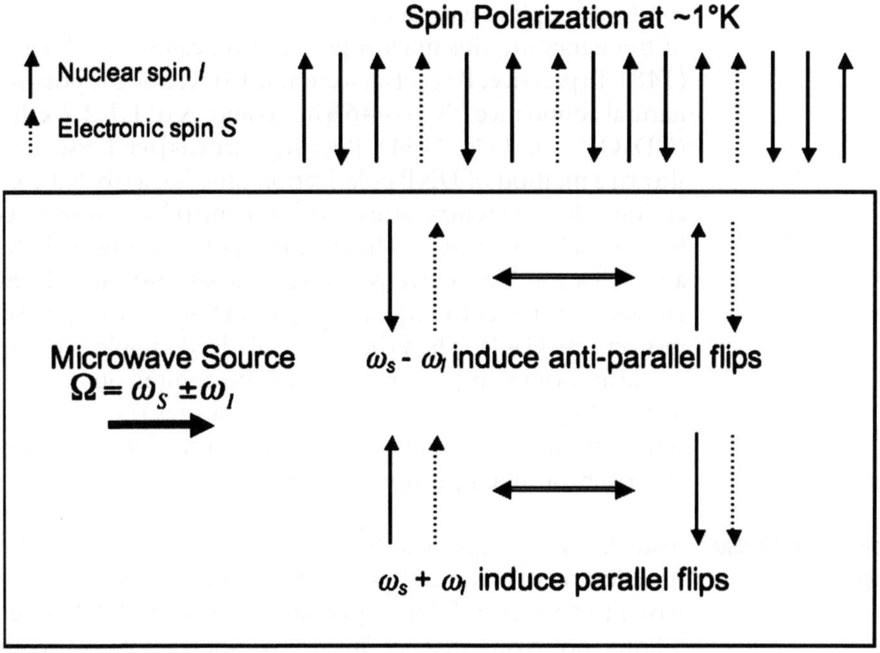

Fig. 13. A graphical representation of spin polarization of the nuclear spin *I* and electron spin *S*.

were originally antiparallel. These spin "flips," which require energy $h(\omega_S \pm \omega_I)$ to occur, are analogous to the spin–lattice relaxation mechanism (T_1 spin relaxation). At low temperatures, the time of this "flip" process for the target nucleus *I* is on the order of 10^3 s, while it is 10^{-3} s for a lone electron spin *S*, as a result of its coupling to the lattice. By providing energy via a laser with frequency $\Omega = \omega_S \pm \omega_I$, these flips can be induced and because the order of electron relaxation is much faster than that of the target nucleus, the spins *S* will bring all of the spins *I* to their "up" position. It has been shown (Abragam 1978) that the case of antiparallel flips is impossible leading to the association of spin change with $\Omega = \omega_S + \omega_I$. When all of the *I* spins are in their "up" position, the target material can be deemed hyperpolarized.

It follows that for a low electronic concentration; each spin *S* must "flip" many nuclear spins. For this to occur, it has been shown that the following condition is required (148):

$$f = \left(\frac{N_I}{T_n}\right)\left(\frac{N_S}{T_e}\right)^{-1} \ll 1$$

where N_I and N_S are the number of respective spins and T_n and T_e are the respective longitudinal relaxation times. With this dipolar coupling as the only means of relaxation, it is assumed that the polarization P_n of the nuclei would reach unity (i.e., that of the electron spins). Due to other mechanisms, such as leakage relaxation as a result of coupling with another species or saturation by microwaves of frequency ω_S, this nuclear polarization can be much less than P_e (148). In practice, Boer et al. were able to increase the polarization of natural abundance ^{13}C to ~46% in a complex of 1,1,2,2-ethanediol-$(CD_2OH)_2$ and Cr^V (154). Recently, Ardenkjaer-Larsen et al. have shown a method of DNP polarization utilizing a labeled compound at liquid helium temperatures with the introduction of an organic-free radical. These studies have shown polarizations of 37% for ^{13}C and 7.8% for ^{15}N, corresponding to a 44,400- and 23,500-fold enhancement over the equilibrium room temperature polarizations, respectively (143), when the hyperpolarized sample is brought to a liquid at room temperature. It should be pointed out, and as shown in Fig. 12, that at liquid helium temperatures (i.e., 1 K) there is a significant increase equilibrium polarization of approximately 300-fold over room temperature (310 K).

6.2. Hardware and Pulse Sequences

Aside from the traditional NMR spectrometer, DNP-NMR requires the addition of a unit composed of multiple components collectively termed a "polarizer." The key components of this DNP system are as follows: polarizing magnet, microwave source, variable temperature insert (VTI), sample holder, dissolution system, control electronics, and solid-state NMR monitor (polarimeter). These elements work in concert to take a sample from its native spin polarization state at room temperature to a highly polarized state at room temperature by way of polarization at liquid helium temperatures.

Figure 14 demonstrates a graphical representation of the polarizer and an adjoining high-field magnet. The method described here is analogous to the method described by Ardenkjaer-Larsen et al. (143) though there are other methods of generating DNP (140, 144). A concentrated mixture of ^{13}C-labeled substrate is mixed with an organic-free radical and placed inside of the sample holder. This sample holder is then lowered into the VTI to the center of the magnet. The sample chamber is filled with liquid helium from the magnet dewar and vacuum pumped to a vapor pressure of ~0.8 mbar, resulting in a temperature of ~1.2 K. The sample is then irradiated for typically 60 min at the microwave frequency associated with the free radical (on the order of 94 GHz). As the electron spins polarize the nuclear spins, the polarimeter monitors the percent polarization. Once the solid-state sample has reached maximum polarization, it is mixed with a super-heated buffer (450 K, 10 bar) through the dissolution system. This process takes less than 2–3 s and brings the sample to room temperature while still preserving the low-temperature nuclear polarization (143). The sample is then injected into the medium of interest and observed in a conventional MRI or NMR spectrometer. Control electronics allow for this process of dissolution and injection to be on the order

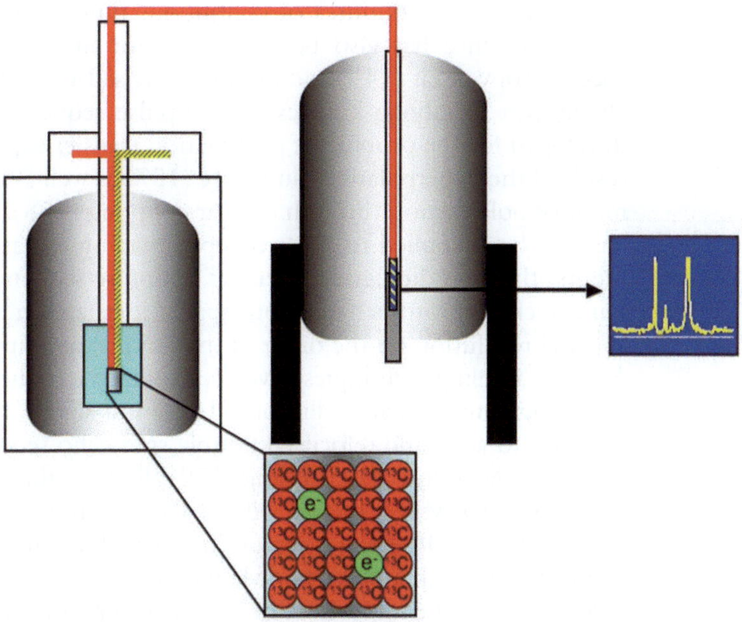

Fig. 14. Schematic of the DNP polarizer/NMR system. DNP (*left*) and high-field NMR system (*center*). The *red line* indicates the flow of the sample after hyperpolarization. The *yellow line* represents the microwave source and its irradiation of the sample chamber. The sample chamber houses the amorphous solid at ~1.2 K. After polarization, the sample is observed in the NMR spectrometer. After exposure to an RF signal at frequency $\Omega = \omega_S \pm \omega_I$, the induced flips are shown.

of seconds. At physiological temperatures, the T_1 value of pyruvate carboxyl carbon is the order 40 s, which implies that the initial polarization in the animal is very close to that at the end of the polarization in the microwave polarizer. The effective experimental time available is around $5T_1$ or ca. 200 s, when the sensitivity has decreased to <1% of its initial value (and see below). Observed magnetization changes can be corrected for the exponential magnetization loss due to relaxation.

Due to the limited lifetime of the substrate polarization, which is proportional to the T_1 relaxation, fast pulse sequences must be implemented in vivo and ex vivo to capture the real-time substrate metabolism. For both ex vivo spectroscopy and in vivo single voxel spectroscopic imaging, the task is fairly simple. Generally, a standard direct detected one-dimensional carbon sequence is used with a very small flip angle (on the order of 5–10°) for a single scan, and by using a low flip angle, the bulk polarization is preserved in the I_z vector. A 10° flip angle preserves 98% of the magnetization along z, and the x component is 17% of the equilibrium value. This allows for multiple scans to be taken as the substrate is metabolized. Recent studies have shown the effectiveness of small flip angles in hyperpolarized tissue culture experiments, with ^{13}C signals lasting for minutes of continuous pulses (50, 151, 155). This procedure has also been adapted for in vivo single voxel spectroscopy in rat (149) and mouse models (147, 156) to explore changes in metabolic kinetics. Other pulse sequences have been developed for the probing of polarization transfer experiments as a result of the hyperpolarized substrate (157) as well as the measurement of polarization through dipolar coupling (158). DNP-NMR has also been applied to spectroscopic imaging (all animal experiments) through the development of fast pulse sequences and sampling techniques to achieve both spatial localization and selective spectral resolution on the order of the DNP experiment. Different *k*-space sampling techniques have been utilized to reduce scan time, including centric (150), ellipsoid (159), and spiral (160). This in addition to adiabatic refocused double spin echo sequences (171) and echo planar fly back encoding (150) allow for the acquisition of a $8 \times 8 \times 16$ MRSI matrix with 0.135 cc spatial resolution in under 14 s (150). Least squares chemical shift imaging has also been applied, with a priori knowledge of resonances of interest, to further reduce the number of necessary data points (159).

6.3. Determination of Flux by DNP

There are many applications of DNP for the study of in vivo processes and mechanisms. A recent advancement is the ability to determine flux, through the real-time metabolism of hyperpolarized substrates. This developing technology has been applied to the study of cell slurries (50), perfused organ (151), and cell bioreactor systems (155). The purpose of these studies has been to create a viable and sustained system where hyperpolarized substrates can be introduced. Monitoring of hyperpolarized substrates over time can then produce an assessment of the dynamic net flux at the time of injection.

Many studies have shown the relationship between tumor metabolism and increased aerobic glycolysis, which has been called the Warburg effect after the original discoveries of Otto Warburg in the 1920s (17). DNP ^{13}C NMR allows for spectroscopy on the order of real-time metabolic reaction kinetics and thus visualization of the kinetics associated with fast reactions, such as glycolysis. To date, $^{13}C_1$-pyruvate has been the only tracer successfully applied to the study of in vivo hyperpolarized kinetics in order to provide a net flux measurement.

This method that determines flux by DNP and hyperpolarized pyruvate has only been performed in a perfused cell bioreactor model, and not in animals or perfused organs. A bioreactor similar to that described by Gamcsik et al. (103), but using alginate encapsulated cells (161), was used. As has been previously discussed, ^{31}P measurements over time can be utilized as a method to monitor cell health and determine cell viability. A recent study of rat hepatoma cell (JM1) encapsulates perfused in a 3D NMR compatible bioreactor (155) and demonstrates the use of this

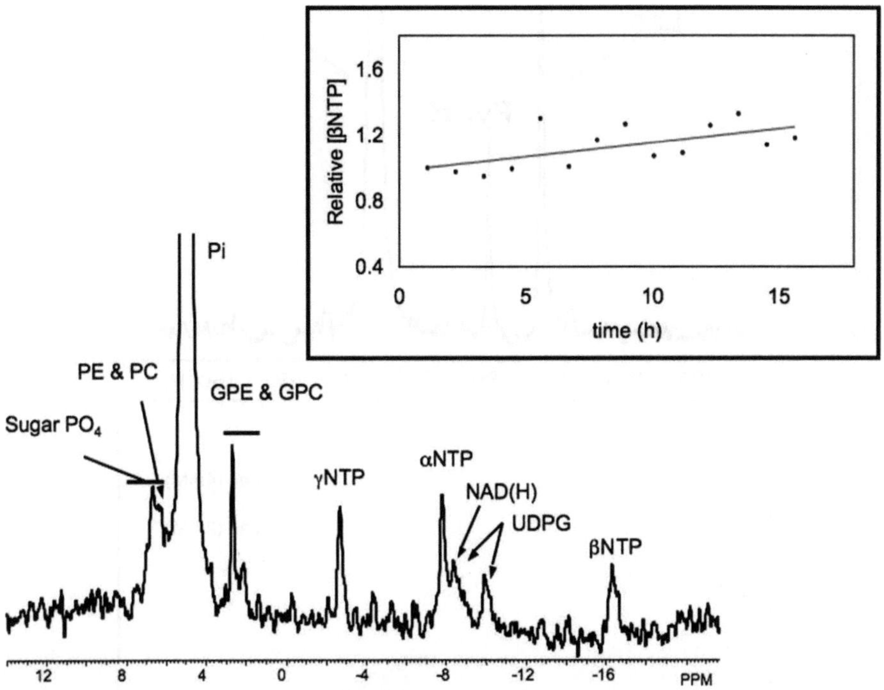

Fig. 15. Representative ^{31}P spectrum of JM1 encapsulated cells after 9 h of perfusion. Peaks corresponding to NTPs demonstrate cell health. The above time course reaffirms the extended cell health over time. Modified from ref. (169).

monitoring and its relationship to DNP. In this study, JM1 cells were monitored using ^{31}P (Fig. 16) to assess cell health and growth. A typical ^{31}P spectrum at 9 h of perfusion shows NTP resonances which imply cells are producing ATP. Increases in these resonances over time demonstrate the growth of these cells (Fig. 15, inset).

After developing a sustainable system, these are then probed using hyperpolarized 1-^{13}C-pyruvate. Figure 16 demonstrates the labeled lactate produced as a result of infusion of hyperpolarized pyruvate. A representative spectrum at 60 s postinjection of 2 mM 1-^{13}C-pyruvate shows a lactate resonance with relatively high signal-to-noise. Time course data of lactate production after injection of 2 and 4 mM hyperpolarized pyruvate demonstrate that these concentrations are below enzyme saturation on the order of the experimental time scale, since there is an increase (i.e., doubling of area under the curve) with a doubling of 1-^{13}C-pyruvate concentration. Taking this data one step further, one can fit the conversion of pyruvate to lactate using a simple two-state model of lactate dehydrogenase (162). This was presented for this study on sequential days of injection of 2 mM pyruvate, as shown in Fig. 17. Though there is a doubling of the apparent rate (k_{app}), when normalized for a doubling of the cell concentration as a result of cell growth (Fig. 15, inset) the flux (V_{app}) is unchanged. This use of

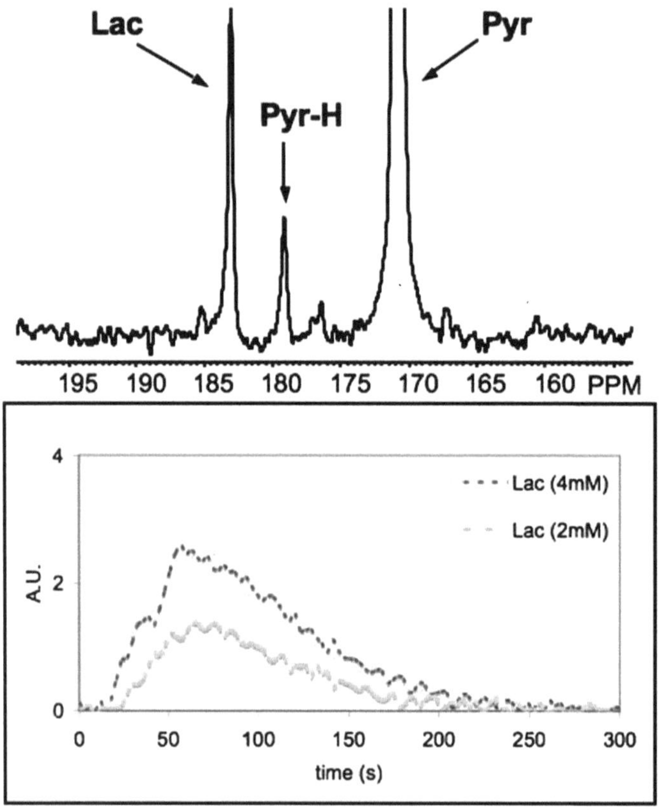

Fig. 16. Representative ^{13}C DNP time courses of JM1 cells. ^{13}C resonances of the carboxylates of pyruvate, lactate, and pyruvate hydrate in JM1 cell encapsulates (*top*). The time course demonstrates the kinetics of pyruvate metabolism (*bottom*). Modified from ref. (169).

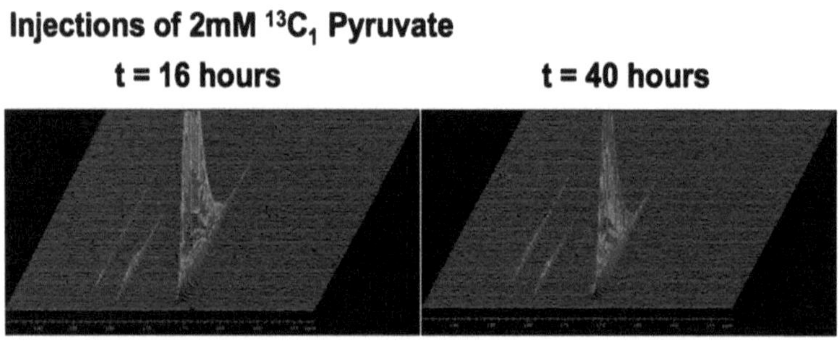

	t = 16 hours	t = 40 hours
max(Lac)/max(pyr)	0.028	0.056
bNTP/P_i	0.059	0.099
k_{app}	0.00077 s^{-1}	0.0015 s^{-1}
V_{app}	11.8 nmols/s/10^8 cells	12.0 nmols/s/10^8 cells

Fig. 17. Stacked plot of the ^{13}C NMR DNP spectra. *Top*, spectra from Fig. 15 bottom the resulting fitted kinetic parameters. Modified from ref. (169).

simple kinetic modeling in conjunction with a reproducible system, the NMR-compatible perfusion system, allows for the application of DNP and net flux to the characterization of systems and the further understanding of changes in metabolism. These studies demonstrate the first applications of hyperpolarized ^{13}C NMR by the DNP in a viable cell culture system and pave the way for the application of flux determination to both animal and potentially human studies. However, this is a single flux measurement and the concentration of substrate is higher so that the steady state is perturbed, but in a similar manner as Michaelis-Menten constants (K_m) are generated so can this be performed in vivo (162). In order to measure multiple flux rates, liver cells with a normal metabolism, or intact animals, multiple hyperpolarized substrates might be used in the future.

7. Translation ^{13}C NMR Fluxomics to Humans

The fluxomic application of in vivo ^{13}C NMRS in humans has been demonstrated using biofluids and analysis of multiple metabolic processes such as gluconeogenesis, anaplerosis, and pyruvate recycling (75). This patented method uses the ^{13}C NMR spectra of the hepatic metabolism of [U-^{13}C]-propionate to measure the rates of these metabolic processes and includes a more recent ingenious use of isotope labels and analysis of glucose in human serum (172). Uniformly labeled propionate was selected to ensure that the ^{13}C NMR spectra would contain multiplets to address cases where the ^{13}C enrichment of metabolic products is low (163). Some technical issues relating to human experimentation are provided in Chap. 3.

Specific metabolite spectra measured in this method include glucose, glutamate, glucuronide, and phenylacetylglutamate. The method presents simple equations that relate these measurements to the relative fluxes through anaplerosis, gluconeogenesis, and oxaloacetate-pyruvate recycling. However, the method is applicable to any pathway that intersects the citric acid cycle of the liver.

In humans, blood and urine samples were collected after ingesting [1,2,3-^{13}C]-propionate, phenylacetate, and acetaminophen to respectively produce the ^{13}C NMR spectrum from glucose and glucuronide or phenylacetylglutamine. The ^{13}C-^{13}C spin-coupled multiplets of gluconate C2, phenylacetylglutamine C2, and β-D-glucuronate C5 were then utilized to provide estimates of net gluconeogenic flux, OAA-pyruvate recycling, and anaplerotic inflow into oxaloacetate.

The use of stable isotopes has been demonstrated for metabolic functions in humans using biofluid analysis, but most rely on mass spectroscopy analysis. For example, a measurement of cytochrome (CYP) P450 activity was developed using ^{14}C-erythromycin (164).

In this study, gas chromatography-selective ion mass spectrometry (GC-MS) was utilized to measure the amount of a common sedative, midazolam, in plasma as a surrogate measure of the rate of CYP P450 activity. It is known that the cytochrome P450 CYP3A enzymes are the major contributors to midazolam metabolism (165) and specifically CYP3A4 is the dominant isozymes of CYP3A that resides in the liver (166). Therefore, this relationship was used to predict the clearance of midazolam by measuring the activity of a specific enzyme, CYP3A4. This enzyme solely catalyzes the *N*-demethylation of [^{14}C-*N*-methyl]erythromycin in liver (167), forming formaldehyde and ultimately $^{14}CO_2$ which is quantified in the breath by GC-MS (168). Although this measures just a single reaction, one could combine this breath test with the fluxomic urine analysis-patented fluxomic method to determine additional metabolic pathways.

8. Conclusions and Future Directions

Fluxomics is in its infancy, and with the advent of isotopomeric analysis of human biofluids, a routine yet robust metabolic diagnostic could be translated to humans. However, at present only a handful of metabolic pathways have simultaneously been determined by both static or dynamic methods. In general, dynamic methods are hindered by a lack of temporal resolution required for accurate description of isotopic incorporation and accurate derivation of kinetic parameter from the time course. This is due to the inherent lack of sensitivity of NMRS. This has been overcome by the introduction of DNP technology, which increases ^{13}C NMR sensitivity four orders of magnitude. Static measurements have the best possibility of translating to humans, since these are convenient and require minimal effort and do not require expensive imaging equipment. Finally, nonsteady state is the typical state of most organisms, in a state of maintaining homeostasis at the expense of increasing flux through metabolic pathways. Simpler analytical models of nonsteady state isotopomeric datasets are required in the future to obtain mass balance in biosystems.

Acknowledgments

Funding for the studies was provided by NIH grants GM075941-01, CA114365-01A1, P30ES10126, and RR-000046.

Glossary

Allosteric modification	Usually refers to an enzyme whose activity is modified by the presence of a ligand that binds reversibly to a site other than the active site. In the context of multisite enzyme, such allosteric effectors change the state of the enzyme to enhance or diminish substrate affinity and/or turnover number.
Cellular compartmentation	In cell biology comprise all closed parts within a cell whose lumen is usually surrounded by a single or double lipid layer membrane. Most organelles are compartments like mitochondria, chloroplasts (in photosynthetic organisms), peroxisomes, lysosomes, the endoplasmic reticulum, the cell nucleus, or the Golgi apparatus. Smaller elements like vesicles, and sometimes even microtubules can also be counted as compartments. In general, there are three main cellular compartments, they are: (1) The nuclear compartment comprising the nucleus; (2) The intercisternal space which comprises the space between the membranes of the endoplasmic reticulum (which is continuous with the nuclear envelope); and (3) The cytosol. Metabolically, the mitochondria comprise a very important compartment, even though they are by volume fraction small (from Wikipedia).
Curve fitting	Finding a curve, which matches a series of data points and possibly other constraints. This section is an introduction to both interpolation (where an exact fit to constraints is expected) and regression analysis. Both are sometimes used for extrapolation. Regression analysis allows for an approximate fit by minimizing the difference between the data points and the curve (from Wikipedia).

Dynamic flux measurement method	The measurement of isotope steady state being reached by a time series measure. In the context of this chapter, it is the serial measurement of an NMR-observable tracer, such as ^{13}C, ^{15}N, ^{19}F, ^{3}H, or ^{2}H, and its incorporation into a metabolite.
Dynamic nuclear polarization (DNP)	Transfer of polarization from electrons to nuclei, which occurs in a magnetic field, close to absolute zero. This is done by inducing transitions, via oscillating microwave RF pulses, between the allowed energy states of the electrons and nuclei, thus transferring polarization from the electrons to the nuclei. This results in more nuclei aligned with the magnetic field, thus resulting in enhancements of the signal-to-noise on the order of several magnitudes.
Flux	The net rate or the difference between the (unidirectional) rates of the forward and reverse reactions.
Helmholtz NMR coil	A volume coil design for an NMR radiofrequency probe consisting of two connecting loops spanning 120° and separated by 60°.
In vivo fluxomics	The measuring of multiple fluxes in live biosystems using noninvasive analytical instrumentation.
Isotope tracer	Use of isotopically labeled compounds administered at levels that do not affect steady state and can be used to trace flow of atoms through reaction networks.
Isotopic balance	The distribution of a single or multiple isotopes within metabolites of a biosystem.
Mass balance	An application of conservation of mass to the analysis of physical systems. By accounting for material entering and leaving a system, mass flows can be identified. The exact conservation law used in the analysis of the system depends on the context of the problem, but all revolve around mass conservation, i.e., that matter cannot

	disappear or be created spontaneously (from Wikipedia).
Metabolic control analysis	A method for modeling metabolism in which equations are used to describe metabolite concentration and flux, signaling pathways, and genetic pathways.
Metabolic flux analysis (MFA)	An analysis where metabolites are measured such that the amount of metabolite formation can be measured over a given period of time. This allows for the calculation of the rate of formation, or flux, of a metabolite.
Multiple component curve-fit	The mathematical curve fitting of residuals in a time series dataset whereby the various components represent time constants for multiple rates. In the context of this chapter, this relates to metabolite turnover rate within the biosystem.
Net flux	Net flux is sometimes used to define the total flux through a metabolic pathway as some of the individual fluxes can be in reverse of the net flux direction for the entire metabolic pathway.
Non-Steady State	
Nonallosteric modification	This is usually a description of covalent modification of proteins (cf. post-translational modification) such as phosphorylation that changes the properties of the target protein, e.g., recognition in signal transduction pathways or in chromatin remodeling.
Pool	Like a compartment, a *pool* is completely defined by the model describing the system. A pool can contain all the members of a particular chemical species for instance, even if they are in several different compartments. A pool can also describe those molecules in a particular physical environment, such as pyruvate in plasma, mitochondria, or cytosol. It can also be a purely theoretical physical space; when a tracer is infused into the bloodstream of an intact animal, the volume of its initial distribution (in plasma, intracellular space, etc.) is thought to describe its pool of entry (20).

Pseudosteady state	A situation in which all state variables remain effectively constant, at least on the macroscopic scale (from Wikipedia).
Quality factor	A dimensionless parameter describing the efficiency of a transceiver, and in context to this chapter, specifically the efficiency of an NMR radiofrequency probe and a measure of the amount of power transmitted to the amount received.
Rate	Speed of a reaction under specified conditions. For simple chemical kinetics, the rate is the first derivative of the product concentration with respect to time, dp/dt, and is equal to a rate constant multiplied by reactant concentrations.
Rate constant	Rate is the product of a rate constant and concentration (strictly, activity). Thus, the units of a rate constant depend on the order of the reaction. For a first order reaction, the rate is $v = k_1 a$, and the first order rate const k_1 has dimensions in seconds. For a second order reaction, $v = ka.b$ and k has dimensions in M/s. Enzymes saturated with substrate show zero order kinetics with respect to the substrate, $v = V_m$.
Redox state	Redox (shorthand for reduction/oxidation reaction) describes all chemical reactions in which atoms have their oxidation number (oxidation state) changed (from Wikipedia).
Signal-to-noise ratio	The ratio of signal peak to the average noise factor. Specifically, the ratio of NMR peak heights of peaks from measurable compounds to noise peaks. To improve the signal-to-noise ratio by a factor of 2, one must acquire a factor of 4 more transients.
Single component curve-fit	The mathematical curve fitting of residuals in a time series dataset whereby a single component represents a time constant for a rate. In the context of this chapter, this relates to metabolite turnover rate within the biosystem.

Solenoid NMR coil	A volume coil design for an NMR radiofrequency probe consisting a wound wire or coil, like a spring, whereby the optimum spacing *f* loops is equal to the wire diameter.
Static flux measurement method	A method of flux analysis whereby 13C fractional enrichment or isotopomers are quantified in a single sample at steady state.
Steady state	A situation in which all state variables are constant in spite of ongoing processes that strive to change them. For an entire system to be at steady state, i.e., for all state variables of a system to be constant, there must be a flow through the system (compare mass balance) (from Wikipedia).
Volume of distribution	A value used to describe the distribution of a xenobiotic between blood plasma and the rest of the body. Xenobiotics with higher volumes of distribution are generally lipid-soluble and thus have low blood plasma concentrations after dosing. Those with lower volumes of distribution are generally more polar and thus have high blood plasma concentrations after dosing.

References

1. Murray RK, Granner DK, Rodwell VW, editors. Harper's illustrated biochemistry, 27th ed. New York: The McGraw-Hill Companies Inc.; 2006.
2. Nelson DL, Cox MM, editors. Lehninger principles of biochemistry, vol. 4. 4th ed. New York: W.H. Freeman & Company; 2004.
3. Wegener G, Krause U. Different modes of activating phosphofrustokinase, a key regulatory enzyme of glycolysis, in working vertebrate muscle. Biochem Soc Trans. 2002;30 (2):264–70.
4. Hunsucker SA, Mitchell BS, Spychala J. The 5′-nucleotidases as regulators of nucleotide and drug metabolism. Pharmacol Ther. 2005;107(1):1–30.
5. Huang M, Graves LM. De novo synthesis of pyrimidine nucleotides; emerging interfaces with signal transduction pathways. Cell Mol Life Sci. 2003;60(2):321–36.
6. Mathews CK. DNA precursor metabolism and genomic stability. FASEB J. 2006;20 (9):1300–14.
7. Yeung M, Thiele I, Palsson BO. Estimation of the number of extreme pathways for metabolic networks. BMC Bioinformatics. 2007;8 (1):363.
8. Vo TD, Palsson BO. Isotopomer analysis of myocardial substrate metabolism: a systems biology approach. Biotechnol Bioeng. 2006;95(5):972–83.
9. Lee DY, Yun H, Park S, Lee SY. MetaFluxNet: the management of metabolic reaction information and quantitative metabolic flux analysis. Bioinformatics. 2003;19:2144–6.
10. Wiechert W, Schweissgut O, Takanaga H, Frommer WB. Fluxomics: mass spectrometry versus quantitative imaging. Curr Opin Plant Biol. 2007;10(3):323–30.

11. Droste P, Weitzel M, Wiechert W. Visual exploration of isotope labeling networks in 3D. Bioprocess Biosyst Eng. 2008;31(3):227–39.
12. Massou S, Nicolas C, Letisse F, Portais JC. NMR-based fluxomics: quantitative 2D NMR methods for isotopomers analysis. Phytochemistry. 2007;68(16–18):2330–40.
13. Ataullakhanov FI, Vitvitsky VM. What determines the intracellular ATP concentration. Biosci Rep. 2002;22(5–6):501–11.
14. Diaz J, Hetzer G, Tello L. An energy balance climate model with hysteresis. Nonlinear Anal. 2006;64(9):2053–74.
15. Hatzianastassiou N, Fotiadi A, Matsoukas C, Pavlakis KG, Drakakis E, Hatzidimitriou D, Vardavas I. Long-term global distribution of Earth's shortwave radiation budget at the top of atmosphere. Atmos Chem Phys. 2004;4:1217–35.
16. Cai M. Dynamical amplification of polar warming. Geophys Res Lett. 2005;32(22):22710.
17. Warburg O, Wind F, Negelein E. The metabolism of turmos in the body. J Gen Physiol. 1927;3:519–30.
18. Gruetter R, Magnusson I, Rothman DL, Avison MJ, Shulman RG, Shulman GI. Validation of 13C NMR measurements of liver glycogen in vivo. Magn Reson Med. 1994;31(6):583–8.
19. Lee K, Berthiaume F, Stephanopoulos GN, Yarmush DM, Yarmush ML. Metabolic flux analysis of postburn hepatic hypermetabolism. Metab Eng. 2000;2(4):312–27.
20. Laughlin MR, Kelleher JK. Tracer theory and ^{13}C NMR. In: Berliner LJ, Robitaille P-M, editors. Biological magnetic resonance: in vivo carbon-13 NMR. New York: Kluwer Academic Publishers; 2002.
21. Sherry AD, Malloy CR. Biological magnetic resonance: in vivo carbon-13 NMR: ^{13}C isotopomer analysis of glutamate. A NMR method to probe metabolic pathways intersecting in the citric acid cycle. In: Berliner LJ, Robitaille PM, editors. Biological magnetic resonance: in vivo carbon-13 NMR. New York: Kluwer Academic Publishers; 2002.
22. Geissler A, Kanamori K, Ross BD. Real-time study of the urea cycle using ^{15}N NMR in the isolated perfused rat liver. Biochem J. 1992;287:813–20.
23. Grunder W, Krumbiegel P, Gersonde K. ^{15}N NMR of glycine metabolism in liver, muscle, and kidney using a new pulsed overhauser technique (POE). Isotopenpraxis Isot Environ Health Stud. 1992;28:81–4.
24. Gabel SA, London RE. A deuterium surface coil nmr study of the metabolism of D-methionine in the liver of the anesthetized rat. Biochemistry. 1988;27(20):7864–9.
25. Nissim I, Lapidot A. Plasma amino acid turnover rates and pools in rabbits: in vivo studies using stable isotopes. Am J Physiol. 1979;237(5):E418–27.
26. Wagenmakers AJ. Tracers to investigate protein and amino acid metabolism in human subjects. Proc Nutr Soc. 1999;58(4):987–1000.
27. Guillet C, Boirie Y, Walrand S. An integrative approach to in-vivo protein synthesis measurement: from whole tissue to specific proteins. Curr Opin Clin Nutr Metab Care. 2004;7(5):531–8.
28. Zawalich WS. Modulation of insulin secretion from beta-cells by phosphoinositide-derived second-messenger molecules. Diabetes. 1988;37(2):137–41.
29. Lodish H, Berk A, Zipursky SL, Matsudaira P, Baltimore D, Darnell J. Molecular cell biology. New York: W.H. Freeman & Company; 1999.
30. Jahoor F, Burrin DG, Reeds PJ, Frazer M. Measurement of plasma protein synthesis rate in infant pig: an investigation of alternative tracer approaches. Am J Physiol. 1994;267(1 Pt 2):R221–7.
31. Berthold HK, Jahoor F, Klein PD, Reeds PJ. Estimates of the effect of feeding on whole-body protein degradation in women vary with the amino acid used as tracer. J Nutr. 1995;125(10):2516–27.
32. Morell P, Ousley AH. Metabolic turnover of myelin glycerophospholipids. Neurochem Res. 1994;19(8):967–74.
33. Rapoport SI. In vivo approaches and rationale for quantifying kinetics and imaging brain lipid metabolic pathways. Prostaglandins Other Lipid Mediat. 2005;77(1–4):185–96.
34. Ritz P, Coward WA. Doubly labelled water measurement of total energy expenditure. Diabete Metab. 1995;21(4):241–51.
35. Damjanovich S, Nagy I, Somogyi B. Application of a molecular enzyme kinetic model for aging cells and tissues. Arch Gerontol Geriatr. 1989;8(1):37–45.
36. Finch CE, Morgan DG. RNA and protein metabolism in the aging brain. Annu Rev Neurosci. 1990;13:75–88.
37. Grimble GK, Malik SB, Boza JJ. Methods for measuring tissue RNA turnover. Curr Opin Clin Nutr Metab Care. 2000;3(5):399–408.
38. Preston CC, Oberlin AS, Holmuhamedov EL, Gupta A, Sagar S, Syed RH, Siddiqui

SA, Raghavakaimal S, Terzic A, Jahangir A. Aging-induced alterations in gene transcripts and functional activity of mitochondrial oxidative phosphorylation complexes in the heart. Mech Ageing Dev. 2008;129(6):304–12.

39. White RJ. RNA polymerases I and III, growth control and cancer. Nat Rev Mol Cell Biol. 2005;6(1):69–78.
40. Kurhanewicz J, Bok R, Nelson SJ, Vigneron DB. Current and potential applications of clinical 13C MR spectroscopy. J Nucl Med. 2008;49(3):341–4.
41. Gadian DG, editor. NMR and its applications to living systems. New York: Oxford University Press; 1995.
42. Mashimo K, Ohno Y. Ethanol hyperpolarizes mitochondrial membrane potential and increases mitochondrial fraction in cultured mouse myocardial cells. Arch Toxicol. 2006;80:421–8.
43. Thurman RG, Kauffman FC, Ji S, Lemasters JJ, Conway JG, Belinsky SA, Kashiwagi T, Matsamura T. Metabolic heterogeneity in the perfused rat liver. Pharmacol Biochem Behav. 1983;18 Suppl 1:415–9.
44. Testa C, Schiavina R, Lodi R, Salizzoni E, Corti B, Farsad M, Kurhanewicz J, Manferrari F, Brunocilla E, Tonon C, Monetti N, Castellucci P, Fanti S, Coe M, Grigioni WF, Martorana G, Canini R, Barbiroli B. Prostate cancer: sextant localization with MR imaging, MR spectroscopy, and 11C-choline PET/CT. Radiology. 2007;244(3):797–806.
45. Macdonald JM, Schmidlin O, James TL. In vivo monitoring of hepatic glutathione in anesthetized rats by ^{13}C NMR. Magn Reson Med. 2002;48(3):430–9.
46. Robbins E. Radiation risks from imaging studies in children with cancer. Pediatr Blood Cancer. 2008;51(4):453–7.
47. Isambert A, Bonniaud G, Lavielle F, Malandain G, Lefkopoulos D. A phantom study of the accuracy of CT, MR and PET image registrations with a block matching-based algorithm. Cancer Radiother. 2008;12 (8):800808.
48. Pichler BJ, Wehrl HF, Judenhofer MS. Latest advances in molecular imaging instrumentation. J Nucl Med. 2008;49 Suppl 2:5S–23.
49. Ikoma Y, Watabe H, Shidahara M, Naganawa M, Kimura Y. PET kinetic analysis: error consideration of quantitative analysis in dynamic studies. Ann Nucl Med. 2008;22(1):1–11.
50. Day SE, Kettunen MI, Gallagher FA, Hu DE, Lerche M, Wolber J, Golman K, Ardenkjaer-Larsen JH, Brindle KM. Detecting tumor response to treatment using hyperpolarized 13C magnetic resonance imaging and spectroscopy. Nat Med. 2007;13(11):1382–7.
51. Szyperski T. ^{13}C-NMR MS and metabolic flux balancing in biotechnology research. Q Rev Biophys. 1998;31(1):41–106.
52. London RE. Carbon-13 labeling in studies of metabolic regulation. Prog Nucl Magn Reson Spectrosc. 1988;20:337–83.
53. Stephanopoulos G, Aristidou A, Nielsen J. Metabolic engineering. San Diego: Academic; 1998.
54. Walker TE, Han CH, Kollman VH, London RE, Matwiyoff NA. ^{13}C nuclear magnetic resonance studies of the biosynthesis by microbacterium ammoniaphilum of L-glutamate selectively enriched with carbon-13. J Biol Chem. 1982;257:1189–95.
55. Beylot M, David MV, Landau BR, Brunengraber H. Tracing hepatic gluconeogenesis relative to citric acid cycle activity in vitro and in vivo. comparisons in the use of [3-^{13}C] lactate, [2-^{13}C] acetate, and α-keto [3-^{13}C] isocaproate. J Biol Chem. 1995; 270:1509–14.
56. Jones JG, Le TH, Storey CJ, Sherry RA, Malloy CR, Burton KP. Effects of different oxidative insults on intermediary metabolism in isolated perfused rat hearts. Free Radic Biol Med. 1996;20:515–23.
57. Jones JG, Sherry RA, Malloy CR. Quantitation of gluconeogenesis by ^{2}H nuclear magnetic resonance analysis of plasma glucose following ingestion of $^{2}H_2O$. Anal Biochem. 2000;277:121–6.
58. Jones JG, Solomon MA, Sherry RA, Jeffrey FM, Malloy CR. ^{13}C NMR measurements of human gluconeogenic fluxes after ingestion of [U-^{13}C] propionate, phenylacetate, and acetaminiophen. Am J Physiol Endocrinol Metab. 1998;275:843–52.
59. Magnusson I, Chandramouli V, Schumann WC, Kumaran K, Wahren J, Landau BR. Pentose pathway in human liver. Proc Natl Acad Sci. 1988;85:4682–5.
60. Magnusson I, Schumann WC, Bartsch GE, Chandramouli V, Kumaran K, Wahren J, Landau BR. Noninvasive tracing of Krebs cycle metabolism in liver. J Biol Chem. 1991; 266:6975–84.
61. Mancuso A, Sharfstein ST, Fernandez EJ, Clark DS, Blanch HW. Effect of extracellular glutamine concentration on primary and secondary metabolism of a murine hybridoma: an in vivo ^{13}C nuclear magnetic resonance study. Biotechnol Bioeng. 1998; 57:172–86.

62. Shulman GI, Rothman DL, Smith D, Johnson CM, Blair JB, Shulman RG, et al. Mechanism of liver glycogen repletion in vivo by nuclear magnetic resonance spectroscopy. J Clin Invest. 1985;76(3):1229–36.
63. Ugurbil K, Brown TR, Hollander JAD, Glynn P, Shulman RG. High-resolution 13C nuclear magnetic resonance studies of glucose metabolism in *Escherichia coli*. Proc Natl Acad Sci U S A. 1978;75(8):3742–6.
64. Sato K, Kashiwaya Y, Keon CA, Tsuchiya N, King MT, Radda GK, Chance B, Clarke K, Veech RL. Insulin, ketone bodies, and mitochondrial energy transduction. FASEB J. 1995;9(8):651–8.
65. Mayevsky A, Nioka S, Chance B. Fiber optic surface fluorometry/reflectometry and 31-p-NMR for monitoring the intracellular energy state in vivo. Adv Exp Med Biol. 1988;222:365–74.
66. Unkefer CJ, London RE. In vivo studies of pyridine nucleotide metabolism in *Escherichia coli* and *Saccharomyces cerevisiae* by carbon-13 NMR spectroscopy. J Biol Chem. 1984;259 (4):2311–20.
67. Chung Y, Jue T. 1H NMR observation of redox potential in liver. Biochemistry. 1992;31(45):11159–65.
68. Willis JA, Schleich T. Oxidative-stress induced protein glutathione mixed-disulfide formation in the ocular lens. Biochim Biophys Acta. 1996;1313(1):20–8.
69. Kreutzer U, Jue T. 1H-nuclear magnetic resonance deoxymyoglobin signal as indicator of intracellular oxygenation in myocardium. Am J Physiol. 1991;261(6 Pt 2):H2091–7.
70. Tran TK, Kreutzer U, Jue T. Observing the deoxy myoglobin and hemoglobin signals from rat myocardium in situ. FEBS Lett. 1998;434(3):309–12.
71. Seagle C, Christie MA, Winnike JH, McClelland RE, Ludlow JW, O'Connell TM, Gamcsik MP, Macdonald JM. High-throughput nuclear magnetic resonance metabolomic footprinting for tissue engineering. Tissue Eng Part C Methods. 2008;14(2):107–18.
72. Todd A. Inclusion of a glycogen regulation mathematical model into a contextual metabolic framework. In: Applied mathematics. Chapel Hill: University of North Carolina; 2007. p. 193.
73. Sherry AD, Malloy CR. Isotopic methods for probing organization of cellular metabolism. Cell Biochem Funct. 1996;14:259–68.
74. Ratcliffe RG, Shachar-Hill Y. Measuring multiple fluxes through plant metabolic networks. Plant J. 2006;45:490–511.
75. Jones JG, Sherry D, Jeffrey FMH, Cottam GL, Malloy CR. Methods for determining gluconeogenesis, anaplerosis, and pyruvate recycling. Patent US6,329,208 B1; 2001.
76. Cohen SM. Simultaneous 13C and 31P NMR studies of perfused rat liver. Effects of insulin and glucagon and a 13C NMR assay of free Mg2+. J Biol Chem. 1983;258 (23):14294–308.
77. Chatham JC, Forder JR. Metabolic compartmentation of lactate in the glucose-perfused rat heart. Am J Physiol. 1996;270(1 Pt 2): H224–9.
78. Chatham JC, Forder JR, Glickson JD, Chance EM. Calculation of absolute metabolic flux and the elucidation of the pathways of glutamate labeling in perfused rat heart by 13C NMR spectroscopy and nonlinear least squares analysis. J Biol Chem. 1995;270 (14):7999–8008.
79. Sandström J. Dynamic N.M.R. spectroscopy. London: Academic; 1982. p. 1226.
80. Cohen SM, Shulman RG, McLaughlin AC. Effects of ethanol on alanine metabolism in perfused mouse liver studied by 13C NMR. Proc Natl Acad Sci U S A. 1979;76 (10):4808–12.
81. London RE. In vivo 2H NMR studies of cellular metabolism. In: Berliner LJ, Reuben J, editors. Biological magnetic resonance: NMR of paramagnetic molecules. New York: Kluwer Academic Publishers; 1998.
82. Thoma WJ, Ugurbil K. Saturation-transfer studies of ATP-Pi exchange in isolated perfused rat liver. Biochim Biophys Acta. 1987;893(2):225–31.
83. Henry PG, Adriany G, Deelchand D, Gruetter R, Marjanska M, Oz G, Seaquist ER, Shestov A, Ugurbil K. In vivo 13C NMR spectroscopy and metabolic modeling in the brain: a practical perspective. Magn Reson Imaging. 2006;24(4):527–39.
84. Henry PG, Tkac I, Gruetter R. 1H-localized broadband 13C NMR spectroscopy of the rat brain in vivo at 9.4 T. Magn Reson Med. 2003;50(4):684–92.
85. Gruetter R, Adriany G, Choi IY, Henry PG, Lei HX, Oz G. Localized in vivo ^{13}C NMR spectoscopy of the brain. NMR Biomed. 2003;16(6–7):313–38.
86. deGraaf RA, Mason GF, Patel AB, Behar KL, Rothman DL. In vivo ^{1}H-[^{13}C]-NMR spectroscopy of cerebral metabolism. NMR Biomed. 2003;313(6–7):339–57.
87. Seymour AML. Imaging cardiac metabolism in heart failure: the potential of NMR

spectroscopy in the era of metabolism revisited. Heart Lung Circ. 2003;12:25–30.

88. Lewandowski ED. Biological magnetic resonance: in vivo carbon-13 NMR: metabolic flux and subcellular transport of metabolites. In: Berliner LJ, Robitaille PM, editors. Biological magnetic resonance: in vivo carbon-13 NMR, vol. 15. New York: Kluwer Academic Publishers; 1998.
89. Weiss RG, Gerstenblith G. Biological magnetic resonance: in vivo carbon-13 NMR. In: Berliner LJ, Robitaille PM, editors. Assessing cardiac metabolic rates during pathologic conditions with dynamic ^{13}C NMR spectra biological magnetic resonance: in vivo carbon-13 NMR, vol. 15. New York: Kluwer Academic Publishers; 1998.
90. Borgias BA, James TL. Two-dimensional nuclear Overhauser effect: complete relaxation matrix analysis. Methods Enzymol. 1989;176:169–83.
91. Mendes P. Emerging bioinformatics for the metabolome. Brief Bioinform. 2002;3(2):134–45.
92. Macdonald JM. Toxicological applications of cell and animal models for in vivo nuclear magnetic resonance spectroscopy. San Francisco: University of California at San Francisco; 1995.
93. Silbernagl S, Volker K, Dantzler WH. Compartmentation of amino acids in the rat kidney. Am J Physiol. 1996;270(1 Pt 2):F154–63.
94. Alger JR, Sillerud LO, Behar KL, Gillies RJ, Shulman RG, Gordon RE, Shaw D, Hanley PE. In vivo carbon-13 nuclear magnetic resonance studies of mammals. Science. 1981;214:660–2.
95. Enderle JD, Blanchard SM, Bronzino JD. Introduction to biomedical engineering. Boston: Elsevier Academic Press; 2005.
96. York MJ, Kuchel PW, Chapman BE, Jones AJ. Incorporation of labelled glycine into reduced glutathione of intact human erythrocytes by enzyme-catalysed exchange. Biochem J. 1982;207:65–72.
97. Roser W, Beckmann N, Wiesmann U, Seelig J. Absolute quantification of the hepatic glycogen content in a patient with glycogen storage disease by 13C magnetic resonance spectroscopy. Magn Reson Imaging. 1996;14(10):1217–20.
98. Gruetter R, Magnusson I, Rothman DL, Avison MJ, Shulman RG, Shulman GI. Validation of 13C NMR measurements of liver glycogen in vivo. Magn Reson Med. 1994;31(6):583–8.
99. Murphy E, Gabel SA, Funk A, London RE. NMR observability of ATP: preferential depletion of cytosolic ATP during ischemia in perfused rat liver. Biochemistry. 1988;27(2):526–8.
100. Masson S, Quistorff B. The 31P NMR visibility of ATP in perfused rat liver remains about 90%, unaffected by changes of metabolic state. Biochemistry. 1992;31(33):7488–93.
101. Kurhanewicz J, Swanson MG, Nelson SJ, Vigneron DB. Combined magnetic resonance imaging and spectroscopic imaging approach to molecular imaging of prostate cancer. J Magn Reson Imaging. 2002;16(4):451–63.
102. Nicholson JK, Timbrell JA, Bales JR, Sadler PJ. A high resolution proton nuclear magnetic resonance approach to the study of hepatocyte and drug metabolism. Application to acetaminophen. Mol Pharmacol. 1985;27(6):634–43.
103. Gamcsik MP, Millis KK, Colvin OM. Noninvasive detection of elevated glutathione levels in MCF-7 cells resistant to 4-hydroperoxycyclophosphamide. Cancer Res. 1995;55(10):2012–6.
104. Tian J, Yin Y, Sun H, Luo X. Magnesium chloride: an efficient 13C NMR relaxation agent for amino acids and some carboxylic acids. J Magn Reson. 2002;159(2):137–44.
105. London RE, Rhee CK, Murphy E, Gabel S, Levy LA. NMR-sensitive fluorinated and fluorescent intracellular calcium ion indicators with high dissociation constants. Am J Physiol. 1994;266(5 Pt 1):C1313–22.
106. Hoener BA, Tzika AA, Englestad BL, White DL. Hepatic transport of the magnetic resonance imaging contrast agent Fe(III)-N-(3-phenylglutaryl)desferrioxamine B. Magn Reson Med. 1991;17(2):509–15.
107. Chance EM, Seeholzer SH, Kobayashi K, Williamson JR. Mathematical analysis of isotope labeling in the citric acid cycle with applications to ^{13}C NMR studies in perfused rat hearts. J Biol Chem. 1983;258(22):13785–94.
108. Novotny EJ, Fulbright RK, Pearl PL, Gibson KM, Rothman DL. Magnetic resonance spectroscopy of neurotransmitters in human brain. Ann Neurol. 2003;54 Suppl 6:S25–31.
109. Waagepetersen HS, Sonnewald U, Schousboe A. Compartmentation of glutamine, glutamate, and GABA metabolism in neurons and astrocytes: functional implications. Neuroscientist. 2003;9(5):398–403.
110. Shen J, Petersen KF, Behar KL, Brown P, Nixon TW, Mason GF, Petroff OA, Shulman GI, Shulman RG, Rothman DL.

Determination of the rate of the glutamate/glutamine cycle in the human brain by in vivo ^{13}C NMR. Proc Natl Acad Sci. 1999;96 (14):8235–40.

111. Sonnewald U, Westergaard N, Hassel B, Muller TB, Unsgard G, Fonnum F, Hertz L, Schousboe A, Petersen SB. NMR spectroscopic studies of ^{13}C acetate and ^{13}C glucose metabolism in neocortical astrocytes: evidence for mitochnodrial heterogeneity. Dev Neurosci. 1993;15(3–5):351–8.
112. Melo TM, Nehlig A, Sonnewald U. Neuronal-glial interactions in rats fed a ketogenic diet. Neurochem Int. 2006;48(6–7):498–507.
113. Hassel B, Sonnewald U, Fonnum F. Glial-neuronal interactions as studied by cerebral metabolism of [2-^{13}C]acetate and [1-^{13}C] glucose: an ex vivo ^{13}C NMR spectroscopic study. J Neurochem. 1995;64(6):2773–82.
114. Snell K, Walker DG. The adaptive behaviour of isoenzyme forms of rat liver alanine aminotransferases during development. Biochem J. 1972;128(2):403–13.
115. Pasternack LB, Laude DA, Appling DR. 13C NMR detection of folate-mediated serine and glycine synthesis in vivo in *Saccharomyces cerevisiae*. Biochemistry. 1992;31(37): 8713–9.
116. Jones JG, Naidoo R, Sherry AD, Jeffrey FM, Cottam GL, Malloy CR. Measurement of gluconeogenesis and pyruvate recycling in the rat liver: a simple analysis of glucose and glutamate isotopomers during metabolism of [1,2,3-(13)C3]propionate. FEBS Lett. 1997; 412(1):131–7.
117. Cohen SM, Rognstad R, Shulman RG, Katz J. A comparison of 13C nuclear magnetic resonance and 14C tracer studies of hepatic metabolism. J Biol Chem. 1981;256(7): 3428–32.
118. Healing G, Smith D. Handbook of pre-clinical continuous intravenous infusion. New York: Taylor & Francis; 2000.
119. Myers R. The radio amateur's handbook: the standard manual of amateur radio communication. Newington: The American Radio Relay League; 1995.
120. Schmidt HC, Gooding CA, James TL. In vivo 31P-MR spectroscopy of the liver in the infant rabbit to study the effect of hypoxia on the phosphorus metabolites and intracellular pH. Invest Radiol. 1986;21(2):156–61.
121. Wald LL, Carvajal L, Moyher SE, Nelson SJ, Grant PE, Barkovich AJ, Vigneron DB. Phased array detectors and an automated intensity-correction algorithm for high-resolution MR imaging of the human brain. Magn Reson Med. 1995;34(3):433–9.
122. Wald LL, Moyher SE, Day MR, Nelson SJ, Vigneron DB. Proton spectroscopic imaging of the human brain using phased array detectors. Magn Reson Med. 1995;34(3):440–5.
123. Benveniste H, Blackband SJ. Translational neuroscience and magnetic-resonance microscopy. Lancet Neurol. 2006;5(6):536–44.
124. Wright SM, Wald LL. Theory and application of array coils in MR spectroscopy. NMR Biomed. 1997;10(8):394–410.
125. Thelwall PE, Yemin AY, Gillian TL, Simpson NE, Kasibhatla MS, Rabbani ZN, Macdonald JM, Blackband SJ, Gamcsik MP. Noninvasive in vivo detection of glutathione metabolism in tumors. Cancer Res. 2005;65 (22):10149–53.
126. Bottomley PA, Edelstein WA, Hart HR, Schenck JF, Smith LS. Spatial localization in ^{31}P and ^{13}C NMR spectroscopy in vivo using surface coils. Magn Reson Med. 1984;1 (3):410–3.
127. Fan TW, Higashi RM. Reproducible nuclear magnetic resonance surface coil fabrication by combining computer-aided design and a photoresist process. Anal Chem. 1989;61 (6):636–8.
128. Mulquiney PJ, Kuchel PW. Modeling metabolism with mathematica. Boca Raton: CRC Press; 2003.
129. Stephanopoulos GN, Aristidou AA, Nielsen J. Metabolic engineering: principles and methodologies. San Diego: Academic; 1998.
130. Palsson BO. Systems biology: properties of reconstructed networks. New York: Cambridge University Press; 2006.
131. Heinrich R, Schuster S. The regulation of cellular systems. New York: Chapman & Hall; 1996.
132. Fell DA. Understanding the control of metabolism. London: Portland Press; 1997.
133. Kacser H, Burns JA. The control of flux. Symp Soc Exp Biol. 1973;27:65–104 (reprinted with modern terms in: Kacser H, Burns JA, Fell DA. Biochem Soc Trans. 1995;23:341–66).
134. Heinrich R, Rapoport TA. A linear steady-state treatment of enzymatic chains. Critique of the crossover theorem and a general procedure to identify interaction sites with an effector. Eur J Biochem. 1974;42:97–105.
135. Heinrich R, Rapoport TA. A linear steady-state treatment of enzymatic chains. General properties, control and effector strength. Eur J Biochem. 1974;42:89–95.
136. Jucker BM, Barucci N, Shulman GI. Metabolic control analysis of insulin-stimulated glucose disposal in rat skeletal muscle. Am J

Physiol Endocrinol Metab. 1999;277: E505–12.
137. Fell DA. MCA: a survey of its theoretical and experimental development. Biochem J. 1992;286:313–30.
138. Klamt S, Stelling J, Ginkel M, Gilles ED. Flux analyzer: exploring structure, pathways and flux distributions in metabolic networks on interactive flux maps. Bioinformatics. 2003;19:261–9.
139. Hoops S, Sahle S, Gauges R, Lee C, Pahle J, Simus N, Singhal M, Xu L, Mendes P, Kummer U. COPASI—a complex pathway simulator. Bioinformatics. 2006;22:3067–74.
140. Golman K, Axelsson O, Johannesson H, Mansson S, Olofsson C, Petersson JS. Parahydrogen-induced polarization in imaging: subsecond (13)C angiography. Magn Reson Med. 2001;46(1):1–5.
141. Goodson BM. Nuclear magnetic resonance of laser-polarized noble gases in molecules, materials, and organisms. J Magn Reson. 2002;155(2):157–216.
142. Golman K, Ardenkjaer-Larsen JH, Petersson JS, Mansson S, Leunbach I. Molecular imaging with endogenous substances. Proc Natl Acad Sci U S A. 2003;100(18):10435–9.
143. Ardenkjaer-Larsen JH, Fridlund B, Gram A, Hansson G, Hansson L, Lerche MH, Servin R, Thaning M, Golman K. Increase in signal-to-noise ratio of >10,000 times in liquid-state NMR. Proc Natl Acad Sci U S A. 2003;100 (18):10158–63.
144. Bowers CR, Weitekamp DP. Parahydrogen and synthesis allow dramatically enhanced nuclear alignment. J Am Chem Soc. 1987;109:5541–2.
145. Canet D, Aroulanda C, Mutzenhardt P, Aime S, Gobetto R, Reineri F. Para-hydrogen enrichment and hyperpolarization. Concepts Magn Reson. 2006;28A(5):321–30.
146. Pravica MG, Weitekamp DP. Net NMR alignment by adiabatic transport of parahydrogen addition products to high magnetic field. Chem Phys Lett. 1998;145(4):255–8.
147. Goldman M, Johannesson H, Axelsson O, Karlsson M. Hyperpolarization of 13C through order transfer from parahydrogen: a new contrast agent for MRI. Magn Reson Imaging. 2005;23(2):153–7.
148. Abragam A, Goldman M. Principles of dynamic nuclear polarization. Rep Prog Phys. 1978;41:396–467.
149. Kohler SJ, Yen Y, Wolber J, Chen AP, Albers MJ, Bok R, Zhang V, Tropp J, Nelson S, Vigneron DB, Kurhanewicz J, Hurd RE. In vivo 13 carbon metabolic imaging at 3 T with hyperpolarized 13C-1-pyruvate. Magn Reson Med. 2007;58(1):65–9.
150. Chen AP, Cunningham CH, Ozturk-Isik E, Xu D, Hurd RE, Kelley DA, Pauly JM, Kurhanewicz J, Nelson SJ, Vigneron DB. High-speed 3 T MR spectroscopic imaging of prostate with flyback echo-planar encoding. J Magn Reson Imaging. 2007;25 (6):1288–92.
151. Merritt ME, Harrison C, Storey C, Jeffrey FM, Sherry AD, Malloy CR. Hyperpolarized 13C allows a direct measure of flux through a single enzyme-catalyzed step by NMR. Proc Natl Acad Sci U S A. 2007;104 (50):19773–7.
152. Overhauser AW. Polarization of nuclei in metals. Phys Rev. 1953;92(2):411–5.
153. Abragam A. Overhauser effect in nonmetals. Phys Rev. 1955;98(6):1729–35.
154. Boer WD, Borghini M, Morimoto K, Niinikoski TO, Udo F. Dynamic polarization of protons, deuterons, and carbon-13 nuclei: thermal contact between nuclear spins and an electron spin-spin interaction resevoir. J Low Temp Phys. 1974;15:249–67.
155. Keshari KR, Kurhanewicz J, Wilson DM, Jeffries RE, Dewar BJ, Van Criekinge M, et al. Hyperpolarized ^{13}C spectroscopy and a novel NMR-compatible bioreactor system for the investigation of real time cellular metabolism. Magn Reson Med. 2010;63:322–9.
156. Chen AP, Albers MJ, Cunningham CH, Kohler SJ, Yen YF, Hurd RE, Tropp J, Bok R, Pauly JM, Nelson SJ, Kurhanewicz J, Vigneron DB. Hyperpolarized C-13 spectroscopic imaging of the TRAMP mouse at 3 T-initial experience. Magn Reson Med. 2007;58 (6):1099–106.
157. Frydman L, Blazina D. Ultrafast two-dimensional nuclear magnetic resonance spectroscopy of hyperpolarized solutions. Nat Phys. 2007;3:415–9.
158. Merritt ME, Harrison C, Mander W, Malloy CR, Sherry AD. Dipolar cross-relaxation modulates signal amplitudes in the (1)H NMR spectrum of hyperpolarized [(13)C]formate. J Magn Reson. 2007;189 (2):280–5.
159. Reeder SB, Brittain JH, Grist TM, Yen YF. Least-squares chemical shift separation for (13)C metabolic imaging. J Magn Reson Imaging. 2007;26(4):1145–52.
160. Levin YS, Mayer D, Yen YF, Hurd RE, Spielman DM. Optimization of fast spiral chemical shift imaging using least squares reconstruction: application for hyperpolarized (13)C metabolic imaging. Magn Reson Med. 2007;58(2):245–52.

161. Macdonald J, Kurhanewicz J, Dahiya R, Espanol MT, Chang LH, Goldberg B, James TL, Narayan P. Effect of glucose and confluency on phosphorus metabolites of perfused human prostatic adenocarcinoma cells as determined by ^{31}P MRS. Magn Reson Med. 1993;29(2):244–8.
162. Zierhut ML, Yen YF, Chen AP, Bok R, Albers MJ, Zhang V, et al. Kinetic modeling of hyperpolarized (13)C(1)-pyruvate metabolism in normal rats and TRAMP mice. J Magn Reson. 2010;202:85–92.
163. Lapidot A, Gopher A. Cerebral metabolic compartmentation. Estimation of glucose flux via pyruvate carboxylase/pyruvate dehydrogenase by ^{13}C nmr isotopomer analysis of D-[U-^{13}C] glucose metabolites. J Biol Chem. 1994;269:27198–208.
164. Lown KS, Thummel KE, Benedict PE, Shen DD, Turgeon DK, Berent S, Watkins PB. The erythromycin breath test predicts clearance of midazolam. Clin Pharmacol Ther. 1995;57:16–24.
165. Kronbach T, Mathys D, Umeno M, Gonzalez FJ, Meyer UA. Oxidation of midazolam and trizaolam by human liver cytochrome P450IIIA4. Mol Pharmacol. 1989;36:89–96.
166. Bork RW, Muto T, Beaune PH, Srivastava PK, Lloyd RS, Guengerich FP. Characterization of mRNA species related to human liver cytochrome P-450 nifedipine oxidase and the regulation of catalytic activity. J Biol Chem. 1989;264:910–9.
167. Watkins PB, Murray SA, Winkelman LG, Heuman DM, Wrighton SA, Guzelian PS. Erythromycin breath test as an assay of glucocorticoid-inducibleliver cytochrome P-450. J Clin Invest. 1989;83:688–97.
168. Baker AL, Kotake AN, Schoeller DS. Clinical utility of breath tests for the assessment of hepatic function. Semin Liver Dis. 1983;3:318–29.
169. Keshari KR, Kurhanewicz J, Wilson DM, Jeffries RE, Dewar BJ, Van Criekinge M, Vigneron DB, Macdonald JM. Hyperpolarized ^{13}C spectroscopy and a novel NMR-compatible bioreactor system for the investigation of real time cellular metabolism. Magn Reson Med. 2010;63:322–9.
170. Kuramitsu S, Inoue K, Kondo K, Aki K, Kagamiyama H. Aspartate aminotransferase isozymes from rabbit liver. Purification and properties. J Biochem. 1985;97(5):1337–45.
171. Cunningham CH, Chen AP, Lustig M, Hargreaves BA, Lupo J, Xu D, et al. Pulse sequence for dynamic volumetric imaging of hyperpolarized metabolic products. J Magn Reson. 2008;193(1):139–46.
172. Jin ES, Jones JG, Merritt M, Burgess SC, Malloy CR, Sherry AD. Glucose production, gluconeogenesis, and hepatic tricarboxylic acid cycle fluxes measured by nuclear magnetic resonance analysis of a single glucose derivative. Anal Biochem. 2004;327(2):149–55.
173. Jue T, Rothman DL, Tavitian BA, Shulman RG. Natural-abundance 13C NMR study of glycogen repletion in human liver and muscle. Proc Natl Acad Sci U S A. 1989;86(5):1439–42.
174. Knüttel A, Kimmich R, Spohn KH. Motion-insensitive volume-selective pulse sequences for direct and proton-detected 13C spectroscopy: detection of glycogen in the human liver in vivo. Magn Reson Med. 1991;17(2):470–82.
175. Magnusson I, Rothman DL, Jucker B, Cline GW, Shulman RG, Shulman GI. Liver-glycogen turnover in fed and fasted humans. Am J Physiol. 1994;266:E796–803.
176. Jehenson P, Canioni P, Hantraye P, Syrota A. Carbon 13 NMR study of glycogen metabolism in the baboon liver in vivo. Biochem Biophys Res Commun. 1992;182(2):900–5.
177. Alger JR, Shulman RG. Metabolic applications of high-resolution 13C nuclear magnetic resonance spectroscopy. Br Med Bull. 1984;40(2):160–4.
178. Vogt JA, Yarmush DM, Yu YM, Zupke C, Fischman AJ, Tompkins RG, et al. TCA cycle flux estimates from NMR- and GC-MS-determined [13C]glutamate isotopomers in liver. Am J Physiol. 1997;272(6 Pt 1):C2049–62.
179. Canioni P, Alger JR, Shulman RG. Natural abundance Carbon-13 nuclear magnetic resonance spectroscopy of liver and adipose tissue of the living rat. Biochemistry. 1983;22(21):4974–80.
180. Cross TA, Pahl C, Oberhänsli R, Aue WP, Keller U, Seelig J. Ketogenesis in the living rat followed by 13C NMR spectroscopy. Biochemistry. 1984;23(26):6398–402.
181. Desmoulin F, Canioni P, Cozzone PJ. Glutamate-glutamine metabolism in the perfused rat liver 13C-NMR study using (2-13C)-enriched acetate. FEBS Lett. 1985;185(1):29–32.
182. Stromski ME, Arias-Mendoza F, Alger JR, Shulman RG. Hepatic gluconeogenesis from alanine: 13C nuclear magnetic resonance methodology for in vivo studies. Magn Reson Med. 1986;3(1):24–32.
183. Kalderon B, Gopher A, Lapidot A. Metabolic pathways leading to liver glycogen repletion

in vivo, studied by GC-MS and NMR. FEBS Lett. 1986;204(1):29–32.

184. Shulman GI, Rossetti L, Rothman DL, Blair JB, Smith D. Quantitative analysis of glycogen repletion by nuclear magnetic resonance spectroscopy in the conscious rat. J Clin Invest. 1987;80(2):387–93.

185. Kalderon B, Gopher A, Lapidot A. A quantitative analysis of the metabolic pathways of hepatic glucose synthesis in vivo with 13C-labeled substrates. FEBS Lett. 1987;213 (1):209–14.

186. Künnecke B, Cerdan S. Multilabeled 13C substrates as probes in in vivo 13C and 1H NMR spectroscopy. NMR Biomed. 1989;2 (5–6):274–7.

187. Shalwitz RA, Reo NV, Becker NN, Hill AC, Ewy CS, Ackerman JJ. Hepatic glycogen synthesis from duodenal glucose and alanine. An in situ 13C NMR study. J Biol Chem. 1989;264(7):3930–4.

188. Chen W, Ackerman JJ. Localized 13C-[1H] NMR of rat liver in vivo using surface-spoiling gradients. NMR Biomed. 1989;2 (5–6):267–73.

189. Zang LH, Laughlin MR, Rothman DL, Shulman RG. 13C NMR relaxation times of hepatic glycogen in vitro and in vivo. Biochemistry. 1990;29(29):6815–20.

190. Cunnane SC. Carbon-by-carbon discrimination of 13C incorporation into liver fatty acids. FEBS Lett. 1992;306(2–3):273–5.

191. Van Cauteren M, Miot F, Segebarth CM, Eisendrath H, Osteaux M, Willem R. Excitation characteristics of adiabatic half-passage RF pulses used in surface coil MR spectroscopy. Application to 13C detection of glycogen in the rat liver. Phys Med Biol. 1992;37 (5):1055–64.

192. Wehmeyer N, Gunderson H, Nauman J, Savage S, Hartzell C. Determination of the glycogen synthesis pathway by 13C nuclear magnetic resonance analysis. Metabolism. 1994;43(1):38–43.

193. Jones JG, Cottam GL, Miller BC, Sherry AD, Malloy CR. A method for obtaining 13C isotopomer populations in 13C-enriched glucose. Anal Biochem. 1994;217(1):148–52.

194. Jucker BM, Lee JY, Shulman RG. In vivo 13C NMR measurements of hepatocellular tricarboxylic acid cycle flux. J Biol Chem. 1998;273(20):12187–94.

195. Küstermann E, Seelig J, Künnecke B. Ascorbic acid, a vitamin, is observed by in vivo 13C nuclear magnetic resonance spectroscopy of rat liver. Am J Physiol. 1998;274(1 Pt 1): E65–71.

196. Likhodii SS, Cunnane SC. Uptake of 13C-tracer arachidonate and gamma-linolenate by the brain and liver of the suckling rat observed using 13C-NMR. J Neurochem. 1998;72 (6):2548–55.

197. Beckmann N, Seelig J, Wick H. Analysis of glycogen storage disease by in vivo 13C NMR: comparison of normal volunteers with a patient. Magn Reson Med. 1990;16 (1):150–60.

198. Petersen KF, West AB, Reuben A, Rothman DL, Shulman GI. Noninvasive assessment of hepatic triglyceride content in humans with 13C nuclear magnetic resonance spectroscopy. Hepatology. 1996;24(1):114–7.

199. Roden M, Perseghin G, Petersen KF, Hwang JH, Cline GW, Gerow K, et al. The roles of insulin and glucagon in the regulation of hepatic glycogen synthesis and turnover in humans. J Clin Invest. 1996;97:642–8.

200. Stevens AN, Iles RA, Morris PG, Griffiths JR. Detection of glycogen in a glycogen storage disease by 13C nuclear magnetic resonance. FEBS Lett. 1982;150(2):489–93.

201. Sillerud LO, Shulman RG. Structure and metabolism of mammalian liver glycogen monitored by carbon-13 nuclear magnetic resonance. Biochemistry. 1983;22 (5):1087–94.

202. Reo NV, Siegfried BA, Ackerman JJ. Direct observation of glycogenesis and glucagon-stimulated glycogenolysis in the rat liver in vivo by high-field carbon-13 surface coil NMR. J Biol Chem. 1984;259(22):13664–7.

203. Siegfried BA, Reo NV, Ewy CS, Shalwitz RA, Ackerman JJ, McDonald JM. Effects of hormone and glucose administration on hepatic glucose and glycogen metabolism in vivo. A 13C NMR study. J Biol Chem. 1985;260 (30):16137–42.

204. Pahl-Wostl C, Seelig J. Metabolic pathways for ketone body production. 13C NMR spectroscopy of rat liver in vivo using 13C-multilabeled fatty acids. Biochemistry. 1986;25 (22):6799–807.

205. Pahl-Wostl C, Seelig J. Ketogenesis in the living rat followed by 13C-NMR spectroscopy. Infusion of [1,3-13C]octanoate. Biol Chem Hoppe Seyler. 1987;368(3):205–14.

206. Cohen SM. Effects of insulin on perfused liver from streptozotocin-diabetic and untreated rats: 13C NMR assay of pyruvate kinase flux. Biochemistry. 1987a;26(2):573–80.

207. Cohen SM. 13C NMR study of effects of fasting and diabetes on the metabolism of pyruvate in the tricarboxylic acid cycle and the utilization of pyruvate and ethanol in

lipogenesis in perfused rat liver. Biochemistry. 1987b;26(2):581–9.

208. Shulman GI, Rothman DL, Chung Y, Rossetti L, Petit Jr WA, Barrett EJ, et al. 13C NMR studies of glycogen turnover in the perfused rat liver. J Biol Chem. 1988;263 (11):5027–9.
209. Cerdan S, Künnecke B, Dölle A, Seelig J. In situ metabolism of 1, omega medium chain dicarboxylic acids in the liver of intact rats as detected by 13C and 1H NMR. J Biol Chem. 1988;263(24):11664–74.
210. Liu KJ, Henderson TO, Kleps RA, Reyes MC, Nyhus LM. Gluconeogenesis in the liver of tumor rats. J Surg Res. 1990;49(2):179–85.
211. David M, Petit WA, Laughlin MR, Shulman RG, King JE, Barrett EJ. Simultaneous synthesis and degradation of rat liver glycogen. An in vivo nuclear magnetic resonance spectroscopic study. J Clin Invest. 1991;86 (2):612–7.
212. Künnecke B, Seelig J. Glycogen metabolism as detected by in vivo and in vitro 13C-NMR spectroscopy using [1,2-13C2]glucose as substrate. Biochim Biophys Acta. 1991;1095 (2):103–13.
213. Liu KJ, Kleps R, Henderson T, Nyhus L. 13C NMR study of hepatic pyruvate carboxylase activity in tumor rats. Biochem Biophys Res Commun. 1991;179(1):366–71.
214. Shulman GI, DeFronzo RA, Rossetti L. Differential effect of hyperglycemia and hyperinsulinemia on pathways of hepatic glycogen repletion. Am J Physiol. 1991;260(5 Pt 1): E731–5.
215. Muller HJ, Lanens D, de Cock Buning TJ, van de Vyver FL, Alderweireldt FC, Dommisse R, et al. Noninvasive in vivo 13C-NMR spectroscopy in the rat to study the pharmacokinetics of 13C-labeled xenobiotics. Drug Metab Dispos. 1992;20(4):507–9.
216. Lanens D, Muller HJ, Van de Vyver F, de Cock-Bunning T, Spanoghe M, Van der Linden A, et al. Noninvasive in vivo 13C-NMR spectroscopy of a 13C-labeled xenobiotic in the rat. Magn Reson Imaging. 1992;10(6):975–81.
217. Petersen KF, Blair JB, Shulman GI. Triiodothyronine treatment increases substrate cycling between pyruvate carboxylase and malic enzyme in perfused rat liver. Metabolism. 1995;44(11):1380–3.
218. Morikawa S, Inubushi T, Takahashi K, Terada Y, Iwata S, Ozawa K. Glucose and energy metabolism in rat liver after ischemic damage assessed by 13 C and 31 P NMR spectroscopy. J Surg Res. 1996;63(2):393–9.
219. Morikawa S, Inubushi T, Takahashi K, Ishii H, Ozawa K. Gluconeogenesis and phosphoenergetics in rat liver during endotoxemia. J Surg Res. 1998;74(2):179–86.
220. Changani KK, Bell JD, Iles RA. 13C-Glycogen deposition during pregnancy in the rat following routine meal feeding. Biochim Biophys Acta. 1998;1380(2):198–208.
221. Yarmush DM, MacDonald AD, Foy BD, Berthiaume F, Tompkins RG, Yarmush ML. Cutaneous burn injury alters relative tricarboxylic acid cycle fluxes in rat liver. J Burn Care Rehabil. 1999;20(4):292–302.
222. Zhaofan X, Jianguang T, Guangyi W, Hongtai T, Shengde G, Horton JW. Effect of thermal injury on relative anaplerosis and gluconeogenesis in the rat during infusion of [U-13C] propionate. Burns. 2002;28(7):625–30.
223. Baillet-Blanco L, Beauvieux MC, Gin H, Rigalleau V, Gallis JL. Insulin induces a positive relationship between the rates of ATP and glycogen changes in isolated rat liver in presence of glucose; a 31P and 13C NMR study. Nutr Metab (Lond). 2005;2:32.
224. Geoffrion Y, Butler K, Pass M, Smith IC, Deslauriers R. Plasmodium berghei: gluconeogenesis in the infected mouse liver studied by 13C nuclear magnetic resonance. Exp Parasitol. 1988;59(3):364–74.
225. Hall JE, Mackenzie NE, Mansfield JM, McCloskey DE, Scott AI. 13C-NMR analysis of alanine metabolism by isolated perfused livers from C3HeB/FeJ mice infected with African trypanosomes. Comp Biochem Physiol B. 1988;89(4):679–85.
226. Nedelec JF, Mégnin F, Patry J, Jullien P, Lhoste JM, Dimicoli JL. Modification of the gluconeogenic/glycolytic balance in isolated perfused liver of myeloproliferative leukemia infected mice: a 13C NMR study. Comp Biochem Physiol B. 1990;95 (3):505–14.
227. Cohen SM, Werrmann JG, Tota MR. 13C NMR study of the effects of leptin treatment on kinetics of hepatic intermediary metabolism. Proc Natl Acad Sci U S A. 1998;95 (13):7385–90.
228. Choi IY, Wu C, Okar DA, Lange AJ, Gruetter R. Elucidation of the role of fructose 2,6-bisphosphate in the regulation of glucose fluxes in mice using in vivo (13)C NMR measurements of hepatic carbohydrate metabolism. Eur J Biochem. 2002;269 (18):4418–26.
229. Cohen SM, Duffy JL, Miller C, Kirk BA, Candelore MR, Ding VD, et al. Direct observation (NMR) of the efficacy of glucagon receptor antagonists in murine liver expressing the human glucagon receptor. Bioorg Med Chem. 2006;14(5):1506–17.

Chapter 12

Compositional Analysis of Phospholipids by Mass Spectrometry and Phosphorus-31 Nuclear Magnetic Resonance Spectroscopy

M. Cecilia Yappert

Abstract

As the roles of phospholipids continue to be unraveled in an expansive list of biological processes, the availability of fast, accurate, and precise analytical approaches becomes of utmost relevance. Traditional methods rely on the separation of phospholipid classes, each with a different polar head group, by either thin-layer or liquid chromatography. The length and degree of unsaturation of the hydrophobic chains are subsequently determined by derivatization and gas chromatography. Although these methods are well developed, they are time-consuming and do not allow for in situ analysis.

The combination of P-31 nuclear magnetic resonance (NMR) spectroscopy and mass spectrometry (MS) provides a powerful alternative for the analysis of phospholipids in complex mixtures. With the use of P-31 NMR spectroscopy, phospholipids can be analyzed quantitatively in either organic solvents or aqueous media containing a detergent. Matrix-assisted laser desorption/ionization (MALDI) and other forms of ionization such as electron-spray ionization (ESI) coupled with mass spectrometry (MS) allow the analysis of intact lipids both in vitro and in situ.

This chapter describes conventional approaches for phospholipid analysis first. The criteria and current options in the choice of matrices for MALDI MS are addressed. The ability of MALDI MS to image phospholipids is then highlighted as well as the remaining challenges. Regarding P-31 NMR, current studies on the measurement of temperature coefficients and pH dependences to improve the accuracy in the assignment of P-31 resonances are described. Finally, the complementary nature of P-31 NMR and MALDI MS is illustrated in the reevaluation of the unusual composition of phospholipids in human lens membranes.

Key words: Phospholipid analysis, mass spectrometry, MALDI, matrices, mass spectral imaging, ^{31}P NMR spectroscopy, bile salts, temperature coefficient

1. Introduction

As the importance of the diversity of lipids continues to be recognized in a wide range of cellular processes, the choice of methods for their analysis is of utmost relevance. This chapter focuses on two current approaches that enable the compositional analysis of

Teresa Whei-Mei Fan et al. (eds.), *The Handbook of Metabolomics*, Methods in Pharmacology and Toxicology,
DOI 10.1007/978-1-61779-618-0_12,

phospholipids (and other lipids) directly in relatively crude extracts and in situ, on intact cells or tissue slices. First, the various types of lipids and phospholipid classes present in biomembranes are described briefly. Then, conventional methods used for the separation and analysis of phospholipids are presented. Then, the application of mass spectrometry to the in vitro analysis and in situ imaging of lipids is illustrated with an example designed to map phospholipids in the lens of the mammalian eye. Finally, the power and limitations of Phosphorus-31 nuclear magnetic resonance (NMR) spectroscopy are highlighted with concrete examples.

1.1. General Classification of Lipids

Lipids may be divided into the following classes: glycolipids (glycoglycerolipids and glycosphingolipids), sterols, and phospholipids (glycerophospholipids and sphingophospholipids). As their name implies, glycolipids contain a sugar moiety. In glycoglycerolipids, the sn-3 position of the glycerol backbone forms a glycosidic link to a carbohydrate such as galactose. These polar lipids are found predominantly in plant chloroplast membranes and are also present in algae and bacteria. Rarely are they found in animals (1). In glycosphingolipids, the glycosidic linkage is to the primary alcohol group of ceramide (see next section). They are classified according to the carbohydrate moiety, which may be a single sugar or complex polymers. They are usually found as minor components on the outer surface of animal cell plasma membranes (1).

Some plant, animal, and microbial membranes contain sterols. Cholesterol, a compact, rigid, hydrophobic molecule with a polar hydroxyl group, is the most common sterol. It makes up about 30% of the mass of the membrane lipids of many animal cell plasma membranes (2).

1.2. Phospholipid Classification

As the number of possible hydrophobic chains is very large, the total number of biologically relevant phospholipids is enormous, and runs into the thousands. For this reason, the most general classification of phospholipids is based on the nature of the interfacial region that connects the polar head group to the nonpolar tails.

1.2.1. Glycerophospholipids

In glycerophospholipids, the most commonly found phospholipids in biomembranes, two of the hydroxyl groups of the glycerol backbone may participate in the formation of two ester linkages that connect to the acyl chains derived from fatty acids. These phospholipids are thus termed diacylglycerophospholipids. Typically, the acyl chain in the sn-2 position of most glycerophospholipids is unsaturated, whereas the acyl chain in the sn-1 position is saturated in most phospholipids (2). By enzymatic hydrolysis by phospholipase A2, these various types of glycerophospholipids may lose the sn-2 chain to become lysoglycerophospholipids. The sn-1 ester bond can also be cleaved by phospholipase A1, but it is less frequent (2).

The linkage at the sn-1 position can also be an ether vinyl, rather than an ester. These species are most often formed when the head group is either a choline or a serine moiety (3–5). These 1-alkenyl, 2-acyl glycerophospholipids are also known as plasmalogens. Even more rare are those glycerophospholipids in which the sn-1 chain is connected to the backbone through an ether linkage. These 1-alkyl, 2-acyl glycerophospholipids appear to play important roles in several pathologies, including cancer (6, 7).

The common feature of all these glycerophospholipids is the presence of a polar phosphate-containing group at the sn-3 position. As shown in Fig. 1, the phosphate is usually linked to a choline (as in phosphatidylcholine, PC), ethanolamine (as in phosphatidylethanolamine, PE), myoinositol (as in phosphatidylinositol, PI), serine (as in phosphatidylserine, PS), or glycerol (as in phosphatidylglycerol, PG). In the case of phosphatidate, the conjugate base of phosphatidic acid, this site is devoid of a head group (X) and deprotonated at physiological pH.

1.2.2. Sphingophospholipids

These lipids also contain a phosphate group but differ from glycerophospholipids in that they derive from a sphingoid base, rather than glycerol. The most common sphingoid base is sphingosine with a *trans* double bond between carbons 4 and 5 (see Fig. 1). However, the saturated base, termed sphinganine or dihydrosphingosine, may also be present in biomembranes (8–11). The addition of an acyl chain through the formation of an amide linkage results in ceramide (with the double bond) or dihydroceramide (with no double bond). The most common sphingolipid present in mammalian cell membranes is sphingomyelin (SM) in which the head group is a choline moiety (Fig. 1). Ethanolamine is the other head group that may be found in sphingophospholipids (2).

2. Conventional Methods for Phospholipid Analysis

The chemical and physical properties of cell membranes are strongly affected by their phospholipid composition. To characterize the phospholipid constituents of membranes, lipids are typically extracted using chloroform–methanol, based on the Folch extraction (12) or with methanol only (13). After this extraction step, the various classes, such as PC, PE, PS, etc. are then separated using chromatographic methods.

2.1. Thin Layer Chromatography (TLC)

This is the most conventional approach for the separation of phospholipid classes. The stationary phase (silica or alumina) interacts with the various polar head groups. Those head groups that are more strongly adsorbed onto the stationary phase do not move as far up the plates as those that are less polar. As a result, the various

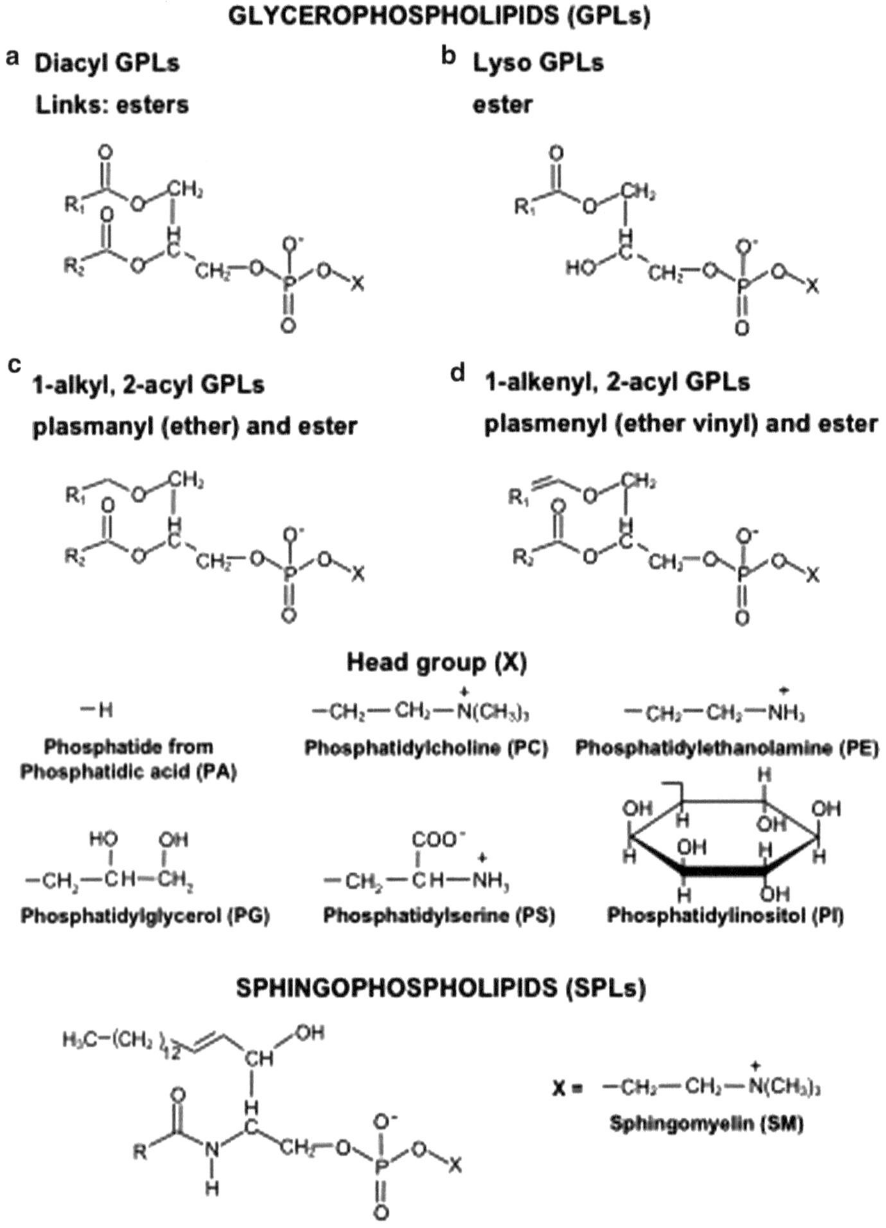

Fig. 1. Structures of various phospholipids found in biomembranes. The degree of protonation/deprotonation shown corresponds to that at pH = 7.4.

classes can be separated from one another. Identification of the separated compounds must then be made by comparing the retention behavior with known standards or preferably by mass spectrometric analysis of the individual spots (see section on mass spectrometry). With the use of thin layer chromatography (TLC), it is very difficult to separate phospholipids that have the same head group but different linkages at the sn-1 and sn-2 positions. Furthermore, the separation of sphingolipids that only differ in the presence or absence of the critical *trans* double bond between C4 and C5 cannot be accomplished with common elution methods.

2.2. High-Performance Liquid Chromatography (HPLC)

High-performance liquid chromatography (HPLC) is another powerful approach for the compositional analysis of lipids (14–16). However, although it is possible to separate the various phospholipids classes, the chromatographic conditions (nature of the stationary and mobile phase, elution profile, etc.) must be carefully chosen depending on the expected composition of the extract. For example, when using a typical set of HPLC conditions (polar silica gel stationary phase, hexane–isopropanol as mobile phase), sphingomyelin and dihydrosphingomyelin (DHSM) coelute. Because of this lack of resolution, the identity of the most abundant phospholipid in membrane of adult human lenses was incorrectly believed to be sphingomyelin for decades (17, 18). In 1991, however, Merchant et al. (19) reported the presence of a phospholipid of unknown identity as its ^{31}P NMR chemical shift did not match that of any common phospholipid. Importantly, this "unknown" lipid made up nearly half of all the phospholipids in adult human lenses. It was through the use of an amino-bound stationary phase that sphingomyelin and the "unknown" could be separated. Once the fraction containing the "unknown" was isolated, multidimensional ^{1}H NMR studies led to the identification of this phospholipid as DHSM, in which the *trans* double bond between C4 and C5 is saturated (9). As with TLC, the acyl chain distribution of each phospholipid class cannot be readily known by HPLC unless a mass spectrometer is used as detector.

2.3. Separation of Molecular Species Within Each Phospholipid Class

Before discussing specific separation techniques, it should be noted that phospholipids may be separated as intact or derivatized species. Both methods have their merits and drawbacks. In general, the derivatization procedure involves enzymatic hydrolysis of the head group with phospholipase C; then, the resulting diacylglycerol moiety is converted to a stable nonpolar derivative. Derivatization of phospholipids offers two main advantages. First, nonpolar derivatives of phospholipids can be resolved better than the intact components because they interact more effectively with the relatively nonpolar stationary phase. If all phospholipid classes are converted to the same type of derivative, they can be analyzed under the same elution conditions. Improved resolution may often be obtained with no requirement for inorganic ions in the mobile phase. Second, UV-absorbing or fluorescent derivatives may be employed, simplifying detection and quantification (20, 21).

On the other hand, analyzing the intact phospholipids is inherently simpler and less time-consuming. In addition, it enables metabolic studies based on isotopic labeling, since the labeled lipids need not be fragmented or derivatized. Finally, artifacts such as the rearrangement of hydrophobic chains that may be introduced by multistep derivatization is not relevant and the risk of oxidative degradation is reduced (21). Using either derivatized or intact phospholipids, the composition of the hydrophobic tails has been investigated by the following methods.

2.3.1. Gas Chromatography

Intact phospholipids are not suitable for GC analysis. The derivatization procedure may entail, for example, hydrolysis with phospholipase C to remove the phosphate and associated head group, and conversion of the resulting 1,2-diacylglycerol (or 1-alkyl, 2-acyl glycerol; or 1-alkenyl, 2-acyl glycerol) into trimethylsilyl (TMS) esters or ethers, tert-butyl dimethylsilyl (t-BDMS) ethers or esters (22). An extensive list of protocols and references for the conversion of fatty acids ester derivatives can be found in the excellent Web site, "The Lipid Library" developed by Professor William W. Christie (http://www.lipidlibrary.co.uk/topics/ester_93/index.htm#H). Compared to HPLC and LC-MS methods, GC with flame ionization detection offers a wider concentration range in which the calibration curve is linear, i.e., great dynamic range.

2.3.2. Reverse Phase HPLC

When solid phases for HPLC composed of alkylated silica particles became available, reverse phase HPLC became one of the most utilized separation methods for characterization of molecular species. The separation of phospholipids by reversed phase chromatography is based not only on the analyte's overall degree of unsaturation but also on differences in chain length. An excellent summary of the different types of mobile and stationary phases and the use of counter ions can be found in Professor Christie's Web site (http://www.lipidlibrary.co.uk/topics/hplc_pl/index.htm).

HPLC of underivatized phospholipids suffers from detection problems. In detection using UV at short wavelengths, the signal intensity is highly influenced by the degree of unsaturation. Calibration becomes a very tedious task since each species needs its own calibration curve; moreover, authentic standards are not always commercially available. Evaporative light-scattering detection (ELSD) is much less sensitive to baseline shift during gradient elution than UV detection and its response is largely independent of the number and configuration of double bonds in the fatty acid chains, thus making quantification more straightforward (22).

One of the most powerful detectors for HPLC is MS. In LC-MS, the separation power of HPLC into either different lipid classes or molecular species within a class together with MS detection makes the simultaneous determination of molecules and the identification of several structural elements possible. An extensive range of applications can be found in the literature and only a few of them are included herein (23–28) to highlight the power of this approach.

3. Mass Spectrometry for Phospholipid Analysis

3.1. Background

Mass spectrometry (MS) offers high speed, selectivity, specificity, and sensitivity. When used independently or coupled with GC or HPLC, it can provide information on the molecular weight, the empirical formula, and structural details on specific phospholipids. In fact, fatty acid methyl esters were the first biological materials to be analyzed using mass spectrometry (29). A detailed introduction to mass spectrometry methods is available in Chap. 4.

For lipids with low molecular weight, such as fatty acids, sterols, and bile acids, electron impact (EI) ionization mass spectrometry has been the traditional mode of ionization. For lipids with higher molecular weight, such as glycerophospholipids and sphingolipids, only their derivatized forms can be analyzed by EI ionization. This conventional approach is relatively more time-consuming and often lacks the sensitivity required for analysis of subcellular membrane lipids.

With the development of soft ionization desorption techniques, it is now possible for relatively large, nonvolatile and thermally labile compounds such as phospholipids to be analyzed in their intact form. Although soft ionization techniques such as field desorption, chemical ionization, plasma ionization, and fast atom bombardment have all been used to analyze phospholipids, this chapter focuses on two relatively new mass spectrometric ionization tools, electrospray ionization (ESI) and, with greater emphasis, matrix-assisted laser desorption/ionization (MALDI). Both forms of ionization emerged in the late 1980s and have led to major breakthroughs in the application of mass spectrometry to biological analysis. With minimal sample preparation, biological fluids and tissues may be analyzed directly using ESI- and MALDI-MS. With sensitivity in the picomole-to-femtomole range, biomolecules such as proteins with molecular weights be greater than 100,000 Da (30) can be detected and further investigated to obtain structural information.

In the area of lipid analysis, ESI-MS has already been used for characterization and quantification of phospholipids. The references listed herein are just a few representative examples of the analysis of phospholipids by ESI-MS and this list is—by no means—exhaustive (23, 24, 26, 28, 31–35).

One of the concerns in the use of ESI-MS for direct analysis of crude biological extracts is the presence of salts that may lead to clogging of the needle where the ionization occurs. Another important limitation in ESI-MS was its inability to perform in situ imaging, since the analytes must be charged in the needle held at high voltages. This drawback was eliminated in 2004, when Cooks and coworkers reported the use of desorption/electrospray ionization or DESI (36). The desorption and ionization of the analytes is induced by a stream of charged water and additives and takes place at atmospheric pressure. The ions are then extracted and introduced in the mass spectrometer. Besides removing the clogging problem just mentioned (37), this approach enables imaging and has been applied to the study of small molecules—including phospholipids—as well as large ones (37–43). The spatial resolution with this imaging approach is limited by the diameter of the water stream and is currently around 250 μm (40). The potential of this imaging approach is just beginning to be realized. With the ability to induce chemical reactions by the inclusion of selective additives in the charged water stream, the selectivity and reactivity-enhanced resolution could be greatly improved.

3.2. MALDI-TOF MS

Matrix-assisted laser desorption-ionization (MALDI) mass spectrometry is an outgrowth of the direct laser desorption (LD) mass spectrometry of small organic molecules that was initially developed in the 1960s and 1970s. In the mid-1980s, Karas, Hillenkamp, and coworkers (30, 44–47), introduced MALDI-MS. They demonstrated that by adding a small molecular weight organic acid matrix to an analyte, molecular photodissociation of the parent ions induced by direct laser irradiation of the sample could be avoided (46).

3.2.1. Theory and Instrumentation

The desorption/ionization process. The MALDI ionization technique (Fig. 2) typically involves the following steps: the sample is allowed to cocrystallize with the matrix on a metal surface, a pulsed UV laser beam is directed to the sample, and a plume of matrix and analyte ions is ejected into the vacuum of the source. The mechanism of MALDI continues to be investigated, but it is believed to involve the following events (48, 49)

1. *Formation of a "solid solution."* Optimal analyte to matrix molar ratio is in the 1:1,000–1:10,000 range. This means

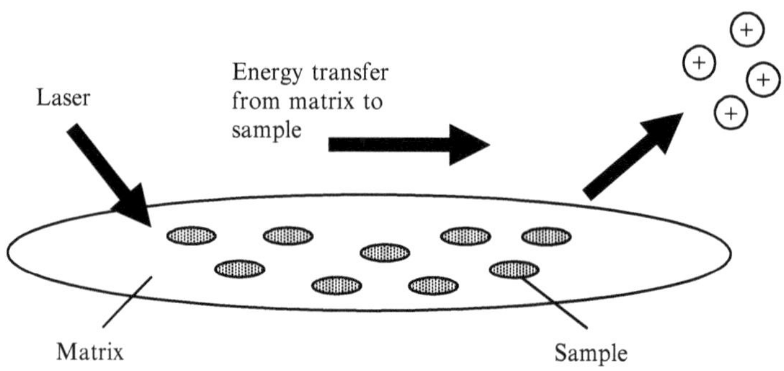

Fig. 2. Diagrammatic matrix-assisted laser desorption ionization. *Source*: Voyager Workstation User's Guide, pp. 1–8.

that analyte molecules are completely isolated from each other and fully surrounded (solvated) by matrix molecules.

2. *Excitation of the matrix and desorption.* The basic criterion for choosing a matrix is for it to be a strong absorber of energy at the chosen laser wavelength. Laser energy absorbed by the matrix causes a chain of events: rapid vibrational excitation of matrix molecules (heating); localized disintegration of the solid solution; formation of clusters of a single analyte molecule surrounded by neutral, excited matrix molecules and/or pseudomolecular radicals; and finally, the evaporation of the matrix molecules from these clusters leaving the excited analyte molecule.
3. *Ionization of analyte.* The desorbed analyte molecules can be protonated and deprotonated by the matrix to form $[M + H]^+$ and $[M - H]^-$. If cations such as sodium or potassium are present in the sample, adducted ion species such as $[M + Na]^+$, $[M + K]^+$ will be detected. Some multiply charged species, dimers, and trimers can also be formed.

Time-of-flight (TOF) mass spectrometry. MALDI is typically used in conjunction with TOF mass analyzers. TOF is well suited to the pulsed nature of laser desorption in MALDI. TOF is a rather simple device with a very high sensitivity and theoretically unlimited mass range. A potential applied across the source extracts and accelerates the ions from the source into the field-free drift zone. Ideally, if all ions leave the source at the same time with the same kinetic energy, then they will arrive at the detector according to the following equation (50–54):

$$t = \left(\frac{m}{2zeV}\right)^{1/2} D \quad (1)$$

where t is the flight time, z is the charge of the ion, e is the elementary charge, V is voltage applied across the source, and D is the length of the drift region.

Equation (1) shows that the flight time of a given ion is proportional to the ratio of its mass (m) and charge (z). The detector records the exact TOF of each ion and a mass spectrum is created. However, not all ions with the same m/z have the same exact time of flight. This leads to peak broadening and the resolution is thus lowered. This is caused primarily by the initial distribution of kinetic energies for ions of the same m/z values. A remarkable invention—the reflectron—was introduced by Mamyrin in 1973 (55–58). Although the reflectron does not change the initial kinetic energy of the ions, it corrects for kinetic-energy differences by allowing those ions with the same m/z but with greater kinetic energy to penetrate farther into the reflectron before they are reflected. Conversely, those ions with lower kinetic energy are bounced sooner. As a result, the differences in times of flight are minimized and spectral resolution is improved. Another approach to enhance spectral resolution is delayed extraction (DE). By introducing a time delay between ion formation and ion extraction from the source, ions are allowed to rearrange their positions according to their initial velocities so that those with higher velocities will gain less energy from the extraction field when it is switched on (53).

Post-source decay (PSD) fragment ion mass analysis. Abundant fragmentation occurs in the mass spectrometer and can provide structural information. Since fragment ions are generally formed in the field-free drift region, after the ions have left the ionization source, this phenomenon is called PSD. This term is also used for the method of observing these fragment ions. In linear-TOF mode, no fragment ions are detected because an intact molecular ion arrives at the detector at the same time as its decay products. With a few modifications, a reflectron TOF-MS can be used to analyze fragment ions. A reflectron separates ions based on their kinetic energy and the kinetic energy of a fragment ion is directly proportional to its fractional mass. Thus, when the ions enter the reflectron, fragment ions are turned around earlier than their respective precursors and arrive at the detector sooner. The product ions are not all in focus. In order to obtain a complete PSD spectrum, spectra are collected at different reflectron voltages. At each reflectron voltage, a narrow mass spectral range is well focused. After acquisition of these multiple spectra, the well-focused ranges are then "stitched" together to produce the PSD spectrum (59). Even though this procedure is time-consuming and requires relatively large amounts of sample to complete the multiple acquisitions, it is a suitable alternative to MS/MS to obtain structural information.

3.3. MALDI MS Applied to Phospholipid Analysis

3.3.1. In Vitro Analysis of Phospholipids in Crude Extracts

A critical step in the analysis of phospholipids by MALDI-MS is the choice of the matrix. Among the various matrices tried in the first applications of MALDI to phospholipid analysis, sinapinic acid, 2,5-dihydroxybenzoic acid (2,5-DHB), α-cyano-4-hydroxycinnamic acid, and esculetin (6,7-dihydroxycoumarin) gave the best results (60–62). Schiller and coworkers reported that 2,5-DHB produced excellent crystallization and signal-to-noise ratio (S/N) (63–65). Since then, 2,5-DHB has become the most popular matrix for phospholipid detection as positive ions. It can be dissolved in methanol or chloroform–methanol (either saturated solutions or 0.50 M).

When analyzing crude biological extracts, the presence of Na^+ and K^+ leads to the formation of at least three possible cationic adducts for a given phospholipid, $[M + H]^+$, $[M + Na]^+$, and $[M + K]^+$. This causes not only loss of sensitivity but also spectral complexity and overlaps. In addition, when acquiring positive-ion spectra, peaks related to sphingomyelins (SMs) and phosphatidylcholines (PCs) tend to overwhelm the traces due to the presence of a permanent positive charge in their choline head group (see Fig. 1). Therefore, the detection of other PL classes without a permanent positive charge is quite difficult. This poses a significant problem for the detection of other lipid species since PCs are the very abundant phospholipids in most biomembranes.

To reduce spectral complexity due to the presence of multiple adducts for the same phospholipid and to enhance sensitivity, either a strong cation-exchange resin (66) or CsCl crystals (66, 67) can be added directly to the crude extract. The quantitative exchange results in virtually only protonated (cation-exchange resin) or Cs^+-adducts (CsCl crystals). Using either approach, the quantification is simplified and the precision is enhanced since only one type of adduct (rather than two or three) is produced.

To enable the detection and identification of PL classes with ionization efficiencies lower than those of SMs and PCs, negative-ion mass spectra can be acquired. Due to its acidity, 2,5-DHB does not produce negative-ion spectra of suitable S/N. After testing several neutral and basic matrices, *para*-nitroaniline (PNA) proved to be an advantageous alternative to the use of 2,5-DHB (66). PNA increases the relative amount of deprotonated species and improves the sensitivity of negative-ion mass spectra. This matrix allowed the detection (in both positive and negative modes) and conclusive identification of species in natural mixtures of PEs and PE plasmalogens (PEps) even in mixtures containing SMs and PCs. Although some cations related to PCs and PEs overlapped in positive-ion spectra, these interferences were eliminated in the negative mode as only the deprotonated forms of PEs and PEps were detectable and those of SMs and PCs were absent due to their neutrality (66).

Our group has applied these two matrices to the analysis of porcine-lens phospholipids, rich in PCs and SMs (68). Although the absolute quantification of the various PL classes detectable in negative-ion spectra was affected by differences in ionization efficiencies, the trends in compositional changes between cortical and nuclear-fiber PLs were in agreement with those obtained by P-31 NMR spectroscopy. For porcine lenses, PCs, PEs and phosphatidylinositols (PIs) exhibited the greatest depletions in going from cortical to nuclear membranes. Among their individual species, those with two or more sites of unsaturation suffered the most significant reduction.

Despite significant progress in the MALDI MS analysis of PLs, improvements in sensitivity are still necessary in the detection of anionic PL classes in the negative mode. High sensitivity cannot be achieved with acidic matrices because deprotonation is hindered, thus precluding sufficient formation of PL negative ions (68–70). Basic matrices lead to improved S/N in negative mode detection. Indeed, a previous report by Fitzgerald et al. evaluated an extensive group of basic organic compounds as MALDI matrices for the detection of acid-sensitive proteins and oligonucleotides (69).

Among them, 2-(2-aminoethylamino)-5-nitropyridine (AAN), showed relatively high basicity (pH ~ 10) and strong absorptivity in the near UV region ($\varepsilon \sim 19{,}000\ M^{-1}\ cm^{-1}$ at 354 nm) (69). For this reason, and to expand the selection of suitable matrices for the study on anionic phospholipids, AAN was tested (71). The detection of phosphatidyl-ethanolamines (PEs), -serines (PSs), -glycerols (PGs), and -inositols (PIs) as anions was possible in simple mixtures and in a crude methanolic soybean extract. The relative ionization efficiency (RIE) was highest for PIs and decreased for PGs, PSs, and PEs. Compared to DHB and PNA, AAN resulted in greater sensitivity than the other tested matrices for the detection of PL classes in the negative mode. AAN also produced more homogeneous spots than DHB or PNA. This enables automation of the data acquisition and improves reproducibility. Relative standard deviations of 1–15% can be achieved with MALDI MS (66, 68, 72, 73).

Overall, over the last decade MALDI MS has become a popular approach for the analysis of phospholipids. However, most of the published applications are of qualitative nature. This is a consequence of the different RIEs for the various phospholipid classes and the tedious nature of the data analysis. The quantification is possible but it requires the use of internal standards that belong to same class as the phospholipids to be quantified but differ in the acyl chain length and/or degree of unsaturation (74). Furthermore, if quantitative data are sought, the control of the laser fluence is critical. We have observed photolytic loss of head groups, particularly for PCs, as the laser fluence is increased (68). For this reason, it is important to establish the minimal fluence needed to desorb/ionize the analytes without causing the loss of the head groups. This can be easily monitored in the low range of m/z, e.g., less than 200.

3.3.2. Imaging of Phospholipids in Tissues and Cells

The first applications of MALDI MS for tissue imaging focused on peptides and proteins in thin tissue slices (74, 75). In this powerful approach first reported by Caprioli et al. (74), the matrix is deposited onto fresh or blotted samples prior to spectral acquisition. Detection of specific proteins throughout the tissue is then accomplished by MALDI-TOF MS (41, 76, 77).

The imaging of phospholipids can be done by TOF-secondary-ion mass spectrometry (SIMS) (78). For example, TOF-SIMS has been applied to image cholesterol and the phosphocholine head group in cells imprinted on a silver surface (79). Although this method provides excellent spatial resolution (~0.5 μm), the detection of phosphocholine does not allow the differentiation of phosphatidylcholines (PCs) from sphingomyelins (SMs) or DHSMs, as they all have the same head group.

In vitro studies of phospholipids in mammalian lenses have revealed interesting correlations between the nonuniform distribution of glycero- and sphingophospholipids and different spatial

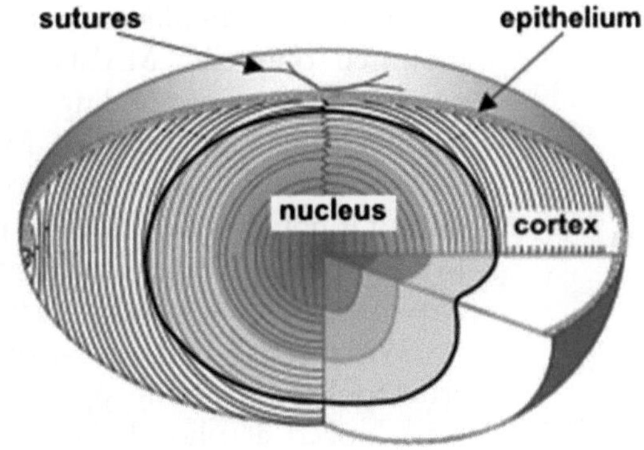

Fig. 3. Diagram of an adult human lens. The oldest fibers are located in the inner nucleus whereas the youngest are in the outer cortical region.

regions where lens cells are present at various stages of differentiation (80, 81). Specifically, for all mammalian lenses investigated, the ratio of PCs to SMs is highest in the superficial cortical fibers and reaches a minimum in the inner nucleus, where the fiber cells are present in a state of senescence (see Fig. 3 for a diagram of an adult lens). This trend is followed regardless of age. The differences between the actual ratios in the outer cortical and inner nuclear fibers are, however, more pronounced in older lenses. Furthermore, greater relative levels of PCs were found in the expanding lateral membranes located in the equatorial annular lens regions, whereas SMs appeared enriched in the fiber terminal ends at the anterior and posterior lens poles, also called sutures (81).

To demonstrate the feasibility of imaging phospholipids in lens tissue, we reported the first in situ profiling of SMs and PCs in bovine lenses using PNA as the matrix (82). Initial trials with 2,5-DHB did not yield spectra of high sensitivity. The quantification of the two phospholipids was carried out and validated by comparison with P-31 NMR results. Clearly, this validation is only applicable to these two lipids that, due to identical nature of their head group (phosphocholine), have comparable RIEs.

Besides the matrix, the thickness of the tissue slice and its consistency affect the ionization step greatly. Thinner slices (less that 50 μm) give the best signals. Due to the significant changes in the protein and lipid content of the lens (much harder nucleus than cortex), it is difficult to obtain whole slices that are thinner than 50 μm. For that reason, we fixed the tissue prior to analysis. Glutaraldehyde led to extensive acidic hydrolysis of the phospholipids. Formaldehyde, on the other hand, did not cause degradation of the lipids. The following protocol gave good results: First, the lens sections were kept in the fixing reagent for only 18 h. After this time period, the tissue, though hardened, allowed for easy slicing and transfer onto the MALDI plate. The typical drying step with ethanol was skipped to preclude the possible loss of lipids. Instead, the tissue was washed with deionized water for only 5 min to minimize cross-linking reversal. Once dry, the slices were mounted onto the MALDI plate using double-sided adhesive tape. Signals corresponding to SMs, DHSMs and PCs could be readily seen. The ability of MALDI-MS to image fixed tissues provides a useful alternative to in situ analysis of phospholipids, since it is not always possible to perform the studies on fresh tissue. In addition, lipid composition may change with fresh tissues due to enzymatic or chemical degradation during prolonged MS analysis.

Without extraction or separation steps, MALDI-MS is a powerful tool for spatial mapping of lipids. Since then, other groups have looked at phospholipids in liver (83), kidneys (84), brain (85–92). There are, however, important challenges to be addressed. Among them is the detection of charged PLs that yield very weak or no signals in positive-ion spectra. Therefore, it is imperative to enhance the sensitivity of negative-ion spectra. The second consideration is the large amount of experimental data generated during the imaging process. Automation of both data acquisition and treatment are now being implemented for PL imaging. Finally, the spatial resolution and precision of the measurements must be improved. Since 2004, important advances in the application of the matrix have improved spatial resolution significantly. For example, Caprioli's group (93) developed an acoustic device that can spot the matrix droplets automatically and with high volume precision. Such challenges are worth pursuing to realize the great potential of MALDI-MS imaging in our pursuit to establish the spatial-specific roles of PLs as relevant participants in complex cell signaling pathways.

4. ^{31}P NMR Analysis of Phospholipids

A general overview of NMR methods is available in many standard textbooks (94–96), and in Chap. 6.

4.1. Background

^{31}P is an attractive nucleus for detecting phospholipid head groups by NMR spectroscopy because it is essentially 100% abundant, and has a high gyromagnetic ratio making it among the most sensitive NMR nuclei. With proton decoupling, a single ^{31}P resonance is seen for each phospholipid class, since most phospholipids have a single ^{31}P nucleus per molecule (exception: cardiolipin with two ^{31}P nuclei). With the proper delay between pulses—3–5 times the value of the longitudinal relaxation time T_1—the integrated area of each resonance can be used for the quantitative evaluation of the relative contribution of each phospholipid class. Furthermore, if an internal standard is added to the sample, the absolute content of each phospholipid can also be determined. This feature makes ^{31}P NMR a relatively fast approach for the quantitative analysis of phospholipids in crude extracts. There exists, however, the possibility of spectral overlap and variability in chemical shifts due to the composition and acidity of the sample. The paragraphs below address these concerns and offer methodologies to increase accuracy in the assignment of resonances and to remove spectral interferences.

4.2. Solvent Systems and Temperature Coefficients

Organic solvents: The analysis of phospholipids by ^{31}P NMR spectroscopy can be performed in either organic or aqueous solvents. However, in a pure organic solvent such as chloroform, the resonances of most phospholipids are very broad and overlap. For this reason, the addition of a polar solvent such as methanol is necessary. A ternary solvent mixture of chloroform, methanol, and 0.2 M Cs-EDTA in water (10:4:1, by volume) was introduced by Meneses and Glonek (97) and is one of the most used systems because it provides high spectral resolution. The mixture forms two phases, a major chloroform phase and a small aqueous phase. EDTA serves to complex and remove divalent cations such as calcium and magnesium, thus reducing line widths. Unfortunately, there are variations in the chemical shift of a given phospholipid class as reported in the literature (98–102). This is a result of the high sensitivity of the ^{31}P nucleus to small stereoelectronic changes (103). Indeed, the type and amount of counterions, the absolute and relative concentration of each lipid, pH, solvent composition, and temperature can and do affect the chemical shift and/or line-width of the resonances.

Regarding solvent composition, variable amounts of water and methanol in the chloroform phase in this ternary system affect the chemical shift (98, 100). The addition of very small amounts of water removed spectral overlap (104). Taking advantage of these effects, the resonances for phosphatidylcholine (PC) and its plasmalogen analog (PCp) were completely resolved by using a single-phase mixture of chloroform, methanol, and water (50:50:15, by volume) (105).

Temperature is another variable that can be easily changed to improve spectral resolution in organic solvents (68, 73, 81, 104, 106–108). For example, in our studies of phospholipids in mammalian lenses, different temperatures allowed the resolution of the resonances corresponding to SM and phosphatidylserine (PS), as well as those due to DHSM and the ether-linked analog of phosphatidylethanolamine (PEe).

Because of the various factors that affect the ^{31}P resonances of PLs in the ternary solvent system, chemical shifts alone can lead to incorrect assignments of PL resonances. For this reason, temperature coefficients can and should be used as additional parameters in the identification of PL resonances in complex biological mixtures.

To evaluate these coefficients, spectra are acquired at three or more temperatures and the rate of change in chemical shift with temperature ($\Delta\delta/\Delta T$) is determined. The temperature coefficients for various glycero- and sphingophospholipids have been reported recently for the chloroform–methanol–0.2 M Cs-EDTA solvent

Table 1
Temperature coefficients ($\Delta\delta/\Delta T$) of PLs using different solvents

PL	MeOH/$CHCl_3$/H_2O pH $\approx$ 6.7 ($\Delta\delta/\Delta T \pm$ SD) ($\times 10^{-3}$ ppm/°C)	NaCho/EDTA (200/10 mM) pH = 7.7 ($\Delta\delta/\Delta T \pm$ SD) ($\times 10^{-3}$ ppm/°C)
PA	−(3.1 ± 0.2)	−(5.75 ± 0.07)
PC	−(0.3 ± 0.2)	0 (reference)
LPC	(2.2 ± 0.3)	0.2
PG	−(0.2 ± 0.1)	−(0.5 ± 0.01)
LPG	2.0	−0.1
PE	(5.5 ± 0.2)	(1.1 ± 0.05)
PEe	(5.6 ± 0.3)	(1.22 ± 0.04)
PEp	(5.8 ± 0.3)	(1.08 ± 0.05)
LPE	(6.5 ± 0.2)	(0.95 ± 0.05)
LPEe	(6.7 ± 0.3)	(1.26 ± 0.04)
LPEp	(6.8 ± 0.4)	(1.25 ± 0.05)
PI	(3.0 ± 0.2)	3.3
LPI	4.3	2.5
PS	(8.0 ± 0.1)	(4.71 ± 0.03)
LPS	(8.7 ± 0.6)	(2.9 ± 0.02)
SM	0 (reference)	(−0.16 ± 0.00)
DHSM	−(1.4 ± 0.1)	−(0.33 ± 0.00)
CL	0.5	N/A
S-1P	N/A	3.1
DHS-1P	N/A	3.3
Cer-1-P		−2.05

system (108). Table 1 incorporates the temperature coefficients reported by Estrada et al. as well as the values measured in aqueous solvents (see next section).

The listed values indicate the strong role played by H-bonds between the phosphate and head groups in the changes of chemical shift with temperature. The smallest temperature coefficients were observed for sphingomyelin (that was chosen as reference), phosphatidylcholine, phosphatidylglycerol, DHSM, and cardiolipin. The resonances for phospholipids with protonated head groups, such as phosphatidylserine and phosphatidylethanolamine, exhibited the highest values, suggesting the presence of a H-bond between the protonated amino group and the phosphate moiety. As the temperature is increased, this H-bond is weakened and the chemical shift increases. Conversely, the lowest and, in fact, negative values were measured for phospholipids with an exposed phosphate group: phosphatide, the conjugate of phosphatidic acid as well as ceramide-1-phosphate and dihydroceramide-1-phosphate. The nature of the interfacial linkages—diacyl, alkyl-acyl, and alkenyl-acyl—did not affect the temperature coefficients significantly for phospholipids with the same head group but led to slight variations in chemical shifts. All lyso analogs, with only one hydrophobic tail at the sn-1 position, exhibited greater temperature coefficients than the corresponding parent phospholipids. This increase was attributed to the presence of an extra OH at the sn-2 position, capable of forming another H-bond with the phosphate group.

Aqueous solvents: When phospholipids are added to water, multilamellar liposomes are formed. The ^{31}P resonances observed for these liposomes are very broad. To alleviate this problem, detergents can be added to form small mixed micelles. Natural bile salts are among the most attractive detergents because of the very small size of the micelles formed by these facial amphiphiles in water (109). At concentrations close to the critical micelle concentration (between 10 and 20 mM), primary micelles are formed. Primary micelles formed by natural bile salts, such as sodium salts of cholate, deoxycholate, taurocholate, deoxytaurocholate are thermodynamically stable and exhibit low aggregation numbers, less than 20 (110–115). As the detergent concentration is increased, secondary micelles are formed (114). Because the phospholipids are not tightly attached to each other within these micelles, very narrow line widths can be achieved and it is possible, in some cases, to resolve phospholipids with the same head group but with different hydrophobic tails (107, 116–120).

Due to the sensitivity of some chemical shifts to temperature and pH, it is possible to alleviate or remove spectral overlaps by changing either or both experimental variables. Indeed, the resolution of resonances for several common phospholipids has been demonstrated (121). Table 1 lists the temperature coefficients evaluated for a selected group of phospholipids and their metabolites. It is important to note that with sodium cholate, the pH cannot be lowered below 6.8 due to the precipitation of the cholic acid. At the higher pH values (pH > 8–9), basic hydrolysis ensues and leads to the generation of lysophospholipids. For that reason, the analysis should be carried out at neutral or near neutral pH values and temperature changes can be applied to remove overlaps. The temperature coefficients measured for mixed micelles of sodium cholate in aqueous media are listed in Table 1.

In addition, the combination of both dependences is valuable in the biophysical characterization of phospholipids. Figure 4 shows the interesting behavior of the temperature coefficients for three

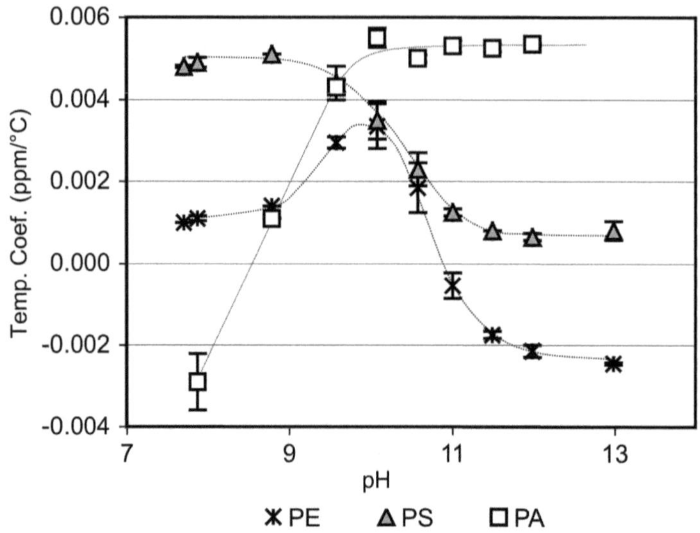

Fig. 4. pH dependence of the temperature coefficients. Coefficients were determined as described in the text for phosphatidylethanolamine (PE), phosphatidylserine (PS), and phosphatide (PA). From ref. (121).

common phospholipids (phosphatide, PA; phosphatidylethanolamine, PE, and phosphatidylserine, PS) as they undergo deprotonation.

In the case of PA, a change from negative to positive coefficients is observed as the final deprotonation occurs. The deprotonation of the NH_3^+ group in PS and PE also affects the temperature coefficients. These trends have been explained in terms of alterations in the H-bonding networks formed in the mixed micelles of sodium cholate (121). Finally, we have used these temperature coefficients and pH dependences to re-evaluate the composition of human lens membranes. Indeed, several of the initial assignments published in 1991 (19) were found to be incorrect (122). The revised composition revealed the preferential age-dependent depletion of diacyl- and alkenyl-acyl phospholipids thus resulting in a relative enrichment of alkyl-acyl phospholipids and their lyso forms (122).

5. Conclusions

The key of any type of thorough and accurate analysis lies in a multifaceted approach that can provide complementary and redundant information. The combination of mass spectrometry and P-31 NMR spectroscopy is such an approach. Whereas P-31 NMR spectroscopy provides little or no information on the composition of the hydrophobic tails, mass spectrometry does. On the other hand, the wide range of ionization efficiencies for the various phospholipid classes makes their quantitative analysis more tedious since the use of internal standards is needed. However, if a semiquantitative analysis is acceptable, relative ionization efficiencies evaluated in model systems may be used.

Mass spectrometry does offer much greater sensitivity than P-31 NMR in the analysis of phospholipids. Indeed, while femtomoles of lipids can be readily detected by MALDI-MS, only nano- to micromoles can be currently analyzed by NMR. Furthermore, the rigorous analysis of the structure of each phospholipid can be achieved by tandem-MS or by the more time-consuming PSD mentioned earlier in this chapter. MALDI-MS and DESI-MS offer the ability to image tissues with high spatial resolution. However, mass spectroscopic approaches are, at this time, destructive. P-31 NMR spectroscopy can be used for in vivo analysis of phospholipids, but the spatial resolution and sensitivity are relatively poor.

Overall, both approaches are individually robust, but their combination is even more powerful. Many challenges remain and are listed below for each of the two methodologies described in this chapter.

For P-31 NMR spectroscopy:

1. Accurate assignment of phospholipid resonances is an overlooked concern that needs to be addressed as we continue to recognize the remarkable variety of types of phospholipids.
2. Improvement in both sensitivity and spatial resolution for in situ or in vivo analysis
3. Development of new solvent systems that allow the resolution of species with different hydrophobic tails corresponding to the same phospholipid class. For MALDI-MS:
   (a) Because the chemical nature of the phospholipids cannot be changed, it is unlikely that the differences in ionization efficiencies can be surmounted. However, it is not completely unreasonable to predict that well designed chemical-derivatization steps could reduce these differences.
   (b) Chemical derivatization could also be paramount for the improvement of spatial resolution in the imaging of phospholipids in tissues. Subcellular imaging would be thus possible.
   (c) Further development of inorganic matrices in the nano- and subnano size range could also improve sensitivity, particularly in the study of small molecules.

Acknowledgments

The ongoing, 25-year collaboration with Professor Douglass Borchman is most deeply appreciated. The discussions and generous donation of animal ocular tissue by the former Director of the Louisville Zoo, Dr. William Foster, and current veterinarians,

Dr. Roy Burns and Dr. Zoole Gymesi are thankfully acknowledged. Professor Donald DuPré's theoretical predictions of P-31 chemical shifts have been most helpful for the interpretation of experimental trends. Without the funding provided by the National Eye Institute many of the studies cited in this chapter would not have been completed. Finally, to the many students in our graduate program that carried out these studies, a heartfelt thank-you.

Glossary

AAN	2-(2-Aminoethylamino)-5-nitropyridine; a basic organic matrix that promotes the generation of anions.
APCI	Atmospheric pressure chemical ionization.
DHB	2,5-Dihydroxybenzoic acid, one of the matrices most commonly used for the MALDI-MS analysis of small molecules, including phospholipids. Its acidic character facilitates the formation of cations.
Electrospray/ nanospray	Mild ionization technique involving nebularization and a high electric field at a metallic nozzle. Compatible with online chromatography as well as direct infusion, and results primarily in molecular ions.
MALDI	Matrix-assisted laser desorption/ionization, a commonly used means of ionizing and vaporizing an analyte for introduction into a mass spectrometer.
PC, PE, PI, PS	Phosphatidylcholine, phosphatidylethanolamine, phosphatidylinositol, phosphatidylserine, common phospholipids (PL) differing at the head group moiety.
Plasmalogens	Ether lipids where the first position of glycerol bears a vinyl residue in an ether linkage rather than an ester. The double bond next to the ether bond.
PNA	*Para*-nitroaniline, a nearly neutral matrix used in the MALDI-MS analysis of phospholipids in both positive and negative modes. It also enables imaging of phospholipids in tissues.
Sphingolipids	Class of lipids based on sphingosine, which has a serine backbone. Different derivatives on the serine hydroxyl give different family members such as ceramide and sphingomyelin (SM).
Temperature coefficient	Variation of, for example, chemical shift with temperature. Often linear, and then defined as $d\delta/dT$. The sign and magnitude may provide clues about interactions, such as hydrogen bonding.

References

1. Gennis R. Biomembranes: molecular structure and function. New York: Springer; 1989.
2. Voet D, Voet JG. Biochemistry. 2nd ed. New York: Wiley & Sons; 1995. p. 1288–90.
3. Brites P, Waterham HR, Wanders RJA. Functions and biosynthesis of plasmalogens in health and disease. Biochim Biophys Acta. 2004;1636(2–3):219–31.
4. Brosche T, Platt D. Mini-review—the biological significance of plasmalogens in defense against oxidative damage. Exp Gerontol. 1998;33(5):363–9.
5. Garg ML, Haerdi JC. The biosynthesis and functions of plasmalogens. J Clin Biochem Nutr. 1993;14(2):71–82.
6. Zimmerman GA, et al. The platelet-activating factor signaling system and its regulators in syndromes of inflammation and thrombosis. Crit Care Med. 2002;30(5):S294–301.
7. Kulikov VI, Muzya GI. Ether lipids and platelet-activating factor: evolution and cellular function. Biochemistry (Mosc). 1997;62(10):1103–8.
8. Greiner JV, et al. Phospholipids in meibomian gland secretion. Ophthalmic Res. 1996;28(1):44–9.
9. Byrdwell WC, et al. Separation and characterization of the unknown phospholipid in human lens membranes. Invest Ophthalmol Vis Sci. 1994;35(13):4333–43.
10. Ferguson SR, Borchman D, Yappert MC. Confirmation of the identity of the major phospholipid in human lens membranes. Invest Ophthalmol Vis Sci. 1996;37(8):1703–6.
11. Kok JW, et al. Dihydroceramide biology. Structure-specific metabolism and intracellular localization. J Biol Chem. 1997;272(34):21128–36.
12. Folch J, Lees M, Sloane Stanley G. A simple method for the isolation and purification of total lipids from animal tissues. J Biol Chem. 1957;226:497–509.
13. Byrdwell WC, et al. 31P NMR quantification and monophasic solvent purification of human and bovine lens phospholipids. Lipids. 2002;37(11):1087–92.
14. Christie WW. Lipid analysis. 3rd ed. Bridgwater: Oily Press; 2003.
15. Christie WW. Separation of phospholipid classes by high-performance liquid chromatography. In: Christie WW, editor. Advances in lipid methodology—three. Dundee: Oily Press; 1996. p. 77–107.
16. Christie WW. The lipid library; 2007. http://www.lipidlibrary.co.uk/topics/hplc_pl/index.htm
17. Broekhuyse RM. Lipids in tissues of the eye. IV. Influence of age and species differences on the phospholipid composition of the lens. Biochim Biophys Acta. 1970;218(3):546–8.
18. Bloemendal H, et al. The plasma membranes of eye lens fibres. Biochemical and structural characterization. Cell Differ. 1972;1(2):91–106.
19. Merchant TE, et al. Human crystalline lens phospholipid analysis with age. Invest Ophthalmol Vis Sci. 1991;32(3):549–55.
20. Christie WW. Recent developments in high-performance liquid and gas-chromatography of lipids. Rev Franc Corps Gras. 1991;38(5–6):155–60.
21. Christie WW. A stable silver-loaded column for the separation of lipids by high-performance liquid-chromatography. J High Res Chromatogr Chromatogr Commun. 1987;10(3):148–50.
22. Olsson NU, Salem N. Molecular species analysis of phospholipids. J Chromatogr B. 1997;692(2):245–56.
23. Hutchins PM, Barkley RM, Murphy RC. Separation of cellular nonpolar neutral lipids by normal-phase chromatography and analysis by electrospray ionization mass spectrometry. J Lipid Res. 2008;49(4):804–13.
24. Whitehead SN, et al. Identification and quantitation of changes in the platelet activating factor family of glycerophospholipids over the course of neuronal differentiation by high-performance liquid chromatography electrospray ionization tandem mass spectrometry. Anal Chem. 2007;79(22):8539–48.
25. Pacetti D, et al. High performance liquid chromatography-tandem mass spectrometry of phospholipid molecular species in eggs from hens fed diets enriched in seal blubber oil. J Chromatogr A. 2005;1097(1–2):66–73.
26. Beermann C, et al. sn-position determination of phospholipid-linked fatty acids derived from erythrocytes by liquid chromatography electrospray ionization ion-trap mass spectrometry. Lipids. 2005;40(2):211–8.
27. Byrdwell WC. Dual parallel liquid chromatography/dual mass spectrometry (LC2/MS2) of bovine brain total lipid extract. J Liq Chromatogr R T. 2003;26(19):3147–81.
28. Kakela R, Somerharju P, Tyynela J. Analysis of phospholipid molecular species in brains

from patients with infantile and juvenile neuronal-ceroid lipofuscinosis using liquid chromatography-electrospray ionization mass spectrometry. J Neurochem. 2003;84(5): 1051–65.

29. Hallgren B, Ryhage R, Stenhagen E. The mass spectra of methyl oleate, methyl linoleate and methyl linolenate. Acta Chem Scand. 1959;13:845–7.
30. Karas M, et al. Laser desorption ionization mass-spectrometry of proteins of mass 100 000 to 250 000 dalton. Angew Chem Int Ed. 1989;28(6):760–1.
31. Hunt AN, et al. Highly saturated endonuclear phosphatidylcholine is synthesized in situ and colocated with CDP-choline pathway enzymes. J Biol Chem. 2001;276(11):8492–9.
32. Hunt AN, et al. Lipidomic analysis of the molecular specificity of a cholinephosphotransferase in situ. Biochem Soc Trans. 2004;32:1060–2.
33. Hunt AN, et al. Use of mass spectrometry-based lipidomics to probe PITP alpha (phosphatidylinositol transfer protein alpha) function inside the nuclei of PITP alpha(+/+) and PITP alpha(−/−) cells. Biochem Soc Trans. 2004;32:1063–5.
34. Burdge GC, Postle AD. Selective changes to phosphatidylcholine and phosphatidylethanolamine molecular species in the developing fetal guinea pig liver and plasma. Reprod Nutr Dev. 2004;44(6):571–82.
35. Han X, et al. Toward fingerprinting cellular lipidomes directly from biological samples by two-dimensional electrospray ionization mass spectrometry. Anal Biochem. 2004;330(2): 317–31.
36. Takats Z, et al. Mass spectrometry sampling under ambient conditions with desorption electrospray ionization. Science. 2004;306 (5695):471–3.
37. Jackson AU, et al. Salt tolerance of desorption electrospray ionization (DESI). J Am Soc Mass Spectrom. 2007;18:2218–25.
38. Cotte-Rodriguez I, Mulligan CC, Cooks G. Non-proximate detection of small and large molecules by desorption electrospray ionization and desorption atmospheric pressure chemical ionization mass spectrometry: instrumentation and applications in forensics, chemistry, and biology. Anal Chem. 2007;79 (18):7069–77.
39. Ifa DR, et al. Development of capabilities for imaging mass spectrometry under ambient conditions with desorption electrospray ionization (DESI). Int J Mass Spectrom. 2007; 259(1–3):8–15.
40. Wiseman JM, et al. Tissue imaging at atmospheric pressure using desorption electrospray ionization (DESI) mass spectrometry. Angew Chem Int Ed. 2006;45(43):7188–92.
41. Wiseman JM, et al. Mass spectrometric profiling of intact biological tissue by using desorption electrospray ionization. Angew Chem Int Ed. 2005;44(43):7094–7.
42. Manicke NE, et al. Desorption electrospray ionization (DESI) mass spectrometry and tandem mass spectrometry (MS/MS) of phospholipids and sphingolipids: Ionization, adduct formation, and fragmentation. J Am Soc Mass Spectrom. 2008;19(4):531–43.
43. Wiseman JM, et al. Ambient molecular imaging by desorption electrospray ionization mass spectrometry. Nat Protoc. 2008;3(3): 517–24.
44. Karas M, et al. Ultraviolet-laser desorption ionization mass-spectrometry of femtomolar amounts of large proteins. Biomed Environ Mass Spectrom. 1989;18(9):841–3.
45. Karas M, Hillenkamp F. Laser desorption ionization of proteins with molecular masses exceeding 10000 daltons. Anal Chem. 1988;60(20):2299–301.
46. Karas M, et al. Matrix-assisted ultraviolet-laser desorption of nonvolatile compounds. Int J Mass Spectrom Ion Process. 1987;78:53–68.
47. Karas M, Bachmann D, Hillenkamp F. Influence of the wavelength in high-irradiance ultraviolet-laser desorption mass-spectrometry of organic-molecules. Anal Chem. 1985;57(14):2935–9.
48. Beavis RC. Matrix-assisted ultraviolet-laser desorption—evolution and principles. Org Mass Spectrom. 1992;27(6):653–9.
49. Beavis RC. Phenomenological models for matrix-assisted laser desorption ion yields near the threshold fluence. Org Mass Spectrom. 1992;27(8):864–8.
50. Cotter RJ. Time-of-flight mass-spectrometry—basic principles and current state. Time Flight Mass Spectrom. 1994;549:16–48.
51. Cotter RJ. Time-of-flight mass-spectrometry for the structural—analysis of biological molecules. Anal Chem. 1992;64(21): A1027–39.
52. Cotter RJ. Time-of-flight mass-spectrometry—an increasing role in the life sciences. Biomed Environ Mass Spectrom. 1989;18(8):513–32.
53. Cotter RJ. The new time-of-flight mass spectrometry. Anal Chem. 1999;71(13): 445A–51.
54. Tabet JC, Cotter RJ. Time-Resolved laser desorption mass-spectrometry. 2. Measurement

of the energy spread of laser desorbed ions. Int J Mass Spectrom Ion Process. 1983;54(1–2): 151–8.

55. Mamyrin BA. Time-of-flight mass spectrometry (concepts, achievements, and prospects). Int J Mass Spectrom. 2001;206(3):251–66.
56. Mamyrin BA. Laser-assisted reflectron time-of-flight mass-spectrometry. Int J Mass Spectrom Ion Process. 1994;131:1–19.
57. Ivanov MA, et al. Mass-reflectron for the study of laser irradiation interaction processes with molecules in an ultrasonic gas-jet. Zh Tekh Fiz. 1983;53(10):2039–44.
58. Mamyrin BA, et al. Mass-reflectron a new nonmagnetic time-of-flight high-resolution mass-spectrometer. Zh Eksp Teor Fiz. 1973;64(1):82–9.
59. Cotter RJ, Iltchenko S, Wang DX. The curved-field reflectron: PSD and CID without scanning, stepping or lifting. Int J Mass Spectrom. 2005;240(3):169–82.
60. Marto JA, et al. Structural characterization of phospholipids by matrix-assisted laser desorption/ionization Fourier transform ion cyclotron resonance mass spectrometry. Anal Chem. 1995;67(21):3979–84.
61. Harvey DJ. Matrix-assisted laser-desorption ionization mass-spectrometry of sphingo-lipids and glycosphingo-lipids. J Mass Spectrom. 1995;30(9):1311–24.
62. Solouki T, et al. Attomole biomolecule mass analysis by matrix-assisted laser desorption/ionization Fourier transform ion cyclotron resonance. Anal Chem. 1995;67(22):4139–44.
63. Schiller J, et al. Lipid analysis by matrix-assisted laser desorption and ionization mass spectrometry: a methodological approach. Anal Biochem. 1999;267(1):46–56.
64. Petkovic M, et al. The signal-to-noise ratio as the measure for the quantification of lysophospholipids by matrix-assisted laser desorption/ionisation time-of-flight mass spectrometry. Analyst. 2001;126(7):1042–50.
65. Benard S, et al. Experiments towards quantification of saturated and polyunsaturated diacylglycerols by matrix-assisted laser desorption and ionization time-of-flight mass spectrometry. Chem Phys Lipids. 1999;100(1–2): 115–25.
66. Estrada R, Yappert MC. Alternative approaches for the detection of various phospholipid classes by matrix-assisted laser desorption/ionization time-of-flight mass spectrometry. J Mass Spectrom. 2004;39: 412–22.
67. Schiller J, et al. CsCl as an auxiliary reagent for the analysis of phosphatidylcholine mixtures by matrix-assisted laser desorption and ionization time-of-flight mass spectrometry (MALDI-TOF MS). Chem Phys Lipids. 2001;113(1–2):123–31.
68. Estrada R, Yappert MC. Regional phospholipid analysis of porcine lens membranes by matrix-assisted laser desorption/ionization time-of-flight mass spectrometry. J Mass Spectrom. 2004;39(12):1531–40.
69. Fitzgerald MC, Parr GR, Smith LM. Basic matrices for the matrix-assisted laser-desorption ionization mass-spectrometry of proteins and oligonucleotides. Anal Chem. 1993;65 (22):3204–11.
70. Schiller J, et al. Recent applications of MALDI-TOF mass spectrometry and P-31 NMR spectroscopy in phospholipid research. Future Lipidol. 2007;1(1):115–25.
71. Lorkiewicz PK, Yappert MC. 2-(2-aminoethylamino)-5-nitropyridine (AAN) as a basic matrix for negative mode matrix-assisted laser desorption/ionization of phospholipids. J Mass Spectrom. 2009;44(1):137–43.
72. Oborina EM, Yappert MC. Effect of sphingomyelin versus dipalmitoylphosphatidylcholine on the extent of lipid oxidation. Chem Phys Lipids. 2003;123:223–32.
73. Rujoi M, et al. Isolation and lipid characterization of cholesterol-enriched fractions in cortical and nuclear human lens fibers. Invest Ophthalmol Vis Sci. 2003;44(4):1634–42.
74. Caprioli RM, Farmer TB, Gile J. Molecular imaging of biological samples: localization of peptides and proteins using MALDI-TOF MS. Anal Chem. 1997;69(23):4751–60.
75. Chaurand P, Stoeckli M, Caprioli RM. Direct profiling of proteins in biological tissue sections by MALDI mass spectrometry. Anal Chem. 1999;71(23):5263–70.
76. Stoeckli M, et al. Imaging mass spectrometry: a new technology for the analysis of protein expression in mammalian tissues. Nat Med. 2001;7(4):493–6.
77. Chaurand P, Caprioli RM. Direct profiling and imaging of peptides and proteins from mammalian cells and tissue sections by mass spectrometry. Electrophoresis. 2002;23(18): 3125–35.
78. Brunelle A, Laprevote O. Recent advances in biological tissue Imaging with time-of-flight secondary ion mass spectrometry: polyatomic ion sources, sample preparation, and applications. Curr Pharm Des. 2007;13 (32):3335–43.
79. Sjovall P, et al. Imaging of membrane lipids in single cells by imprint-imaging time-of-flight secondary ion mass spectrometry. Anal Chem. 2003;75(14):3429–34.

80. Yappert MC, Borchman D. Sphingolipids in human lens membranes: an update on their composition and possible biological implications. Chem Phys Lipids. 2004;129:1–20.
81. Yappert MC, et al. Glycero- versus sphingo-phospholipids: correlations with human and non-human mammalian lens growth. Exp Eye Res. 2003;76(6):725–34.
82. Rujoi M, Estrada R, Yappert MC. In situ MALDI-TOF MS regional analysis of neutral phospholipids in lens tissue. Anal Chem. 2004;76(6):1657–63.
83. Shimma S, et al. MALDI-based imaging mass spectrometry revealed abnormal distribution of phospholipids in colon cancer liver metastasis. J Chromatogr B Analyt Technol Biomed Life Sci. 2007;855(1):98–103.
84. Herring KD, Oppenheimer SR, Caprioli RM. Direct tissue analysis by matrix-assisted laser desorption ionization mass spectrometry: application to kidney biology. Semin Nephrol. 2007;27(6):597–608.
85. Jackson SN, et al. MALDI-ion mobility-TOFMS imaging of lipids in rat brain tissue. J Mass Spectrom. 2007;42(8):1093–8.
86. McLean JA, Ridenour WB, Caprioli RM. Profiling and imaging of tissues by imaging ion mobility-mass spectrometry. J Mass Spectrom. 2007;42(8):1099–105.
87. Jackson SN, Wang HYJ, Woods AS. In situ structural characterization of glycerophospholipids and sulfatides in brain tissue using MALDI-MS/MS. J Am Soc Mass Spectrom. 2007;18(1):17–26.
88. Woods AS, Jackson SN. Brain tissue lipidomics: direct probing using matrix-assisted laser desorption/ionization mass spectrometry. AAPS J. 2006;8(2):E391–5.
89. Jones JJ, et al. Characterizing the phospholipid profiles in mammalian tissues by MALDI FTMS. Anal Chem. 2006;78(9):3062–71.
90. Jackson SN, Wang HYJ, Woods AS. In situ structural characterization of phosphatidylcholines in brain tissue using MALDI-MS/MS. J Am Soc Mass Spectrom. 2005;16(12):2052–6.
91. Jackson SN, Wang HYJ, Woods AS. Direct profiling of lipid distribution in brain tissue using MALDI-TOFMS. Anal Chem. 2005;77(14):4523–7.
92. Jackson SN, Wang HYJ, Woods AS. Direct tissue analysis of phospholipids in rat brain using MALDI-TOFMS and MALDI-ion mobility-TOFMS. J Am Soc Mass Spectrom. 2005;16(2):133–8.
93. Aerni HR, Cornett DS, Caprioli RM. Automated acoustic matrix deposition for MALDI sample preparation. Anal Chem. 2006;78(3):827–34.
94. Claridge TDW. High-resolution NMR techniques in organic chemistry. San Diego: Elsevier; 1999.
95. Pochapsky TC, Pochapsky SS. NMR for physical and biological scientists. New York: Taylor & Francis; 2007.
96. Sanders JKM, Hunter BK. Modern NMR spectroscopy. A guide for chemists. Oxford: Oxford University Press; 1987.
97. Meneses P, Glonek T. P-31 NMR lipid analysis from biological sources. Biophys J. 1988; 53(2):A200.
98. Branca M, et al. ^{31}P nuclear magnetic resonance analysis of phospholipids in a ternary homogeneous system. Anal Biochem. 1995; 232(1):1–6.
99. Bosco MC, Culeddu N, Toffanin R, Pollesello P. Organic solvent systems for 31P nuclear magnetic resonance analysis of lecithin phospholipids: applications to two-dimensional gradient-enhanced 1H-detected heteronuclear multiple quantum coherence experiments. Anal Biochem. 1997;245(1):38–47.
100. Edzes HT, et al. Analysis of phospholipids in brain tissue by ^{31}P NMR at different compositions of the solvent system chloroform-methanol-water. Magn Reson Med. 1992;26(1):46–59.
101. Culeddu N, et al. ^{31}P NMR analysis of phospholipids in crude extracts from different sources: improved efficiency of the solvent system. Magn Reson Chem. 1998;36(12): 907–12.
102. Pearce JM, Komoroski RA. Analysis of phospholipid molecular species in brain by ^{31}P NMR spectroscopy. Magn Reson Med. 2000;44(2):215–23.
103. Gorestein DG, editor. Phosphorus-31 NMR: principles and applications. San Francisco: Academic; 1984. p. 7–36.
104. Sotirhos N, Herslof B, Kenne L. Quantitative analysis of phospholipids by ^{31}P-NMR. J Lipid Res. 1986;27(4):386–92.
105. Baumann CG, et al. Lipid differentiation in MP26 junction enriched membranes of bovine lens fiber cells. Biochim Biophys Acta. 1996;1303(2):145–53.
106. Estrada R, Borchman D, Yappert MC. Tracking phospholipid biogenesis by MALDI-TOFMS. Biophys J. 2005;88(1):354A.
107. Pearce JM, Komoroski RA. Analysis of phospholipid molecular species in brain by P-31 NMR spectroscopy. Magn Reson Med. 2000;44(2):215–23.

108. Estrada R, Stolowich N, Yappert MC. Influence of temperature on P-31 NMR chemical shifts of phospholipids and their metabolites. I. In chloroform-methanol-water. Anal Biochem. 2008;380(1):41–50.
109. Chen Y, et al. Facial amphiphiles. J Am Chem Soc. 1992;114(18):7319–20.
110. Hildebrand A, et al. Solubilization of negatively charged DPPC/DPPG liposomes by bile salts. J Colloid Interface Sci. 2004;279 (2):559–71.
111. Hildebrand A, et al. Thermodynamics of demicellization of mixed micelles composed of sodium oleate and bile salts. Langmuir. 2004;20(2):320–8.
112. Hildebrand A, et al. Temperature dependence of the interaction of cholate and deoxycholate with fluid model membranes and their solubilization into mixed micelles. Colloid Surf B. 2003;32(4):335–51.
113. Hildebrand A, et al. Bile salt induced solubilization of synthetic phosphatidylcholine vesicles studied by isothermal titration calorimetry. Langmuir. 2002;18(7):2836–47.
114. Garidel P, et al. Thermodynamic characterization of bile salt aggregation as a function of temperature and ionic strength using isothermal titration calorimetry. Langmuir. 2000;16 (12):5267–75.
115. Santhanalakshmi J, et al. Small-angle neutron scattering study of sodium cholate and sodium deoxycholate interacting micelles in aqueous medium. Proc Indian Acad Sci (Chem Sci). 2001;113(1):55–62.
116. Komoroski RA, et al. Phospholipid abnormalities in postmortem schizophrenic brains detected by P-31 nuclear magnetic resonance spectroscopy: a preliminary study. Psychiat Res Neuroim. 2001;106(3):171–80.
117. Pearce JM, et al. Analysis of saturated phosphatidylcholine in amniotic-fluid by P-31 NMR. Magn Reson Med. 1993;30(4):476–84.
118. Pearce JM, et al. Analysis of phospholipids in human amniotic fluid by ^{31}P NMR. Magn Reson Med. 1991;21(1):107–16.
119. Pearce JM, Komoroski RA. Resolution of phospholipid molecular species by ^{31}P NMR. Magn Reson Med. 1993;29(6):724–31.
120. Schiller J, Arnold K. Application of high resolution ^{31}P NMR spectroscopy to the characterization of the phospholipid composition of tissues and body fluids—a methodological review. Med Sci Monit. 2002;8(11):205–22.
121. Puppato A, et al. Effect of temperature and pH on P-31 nuclear magnetic resonances of phospholipids in cholate micelles. Chem Phys Lipids. 2007;150(2):176–85.
122. Estrada R, et al. Re-evaluation of the phospholipids composition in membranes of adult human lenses. Biochim Biophys Acta- Biomembranes. 2010;1798(3):303–311.

Chapter 13

The HumanCyc Pathway-Genome Database and Pathway Tools Software as Tools for Imaging and Analyzing Metabolomics Data

Pedro Romero

Abstract

Metabolomics analysis provides a window to the phenotypic responses to stimuli, including disease states and drug interventions. These responses are the end result of complex processes encoded by the organism's genome. This chapter describes a computational set of tools that can be of great assistance in all kinds of studies related to the metabolic network of an organism in the context of genomic information. These tools comprise (1) Pathway/Genome Databases (PGDBs) a high-level, last-generation database that relates metabolic information to an organism's genome and (2) Pathway Tools, a software suite designed to access and facilitate analysis on the PGDB information. In particular, we describe HumanCyc, the human PGDB, and explore its usefulness in analyzing and extracting knowledge from the data produced by metabolomics, transcriptomics, and other systemic experiments. In the so-called postgenomic era, the lack of sophistication of many biological databases and resources has become a hurdle for the development of complex analytical tools, especially at the systems biology level, and a common complaint by computational molecular biologists. Resources such as HumanCyc and Pathway Tools can change this situation by providing the developer with a computable encoding of biological knowledge and a sophisticated collection of computational tools to access it.

Key words: HumanCyc, Pathway-genome databases, systems biology

1. Pathway-Genome Databases and the Pathway Tools Software

Metabolomics is one of the experimental tools we can use to understand and analyze the complex processes encoded by an organism's genome. In general, to carry out systemic studies at the molecular level it is advantageous to assign the genome's protein products to biological networks such as the system of biochemical reactions and pathways that comprise an organism's metabolism, or the complex net of protein–protein interactions involved in signaling or regulatory processes. These assignments relate genes within a systemic context which facilitates the analysis of causal relationships when

Teresa Whei-Mei Fan et al. (eds.), *The Handbook of Metabolomics*, Methods in Pharmacology and Toxicology,
DOI 10.1007/978-1-61779-618-0_13, © Springer Science+Business Media New York 2012

studying the potential effects of specific changes to any element of the system, from the knockout of a gene to mutations, to environmental effects at the molecular level.

This chapter describes a computational set of tools that can be of great assistance in all kinds of studies related to the metabolic network of an organism in the context of genomic information. These tools comprise (1) Pathway/Genome Databases (PGDBs) a high-level, last-generation database that relates metabolic information to an organism's genome, and (2) Pathway Tools, a software suite designed to access and facilitate analysis on the PGDB information. In particular, we describe HumanCyc, the human PGDB, and explore its usefulness in analyzing and extracting knowledge from the data produced by metabolomics and other systemic experiments.

2. Pathway-Genome Databases

A PGDB is a type of Model Organism Database (MOD) that integrates information about the genes, proteins, metabolic network and genetic network of an organism. A PGDB describes the following:

- The genome of an organism—its chromosome(s), genes, and genome sequence
- The product of each gene
- The metabolic network of the organism—its pathways, reactions, enzymes, and metabolites

A PGDB can also include:

- The transporter complement of the organism
- The genetic network of the organism, including its operons (prokaryotes), transcription factors, and the interactions among transcription factors and their small-molecule ligands and with the DNA binding sites
- Signal transduction pathways

Figure 1 shows the organization of the data in a PGDB. The data enclosed by the green rectangle corresponds to the information found in a typical genomic database such as GenBank (1) or Ensembl (2), that is, the genomic maps (i.e., the location of genes in the organism's replicons—chromosomes or plasmids); information on the genes themselves, and information on the genes' products, mainly proteins.

A PGDB ties the genomic information to the organism's metabolic network through the gene products that catalyze biochemical reactions, that is, the organism's enzymes. This adds an extra layer of information to the organism's genome and allows for the study of metabolism not only as a network of biochemical reactions, but

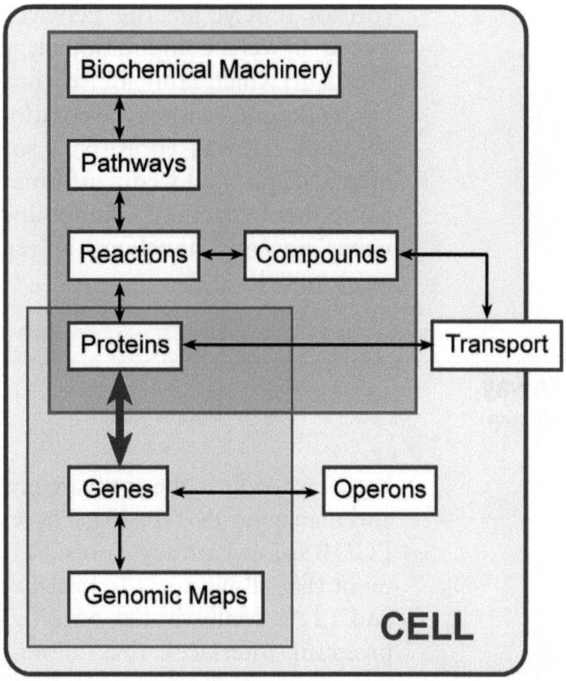

Fig. 1. Schematic representation of the data in a PGDB. Proteins, more specifically enzymes, provide the link between the genome of an organism and its metabolic network, as well as its genetic and (not shown) signaling networks.

also from a genomics perspective. Additionally, prokaryotic PGDBs are capable of holding both genetic (regulatory) and signaling networks, which augment the information available for systemic analyses.

PGDBs are built using an object-oriented database called a Frame Representation System (FRS) (3). In short, every biological object (such as a compound or gene) is stored in a frame bearing a unique ID. A frame has slots, in which attributes and connections to other frames can be stored as values. Slots can store single or multiple values, and individual values can be annotated with comments or literature references. As is the case in object-oriented databases in general, frames are organized in a class hierarchy.

A PGDB can be thought of as a symbolic computational theory of a species' metabolic functions and genetic interactions (4), encoding knowledge in a manner suitable for computational analysis. Indeed, encoding an organism's genome and biochemical network within the schema of a PGDB opens up new possibilities for computational analysis, because many important semantic relationships are described in a computable fashion.

BioCyc (see http://BioCyc.org/), a resource led by Peter Karp and his group at SRI International, is a collection including, as of Fall 2007, 371 PGDBs. The highly curated Tier 1 PGDBs at the core of BioCyc are the EcoCyc and MetaCyc DBs (5, 6). Tiers 2 and 3 were computationally predicted using Pathways Tools. Tier 2, to which HumanCyc, the PGDB described herein, belongs, has undergone moderate curation. PGDBs are viewed and edited through Pathway Tools (5), a software environment developed to query, display, and edit information about each pathway and its component reactions, compounds, enzymes, protein complexes, genes, operons, signaling, and regulation at the substrate and transcriptional level.

3. The Pathway Tools Software

Pathway Tools is the software environment developed for creating and managing PGDBs (5). There are two ways of interacting with a PGDB using Pathway Tools: (1) An interactive graphical environment that allows users to visualize and update the data in a PGDB and (2) a sophisticated ontology and database API (application program interface) that allow programs to perform complex queries, symbolic computations, and data mining on the contents of a PGDB. This API turns a Pathway Tools-managed PGDB into an extremely useful tool for analyzing metabolomics and other systemic data, as explained later, in the context of the HumanCyc PGDB.

The following high-level capabilities are provided by the main software components of the Pathway Tools (5).

3.1. The Pathway-Genome Navigator

The Navigator software provides a scientist user with the ability to interrogate a PGDB and visualize the results of a query in an intuitive, graphical fashion. It also provides analysis operations, such as whole metabolic-map comparisons across multiple organisms. The Navigator contains several visualization tools, each of which has been carefully crafted to generate a window of information for a given bioinformatics data type, such as operons or metabolic pathways. These visualization tools include:

- The pathway visualization, which produces automated layouts of metabolic pathways at multiple levels of detail (Fig. 2).
- The reaction visualization, which displays a biochemical transformation, such as enzymatic, transport, and signal-transduction reactions, including, for example, the subunit structure, cofactors, activators, and inhibitors of the catalyzing enzyme(s) (Fig. 3).
- The gene visualization, which lists the nucleotide position of the gene, the chromosome on which the gene is present, the gene product, and the pathway(s) in which that product is involved. In this view, the user can retrieve the nucleotide

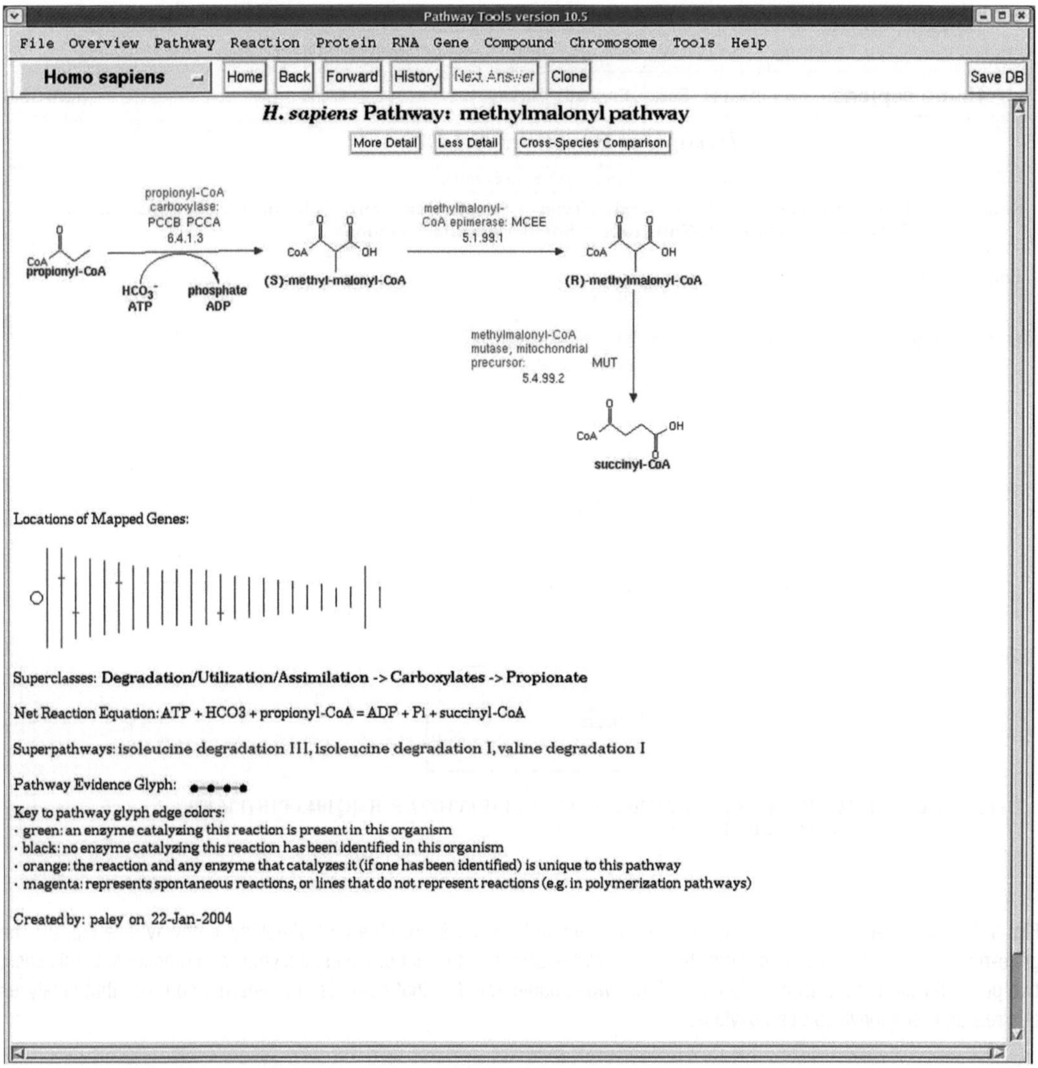

Fig. 2. Pathway visualization. The figure depicts the methylmalonyl pathway from the Human PGDB, HumanCyc. This detailed view shows the metabolites' structures and connections to other pathways in the metabolic network. Other information include the enzymes, EC numbers and genes related to each reaction. Clicking on any of the objects shown (reactions, genes, enzymes) will take the user to its corresponding page.

sequence of the gene and the amino-acid sequence of its product (Fig. 4).

- The chromosome viewer, which allows browsing of chromosomes and other replicons at multiple levels of resolution, showing genes, promoters, transcription factor binding sites, and transcription terminators (Fig. 5).
- The cellular overview visualization and the "omics" viewer, described later in the chapter.

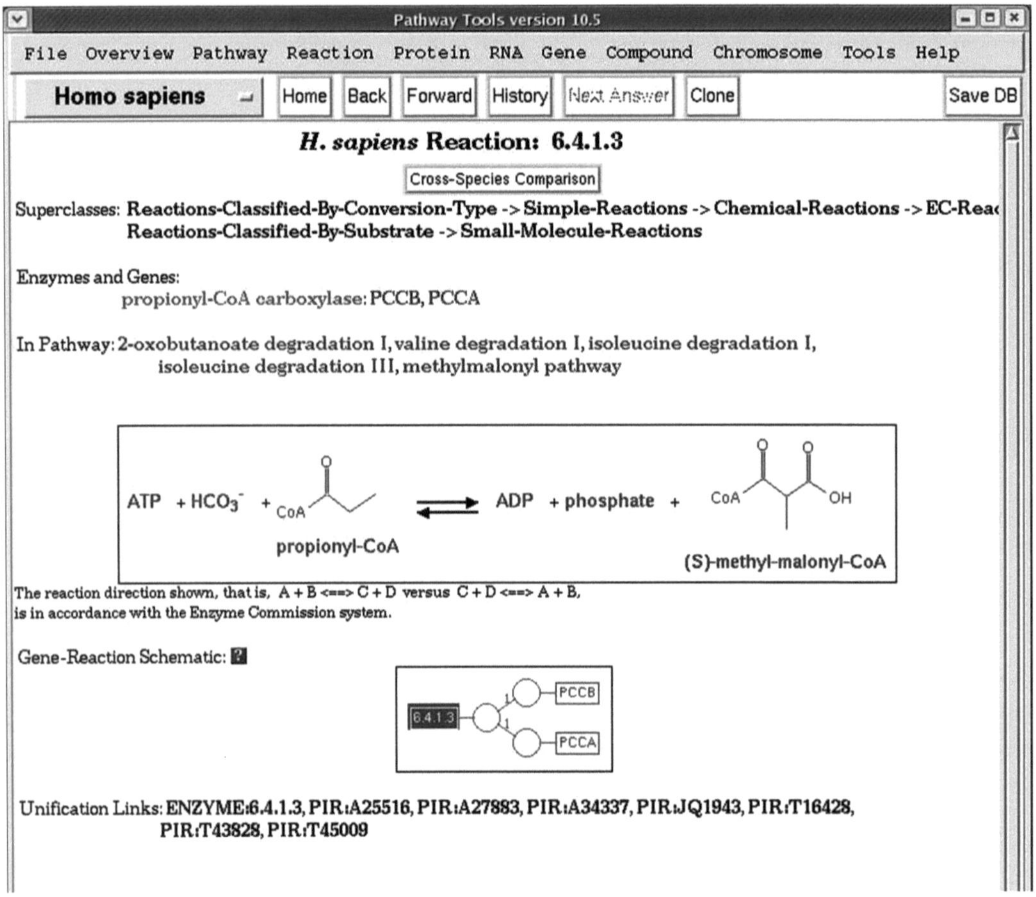

Fig. 3. Reaction visualization. This is the page for reaction EC 6.4.1.3 from the methylmalonyl pathway (see Fig. 2). The gene-reaction schematic at the *bottom* shows the relationship among a set of genes, enzymes and reactions. In this case, two genes (PCCA and PCCB) encode each of the two subunits (*circles*) that comprise the enzyme complex that catalyzes this reaction, propionyl-CoA carboxylase.

Queries supported by the navigator include (1) query objects by exact or substring match to a synonym for the object name, (2) query genes, reactions, pathways, and compounds using stored classification hierarchies, and (3) show a gene's position on the genomic map.

The elements in a Pathway Tools view are hyperlinked to other objects in the PGDB. For example, clicking on a compound in a reaction or pathway view will take the user to that compound's corresponding view. The same effect occurs when clicking enzyme or gene names, reaction arrows within a pathway, genes in a genomic map, and the like.

3.2. The PathoLogic Pathway Predictor

The PathoLogic program creates a new PGDB from an input file that describes the annotated genome of an organism, such as a

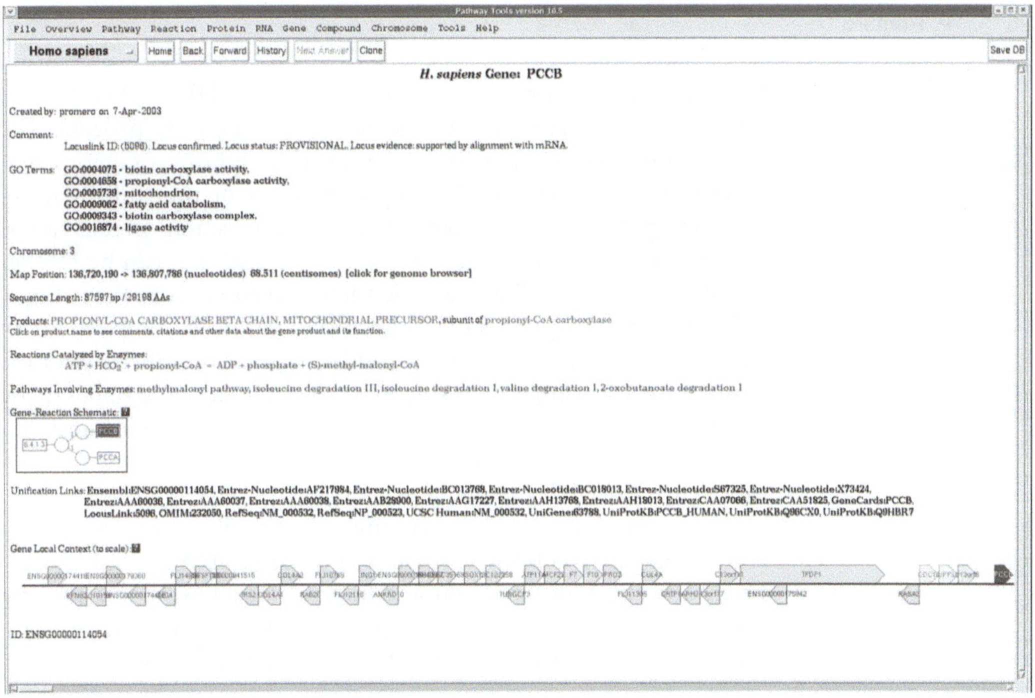

Fig. 4. Gene visualization. This figure shows the gene page for the PCCA gene in HumanCyc. The gene encodes for one of the subunits of propionyl-CoA carboxylase (see Fig. 3). Notice again the gene-reaction schematic at the *bottom*, along with a schematic depicting the exon/intron organization of the gene. The gene-reaction schematic appears in the reaction (Fig. 3), protein and gene visualizations.

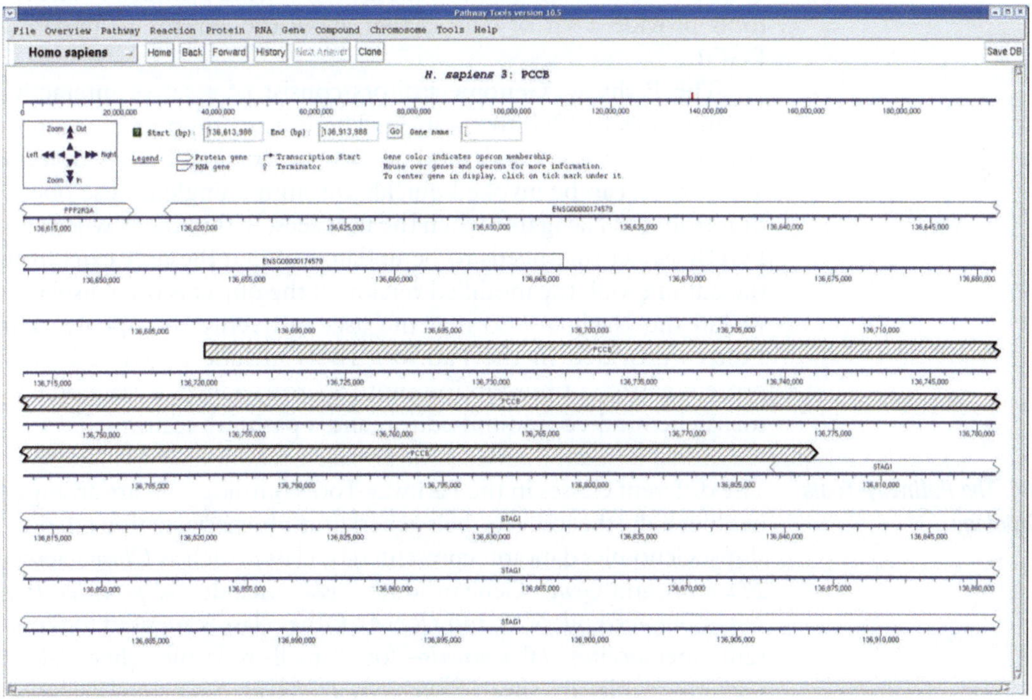

Fig. 5. Chromosome viewer or genome browser. Shown here is the human mitochondrion from HumanCyc, with a short region (presented as a *red region* in the *top diagram*) presented *below* at a greater level of magnification. Notice the zooming controls and the way genes are represented. Clicking on any gene shown in this view will take the user to the corresponding gene page.

GenBank file. PathoLogic generates a PGDB through two phases: (1) a conversion process and (2) an inference process. The conversion process transforms flatfile descriptions of genes and gene products into a PGDB representation of that information, converting the genome annotation into a representation that can be queried and displayed using the Navigator and that can be further updated using the Pathway/Genome Editors. The PathoLogic inference process predicts the metabolic pathway complement of an organism from the protein products described in its genome annotation by comparison to a reference metabolic database, the MetaCyc pathway DB (7). MetaCyc currently contains around 900 nonredundant, experimentally elucidated metabolic pathways from more than 900 different organisms.

In essence, researchers working on a specific organism whose entire genome has been sequenced and annotated can use PathoLogic and the annotated genome to generate a PGDB as a starting point for metabolomics and pathway reconstruction studies. Details of the PathoLogic algorithm can be found in ref. (8).

3.3. The Pathway-Genome Editors

New information about the organism modeled in a PGDB that comes to light from experimental studies and pathway reconstruction analyses will require updates of the PGDB to reflect changes such as additional functions for some genes, changes in the metabolic network or the identification of new gene products. Pathway tools provide a set of editors that allow the curator to update a PGDB.

The Pathway/Genome Editors consist of a set of interactive editing tools for PGDB curation. The Editors support creation of new PGDB objects and modification of existing PGDB objects. These tools can be invoked quickly through a single mouse operation from the Navigator when the user sees, within the Navigator, a PGDB object that needs to be updated. When the user exits from the editing tool, the modified version of the object is then displayed within the Navigator so that the user can verify the update. The Editors provided in the Pathway Tools include a gene editor, a protein editor, a transcription-unit (operon) editor, a reaction editor, a chemical-compound editor, and a pathway editor.

3.4. The Pathway-Tools Ontology

The different classes in the Pathway Tools ontology (3) are arranged in a hierarchy that reflects their generalization-specialization relationships. Genomics data are represented by classes such as *Chromosomes*, *Plasmids*, and *Genes*. Gene product classes include *Polypeptides*, *Protein-Complexes*, *rRNAs*, and *tRNAs*. Other classes are used to represent metabolites (*Chemicals*—for "small-molecule chemicals"), Genetic regulatory sites (*Promoters*, *DNA binding sites*, *Terminators*), and molecular interactions (*Reactions* and *Pathways*).

The ontology associates, with each class, slots used to encode attributes of a biological object, and relationships among those objects. For example, the class *Reactions* has slots that specify the reactants and products of a reaction. These reaction substrates can be tagged with information about their cellular location, allowing for the description of transport events. Other slots of the class *Reactions* define, for example, the enzyme(s) that catalyze the reaction, the corresponding EC number, if any, pathways that include the reaction, and an equilibrium constant of the reaction, when known.

3.5. The Ocelot Object Database

Ocelot (9) is a mature and stable database manager combining the expressive power of frame knowledge representation systems with the scalability, multiuser access capabilities, and robust operation of relational database systems. The FRS object data model is far superior to the relational data model for representing biological data.

Ocelot DBs can be queried using short Lisp programs that employ the Ocelot API, which is called GFP (Generic Frame Protocol). API for Perl and Java are also available. Using APIs allows the user to create not only complex queries, but also complete programs for complex analyses involving metabolomics, proteomics and transcriptomics data. Indeed, it is not difficult to map an entire protein interaction network on top of a PGDB with the appropriate program. The possibilities for realizing complex analyses are enormous when the entire known genome, proteome and metabolome are available, encoded in a computable fashion. An interesting example of such a study analyzed the *Escherichia coli* metabolic network from the point of view of nutrient utilization (10). The additional information layered on top of the annotated genome in a PGDB can also help improve computational tools that rely only on genomic information. An example of such an application is the improvement of an operon predictor based on intergenic distance by using metabolic pathway and protein complex information available in a PGDB (11).

4. HumanCyc: The Human PGDB

The advantages of Pathway Tools-managed PGDBs (including the overview visualization and the "omics" viewer, described later) for systemic analyses can be applied to human data through HumanCyc, the *Homo sapiens* PGDB (http://humancyc.org) (12). HumanCyc contains the complete genome sequence of *H. sapiens*, as presented in Build 31 and describes the nucleotide position and function of every *H. sapiens* gene, as well as their products and predicted metabolic network.

HumanCyc is linked to many biological databases:

- Genomic
  - Ensembl
  - GenBank (Entrez)

  - LocusLink
  - RefSeq
  - Unigene
  - GeneCards
  - UCSC Human Genome DB
- Protein
  - SwissProt
  - RefSeq
  - Entrez
- Disease
  - OMIM
- Other
  - GO (Gene Ontology)
  - PubMed

Data on the human genome from Ensembl, LocusLink, and GenBank were carefully parsed computationally, and then merged, in order to create a minimally redundant human gene set to serve as an input to the PathoLogic software, which generated the database and predicted *H. sapiens* metabolic pathways as explained before. The resulting PGDB includes information on 28,783 genes, their products and the metabolic reactions and pathways they catalyze. Also included are many links to other databases and publications.

HumanCyc was generated by combining the gene sets from the Ensembl and LocusLink databases. LocusLink gene entries were merged into Ensembl genes when appropriate, based on equivalence of gene names and links to other databases, in order to obtain as nonredundant a gene set as possible. However, some duplicate genes may remain, as merging was avoided when the correspondence between Ensembl and LocusLink genes was not clear. GenBank genomic data were used for the mitochondrion.

HumanCyc has undergone a limited curation effort that includes an assessment and correction of the computationally generated metabolic network, and some curation of metabolic pathways and enzymes. The list of curated pathways is available on the Release Notes page at the humancyc.org Web site. Table 1 shows some statistics of version 14.5 (released in October 2010).

Currently, HumanCyc does not contain signaling pathways. Some data, such as alternative splicings and tissue specificity, are not yet supported, whereas other types of information, such as transporters and cellular compartments, although supported by the software, have yet to be added. As for all other biological databases, HumanCyc is a work in progress, but despite these limitations,

Table 1
HumanCyc vers. 14.5 statistics

Class	Number
Pathways	247
Enzymatic reactions	1,831
Transport reactions	20
Polypeptides	20,891
Protein complexes	108
Enzymes	3,332
Transporters	75
Compounds	1,189
Transcription units	0
tRNAs	53

the PGDB can be a powerful tool for analyzing metabolomics and other systemic data from a genomics perspective.

We now describe one of the most useful visualization tools available to HumanCyc and other PGDBs through the Pathway Tools software, and finally show some examples of potential metabolomics applications.

5. Visualizing Systems Biology Measurements in Pathway Tools: The Cellular Overview Diagram and the Omics Viewer

Pathway Tools can automatically generate, from an organism PGDB, a cellular overview diagram which can be used for interpreting systems-biology studies of that organism. As a PGDB such as HumanCyc is revised to reflect evolving scientific knowledge of the organism, its overview is automatically updated to reflect those changes. The cellular overview includes metabolic, transport and signaling pathways, as well as transport reactions, and can be displayed at different levels of magnification. Using the cellular overview diagram, the Omics Viewer can produce static or animated visualizations of whole-organism datasets, such as transcriptomics or metabolomics experiments and it allows the user to zero in on specific pathways at high resolution. When time course data is available, the Omics viewer can present it in an animated visualization that dynamically depicts the changes across the entire network.

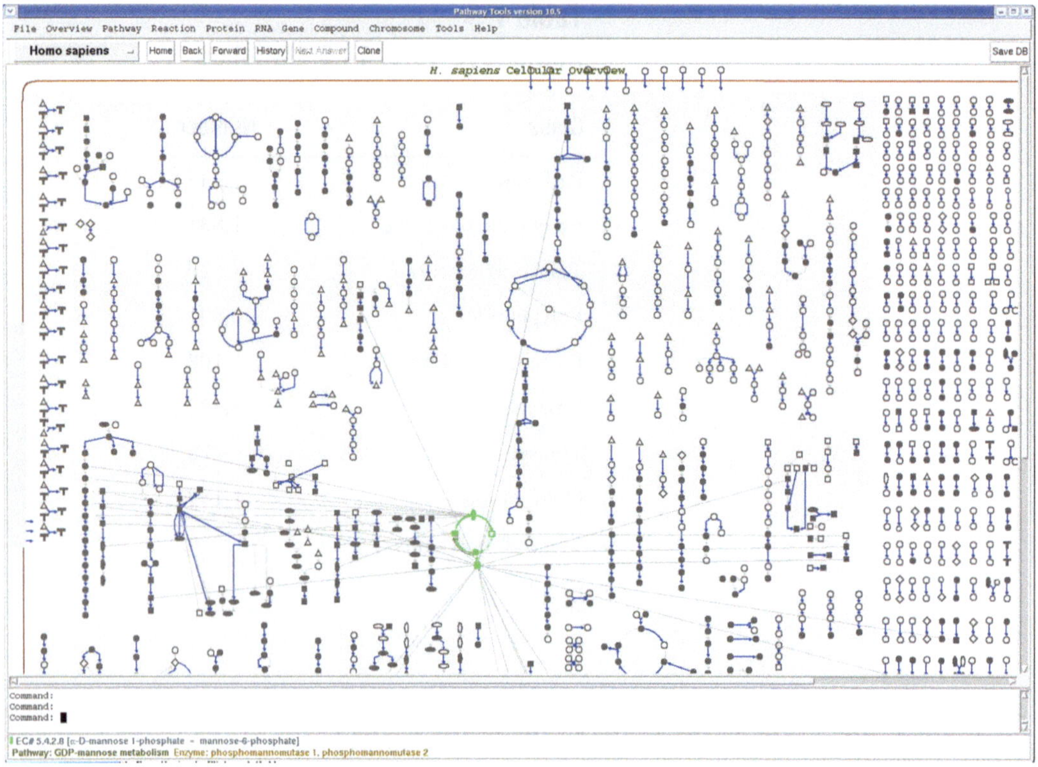

Fig. 6. A portion of the cellular overview diagram from HumanCyc. The pathway at the *center* is ketogluconate metabolism. The diagram shows all connections from metabolites in this pathway to other pathways or reactions.

5.1. Organization of the Cellular Overview Diagram

The cellular overview diagram is a graph that depicts many aspects of the cellular biochemical network, including metabolic and transport reactions and pathways, bacterial signaling pathways, and periplasmic and membrane proteins. A sample cellular overview diagram is shown in Fig. 6. Visual elements of the diagram encode the following aspects of the biochemical network. Nodes in the overview represent biochemical species, including small-molecule metabolites and proteins. The shape of a node indicates the type of chemical compound (e.g. triangles depict amino acids, squares depict carbohydrates and diamonds depict proteins). Filled nodes (as opposed to outline shapes) represent phosphorylated molecules.

Biochemical or transport reactions are represented by lines connecting nodes. Transport reactions are shown as lines that span a membrane. Directionality of transport is indicated by arrowheads. Most pathways flow in the downward direction in the diagram. Pathways with related biological functions are grouped together in the diagram within shaded background boxes, and these groupings are positioned so that biosynthetic pathways appear to the left of the overview, with degradation pathways situated on the right and energy metabolism pathways in the middle. Reactions in the PGDB that are not members of pathways appear to the far right of the diagram. Any signal transduction pathways included in the PGDB will appear at the bottom.

5.2. Querying the Overview

The Cellular Overview provides interactive querying capabilities for the analysis and exploration of the metabolic and signaling networks it depicts. Pointing to any part of the diagram generates a description of the object (pathway, reaction, compound) the mouse pointer is over. Clicking on an object produces a menu of links to the selected pathway, reaction, or metabolite. The user also controls the magnification of the entire diagram. Clicking on a pathway pops up an enlarged view of that pathway, including the individual metabolite and gene names, so that the user can easily focus in on pathways of interest.

Many types of relationships can be explored in the Cellular Overview. The overview provides for menu driven predefined queries whose results can be highlighted so that users can visualize them in the context of the cellular networks encoded by the PGDB. But highlighting not only works for results from predefined queries, as highlighting is easily accomplished from within programmatic queries written by the user. In this way, users can search for and highlight, for example, all proteins with a particular cellular location, all reactions whose enzymes are activated or inhibited by a particular compound, all enzymes whose expression is regulated by a particular transcription factor (see Fig. 8), all reactions catalyzed by the same enzyme(s), and even the results of complex analyses of the metabolic network carried out by a user-developed program. Highlighting can be also applied to a list of objects (genes, reactions, compounds and so on) imported from a user-supplied file. A zooming capability allows the diagram to be shown at different levels of magnification, which can make highlights easier to see.

The cellular overview diagram can also be used for comparative analyses of the complete metabolic networks of two or more organisms or strains highlighting all reactions that are either shared or not shared within a set of organisms for which PGDBs are available.

5.3. The Omics Viewer

The Omics Viewer uses the cellular overview diagram to project data from high-throughput experiments onto the metabolic network encoded in a PGDB. The Omics viewer is so named because it supports overview-based visualizations— both static and animated—of data from a variety of different kinds of "-omics" experiments, such as gene expression data, metabolomics data, proteomics data, or any other kind of experimental data in which numerical data values are assigned to many individual genes, proteins, reactions, or metabolites.

Experimental data are visualized in the Omics Viewer through a special kind of highlighting in which different values are assigned corresponding colors from a customizable palette. Nodes and lines in the cellular overview are drawn in the color corresponding to the value for the particular gene, protein, or metabolite. The result is a color-coded metabolic chart that enables the user to see which metabolites or reactions are significantly affected by a given set of experimental conditions. An example display can be seen at http://biocyc.org/expr-examples/single-expt.html.

The Omics Viewer offers the ability to view time-series experiments dynamically, as animations. Each time step in the series corresponds to one animation frame. The animation can be run continuously or viewed in a frame by frame fashion.

Data input files for the omics viewer are easily constructed as tabular, tab-delimited text files. In the case of microarray data, the Omics Viewer can also accept as input the output file generated by SAM (13), a plug-in for the Microsoft Excel spreadsheet program that combines the results of multiple repetitions of a single microarray experiment to produce lists of statistically significant regulated genes.

It is also possible to combine multiple types of data into a single file. This allows for the simultaneous visualization of metabolomics and transcriptomics data obtained from the same sample or experiment, by coloring nodes (metabolites) according to their metabolic profile values and lines (reactions) according to the transcription levels of their corresponding enzymes' genes.

If a reaction has multiple isozymes, then multiple genes or proteins will be associated with a single reaction line, each with its own associated data value. Whereas these multiple data values are not visible in the full overview diagram (only the most extreme values are shown), they can be visualized in the zoomed-in or enlarged version of a pathway, where the different isozymes are represented by parallel lines, each with its own color depending on their associated experimental values, as seen in Fig. 7. The software can also generate a table of magnified views of all pathways that have one or more experimental values exceeding a specified threshold, with omics data painted onto the pathway.

The Omics Viewer potential as a tool for analyzing metabolomics experiments, especially when combined or related to transcriptomics data, is evident. The capability for overlaying multiple kinds of profile data onto a metabolic network, allowing for visualization in a cellular context, provides scientists with a set of visual tools that helps them derive biologically meaningful insights from their data. Example uses of the Omics Viewer by life sciences researchers include analyzing time series and gene knockout gene expression in order to assess the relative significance of individual metabolic pathways for the colonization of *E. coli* in the mouse intestine (14), and combining gene expression and metabolite profiling data to identify and analyze changes in the metabolism of *Arabidopsis thaliana* under conditions of sulfur starvation (15).

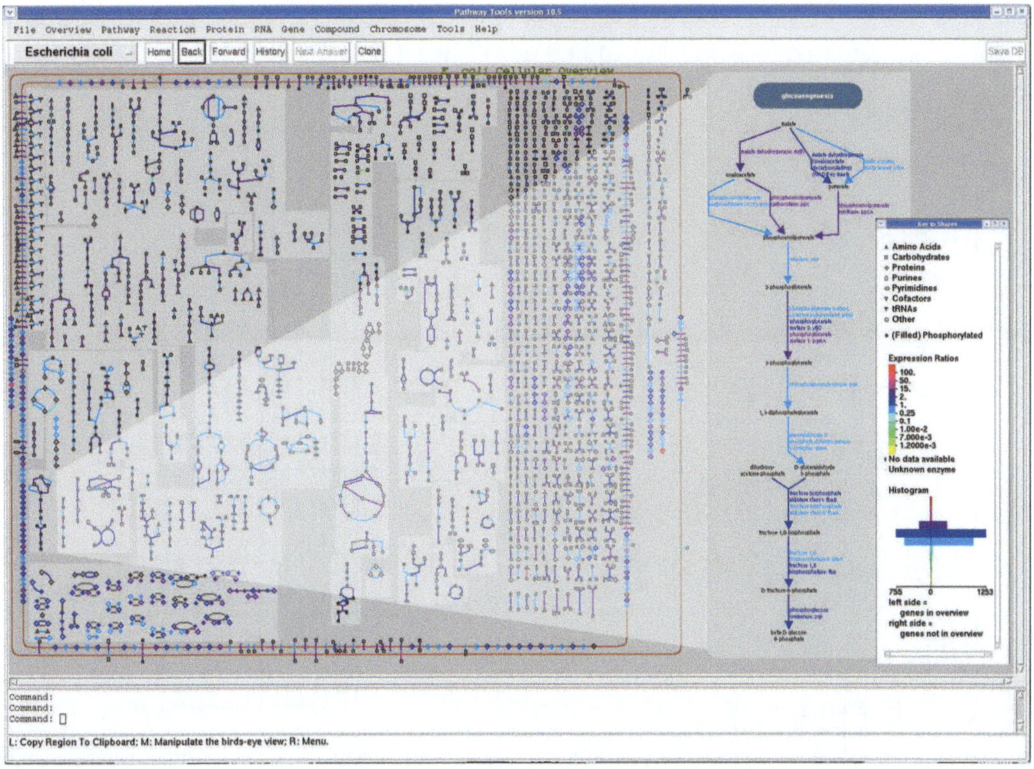

Fig. 7. The Omics Viewer. The figure shows part of the Cellular overview overlaid with data from a gene expression experiment, showing a magnified view of the gluconeogenesis pathway. Notice that in this magnified view, isozymes are distinguished as *parallel lines*.

6. Taking HumanCyc to Its Full Potential: The Pathway Tools API

As useful as the visualization tools are, the part of Pathway Tools that help realize the potential of a PGDB is the API. From complex queries to entire programs, the user can build all kind of utilities around Pathway Tools using the Generic Frame Protocol primitives, as well as Pathway Tools own functions. Among the possible applications that can be developed are:

- Traverse the PGDB's metabolic network and apply different graph-theoretical analyses. All kinds of connections can be analyzed as graph data structures: Reactions connect metabolites; pathways connect enzymes and their corresponding genes; common metabolites, as well as enzymes, connect pathways; protein complexes connect proteins and genes. All these connections are directly accessible through the API.
- Associate values or labels to any object in the PGDB beyond the information stored in the objects' slots. This allows for the

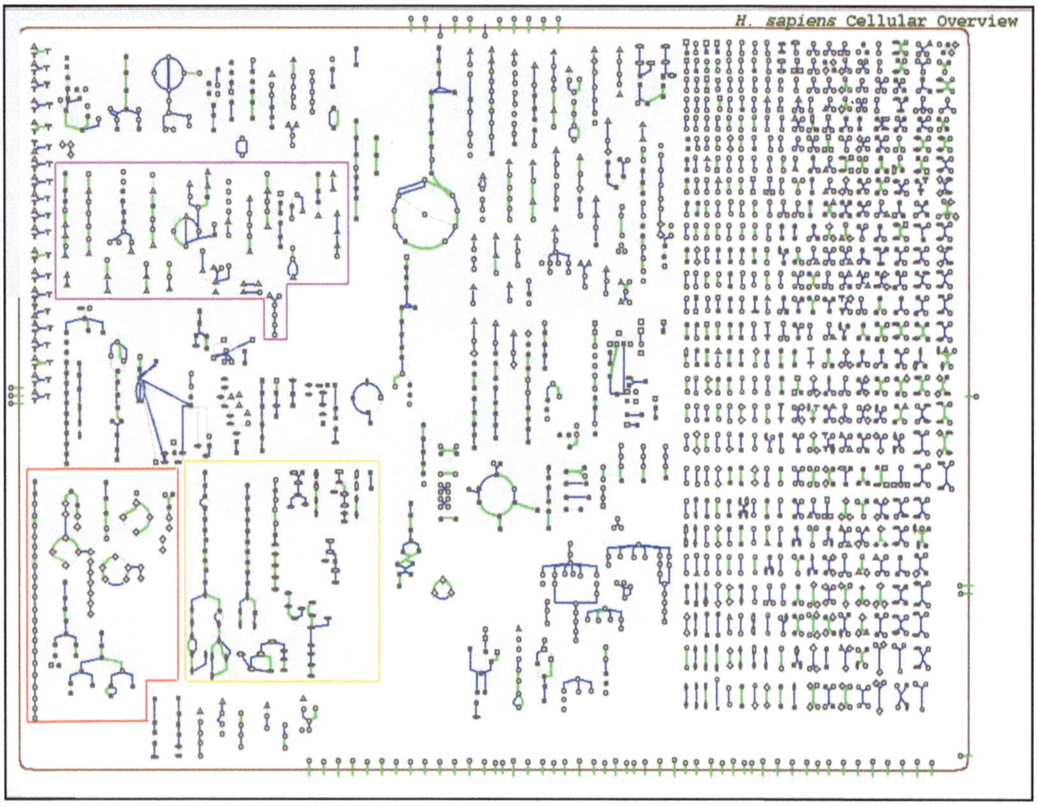

Fig. 8. HumanCyc metabolic overview diagram, showing reactions whose enzymes are affected by the cMyc transcription factor. *Lines* in this diagram correspond to reactions, with highlighted reactions shown in *green*. The *shaded areas* represent different classes of metabolic pathways, with anabolic pathways placed to the *left* of the diagram and catabolic ones placed to the *right*. Some of these classes have been highlighted with color borders as follows: *Red*: Fatty acids biosynthesis, *Orange*: Nucleotides and nucleosides biosynthesis, and *Purple*: Amino acids biosynthesis. The big circular pathway at the *top center* of the figure is the TCA cycle, connected above to the glycolysis pathway.

use of systemic data like that used by the omics viewer in more complex analyses than those carried out through visualization. Causally relating transcriptomics and metabolomics profiles is an example of this application.

- Carry out symbolic simulations, as, for example, those performed to analyze nutrient transformation through the *E. coli* metabolic network in (10). In this work, nutrients where "fed" to the cell by means of the corresponding transport reactions, then transformed and their products propagated through the different metabolic pathways. The analysis provided validation for the PGDB and was helpful for the detection of gaps in the metabolic network.
- Perform flux balance analyses. Indeed, PGDBs have been used to generate the stoichiometry matrices used in FBA (see, for example (16, 17)).

- Produce customized highlighting of the cellular overview according to the results of some analysis (see cMyc example below).
- Build predictors based on PGDB information. An example of a PGDB-based predictor is the operon predictor described in ref. (11).
- Perform pathway reconstruction analyses. A Bayesian network methodology was used to fill "pathway holes" (i.e., reaction with no assigned enzyme in the organism's genome) in HumanCyc by using homology, contextual and functional evidence obtained from the PGDB (18, 19).
- Link isotopomer-based metabolomics data to the metabolic network at large. The main difficulty in mapping metabolic profiles of labeled compounds to a metabolic network is the fact that metabolic databases do not carry separate isotopomer species. This is easily solved through Pathway Tools' API by assigning a data structure to each metabolite capable of carrying different values for the different isotopomer species.

These are but a few examples of the kinds of software that can be built around a PGDB using the Pathway Tools API. Evidently, the potential for metabolomics applications is considerable. Furthermore, many of the analyses performed on PGDBs such as HumanCyc will in turn result in new information about the organism's metabolic network, information that is easily added to the PGDB through the Pathway Tools editors.

7. Integrating Metabolomics and Gene Expression to Probe Metabolic Networks and Regulation

As stated above, the combined analysis of transcriptomics and metabolomics data holds great promise for helping us understand the complex systemic relationships that give rise to an organism's phenotype. Indeed, gene expression and metabolic networks are linked in multiple ways: The dynamics of metabolic networks is directly regulated by the participating enzymes, which can in turn be modulated by their gene expression and the expression of transcription factors. It is also common to have metabolites that act as second messengers (e.g., cAMP, phosphoinositides) elicit a cascade of signaling events leading to gene expression. Moreover, several intermediary metabolic enzymes including glyceraldehyde-3-phosphate dehydrogenase (GAPDH) and lactate dehydrogenase (LDH) have been found to be involved in the transcriptional activation of histone proteins, providing yet another linkage of metabolism to gene expression (20). The complex web of the cancer metabolome and regulation can be much better resolved by integrating isotopomer-based metabolomics with gene expression patterns than by either approach alone. A few studies have emerged in the past several years to illustrate this advantage (21, 22) (and see Chap. 14 by Fan in this volume).

The technical difficulty for "translating" the vast metabolite and isotopomer dataset into metabolic networks for global linkage to metabolic gene expression is indeed a key barrier to this integration. It is clear that computational approaches are needed to facilitate the process, and such computational procedures will need to be applied to metabolic databases that include genomic information, such as HumanCyc.

Figure 8 not only demonstrates the usefulness of this linkage of genomic and metabolic information, but also shows how a simple query can provide immediate insight on the potential effects of regulatory elements on an organism's metabolism. For example, a query on genes that are directly affected by the cMyc transcription factor involved reading a list of more than 4,000 genes, and then highlighting reactions catalyzed by the products of any metabolic genes in the list. The query found 413 metabolic genes affecting 215 reactions. The 215 highlighted reactions are shown as green lines in the diagram (Fig. 8). The image dramatically shows the widespread effect of cMyc on the entire metabolic network, as it can be seen in three classes of pathways highlighted in the figure: Fatty acids (red), amino acids (purple), and nucleotides/nucleosides (orange) biosynthesis. The experimental aspects of linking omics data are treated in Chap. 14.

8. Conclusions

This chapter outlines the features of PGDB's such as HumanCyc, as well as some potential applications of such a high-level specialized database to the kind of analyses prompted by metabolomics data of ever increasing complexity and other systemic data. Some of the applications described here are currently in development, and the Pathway Tools platform is ideally suited for this kind of work.

The lack of sophistication of many biological databases and resources is a hurdle for the development of complex analytical tools and a common complaint by molecular biologists. Resources such as HumanCyc and Pathway Tools can change this situation by providing the developer with a computable encoding of biological knowledge and a sophisticated collection of computational tools to access it.

In the era of systems biology, next-generation results require the application of next-generation computational resources.

9. Important Resources

BioCyc (see http://BioCyc.org/)

http://humancyc.org/

http://www.arabidopsis.org/biocyc/perlcyc/index.jsp (PerlCyc and JavaCyc APIs)

KEGG (Kyoto Encyclopedia of Genes and Genomes)

http://www.genome.jp/kegg/

http://www.metabolome.jp/

Glossary

API	Application program interface
DB	Data base
FRS	Frame representation system
GFP	Generic frame protocol
Isozyme	Variant form of an enzyme coded for by a separate allele. There is often tissue specific expression of isozymes, which may have significantly different kinetic properties from one another. In multisubunit enzymes, such as LDH two alleles give rise to a (statistical) mixture of enzymes, viz L4, L3M, L2M2, LM3, and M4, where L and M are the products of the two LDH genes.
MOD	Model organism database
Omics	The group of biological sub specialties whose descriptors end in “omics” such as genomics, proteomics and metabolomics spuriously described by adding this suffix to a field name such as gene → gene → genomics. The Omics refers to the systematic study of the phenomena: metabolomics is the study of the metabolome. Many possible subfields have been “omicized” (http://omics.org/index.php/Main_Page#Definition_of_Omics). A challenge is to integrate information and concepts obtained from these areas that frequently used very different platforms.
Ontology	The study of existence (philosophy). In informatics, and ontology is a data model that represents a set of concepts within a domain and the relationships between those concepts. It is used to reason about entities within that domain
PGDB	Pathway/genome database

References

1. Benson DA, Karsch-Mizrachi I, Lipman DJ, Ostell J, Wheeler DL. GenBank. Nucleic Acids Res. 2006;34(Database issue):D16–20.
2. Birney E, Andrews D, Caccamo M, Chen Y, Clarke L, Coates G, Cox T, Cunningham F, Curwen V, Cutts T, et al. Ensembl 2006. Nucleic Acids Res. 2006;34(Database issue):D556–61.
3. Karp PD. An ontology for biological function based on molecular interactions. Bioinformatics. 2000;16(3):269–85.
4. Karp PD. Pathway databases: a case study in computational symbolic theories. Science. 2001;293(5537):2040–4.
5. Karp PD, Paley S, Romero P. The pathway tools software. Bioinformatics. 2002;18 Suppl 1:S225–32.
6. Karp PD, Riley M, Paley SM, Pellegrini-Toole A. The MetaCyc database. Nucleic Acids Res. 2002;30(1):59–61.
7. Caspi R, Foerster H, Fulcher CA, Hopkinson R, Ingraham J, Kaipa P, Krummenacker M, Paley S, Pick J, Rhee SY, et al. MetaCyc: a multiorganism database of metabolic pathways and enzymes. Nucleic Acids Res. 2006;34 (Database issue):D511–6.
8. Paley SM, Karp PD. Evaluation of computational metabolic-pathway predictions for *Helicobacter pylori*. Bioinformatics. 2002;18(5):715–24.
9. Karp PD, Krummenacker M, Paley S, Wagg J. Integrated pathway-genome databases and their role in drug discovery. Trends Biotechnol. 1999;17(7):275–81.
10. Romero PR, Karp P. Nutrient-related analysis of pathway/genome databases. Pac Symp Biocomput. 2001;6:471–82.
11. Romero PR, Karp PD. Using functional and organizational information to improve genome-wide computational prediction of transcription units on pathway-genome databases. Bioinformatics. 2004;20(5):709–17.
12. Romero P, Wagg J, Green ML, Kaiser D, Krummenacker M, Karp PD. Computational prediction of human metabolic pathways from the complete human genome. Genome Biol. 2005;6(1):R2.
13. Tusher VG, Tibshirani R, Chu G. Significance analysis of microarrays applied to the ionizing radiation response. Proc Natl Acad Sci U S A. 2001;98(9):5116–21.
14. Chang DE, Smalley DJ, Tucker DL, Leatham MP, Norris WE, Stevenson SJ, Anderson AB, Grissom JE, Laux DC, Cohen PS, et al. Carbon nutrition of *Escherichia coli* in the mouse intestine. Proc Natl Acad Sci U S A. 2004;101 (19):7427–32.
15. Nikiforova VJ, Kopka J, Tolstikov V, Fiehn O, Hopkins L, Hawkesford MJ, Hesse H, Hoefgen R. Systems rebalancing of metabolism in response to sulfur deprivation, as revealed by metabolome analysis of *Arabidopsis* plants. Plant Physiol. 2005;138(1):304–18.
16. Kayser A, Weber J, Hecht V, Rinas U. Metabolic flux analysis of *Escherichia coli* in glucose-limited continuous culture. I. Growth-rate-dependent metabolic efficiency at steady state. Microbiology. 2005;151(Pt 3):693–706.
17. Weber J, Kayser A, Rinas U. Metabolic flux analysis of *Escherichia coli* in glucose-limited continuous culture. II. Dynamic response to famine and feast, activation of the methylglyoxal pathway and oscillatory behaviour. Microbiology. 2005;151(Pt 3):707–16.
18. Green ML, Karp PD. A Bayesian method for identifying missing enzymes in predicted metabolic pathway databases. BMC Bioinformatics. 2004;5:76.
19. Green ML, Karp PD. Using genome-context data to identify specific types of functional associations in pathway/genome databases. Bioinformatics. 2007;23(13):i205–11.
20. McKnight S. Gene switching by metabolic enzymes—how did you get on the invitation list? Cell. 2003;114(2):150–2.
21. Wong MS, Raab RM, Rigoutsos I, Stephanopoulos GN, Kelleher JK. Metabolic and transcriptional patterns accompanying glutamine depletion and repletion in mouse hepatoma cells: a model for physiological regulatory networks. Physiol Genomics. 2004;16(2): 247–55.
22. Fan TW, Higashi RM, Lane AN. Integrating metabolomics and transcriptomics for probing SE anticancer mechanisms. Drug Metab Rev. 2006;38(4):707–32.

Chapter 14

Metabolomics-Edited Transcriptomics Analysis (META)

Teresa Whei-Mei Fan

Abstract

The study of the metabolome or systems biochemical functions in response to external agents such as drugs or toxicants is made possible by recent advances in NMR and mass spectrometry. By coupling the analytical technologies with the stable isotope tracer approach, it is also practical to map changes in metabolic networks with atomic resolution such that metabolic perturbations can be discerned at the enzyme reaction level. This information readily lends its use in guiding transcriptomic analysis for metabolic regulations at the transcriptional level—an approach called "*M*etabolomics-*E*dited *T*ranscriptomic *A*nalysis" or META. Two example studies are given to illustrate the use of uniformly ^{13}C-labeled glucose tracer, ^{13}C-isotopomer-based metabolomic analysis, and META for reconstructing metabolic pathways and for discerning their regulatory pathways. The first example describes a hypothetical investigation on the role of a "master" metabolic switch (AMP-activated protein kinase or AMPK) in regulating nucleic acid, lipid, and protein-related metabolism. NMR and GC-MS are complementarily used to obtain quantitative changes in metabolite and ^{13}C-isotopomer profiles in a model cancer cell in response to AMPK activation (induced by AICAR, an adenosine analogue) or AMPK inactivation via siRNA knockdown. Expected findings from META that are consistent with known AMPK-mediated regulations include downregulation or phosphorylation of key proteins involved in the synthesis of fatty acids, phospholipids, and proteins. Scenarios for uncovering metabolic regulations previously unknown or contradictory to known AMPK actions are also given. The second example illustrates a real-world investigation on defining the multitargeted action of selenite in human lung adenocarcinoma A549 cells. The META approach revealed AMPK-mediated downregulation of fatty acid and protein synthesis, in addition to negative regulation of glycolysis, pentose phosphate pathway, Krebs cycle, glutathione synthesis, and nucleotide synthesis, as well as positive regulation of Gln metabolism. The complexity of the selenite action including the induction of opposing regulatory events was resolvable with the integrated metabolomics and transcriptomics approach, which is also generally applicable to any living system including the human body.

Key words: META, metabolomics, isotopomer analysis, AMPK, AICAR, selenite, A549, lung adenocarcinoma

Abbreviations

ACC	Acetyl CoA carboxylase
ACLY	ATP citrate lyase
aG3P	α-Glycerol-3-phosphate

Teresa Whei-Mei Fan et al. (eds.), *The Handbook of Metabolomics*, Methods in Pharmacology and Toxicology, DOI 10.1007/978-1-61779-618-0_14, © Springer Science+Business Media New York 2012

AICAR	5-Aminoimidazole-4-carboxamide ribonucleoside
aKG	α-Ketoglutarate
AMPK	AMP-activated protein kinase
AXP	Adenine nucleotides
ChREBP	Carbohydrate-response-element-binding protein
CT	Choline transporter
CXP	Cytosine nucleotides
DAG	Diacylglycerol
DAGK	Diacylglycerol kinase
DHAP	Dihydroxyacetone phosphate
eEF2	Eukaryotic elongation factor 2
eIF4E-BP	Eukaryotic initiation factor 4E binding protein
FAS	Fatty acid synthase
FBPase	Fructose bisphosphatase
G6Pase	Glucose-6-phosphatase
G6PDH	Glucose-6-phosphate dehydrogenase
GAP	Glyceraldehyde-3-phosphate
GCL	Glutamyl-cysteinyl ligase
GDH	Glutamate dehydrogenase
Glnase IP	Glutaminase interacting protein
GLU4	Glucose transporter 4
GPAT	Glycerol phosphate acyl transferase
GPC	Glycerophosphorylcholine
GPDH	Glycerol-3-phosphate dehydrogenase
GS	Glycogen synthase
GSH	Reduced glutathione
GSSG	Oxidized glutathione
GXP	Guanine nucleotides
HMGR	3-Hydroxy-3-methylglutaryl-coenzyme A reductase
HSQC	Heteronuclear single quantum coherence spectroscopy
iPFK2	Inducible phosphofructokinase 2
KD	Knockdown
LDH	Lactate dehydrogenase
LysoPlase	Lysophospholipase
MCT1	Monocarboxylic acid transporter 1
MDH	Malate dehydrogenase
ME	Malic enzyme
META	Metabolomics-edited transcriptomic analysis
METPA	Metabolomics-edited transcriptomics and proteomics analysis
mTOR	Mammalian target of rapamycin
N transporter	Neutral amino acid transporter
OAA	Oxaloacetate
PABP	Poly(A)-binding protein
PC	Phosphatidylcholines
PCase	Pyruvate carboxylase
P-choline	Phosphorylcholine
PDH	Pyruvate dehydrogenase

PDK	1,3-Phosphoinositide-dependent protein kinase
PE	Phosphatidylethanolamines
PEP	Phosphoenolpyruvate
PEPCK	Phosphoenolpyruvate carboxykinase
PFK	6-Phosphofructo-2-kinase
PI3K	Phosphoinositide-3 kinase
PK	Pyruvate kinase
PKB	Protein kinase B
PKC	Protein kinase C
PL	Phospholipids
PLase	Phospholipase
PPP	Pentose phosphate pathway
S6K	S6 protein kinase
SDH	Succinate dehydrogenase
SREBP	Steroid-regulated-element binding protein
TCA	Trichloroacetic acid
TOCSY	Total correlation spectroscopy
TOP	5′-Tract of oligopyrimidine
TPI	Triosephosphate isomerase
TSC2	Tuberous sclerosis component 2
[U-^{13}C]-Glc	^{13}C labeled glucose
UXP	Uracil nucleotides

1. Introduction

The metabolome can be considered as a full description of biochemical phenotypes that interfaces genome and proteome to the macroscopic physical phenotypes of living organisms. It encompasses the actual biochemical functions, whereas genome or proteome provides the "blueprint" or "scaffolding" for biochemical functions. Thus, unraveling the metabolome is understandably the key to translating molecular regulations at the gene and protein levels into physical phenotypes such as individual variations in drug susceptibility or sensitivity to disease vectors.

The immense task of defining the metabolome in its entirety is beyond the limits of present analytical technologies as described in Chaps. 6 and 4 by Lane and Higashi. However, from the standpoint of deciphering a given phenotypic manifestation such as disease development or drug action, only a small fraction of the metabolome is expected to be altered, which is within the realm of investigations using current metabolomic technologies. Many examples of such investigations can be found in the literature (1–36). In particular, the coupled use of stable isotope tracers and isotopomer-based metabolomic analysis is most powerful in linking altered biochemical phenotypes to changes in molecular regulations occurring at the transcriptional or translational levels.

As illustrated below, stable isotope tracers such as uniformly ^{13}C labeled glucose ([U-^{13}C]-Glc) can be used to trace metabolic pathways or networks in cells or tissues that respond to a given perturbation such as the administration of a growth inhibitor. By profiling the extent and atomic position of stable isotope incorporation into relevant metabolites, the set of enzymes that are involved in the biochemical conversion of parent tracers into these metabolites can be identified along with their possible regulation by allosteric metabolites. This information can then be used in targeted interrogation of global gene microarray data for up- or downregulation of these enzyme genes. The same information is also useful for targeted proteomic analysis of the responsive enzyme(s) for protein expression or posttranslational modification. Furthermore, the enzyme target(s) revealed can serve as a "beacon" for linkage to altered regulatory pathways that involve signal transduction or activation of transcription factors. Thus, such metabolomics-edited transcriptomic or proteomic analysis can transcend the inherent limitations of functional genomics and proteomics in providing clues to all levels of biochemical regulation, i.e., transcriptional, posttranscriptional, translational, posttranslational, and enzyme levels.

In the following two sections, the use of metabolomics-edited transcriptomic analysis (META) in linking phenotypic and metabolic changes to molecular regulation network is illustrated first as a hypothetical and second a real experimental case study.

2. Illustration of META: Deciphering AMPK-Regulated Metabolic Networks

In this hypothetical example, the energy-sensing regulatory enzyme, AMP-activated protein kinase (AMPK), is investigated for its role in regulating lipid and protein metabolism via the mTOR (mammalian target of rapamycin) regulatory pathway in human cancer cells.

2.1. AMPK Regulation and Signaling Cascades

AMPK is known as a nutrient/energy-sensing protein and a "metabolic master switch" that can control a number of metabolic processes such as fatty acid oxidation, glucose uptake and metabolism, as well as synthesis of protein, fatty acid, and cholesterol (37). AMPK is activated by both AMP-dependent and independent mechanisms. The AMP-dependent mechanism involves the binding of 5′-AMP to the regulatory γ-subunit of AMPK, thereby activating the enzyme allosterically (38). ATP competes with AMP for binding to the allosteric site, which can account for the sensitivity of AMPK to the AMP/ATP ratio rather than just the AMP concentration alone (39). Thus, stress conditions such as hypoxia, ischemia, low blood glucose, or muscle

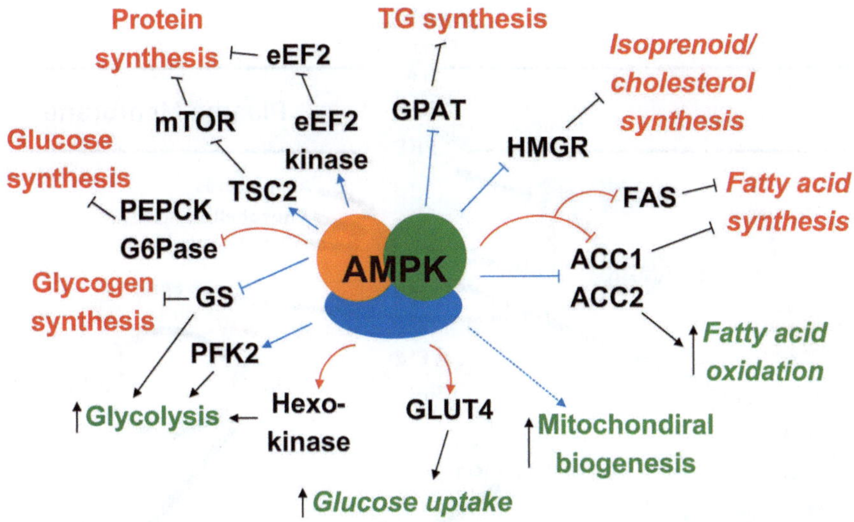

Fig. 1. AMPK-regulated metabolic processes (adapted from ref. (37)). A subset of proteins and processes are shown. *Blue straight lines* and *dashed lines* denote direct protein phosphorylation and unknown mechanism, respectively; *curved red lines* indicate transcriptional induction or suppression. *Green* and *red texts* highlight metabolic processes stimulated or inhibited upon AMPK activation. *ACC* acetyl CoA carboxylase; *GLU4* glucose transporter 4; *PFK2* 6-phosphofructo-2-kinase 2; *GS* glycogen synthase; *PEPCK* phosphoenolpyruvate carboxykinase; *G6Pase* glucose-6-phosphatase; *TSC2* tuberous sclerosis component 2; *mTOR* mammalian target of rapamycin; *eEF2* eukaryotic elongation factor 2; *GPAT* glycerol phosphate acyl transferase; *HMGR* 3-hydroxy-3-methylglutaryl-coenzyme A reductase; *FAS* fatty acid synthase.

contraction that increases the AMP/ATP ratio activate AMPK. The AMP-independent mechanism is triggered by phosphorylation of a threonine residue in the activation loop of the α-subunit of AMPK by an upstream kinase such as LKB1, also known as a tumor suppressor (40).

Once activated, AMPK can influence a number of protein functions either by direct phosphorylation or by transcriptional induction/repression, which can lead to stimulation or inhibition of metabolic processes, as illustrated in Fig. 1. The outcome of AMPK activation is tissue and cell-dependent. For example, transcriptional induction of the glucose transporter GLUT4 and/or its redistribution to the plasma membrane occurs in muscle to increase its glucose uptake (41) while liver is the site for transcriptional suppression of phosphoenolpyruvate carboxykinase (PEPCK) and glucose-6-phosphatase (G6Pase) to block gluconeogenesis (42). In human lung cancers, recent reports reveal the role of AMPK, its upstream regulatory kinase LKB1, and downstream mTOR signaling pathways in tumor development (43–48). The postulated signaling network involving AMPK, mTOR, and protein kinase B (PKB) or Akt is illustrated in Fig. 2, where the outcome of AMPK and PKB activation is, respectively, inhibition and initiation of 5′-cap and 5′-TOP-dependent protein biosynthesis.

In addition to the complex modulation of protein biosynthesis, AMPK can regulate glucose metabolism, lipogenesis, and cholesterol

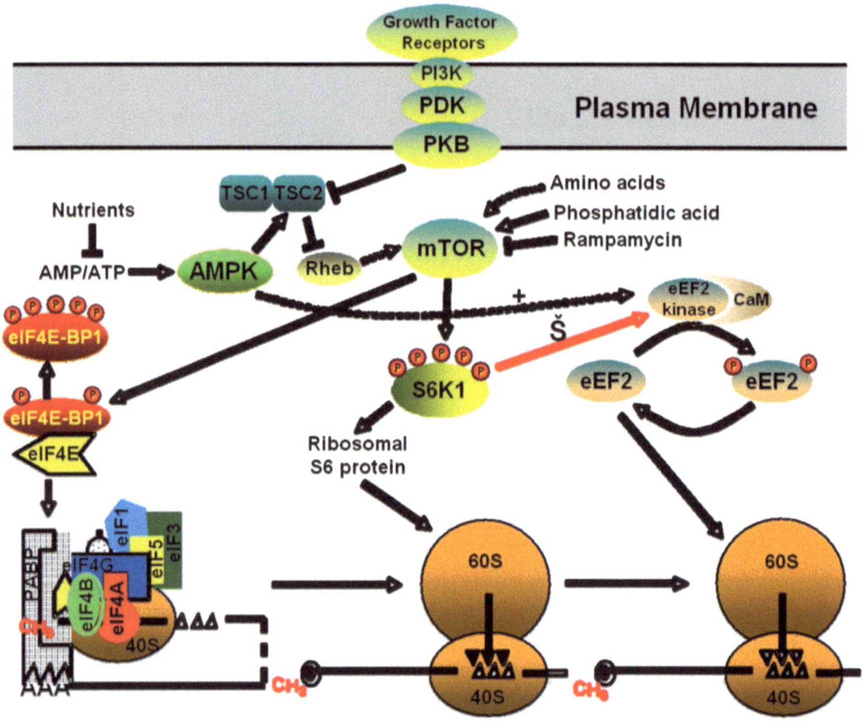

Fig. 2. Postulated AMPK, PKB, and mTOR signaling networks. Poor nutrient status increases AMP/ATP ratio, which activates AMPK. Active AMPK phosphorylates TSC2, which causes GTP hydrolysis in Rheb, thereby blocking Rheb activation of mTOR. PKB or Akt is activated by the signaling cascade mediated via growth factors interacting with receptors, and subsequent activation of phosphoinositide-3 kinase (PI3K) and 1,3-phosphoinositide-dependent protein kinase (PDK). Active PKB phosphorylates TSC2 at a site different from the AMPK site to block GTP hydrolysis in Rheb, thereby activating mTOR. Active mTOR phosphorylates eukaryotic initiation factor 4E binding protein 1 (eIF4E-BP1) and S6K1, which leads to the release of eIF4E and phosphorylated ribosomal S6 protein, respectively. Free eIF4E forms a complex with eIF4G, eIF4A, eIF4B, poly(A)-binding protein (PABP), and 5′-cap of mRNA, which recruits 40S subunit of the ribosome, followed by the binding of eIF2 complexed with Met-tRANi, eIF1, eIF3, and eIF5. After scanning and positioning the translation initiation complex for the start codon AUG, the initiation factors are released along with the joining of the ribosomal 60S subunit, where translation elongation begins. Phosphorylated S6 protein activates the translation of 5′-tract of oligopyrimidine (TOP) mRNA which synthesizes the translation apparatus. Both AMPK and S6K1 can phosphorylate eukaryotic elongation factor 2 (eEF2) kinase, thereby activating or inhibiting its activity, respectively. Active eEF2 kinase inhibits eEF2 in mediating chain elongation. Amino acids and phosphatidic acid can activate mTOR directly while rapamycin inhibits it (adapted from ref. (37) and http://www.mun.ca/biochem/courses/3107/Topics/Euk_prot_synth.html).

biosynthesis (Fig. 1 and (49)). Although the exact transcriptional mechanism(s) is still unclear, AMPK inhibition of lipid and cholesterol biosynthesis may be mediated by interfering with the transcription factor steroid-regulated-element binding protein-1c (SREBP-1c). This then leads to decreased gene expression of a number of enzymes (e.g., ATP citrate lyase or ACLY, acetyl CoA carboxylase or ACC, fatty acid synthase or FAS, HMG CoA reductase) involved in lipid and cholesterol biosynthesis (50). The inhibition of glucose-responsive gene expression by AMPK may involve another transcription factor carbohydrate-response-element-binding protein (ChREBP), which coordinates the expression of genes governing both glucose utilization (e.g., liver pyruvate kinase (PK), malic enzyme [ME]) and lipid synthesis (e.g., ACLY, FAS, ACC) (51).

The many implications of AMPK in regulating lipid, protein, and glucose metabolism are inferred from evidence acquired at the protein and/or gene levels. As indicated above, gene or protein-level effects are not necessarily translated into metabolic activities due to numerous possible regulatory processes. These include posttranslational modifications, presence or induction of inhibitor proteins, allosteric regulation by effector metabolites, alternative gene functions, or compartmentalization. Moreover, the majority of the AMPK-associated regulatory network has been demonstrated in liver, muscle, or pancreatic β-cells, relatively little is known in other tissue context or diseased state, such as human cancers. In the hypothetical example below, we illustrate the use of ^{13}C-labeled glucose tracers and ^{13}C-isotopomer analysis by NMR and MS to map the many metabolic pathways that can be regulated by AMPK activation in a model human adenocarcinoma cancer cell.

2.2. Hypothetical Investigation of AMPK-Related Metabolic Networks in Human Cancer Cells

2.2.1. Approach

Metabolic networks in cancer cells that may be governed by AMPK are probed by two approaches, i.e., via AMPK activation and attenuation. AMPK in cultured cancer cells is activated by treatment with an experimental anticancer drug, 5-aminoimidazole-4-carboxamide ribonucleoside (AICAR, an adenosine analogue) at 1 mM. AICAR is converted in vivo to the AMP analogue, ZMP, which activates AMPK. At 1 mM, maximal AMPK activity, relative to the control treatment, is attained in 2 h of AICAR treatment, as assayed by radioactive ^{32}P incorporation from [γ-^{32}P]-ATP into a synthetic SAMS peptide substrate (52).

The AICAR treatment is done in the presence of 10 mM uniformly [U-^{13}C]-Glc. Medium samples are collected after 0, 1, 2, 4, 8, and 24 h of incubation at 37°C, 5% CO_2 for metabolite analysis. Cells are also harvested for metabolite profiling at the end of the treatment (24 h). A parallel cell growth without AICAR treatment is performed as control. Each cell sample containing a minimum of 2×10^6 cells (ca. 1 mg dry weight) is washed with-ice-cold PBS to remove growth medium components while minimizing metabolic activity during harvest (see Chap. 2 by Fan on sample preparation). The final cell pellets are flash-frozen in liquid N_2 before lyophilization.

The physical phenotypic effect of AICAR on cancer cells is investigated in parallel, including growth, viability, colony formation, and apoptosis for comparison with the metabolic effect. Moreover, global gene expression profile is obtained for both control and AICAR-treated cells after 24 h of treatment when significant changes in gene and protein expression as well as lipid biosynthesis is expected to occur.

Inactivation of AMPK is achieved by transducing cancer cells with adenovirus containing tetracycline-inducible siRNA vectors for AMPKα1 and α2 (AGCCCTAGGTAGTCGTTGA and CGCTCGTTGATAGTTTCTG, respectively) (53). AMPK knockdown (KD) is induced by incubating the transduced cells with tetracycline in the presence of 10 mM [U-^{13}C]-Glc. Cells are harvested at 24 h after the induction, flash-frozen, and lyophilized, as described above.

Polar and lipophilic metabolites in treated cells are extracted with 10% trichloroacetic acid (TCA) and methanol, respectively, before NMR and MS analysis. Metabolites and their ^{13}C-labeled positional isotopomers are identified by 2D NMR (i.e., 2D ^{1}H total correlation spectroscopy [TOCSY] and ^{1}H-^{13}C heteronuclear single quantum coherence spectroscopy [HSQC]) (cf. Chap. 6) while GC-MS is employed to quantify metabolites and ^{13}C-labeled mass isotopomers (cf. Chap. 4).

2.2.2. Example Observation

Phenotypic Effect of AICAR

The ability of AICAR to activate AMPK is confirmed by Western blot analysis with an antibody against Thr172-phosphorylated AMPKα. Increased phosphorylation is detected as early as 15 min after addition of AICAR. Activation of AMPK is demonstrated by assessing the in vitro phosphorylation of a synthetic SAMS peptide by cell lysates and in intact cells by Western blot analysis with an antiserum against phospho-Ser-79 ACC. Counting of trypan blue excluded cells reveals that whereas the number of cells in control conditions increases exponentially as a function of the incubation time, AICAR causes a stagnation of the number of living cells. Differences in growth curves are noticeable 2 days after addition of AICAR. On day 3, cell death can be observed in a substantial fraction (30–50%) of the cells. Cells also display typical signs of apoptosis (DNA condensation and nuclear fragmentation) as revealed by staining with the DNA intercalating dye Hoechst 33342 and as confirmed staining with Annexin V-FITC as well as by Western blot analysis of cleaved PARP. Moreover, cells show signs of autophagy as revealed by staining with monodansylcadaverine and conversion of cytosolic LC3-I to LC3-II (by Western blot analysis). The inhibition of cell proliferation and the partial induction of cell death is reflected also in the reduced ability of cancer cells to form colonies, when plated at a low density. AICAR decreases the size of the colonies and causes a marked reduction of their number. AICAR also blocks cell migration and invasiveness as assessed using a modified two-well Boyden chamber without or with Matrigel coating, respectively. Together, these experiments indicate that mimicry of a low energy status in cancer cells by AICAR treatment leads cancer cells into blocking typical cancer cell-associated processes, including cell proliferation, colony formation, migration and matrix invasion.

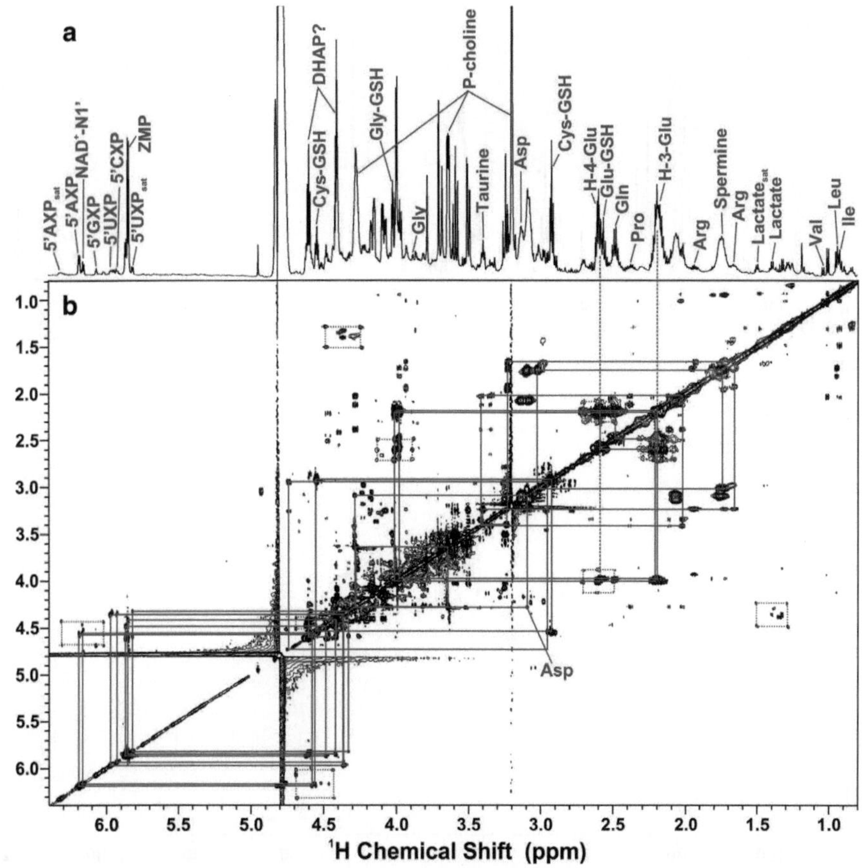

Fig. 3. ^{1}H NMR identified polar metabolites in TCA extract of cancer cells. The 2D ^{1}H TOCSY contour map (**b**) is shown along with the corresponding 1D high-resolution ^{1}H spectrum (**a**). The metabolites are assigned based on their ^{1}H chemical shifts, ^{1}H spin-coupling patterns, and covalent connectivity (traced by *solid rectangular boxes*). Their ^{13}C-labeled isotopomers are identified based on the 2D cross-peak pattern of the ^{13}C-satellites (traced by *dashed rectangular boxes*). For example, the satellite cross-peak pattern for the 4-protons of Glu (H-4-Glu) indicates a mixture of ^{13}C-Glu isotopomers labeled at C-4, C-2, and C-2,4 positions with ^{13}C-4 the dominant species (cf. Chap. 6). Similarly, the H-3-Glu satellite cross peak pattern reveals the presence of ^{13}C-Glu isotopomers labeled at C-3, C-4, and C-3,4 positions again with dominant contribution from ^{13}C-4. Except for DHAP, TOCSY assignment is confirmed and complemented by the 2D HSQC analysis (cf. Fig. 4). *P-choline* phosphorylcholine; *DHAP* dihydroxyacetone phosphate; *UXP* uracil nucleotides; *CXP* cytosine nucleotides; *GXP* guanine nucleotides; *AXP* adenine nucleotides; *metabolite$_{sat}$* ^{13}C satellites of metabolites.

NMR Identification and Semi-quantification of Metabolites and ^{13}C-Isotopomer Profiles

Polar metabolites in the TCA extract of cancer cells are analyzed by 1D high-resolution ^{1}H and 2D ^{1}H TOCSY, as illustrated in Fig. 3. Metabolites assigned include Ile, Leu, Val, lactate, Arg, spermine, Glu, Pro, Gln, reduced glutathione (GSH), oxidized glutathione (GSSG), Asp, phosphorylcholine (P-choline), taurine, Gly, dihydroxyacetone phosphate (DHAP, tentative assignment), and nucleotides of uracil, cytosine, guanine, and adenine. In addition, a number of ^{13}C-labeled positional isotopomers of lactate, Glu, and adenine nucleotides (AXP) are found, including [^{13}C-2,3]-lactate, [^{13}C-2]-Glu, [^{13}C-3]-Glu, [^{13}C-4]-Glu, [^{13}C-2,4]-Glu, [^{13}C-3,4]-Glu, [^{13}C-1′,2′]-5′AXP.

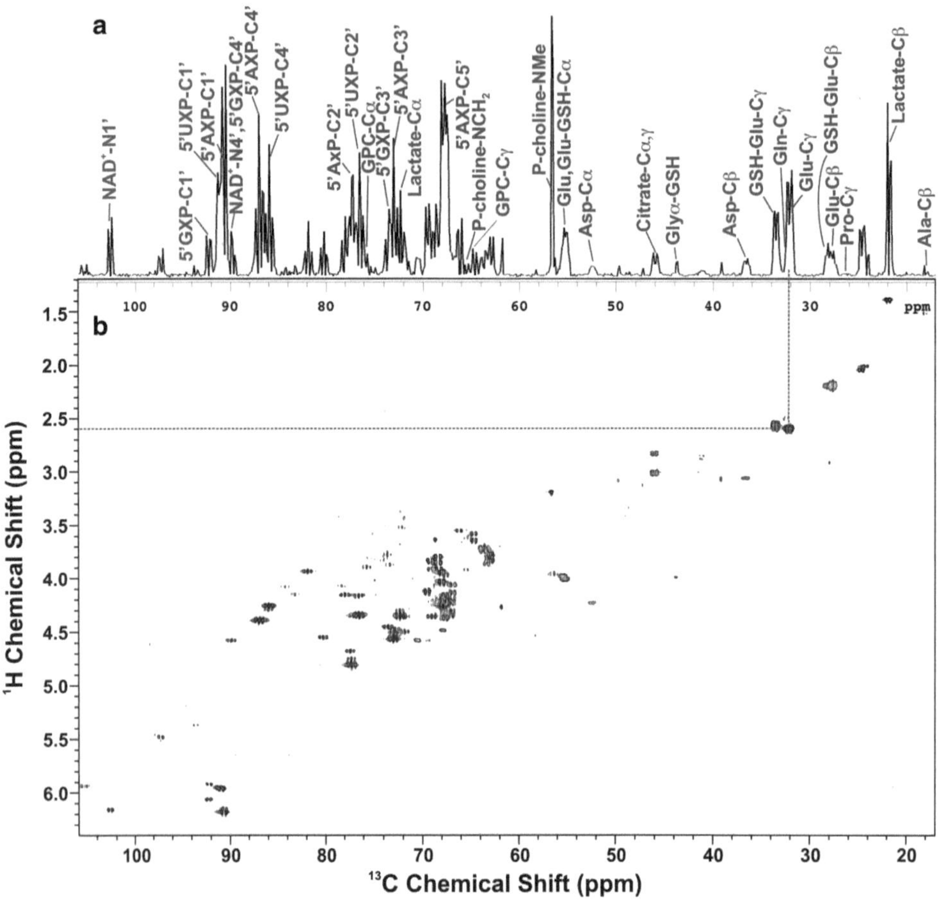

Fig. 4. 2D ^{1}H-^{13}C HSQC identified polar metabolites in TCA extract of cancer cells. The 2D HSQC contour map (**b**) is shown along with the corresponding 1D ^{13}C projection spectrum (**a**). Metabolites are assigned based on their ^{1}H and ^{13}C chemical shifts, ^{13}C spin-coupling patterns, and ^{1}H-^{13}C covalent connectivity. Their ^{13}C-labeled isotopomers are identified based on the 2D cross-peak and ^{13}C spin coupling pattern. For example, the cross-peak of ^{1}H-^{13}C has ^{1}H and ^{13}C chemical shifts at 2.61 and 32.2 ppm, respectively, which matches with those of Glu at the 4 position (Glu-Cγ). The doublet appearance of the ^{13}C resonance indicates the dominance of spin coupling to ^{13}C at Cβ (C-3) or C-5 (carboxylate) positions but not both. Similarly, the doublet nature of Glu-Cβ (C-3) suggests a major contribution from dual ^{13}C labeling at Cβ and Cα (C-2) or Cγ (C-4). The ^{13}Cβ and ^{13}Cγ coupling (which exists based on the TOCSY data, Fig. 3) is a minor component in both cases, since such coupling gives rise to a triplet pattern for Cβ, not doublet. Thus, the dominant ^{13}C positional isotopomers of Glu are [^{13}C-2,3]-Glu and [^{13}C-4,5]-Glu.

The same extract from Fig. 3 is also analyzed by 2D high-resolution ^{1}H-^{13}C HSQC for additional ^{13}C-labeled positional isotopomers, as shown in Fig. 4. The isotopomers assigned include [U-^{13}C]-Ala, [U-^{13}C]-lactate, [^{13}C-2,3]-Glu, [^{13}C-4,5]-Glu, [^{13}C-2,3-Glu]-GSH, [^{13}C-4,5-Glu]-GSH, [^{13}C-2,3]-, [^{13}C-3,4]-, [^{13}C-1,2], [^{13}C-1,2,3]-, [^{13}C-2,3,4]-, and/or [^{13}C-1,2,3,4]-Asp, [U-^{13}C-ribose]-5′AXP, [U-^{13}C-ribose]-5′UXP, [U-^{13}C-ribose]-5′GXP, and [U-^{13}C-nicotinamide-ribose]-NAD$^+$, [^{13}C-5,6] uracil nucleotides (UXP) (data not shown), and [^{13}C-1,2]- or [^{13}C-5,6]-citrate.

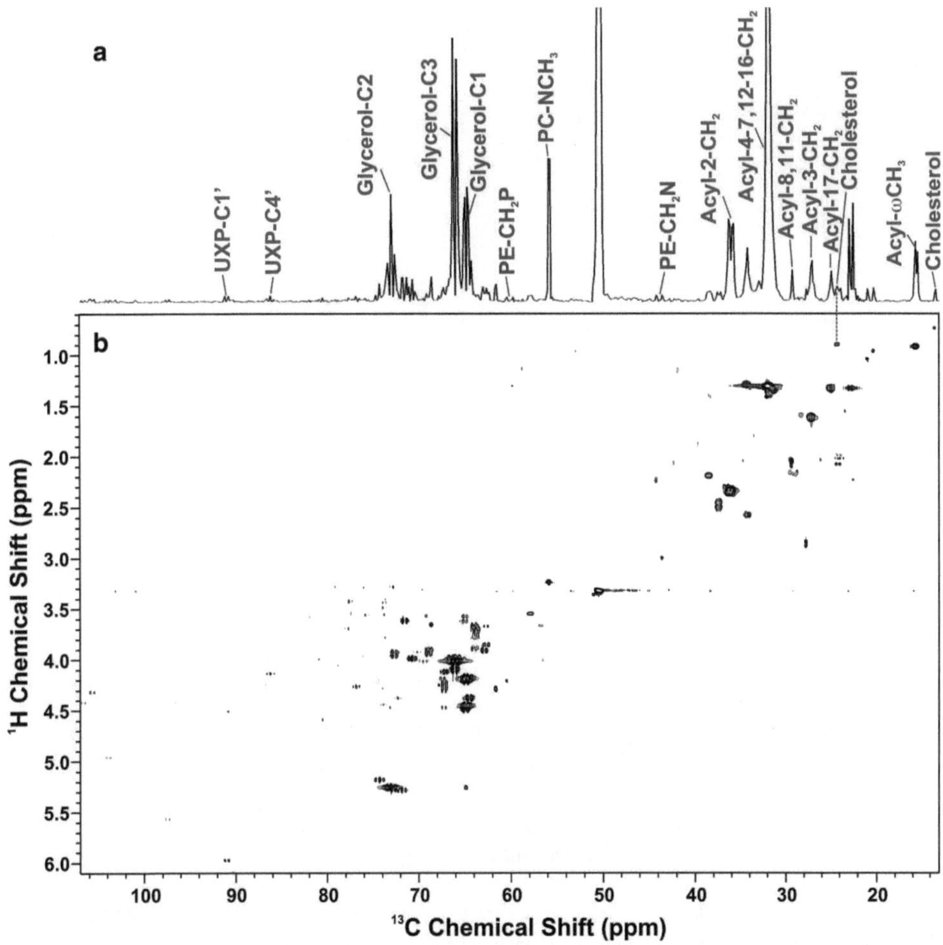

Fig. 5. 2D ^{1}H-^{13}C HSQC analysis of methanolic extract of cancer cells reveals ^{13}C-labeled isotopomers of phospholipids (PL). The 2D contour map (**b**) is shown along with its 1D projection spectrum along the ^{13}C dimension (**a**). The most abundant ^{13}C resonance of PL, i.e., that of [^{13}C-4-7,12-16]-acyl chain, is plotted off-scale to better illustrate the less abundant resonances such those of cholesterol. The resonances of the terminal carbon of acyl chains (Acyl-ωCH_3) and [^{13}C-2-CH_3-]-acyl chain (methylene carbon next to the carbonyl carbon) have a doublet appearance, which is consistent with dual ^{13}C labeling each at ω and ω-1 as well as carbonyl and C-2 carbons. The C-1, C-2, and C-3 carbons of glycerol backbone of PL are doublet, doublet, and triplet, respectively, which indicates the presence of [U-^{13}C]-glyceryl residue. One of the methyl resonances of cholesterol at 24.2 ppm (denoted by *dashed line*) is also doublet in nature, which is consistent with its origin from [U-^{13}C]-acetyl CoA. *PC* phosphatidylcholines; *PE* phosphatidylethanolamines.

In addition to polar metabolites, lipophilic metabolites and their ^{13}C isotopomers are analyzed by 2D ^{1}H TOCSY (data not shown) and ^{1}H-^{13}C HSQC (Fig. 5). Figure 5 reveals the presence of the following ^{13}C-positional isotopomers of phospholipids (PL): [^{13}C-ω,ω-1]-acyl chains, [^{13}C-1,2]-acyl chains, [U-^{13}C]-glyceryl backbone, and [^{13}C-one of the methyl plus its adjacent carbons]-cholesterol.

Based on the above assignment, changes in the polar metabolite profiles induced by AICAR are obtained from 1D ^{1}H (Fig. 6) and ^{13}C HSQC projection (Fig. 7) spectral comparison of control

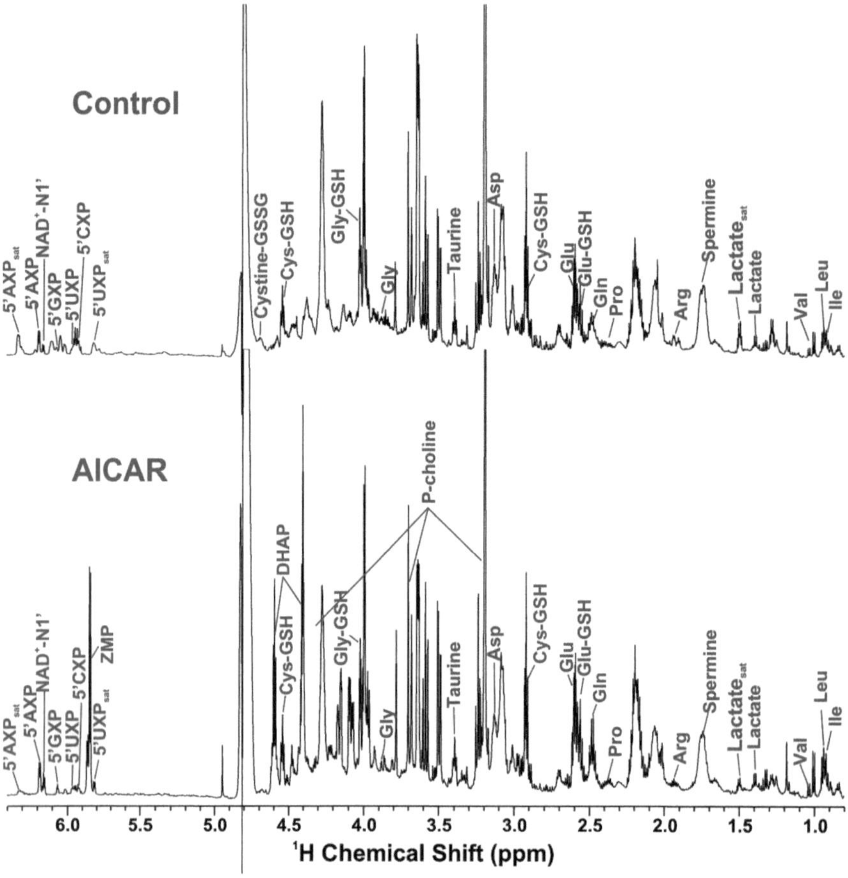

Fig. 6. Changes in the polar metabolite profile induced by AICAR in cancer cells as analyzed by 1D ^{1}H NMR. Metabolites and ^{13}C-isotopomers are assigned as in Fig. 3. Note the absence of significant glucose or glucose-6-phosphate in these cells. Spectra are normalized to cell dry weight for direct comparison.

vs. AICAR-treated cells. From Fig. 6, it is evident that AICAR causes the accumulation of amino acids including Val, Leu, Ile, Pro, and Gln along with the metabolic product of AICAR, ZMP. Metabolites that are depleted by the AICAR treatment include Asp, 5′UXP, and 5′CXP. Also depleted are the ^{13}C-isotopomers of lactate, 5′AXP and 5′UXP. More detailed changes in ^{13}C-isotopomer profile induced by AICAR are obtained from the ^{13}C HSQC projection spectral data in Fig. 7. Depletion of the following ^{13}C-isotopomers is evident: [U-^{13}C]-Ala, [U-^{13}C]-lactate, [^{13}C-4,5]-Glu, [^{13}C-4,5-Glu]-GSH, [^{13}C-1,2-Gly]-GSH, combinations of ^{13}C-isotopomers of Asp, [^{13}C-1,2, or 5,6]-citrate, [U-^{13}C-ribose]-5′AXP, [U-^{13}C-ribose]-5′UXP, [U-^{13}C-ribose]-5′GXP, and [U-^{13}C-nicotinamide-ribose]-NAD$^+$. These changes could be related to perturbations of glycolysis, pentose phosphate pathway (PPP), Krebs cycle, nucleotide synthesis, and glutathione metabolism.

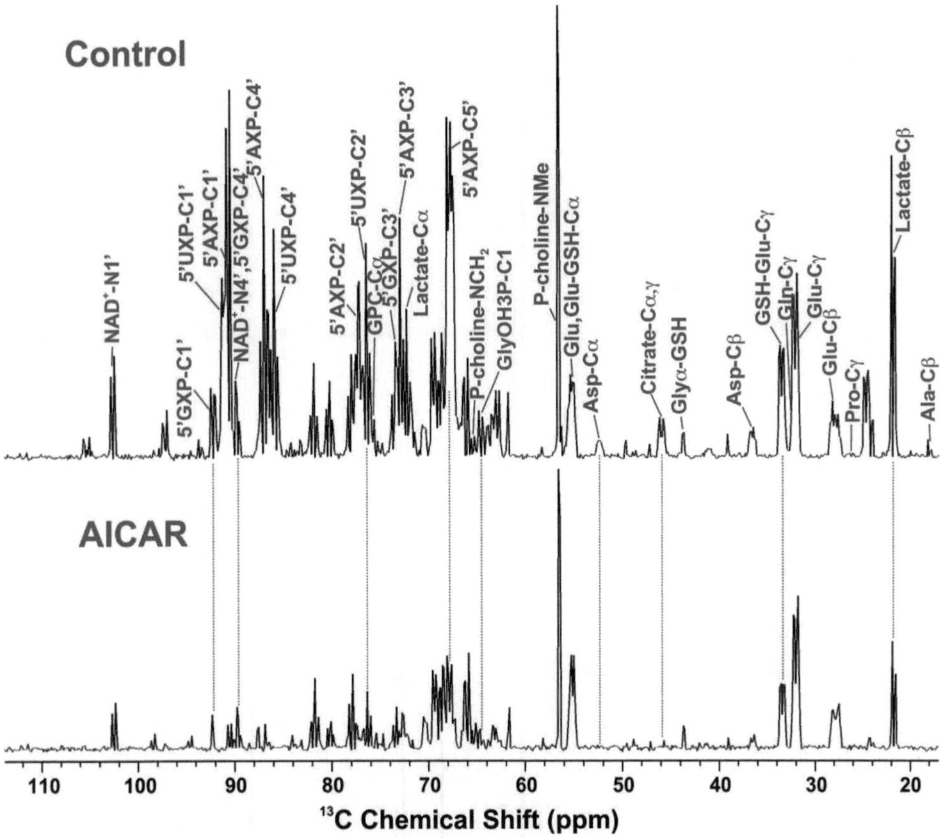

Fig. 7. Changes in the polar metabolite profile induced by AICAR in cancer cells as revealed by 1D ^{13}C projection spectra of HSQC. Metabolites and ^{13}C-isotopomers are assigned as in Fig. 4. *Metabolite-Cβ* C-3 of metabolite; *Metabolite-Cγ* C-4 of metabolite; *Metabolite-Cα* C-2 of metabolite; *Citrate-Cα,γ* C-2,5 of citrate.

Similarly, the changes in lipophilic metabolite profiles induced by AICAR are evident from the ^{13}C HSQC projection spectral comparison of control vs. AICAR-treated cells (Fig. 8). A large reduction in the intensity of ^{13}C resonances of acyl chain (ωCH_3, 2-CH_2) and glyceryl backbone (C-1,2,3) is evident with AICAR treatment. This indicates a substantial decrease in the synthesis of acyl chains and glycerol incorporation into PL. A much smaller effect of AICAR on ^{13}C enrichment in cholesterol is also observed from a small decrease in the intensity of the CH_3 resonance of cholesterol at 24.2 pm (Fig. 8).

Furthermore, 2D HSQC analysis is useful for probing AICAR effect on the incorporation of ^{13}C label from [U-^{13}C]-Glc into cellular proteins. This is done by acid hydrolysis of extracted proteins to release free amino acids before HSQC analysis. Figure 9 shows the 1D ^{13}C HSQC projection spectra of acid-released amino acid profiles for control vs. AICAR-treated cells. The ^{13}C splitting patterns observed for both control and AICAR treatments indicate

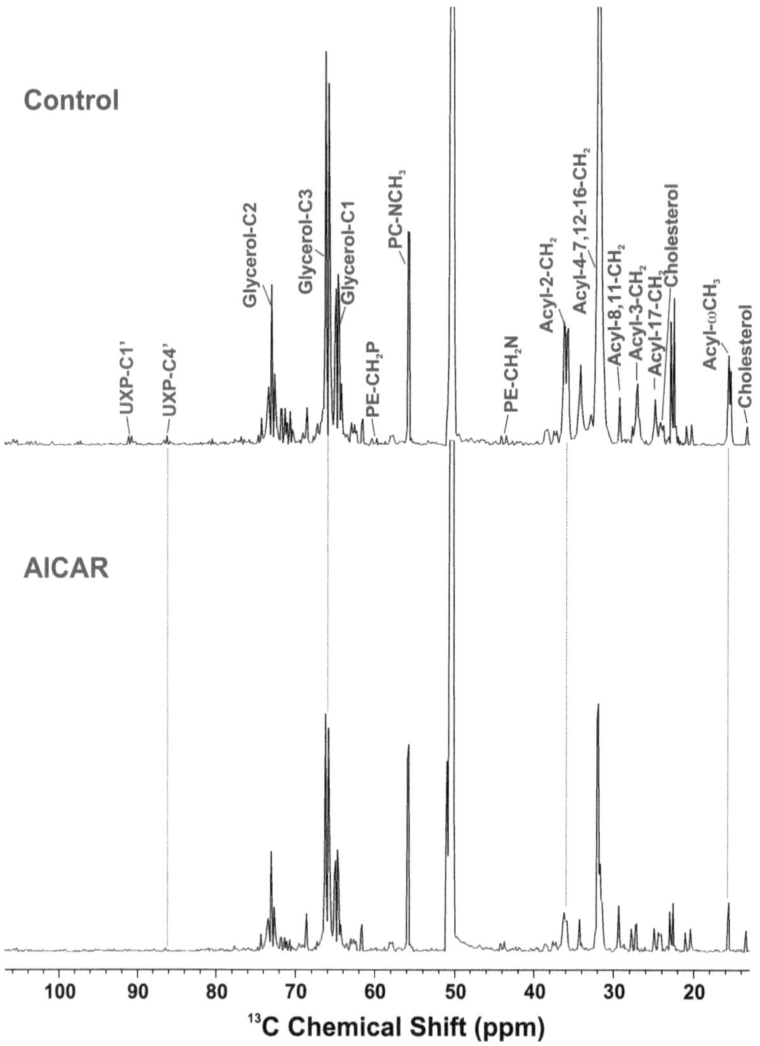

Fig. 8. Changes in lipophilic metabolite profiles of cancer cells induced by AICAR. The 1D ^{13}C-projection spectra of HSQC are shown for example methanolic extracts of control and AICAR-treated cells. ^{13}C resonances are assigned as in Fig. 5. A large AICAR-induced reduction in the intensity of ωCH_3, 2-CH_2 resonances of acyl chain of PL as well as 3-CH_2 resonance of glyceryl backbone of PL is noted with *dashed lines*.

the presence of [U-^{13}C]-Ala and ^{13}C labeling at more than 2 carbons of Glu and Asp. For all three amino acids, a significant reduction in ^{13}C enrichment is evident in response to AICAR, which is consistent with a reduced de novo protein synthesis.

Quantification of Metabolite and ^{13}C-Isotopomer Profiles by NMR and GC-MS

Changes in the concentrations of metabolites and their ^{13}C-isotopomers are quantified for both medium and cell extracts from control and AICAR treatments by ^{1}H NMR and GC-MS. Figure 10 shows the time courses of ^{12}C-lactate and [U-^{13}C]-lactate excreted by control or AICAR-treated cells into the growth medium. This figure demonstrates that in both control and treated

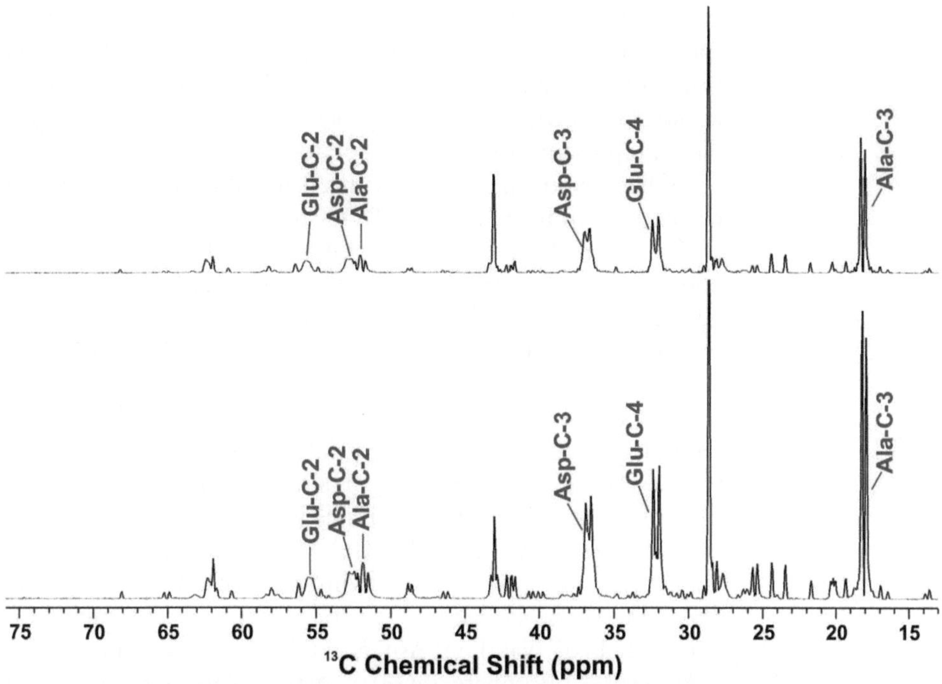

Fig. 9. 1D ^{13}C HSQC projection spectra of acid hydrolysates of proteins extracted from control (*bottom panel*) and AICAR-treated (*top panel*) cancer cells. Protein extracts are hydrolyzed in 6 N HCl at 110°C for 24 h to liberate free amino acids. The hydrolyzed amino acids are analyzed by 2D ^{1}H-^{13}C HSQC for identification of ^{13}C enrichment, as in Fig. 4. The doublet and triplet patterns of C-3- and C-2-Ala, respectively, indicate [U-^{13}C]-Ala while the doublet for C-4-Glu and C-3-Asp as well as complex ^{13}C splitting pattern for C-2 of Glu and Asp represent ^{13}C labeling at more than 2 carbons.

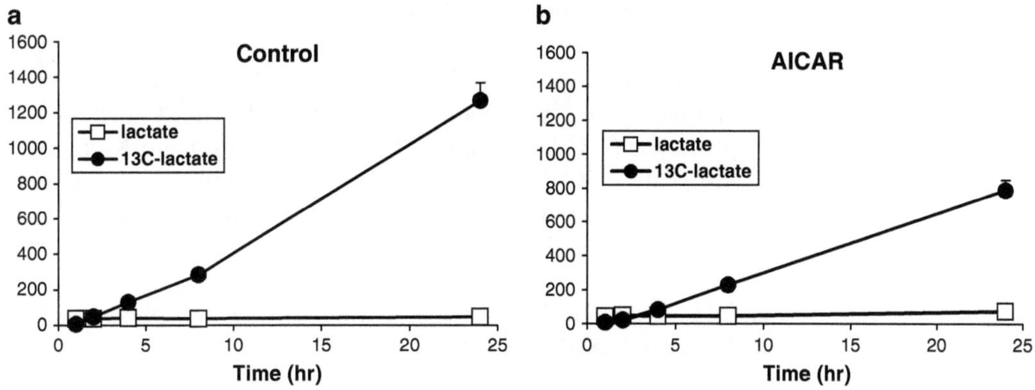

Fig. 10. Time courses of lactate excretion into growth medium by control and AICAR-treated cancer cells. Concentrations of ^{12}C-lactate (lactate) and [U-^{13}C]-lactate (^{13}C-lactate) are determined from 1D ^{1}H NMR spectra of three replicate medium samples, as described in Chap. 6. Each value is an average of the three replicates.

cells, most of the secreted lactate is derived from labeled glucose, while the contribution from nonglycolytic sources (^{12}C-lactate) is <1%. It is clear that AICAR inhibits the production and release of [U-^{13}C]-lactate into the medium as early as 1 h after the treatment. AICAR also decreases the rate of glucose uptake from the medium, by about the same factor as the lactate inhibition (data not shown). The amount of [U-^{13}C]-lactate excreted constitutes about 25% of the [U-^{13}C]-Glc consumed after 24 h of cell growth, which represents a significant sink for glucose carbon.

Changes in unlabeled and total metabolite concentrations of cell extracts induced by AICAR are shown respectively in panels a, b (from ^{1}H NMR) and d, e (from GC-MS) in Fig. 11. Relative to the control, AICAR-treated cells show a large buildup of the unlabeled AICAR metabolite (ZMP) and depletion of unlabeled P-choline in the order of 10 μmole/g cell dry weight (Fig. 11a). Unlabeled Tyr accumulates significantly in response to AICAR (Fig. 11b). AICAR-induced depletion of unlabeled 5′UXP is also substantial, while the decrease in unlabeled 5′AXP and NAD^{+} concentrations is to a lesser extent (Fig. 11b). There was no significant difference in unlabeled GSH and taurine levels of AICAR-treated vs. control cells (Fig. 11a). The GC MS analysis of total metabolite concentrations show the following distinction of AICAR-treated relative to control cells: accumulation of amino acids including Gly, Pro (Fig. 11d), Val, Leu, Asn, and Gln (Fig. 11e) and depletion of α-glycerol-3-phosphate (aG3P), Asp, malate, citrate (Fig. 11d), fumarate, and α-ketoglutarate (aKG) (Fig. 11e).

NMR quantification of [U-^{13}C]-lactate, [U-^{13}C-ribose]-5′UXP, and [U-^{13}C-ribose]-5′AXP in response to AICAR is shown in Fig. 11c. In all cases, a large depletion is observed. [U-^{13}C]-lactate is derived mainly from glycolysis and to a much lesser extent, from the PPP while [U-^{13}C]-ribosyl residue of nucleotides is synthesized from PPP only. GC-MS quantification of metabolite changes in total concentrations of ^{13}C-mass isotopomers elicited by AICAR is displayed in Fig. 11f, g. Except for a small accumulation of ^{13}C-Ala and ^{13}C-Gly (Fig. 11g), ^{13}C-metabolites of glycolysis (^{13}C-lactate and ^{13}C-aG3P, Fig. 11f) and Krebs cycle (^{13}C-malate, ^{13}C-citrate, ^{13}C-aKG, ^{13}C-fumarate, and ^{13}C-Asp, Fig. 11f, g) show depletion to a varying extent. Among the mass isotopomers, the dominant species and the largest change comes from the $m + 3$ species of lactate and αG3P (i.e., [U-^{13}C]-lactate and [U-^{13}C]-aG3P), $m + 2$ of citrate, and $m + 2$ plus $m + 3$ of malate and Asp (data not shown).

Confirmatory and Complementary Nature of NMR and MS Analysis

It should be noted that the GC-MS quantification confirms the semi-quantitative observation by NMR in Figs. 6 and 7. Such independent check greatly improves the confidence in metabolomic data, which can be fraught with analytical errors. The two techniques also complement each other in at least two ways.

First, they extend each other in the range of metabolites that can be analyzed, e.g., non-gas-chromatographable nucleotides, P-choline, and GSH by NMR; low abundance or poorly

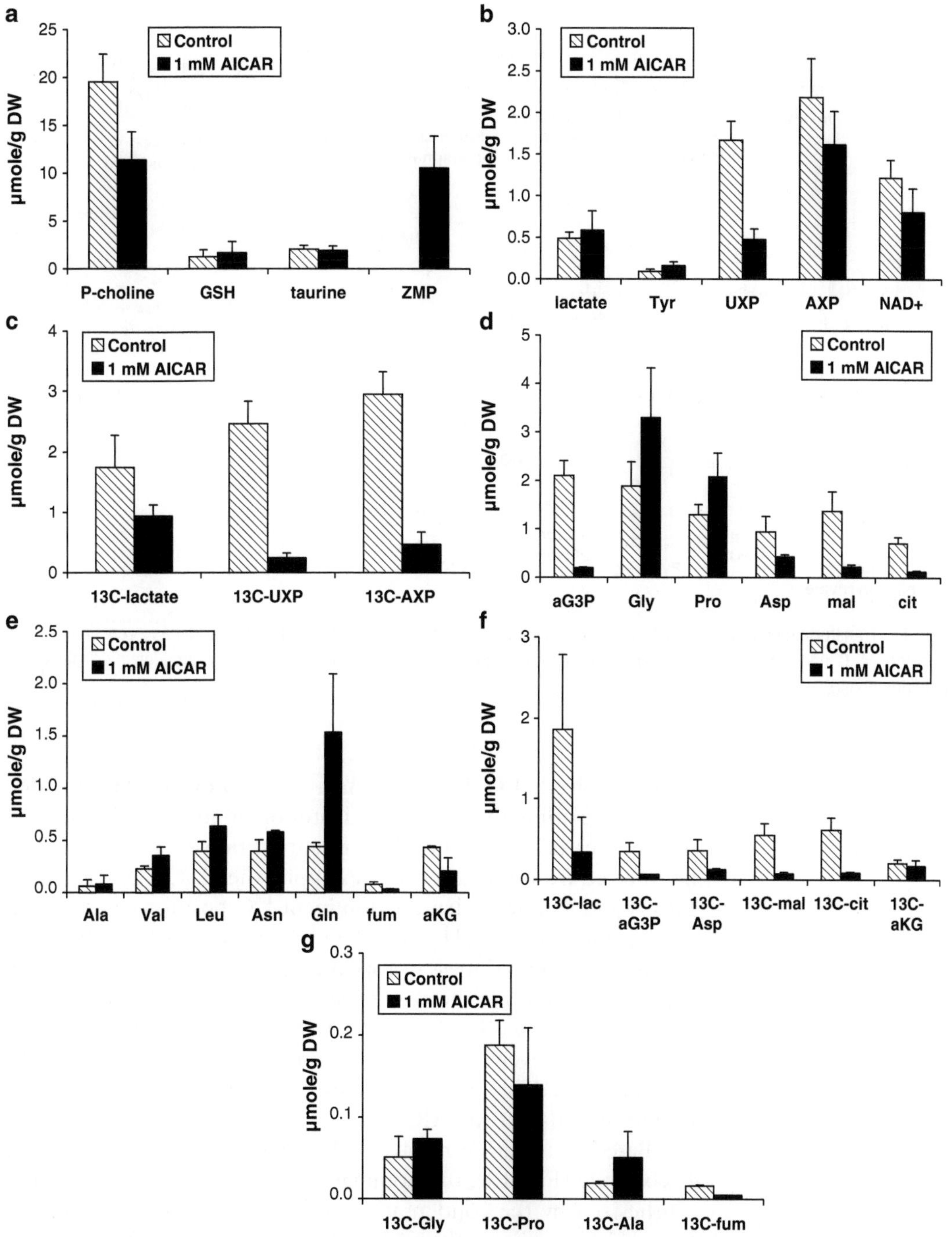

Fig. 11. Quantification of polar metabolites and ^{13}C-isotopomers in control and AICAR-treated cancer cells. (**a–c**) are obtained from 1D ^{1}H NMR analysis, where concentrations in (**a**, **b**) are those of the all ^{12}C isotopomers (unlabeled) and concentrations in (**c**) are those of [U-^{13}C]-lactate, [U-^{13}C-ribose]-5′UXP, and [U-^{13}C-ribose]-5′AXP. (**d–g**) are analyzed by GC-MS, where (**d**, **e**) report total metabolite concentrations and (**f**, **g**) show the sum of all ^{13}C-mass isotopomer concentrations. Each value is an average of three replicates. *P-choline* phosphorylcholine; *GSH* reduced glutathione; *aG3P* α-glycerol-3-phosphate; *mal* malate; *cit* citrate; *fum* fumarate; *aKG* α-ketoglutarate.

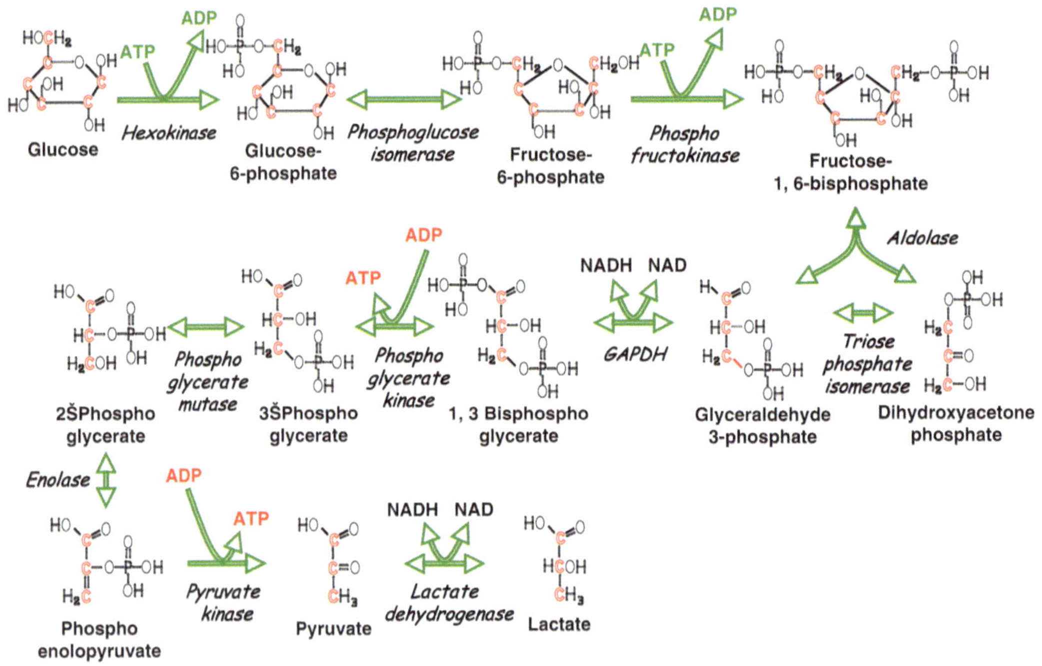

Fig. 12. Transformations of [U-^{13}C]-Glc to [U-^{13}C]-lactate via glycolytic and lactate dehydrogenase reactions. ^{13}C is denoted as **C** and *double-headed arrows* represent freely reversible reactions. *GAPDH* glyceraldehyde-3-phosphate dehydrogenase.

NMR-resolved aKG, fumarate, Asn, and Leu by GC-MS. In addition, by relating the positional isotopomer from NMR to mass isotopomer data from GC-MS, quantification of the former can be inferred from the latter. For example, the HSQC NMR data in Figs. 4 and 7 indicate that the dominant ^{13}C-positional isotopomer (s) of citrate is [^{13}C-1,2]-, or [^{13}C-5,6]-citrate, which is relatable to the dominant $m + 2$ mass isotopomer species observed by GC-MS. The concentration of the $m + 2$ species for the control and AICAR-treated cells is 0.39 ± 0.03 and 0.05 ± 0.01 μmole/g cell dry weight, respectively. Thus, it is reasoned that [^{13}C-1,2]-, or [^{13}C-5,6]-citrate is depleted by 0.34 μmole/g cell dry weight or eight-fold in response to AICAR.

Based on the atom-resolved schemes of glycolysis (Fig. 12) and Krebs cycle (Fig. 13), the dominant $^{13}C_2$-citrate species should be synthesized by the condensation of [U-^{13}C]-acetyl CoA (derived from [U-^{13}C]-Glc) with unlabeled oxaloacetate (OAA) in the first turn of the Krebs cycle. Due to the structural symmetry of citrate, [^{13}C-1,2]-citrate is indistinguishable from [^{13}C-5,6]-citrate by NMR. However, the enzymes citrate synthase and aconitase exhibit chiral recognition of citrate such that the dehydration and rehydration reactions of aconitase occur stereospecifically and away from the newly incorporated acetyl moiety of citrate to form isocitrate.

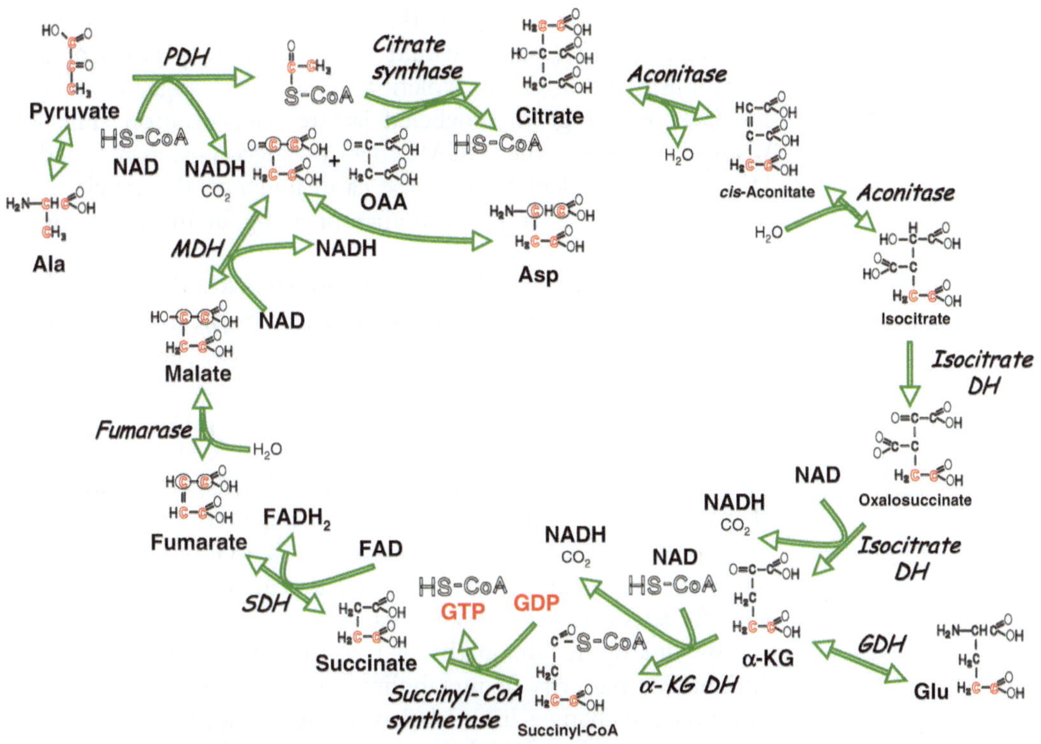

Fig. 13. Transformations of glycolytic end product [U-^{13}C]-pyruvate through the Krebs cycle sequence. **C** denotes ^{13}C and *double-headed arrows* represent freely reversible reactions. The scrambling of ^{13}C at fumarate, malate and OAA is indicated by circled **C**. *PDH* pyruvate dehydrogenase; *OAA* oxaloacetate; *GDH* glutamate dehydrogenase; *α-KG* α-ketoglutarate; *SDH* succinate dehydrogenase; *MDH* malate dehydrogenase.

It should also be noted that the enzyme succinate dehydrogenase (SDH) does not recognize succinate chirally such that the ^{13}C label of succinate becomes scrambled at the subsequent dehydration step (fumarase reaction) leading to a 50:50 mixture of [^{13}C-1,2]- or [^{13}C-3,4]-malate and OAA (Fig. 13).

Metabolomics-Edited Transcriptomics Analysis (META) of AICAR Effect

The AICAR-induced changes in metabolite profile, particularly in terms of the ^{13}C-isotopomers, provide valuable information on the metabolic pathways in cancer cells altered by AICAR. The depletion of [U-^{13}C]-lactate, [U-^{13}C]-Ala, and [U-^{13}C]-aG3P (Figs. 7, 10, and 11) indicates a reduced flow of carbon through glycolysis and/or PPP. Attenuation of the Krebs cycle activity is evident from the reduced synthesis of ^{13}C-citrate, ^{13}C-aKG, ^{13}C-fumarate, ^{13}C-malate, and ^{13}C-Asp (a surrogate marker of OAA and precursor to pyrimidine ring synthesis) (Figs. 7 and 11). The depletion of [U-^{13}C-ribose]-nucleotides (Figs. 7 and 11), ^{13}C label in the pyrimidine nucleobases, and ^{13}C-Asp supports the disruption of nucleotide biosynthesis and the PPP. Decreased ^{13}C enrichment in the antioxidant GSH (Fig. 7) can be related to diminished synthesis of GSH.

It is important to note that the unlabeled GSH does not deplete (Fig. 11), which would fail to indicate perturbed GSH metabolism, if not for the depletion of ^{13}C-GSH (Fig. 7). Similarly, the lack of change in unlabeled lactate concentration (Fig. 11) would not capture the AICAR effect on glycolysis, as revealed by [U-^{13}C]-lactate depletion. These cases illustrate the crucial need for labeled tracers and isotopomer profiling in mapping altered metabolic networks.

^{13}C isotopomer profiling also reveals AICAR-induced reduction of de novo protein biosynthesis, as evidenced by the decreased incorporation of [U-^{13}C]-Ala, ^{13}C-Glu, and ^{13}C-Asp into cancer cell proteins (Fig. 9). Attenuated fatty acid biosynthesis, acyl incorporation into PL, and cholesterol biosynthesis are supported respectively by the depletion of [^{13}C-ω,ω-1]-acyl chains, [^{13}C-1,2]-acyl chains, [U-^{13}C]-glyceryl backbone of PL, and ^{13}C-labeled cholesterol (Fig. 8). These ^{13}C-positional isotopomer patterns of PL are also consistent with the transformations of [U-^{13}C]-Glc via glycolysis and Krebs cycle to generate the respective precursors, aG3P and acetyl CoA for fatty acid and PL synthesis.

By linking to the pathway information afforded from ^{13}C enrichment patterns of metabolites, it is also practical to better interpret the changes in unlabeled or total concentration of metabolites induced by AICAR. For example, since PL synthesis is attenuated, the decrease in unlabeled P-choline concentration (Fig. 11) is not related to PL synthesis, rather it is a result of reduced choline uptake or choline kinase activity, or decreased lipid catabolism. Mammalian cells are not capable of de novo synthesis of P-choline from glucose, which accounts for the lack of ^{13}C labeling in this metabolite. Likewise, the observed decrease in protein synthesis should contribute to the buildup of unlabeled amino acids (Val, Leu, Gln, Asn, Tyr, and Pro in Fig. 11) Val, Leu, and Tyr. However, this does not rule out the possibility that the amino acids accumulated also come from increased amino acid uptake or protein degradation. Furthermore, unlabeled 5′AXP is depleted to a much lesser extent than ^{13}C-labeled 5′AXP (Fig. 11), which implicates decreased utilization, in addition to reduced synthesis, of 5′AXP with AICAR treatment. The former is consistent with the attenuation in protein and lipid biosynthesis.

All of the above effects of AICAR on metabolic pathways are associated with the ZMP buildup resulting from AICAR metabolism. ZMP activates AMPK, which in turn modulate metabolism via protein phosphorylation and/or transcriptional suppression (37). The altered metabolic processes revealed from the metabolomic analysis provide strong clues to the molecular regulation underlying these changes, as mediated by AMPK activation. Regulation via transcriptional suppression is obtained from querying global gene expression profiles while modulation via protein phosphorylation is probed by Western blot and targeted proteomics.

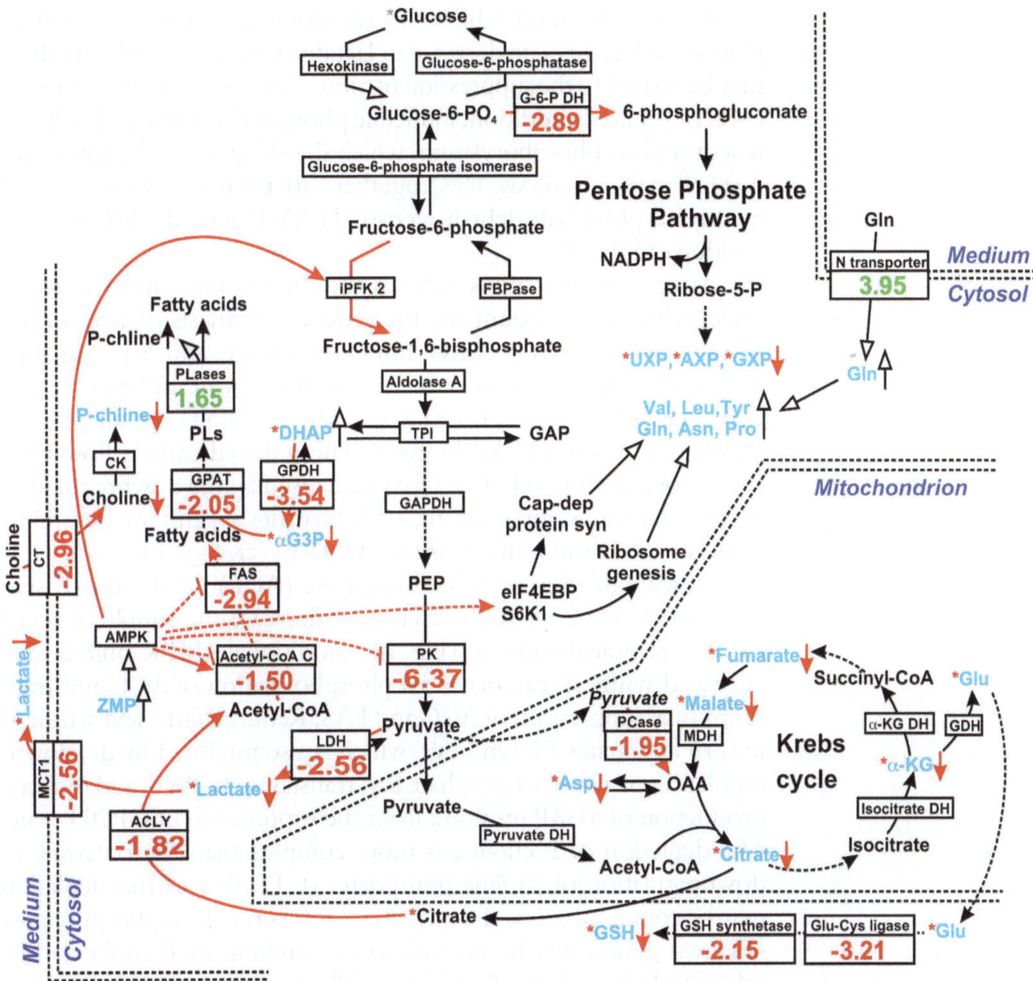

Fig. 14. Metabolomics-edited transcriptomics and proteomics analysis of AICAR effect. Based on the changes in metabolite and ^{13}C-isotopomer changes, expected gene expression and protein phosphorylation events impacted by AICAR are shown. *Red* and *open arrows* denote negative and positive changes, respectively; *dashed arrows* trace multistep or postulated processes; *blue text*, *dotted line* and * indicate measured metabolites, transcriptional suppression and ^{13}C labeling, respectively. *AMPK* AMP-activated protein kinase; *Acetyl-CoA C* acetyl CoA carboxylase; *ACLY* ATP citrate lyase; *LDH* lactate dehydrogenase; *PCase* pyruvate carboxylase; *OAA* oxaloacetate; *MDH* malate dehydrogenase; *α-KG* α-ketoglutarate; *GDH* glutamate dehydrogenase; *SDH* succinate dehydrogenase; *TPI* triosephosphate isomerase; *iPFK2* inducible phosphofructokinase; *FBPase* fructose bisphosphatase; *DHAP* dihydroxyacetone phosphate; *αG3P* α-glycerol-3-phosphate; *GAPDH* glyceraldehyde-3-phosphate dehydrogenase; *PEP* phosphoenolpyruvate; *PK* pyruvate kinase; *GPAT* glycerol phosphate acyl transferase; *GPDH* glycerol-3-phosphate dehydrogenase; *FAS* fatty acid synthase; *PLases* phospholipases; *P-choline* phosphorylcholine; *MCT* monocarboxylic acid transporter; *N transporter* neutral amino acid transporter; *CT* choline transporter; *CP* choline kinase; *eIF4EBP* eukaryotic initiation factor 4E binding protein; *S6K* S6 protein kinase.

Figure 14 displays a possible outcome of the metabolomics-edited transcriptomics and proteomics analysis (METPA) of AICAR effect, where multiple gene expression and protein phosphorylation events occur. By querying the expression of the full suite of genes for glycolytic enzymes, the large suppression of PK and lactate dehydrogenase

(LDH) genes is found, which may account for the reduced flow from glucose to lactate. The decrease in lactate excretion into the medium may be related to the suppression of monocarboxylic acid transporter 1 (MCT1) gene. In addition, inducible phosphofructokinase 2 (iPFK2) is activated via phosphorylation, which should increase the flow in the first half of the glycolysis. This, together with the reduced expression of glycerol-3-phosphate dehydrogenase (GPDH) gene, could lead to the buildup of DHAP.

Attenuated glycolysis reduces the carbon flow into the Krebs cycle, which can account for the reduced synthesis of Krebs cycle metabolites, i.e., citrate, aKG, fumarate, malate, and Asp (Fig. 14). Also contributed to this reduction is the downregulation of the pyruvate carboxylase (PCase) gene, which inhibits the anaplerotic carbon input into the Krebs cycle. The reduced carbon flow from the Krebs cycle's Glu to GSH may be caused by the downregulation of two enzymes involved in GSH synthesis (glutamyl-cysteinyl ligase or GCL and glutathione synthetase) (cf. Fig. 14).

Downregulation of ATP-citrate lyase (ACLY) and reduced synthesis of citrate from Krebs cycle may decrease the supply of acetyl CoA for fatty acid synthesis (Fig. 14). Additional AMPK inhibition of fatty acid synthesis can occur via phosphorylation of ACC and transcriptional suppression of ACC and FAS. Reduced fatty acid synthesis in turn attenuates PL synthesis, which is also inhibited by the downregulation of glycerol phosphate acyl transferase (GPAT) and reduced production of αG3P resulting from the suppression of GPDH gene. The depletion of P-choline is more complex than the outcome of downregulation of choline transporter (CT). Part of this depletion may be counteracted by the increased expression of the phospholipase (PLases) genes, which can lead to the buildup of P-choline while releasing fatty acids for β-oxidation. The latter process may occur to a lesser extent than the former to account for a net decrease in P-choline level. In this case, transcriptomic analysis aids in the resolution of two opposing metabolic events involving the same metabolite pool.

AMPK activation can also inhibit the phosphorylation of eukaryotic initiation factor 4E binding protein (eIF4E-BP) and S6 protein kinase 1 (S6K1) via the mTOR pathway, which can lead to a reduction of protein translational machinery involved in the synthesis of cap-dependent and ribosomal proteins (Fig. 14). This effect of AICAR is consistent with the observed accumulation of protein amino acids. The upregulation of neutral amino acid transporter (N transporter) may also contribute to the buildup of the Gln pool (Fig. 11), which is in excess of other amino acids.

Furthermore, the downregulation of the entry enzyme to PPP, glucose-6-phosphate dehydrogenase (G6PDH), is expected to inhibit ribose-5-phosphate synthesis and NADPH production, thereby reducing the incorporation of newly synthesized ribose into nucleotides. ZMP is an intermediate in purine biosynthesis, which could compete with de novo purine nucleotide synthesis. Additional inhibition of pyrimidine nucleotide synthesis could come from reduced supply of the Asp precursor, as a result of carbon shortage in the Krebs cycle (see above).

In the scenario depicted in Fig. 14, many of the transcriptional and protein phosphorylation events are consistent with known AMPK regulations reported for liver, muscle, or pancreatic β-cells (cf. Figs. 1 and 2). However, the inhibition of glycolysis observed for cancer cells is contrary to the recognized stimulation of glycolysis by activated AMPK (cf. Fig. 1). This inconsistency suggests that glycolytic regulation by AMPK differs between cancer and noncancerous cells, or alternatively, the glycolytic effect in cancer cells is not mediated by AMPK. Equally intriguing is the discovery of many regulatory processes not known to be associated with AMPK activation. These include the upregulation of N transporter and PLases, as well as downregulation of G6PDH, GPDH, LDH, GCL, glycogen synthase (GS), PC, CT, and MCT1 (cf. Fig. 14). Without the guidance from metabolomic data, these gene expression modulations may not be readily discerned through de novo gene pathway association analysis of transcriptomic data.

META of Effect of AMPK-Knockdown in Cancer Cells

Whether the regulatory events in Fig. 14 are mediated by AMPK activation or by AMPK-independent effect of AICAR can be addressed by applying the same META approach to characterize cancer cells with AMPK KD. If AMPK activation underlies all processes summarized in Fig. 14, then no significant or much smaller differences in metabolite and ^{13}C-isotopomer profiles (cf. Figs. 6–11) are expected between KD cells with and without AICAR treatment. Likewise, the gene expression and protein phosphorylation events in Fig. 14 would not be as significantly induced by AICAR in KD cells.

On the other hand, if inhibition of glycolysis, GSH synthesis, and choline transport is independent of AMPK activation, we would expect only the following metabolic changes: reduced production of [U-^{13}C]-lactate and [^{13}C-Glu]-GSH as well as choline depletion in KD cells in response to AICAR. We would also expect the corresponding downregulation of PK, CT, GCL, and GSH synthetase from the transcriptomic analysis.

Thus in the example illustrated above, the META approach can greatly accelerate de novo generation of highly testable hypotheses for AMPK's role in regulating metabolic networks of a given cell system. By coupling with complementary manipulations of AMPK activity, this approach can also be powerful in deciphering AMPK-dependent and independent regulations. As such, the potential for hypothesis-generation as well as hypothesis-driven research is not to be underestimated.

3. Deciphering Anticancer Selenite Action in Lung Cancer Cells

3.1. Anticancer Role of Selenium Agents

The trace element selenium (Se) has received increasing attention in chemoprevention for the past decade, as reflected by many clinical trials conducted using different Se agents (54–60). Se is an essential nutrient that serves a number of vital cellular functions involved in proliferation, survival, and differentiation (61–63). It is incorporated as selenocysteine (Se-Cys) posttranscriptionally into at least 25 mammalian proteins including thioredoxin reductase (TrxR), glutathione peroxidase, and iodothyronine 5′-deiodinase (64, 65). Clinical trials and laboratory research have shown that at supranutritional levels, some selenium compounds possess chemopreventive activity against a number of cancers including lung, prostate, breast, and colorectal (the four most lethal human cancers) (54–56, 61, 66–70). However, the efficacy of Se depends on the chemical form and the tissue type, suggesting the involvement of metabolic transformation into active cytotoxic form(s). For example, selenite, selenomethionine (SeM), methylseleninic acid (MSA), and methylselenocysteine show varied toxicity to different cancer cells and tumors including those of pulmonary origin (71–73). Se supplementation has also been shown to reduce anticancer drug resistance or toxicity, or synergize with anticancer drug therapy by inhibiting both tumor growth and metastasis (74–81).

Despite the promising beneficial effects of Se in chemoprevention and therapy, the underlying molecular mechanisms are still unclear. For example, a wide range of Se effects on cellular functions has been reported, including apoptosis, necrosis, inhibition of cell motility/migration/adhesion, cell cycle arrest, disruption of Ca^{2+} homeostasis, as well as modulation of matrix metalloproteinase expression, cell surface receptors, signaling protein kinases, growth factors, transcription factors, tumor suppressors, and DNA damage (55, 61, 71, 82–89). How these effects relate to metabolic functions and molecular regulations in different tissue and cell contexts is unclear. In particular the mechanism(s) of how Se compounds can block lung cancer progression have not been studied in detail (90).

Many of these effects are involved in carcinogenesis and metastasis, which may be mediated via antioxidative selenoproteins such as TrxR. TrxR has been implicated in cancer cell resistance to cisplatin (91), redox control of cell cycle proteins (61, 83), modulation of growth-, survival- and mobility-regulating transcription factors NFκB, p53, AP-1 (fos-jun), HIF-1, and thioredoxin peroxidases (92–98), as well as suppression of apoptosis signaling kinase ASK-1 (99). In particular, the modulation of transcription factors such as HIF-1 (a "master switch" for metabolic genes) is expected to alter many aspects of cellular and extracellular metabolism.

Clearly, Se in its different chemical forms has a complex and varying impact on cancer cells and tumors. This complexity will be extremely challenging to resolve without a systematic means for characterizing metabolic dysfunctions induced by different Se forms, and how such dysfunctions are linked to perturbed gene regulatory events. Thus, we developed the META approach to overcome this difficulty. Described below is how META was used to probe into the complex action of two anticancer Se agents in human lung cancer cells

3.2. Metabolomics-Edited Transcriptomic Analysis of Anticancer Se Action in Human Lung Adenocarcinoma A549 Cells

3.2.1. Approach

In this real-world example (15, 100), a similar approach as described for the hypothetical AMPK investigation above was employed. Briefly, the phenotypic effects and effective concentration (EC) for two Se agents, selenite and selenomethionine (SeM), on A549 cells was defined. These include cell proliferation, apoptosis, mitochondrial redox potential, and cytoskeleton integrity. The EC_{50-70} dose for each Se agent was used for subsequent metabolomic analysis, which included metabolite profiling and use of [U-^{13}C]-Glc tracer coupled with ^{13}C-isotopomer profiling. Transcriptomic analysis using Affymetrix human gene microarray was conducted for the selenite treated cells, in parallel to the metabolomics analysis.

3.2.2. Actual Observation

Phenotypic Effect of Selenite and SeM

The phenotypic changes in human lung adenocarcinoma A549 cells induced by selenite or SeM is shown in Figs. 15 and 16. Figure 15 shows the dose- and time-dependent effect of selenite and SeM on the growth of A549 cells (101). For selenite (Fig. 15a), growth inhibition was evident after 48 h of incubation at 0.2 ppm and the degree of inhibition increased with higher doses and longer incubation (e.g., $\geq$70% growth inhibition with 0.5 ppm selenite after 48 h). This growth inhibition was accompanied by alterations in cell morphology and cytoskeleton structures, as well as inhibition of mitochondrial redox activity, as illustrated in Fig. 16 for the 0.5 ppm selenite/48 h treatment. Moreover, selenite exposure enhanced apoptosis in A549 cells, as evidenced by an increase in DNA fragmentation and caspase activity (15, 100).

In contrast, A549 cell growth was not inhibited by SeM at an order of magnitude higher concentration (Fig. 15b). Growth inhibition only occurred when concentration reached 40 mg Se/L or 40 ppm (500 μM) and to a lesser extent, ca. 40% after 48 h (data not shown). Neither did 20 ppm of SeM induce significant changes in cell morphology, cytoskeleton structure, mitochondrial redox potential (Fig. 16), or apoptosis after 48 h of treatment.

NMR Identification and Semi-quantification of Metabolites and ^{13}C-Isotopomer Profiles

Polar metabolites in the TCA extracts of A549 cells were identified based on 2D ^{1}H TOCSY (Fig. 17) and high resolution ^{1}H-^{13}C HSQC (Fig. 18) analysis, as described in 2.2.2. A similar set of metabolites and ^{13}C-positional isotopomers as in Figs. 3 and 4 was

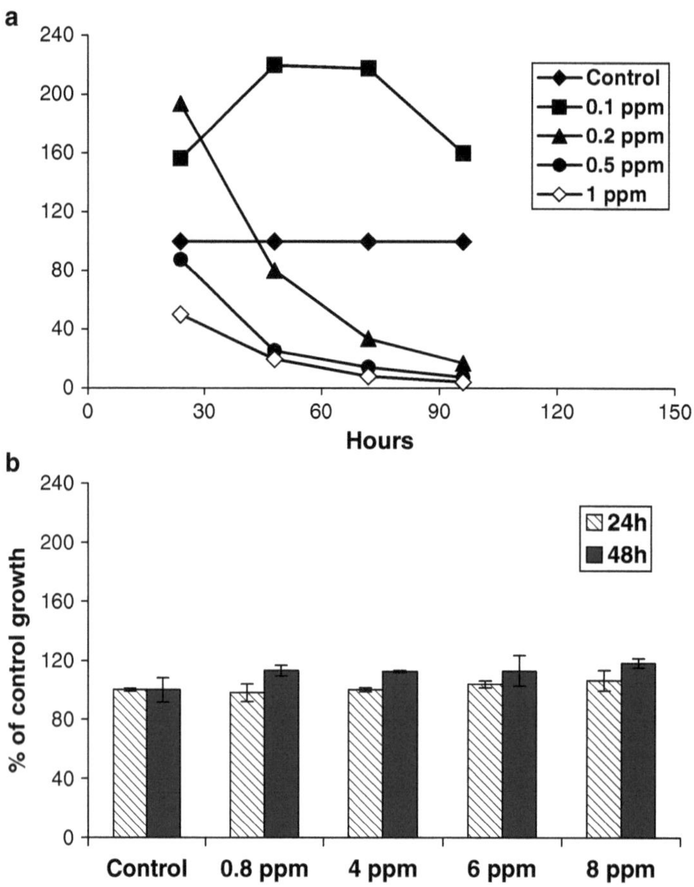

Fig. 15. Effect of selenite (**a**) or selenomethionine (**b**) on A549 cell growth as a function of time and dose. The cells were incubated with various doses of selenite or SeM for up to 96 h and daily growth measurement was performed using the MTT test. Each value was an average of quadruplicate measurements. All growth data were normalized to that under serum-deprived conditions (15).

observed in A549 cell extracts. These include Ala, [U-^{13}C]-Ala, lactate, [U-^{13}C]-lactate, Pro, Glu, [^{13}C-2,3]-Glu, [^{13}C-4,5]-Glu, GSH, [^{13}C-2,3-Glu]-GSH, [^{13}C-4,5-Glu]-GSH Asp, [^{13}C-1,2 or 3,4, or 2,3]-Asp, citrate, [^{13}C-1,2 or 5,6]-citrate, 5′AXP, [^{13}C-ribose]-5′AXP, 5′UXP, [U-^{13}C-ribose]-5′UXP, 5′GXP, [U-^{13}C-ribose]-5′GXP, NAD^+, and [U-^{13}C-nicotinamide-linked ribose]-NAD^+.

Using the ^{1}H and ^{13}C assignments above, a semi-quantitative evaluation of Se-induced changes in metabolite and their ^{13}C-positional isotopomer profiles was made. Figure 19 compares the metabolite profiles of control, selenite, and SeM-treated A549 cells. Selenite treatment caused a prominent accumulation of essential protein amino acids (Ile, Leu, Val, Arg, Gln, Tyr, and Phe) along with a moderate increase in spermine concentration. Other significant changes induced by selenite included large

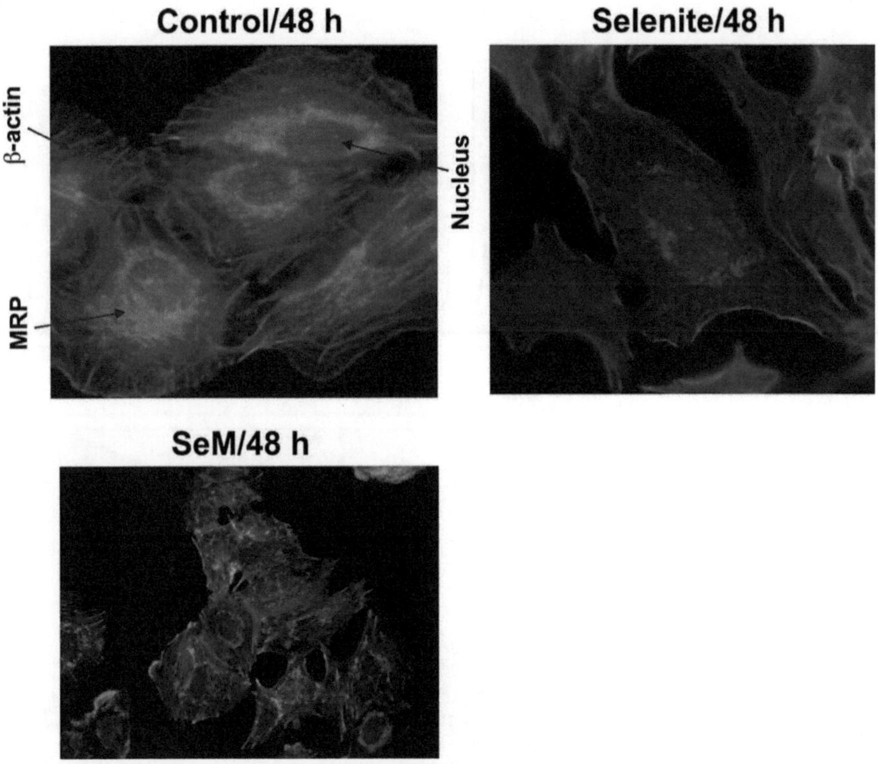

Fig. 16. Effect of selenite or selenomethionine on cytoskeleton structure and mitochondrial redox potential (MRP) in A549 cells. The cells were incubated with 0.5 ppm selenite or 20 ppm SeM for 48 h on microslides before staining for β-actin, MRP, and nucleus, as described in ref. (15).

depletion of Glu, GSH, Asp, and taurine. Relative to selenite, the SeM-induced metabolite changes were much less significant, except for P-choline (Fig. 19). P-choline was almost completely depleted by SeM treatment.

Changes in ^{13}C-positional isotopomers of polar metabolites induced by selenite or SeM are shown in Figs. 20 and 21, where respectively the 1D ^{1}H or ^{13}C projection spectra of 2D ^{1}H HCCH-TOCSY or HSQC analysis for control, selenite, or SeM treatments were compared. For the 24 h selenite treatment, a substantial depletion of the following isotopomers was evident: [U-^{13}C]-Ala, [U-^{13}C]-lactate, [^{13}C-2,3 or 4,5]-Glu, [^{13}C-2,3 or 4,5-Glu]-GSH, [^{13}C-1,2 or 2,3 or 3,4]-Asp, [U-^{13}C-ribose]-5′AXP, [U-^{13}C-ribose]-5′UXP, [U-^{13}C-ribose]-5′GXP, and [U-^{13}C-nicotinamide-linked ribose]-NAD^{+} (Fig. 21). Longer selenite treatment (48 h) also led to the accumulation of [U-^{13}C-glycerol]-GPC (Fig. 20). The SeM treatment, on the other hand, showed a much lesser extent of depletion in these isotopomers in 24 h of treatment (Fig. 21). The large attenuation in the ^{13}C intensity of the *N*-methyl resonance of P-choline (P-choline-NMe) was a result of depletion in P-choline at natural abundance. These changes in ^{13}C-positional isotopomer

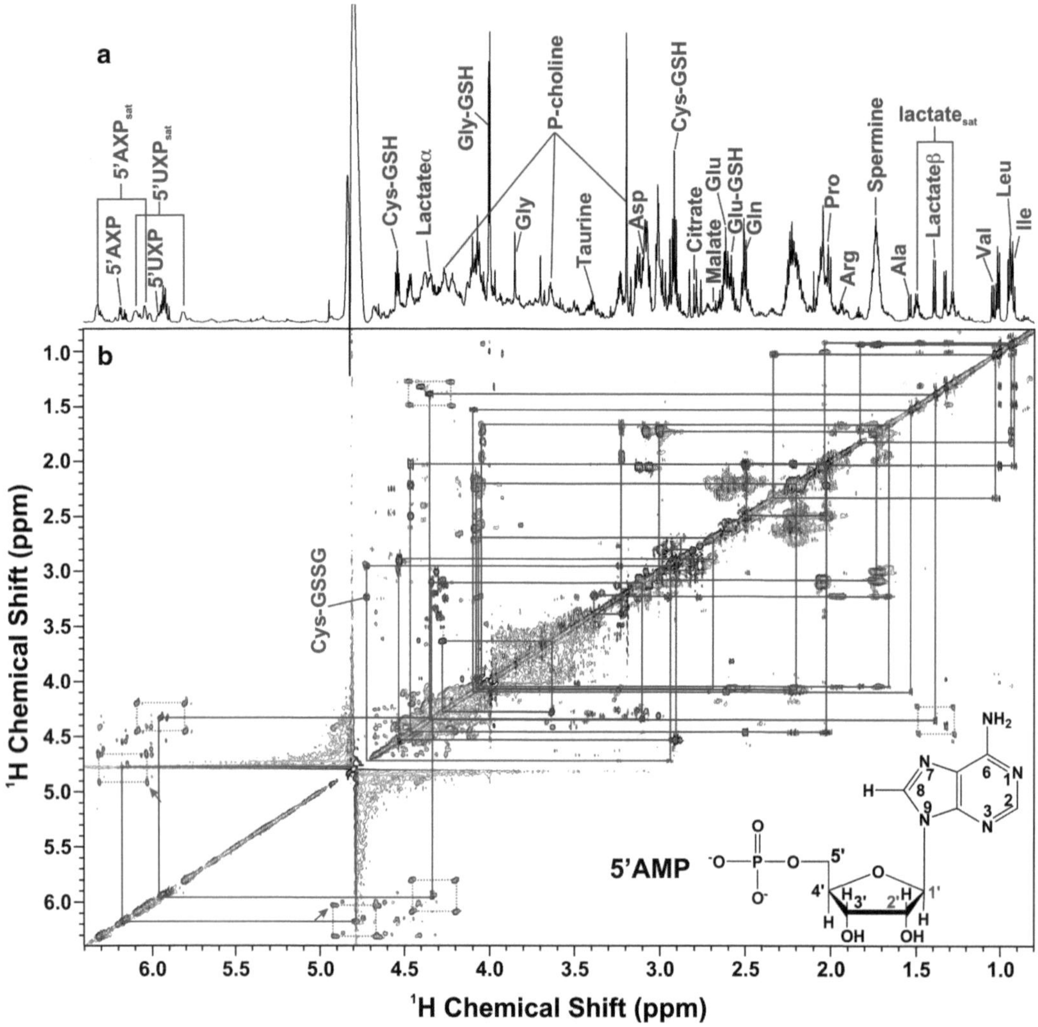

Fig. 17. ¹H NMR identified polar metabolites in example TCA extract of A549 cells. The extract was obtained from 40 ppm SeM-treated cells. The 2D ¹H TOCSY contour map (**b**) is shown along with the corresponding 1D high-resolution ¹H spectrum (**a**). The metabolites and their ¹³C-labeled isotopomers are assigned as described in Fig. 3. The *two arrows* indicate the ¹³C-satellite cross-peaks for the 1′ and 2′ protons of 5′AXP, as illustrated in the structure of 5′AMP.

profiles implicated a substantial reduction in carbon flow through glycolysis, PPP, Krebs cycle, GSH synthesis, and nucleotide synthesis as well as increase in lipid catabolism in response to selenite. In addition, these pathways were much less impacted by SeM.

Similar comparison of 1D ^{13}C HSQC projection spectra of lipophilic metabolites extracted from control and selenite treatments revealed changes in ^{13}C-positional isotopomers of PL induced by selenite (Fig. 22). [^{13}C-ω, ω-1]-acyl chains and [^{13}C-1,2]-acyl chains were depleted by selenite but not [U-^{13}C]-glycerol backbone of PL. This result indicated the specific

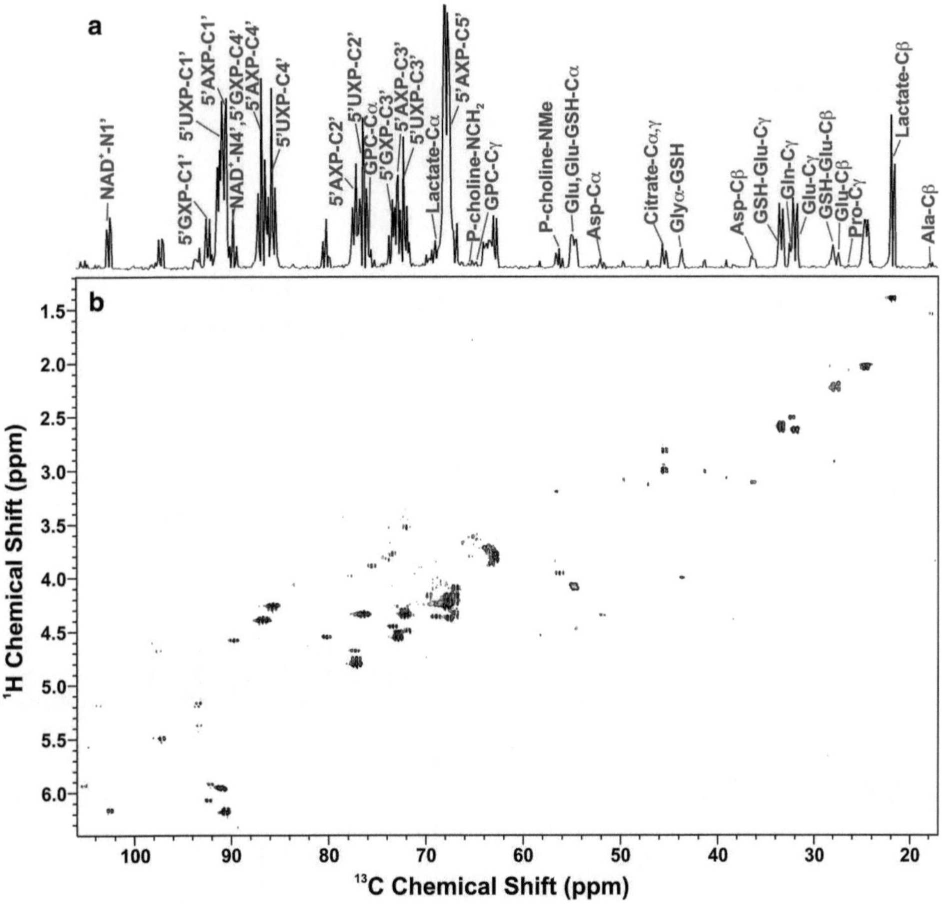

Fig. 18. 2D ^{1}H-^{13}C HSQC identified polar metabolites in the same extract of A549 cells as in Fig. 17. The 2D HSQC contour map (**b**) is shown along with the corresponding 1D ^{13}C projection spectrum (**a**). The metabolites and ^{13}C-positional isotopomers were assigned as in Fig. 4.

action of selenite in attenuating fatty acid biosynthesis but not the glycerol backbone incorporation into PL.

Quantification of Metabolite and ^{13}C-Isotopomer Profiles by ^{1}H NMR, GC-MS, and HPLC

Quantitative changes in metabolite profiles of A549 cells in response to selenite was obtained by GC-MS and HPLC analysis (Fig. 23a), which not only verified the NMR observation (Fig. 19) but also extended the range of metabolite changes quantified. Metabolites that accumulated to >10 μmole/g cell dry weight were spermine, P-choline, and OHPro, those accumulated to 1–10 μmole/g cell dry weight included taurine, Ser, Thr, Gln, Ala, Gly, Val, Leu, Ile, Phe, Tyr, Pro, Arg, NAD^+, ornithine, and Lys, while AMP, Met and Asn accumulated to <1 μmole/g cell dry weight. Except for UDP, metabolites (lactate, Glu, GSH, Asp, UTP, and ATP) that depleted were in the range of 1–10 μmole/g cell dry weight.

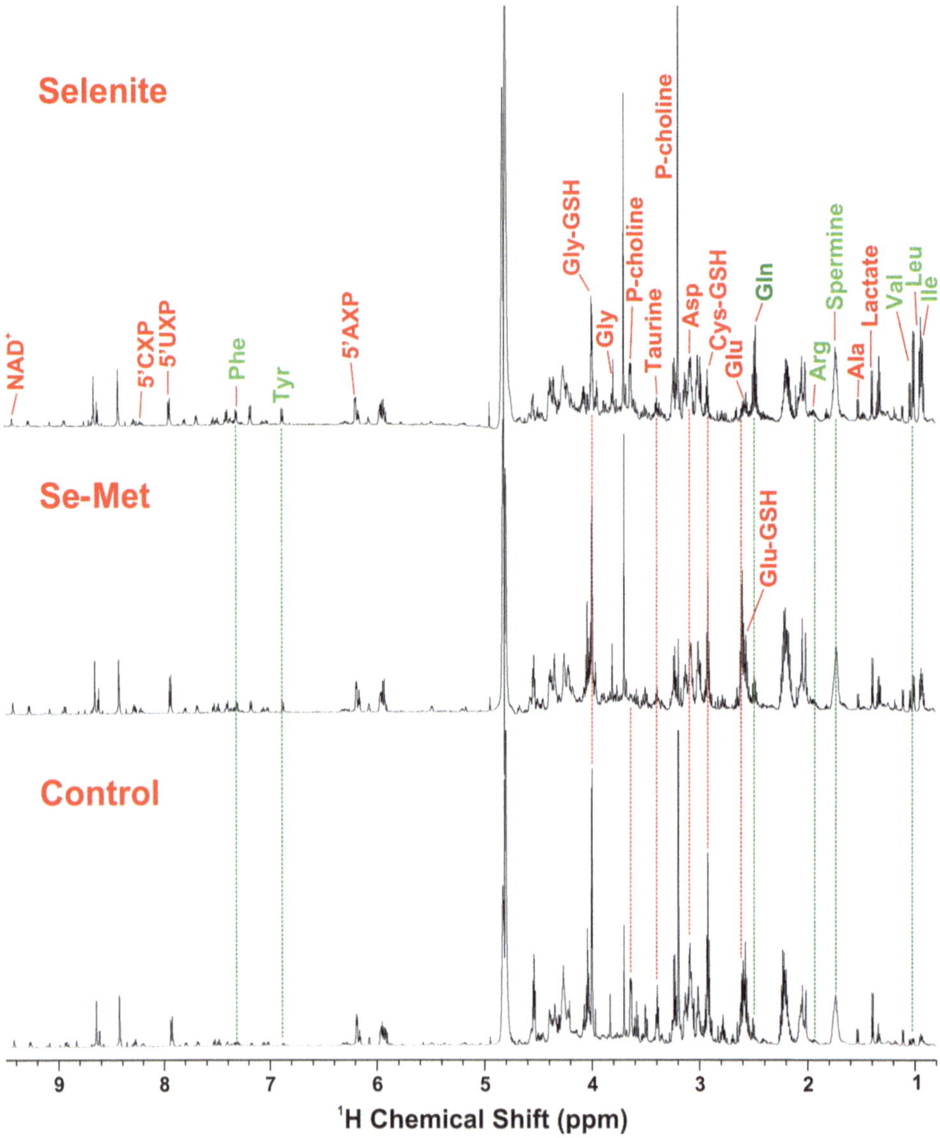

Fig. 19. 1D ^{1}H NMR comparison of TCA extracts of control, selenite, and SeM–treated A549 cells (adapted from ref. (100)). The cells were treated for 24 h without ^{13}C enrichment. Metabolite assignments were as in Fig. 17. *Dashed green* and *red lines* follow metabolites that accumulated and depleted, respectively, in response to Se treatments.

The quantitative changes in ^{13}C-mass isotopomers of selected metabolites are shown in Fig. 23b. For mass balance, the concentration of each mass isotopomer series (e.g., $m + 0$, $m + 1$, $m + 2$, etc.) is displayed along with the total concentration of a given metabolite. It is clear that selenite-induced depletion of total lactate was mostly attributed to [U-^{13}C]-lactate (lactate + 3) depletion. Change in total Ala concentration in response to selenite was largely due to the increased concentration of unlabeled Ala (Ala + 0). A similar case also applied to Pro and Ser, implicating

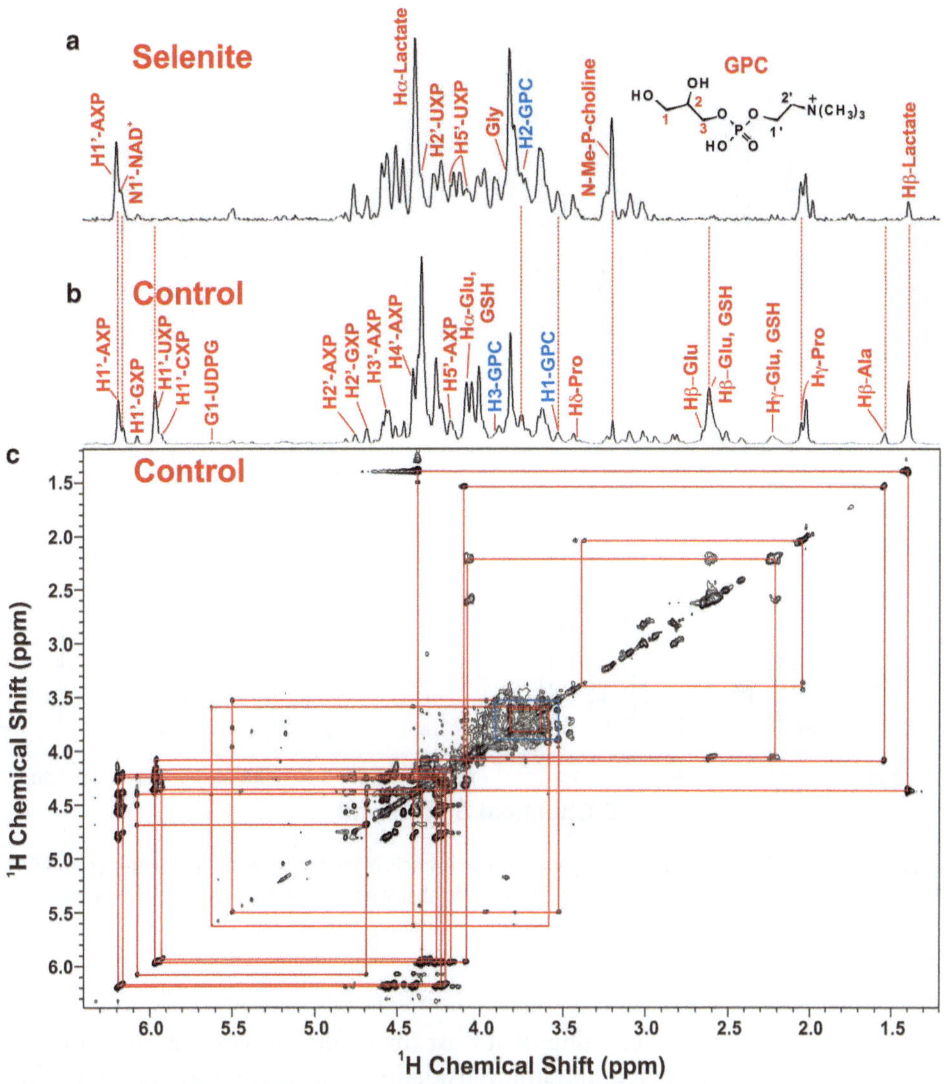

Fig. 20. 2D ^{1}H HCCH-TOCSY of TCA extracts better resolved accumulation of ^{13}C-GPC in response to selenite (adapted from ref. (15)). Cells were treated for 48 h in the presence of [U-^{13}C]-Glc. The 2D contour map of HCCH-TOCSY for control (**c**) is shown along with the 1D ^{1}H projection spectra of control (**b**) and selenite-treated (**a**) extracts. The HCCH-TOCSY analysis revealed only those ^{13}C-isotopomers which had consecutively labeled carbons in the structure (cf. Chap. 6). This greatly reduced spectral overlap in standard ^{1}H spectra (cf. Figs. 17 and 19) to highlight consecutively ^{13}C-labeled isotopomers present at low abundance. For example, The ^{1}H covalent connectivity (traced by *blue rectangle*) for [U-^{13}C-glycerol]-GPC was clearly seen in C but not discernable in Fig. 17. Metabolite assignments were based on Figs. 17 and 18. *Dashed lines* follow metabolites that changed in ^{13}C enrichment (e.g., [U-^{13}C-glycerol]-GPC accumulation) in response to selenite.

the origin of these changes from non-^{13}C-labeled sources such as uptake from medium or degradation of unlabeled proteins. The depletion of total Glu by selenite was a combination of decrease in concentrations of unlabeled, singly (Glu + 1), doubly (Glu + 2), and triply labeled (Glu + 3) Glu. This result pointed to the

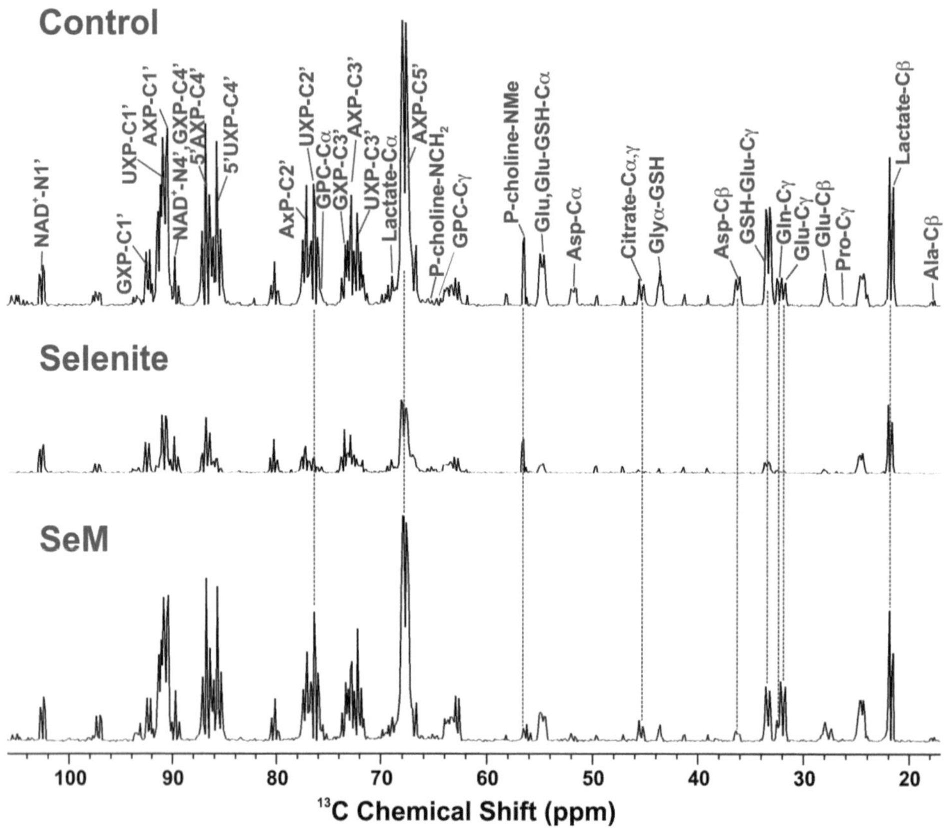

Fig. 21. Comparison of 1D ^{13}C HSQC projection spectra of TCA extracts of control, selenite, and SeM–treated A549 cells. The cells were treated for 24 h in the presence of [U-^{13}C]-Glc. Metabolite assignments are as in Fig. 18. *Dashed lines* trace metabolites that depleted in response to Se treatments.

malfunctioning of at least three Glu sources, e.g., medium uptake, unlabeled glutamine oxidation, and the Krebs cycle (cf. Fig. 13). The accumulation of total malate or depletion of total fumarate by selenite had the opposite contribution of unlabeled (accumulation) and labeled (depletion) mass isotopomers. As depicted in Fig. 13, the depletion of ^{13}C-malate (e.g., $^{13}C_2$ or $m + 2$ species) in Fig. 23b can be related to a reduced flux through the Krebs cycle, which could also lead to the depletion of ^{13}C-[1,2 or 5,6]-citrate and ^{13}C-[4,5]-Glu (Fig. 21). The accumulation of unlabeled malate could result from an increased oxidation of Gln (glutaminolysis) in response to selenite (cf. Fig. 24).

Again, the above results illustrate the value of isotopomer profiling by NMR and GC-MS in delineating drug or toxicant-induced perturbations of multiple pathways, particularly those commonly participating in the metabolism of the same metabolite. This is a task not practical to accomplish from total metabolite profiles alone.

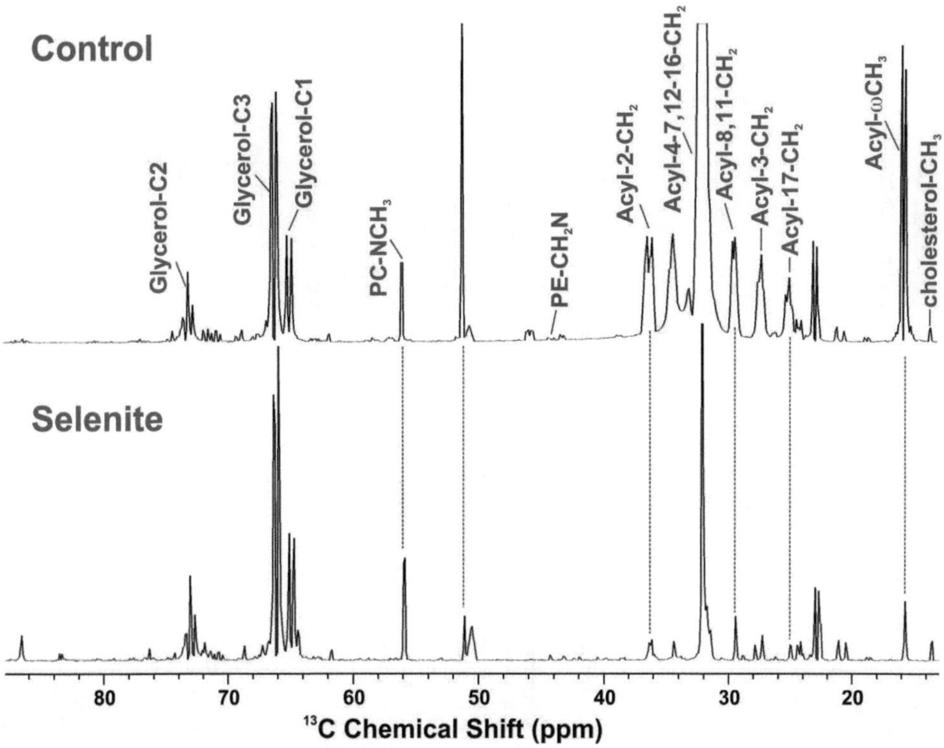

Fig. 22. Comparison of 1D ^{13}C HSQC projection spectra of methanolic extracts of control and selenite–treated A549 cells. The cells were treated for 48 h in the presence of [U-^{13}C]-Glc. Phospholipid (PL) assignments are as in Fig. 8. *Dashed lines* trace ^{13}C resonances of PL that decreased in intensity in response to selenite.

Metabolomics-Edited Transcriptomics Analysis (META) of Se Action in A549 Cells

The metabolite and ^{13}C isotopomer change patterns from above indicated perturbations to the following metabolic pathways. Reduced glycolysis and PPP activity was related to the depletion of [U-^{13}C]-lactate and [U-^{13}C-ribose]-nucleotides while disruption to the Krebs cycle was associated with the decreased ^{13}C incorporation into citrate, malate, Glu, and Asp (Figs. 21 and 23b). Inhibition of GSH synthesis was indicated by the depletion of ^{13}C-GSH isotopomers (Figs. 20 and 21). Decreased nucleotide biosynthesis could be inferred from the depletion of [U-^{13}C-ribose]-nucleotides and [^{13}C-5,6-ring]-UXP and UDPG (data not shown). Attenuation in fatty acid synthesis was indicated by the depletion of [^{13}C-ω,ω-1]-acyl chains and [^{13}C-1,2]-acyl chains of PL while stimulation of lipid degradation could be related to the accumulation of [U-^{13}C-glycerol]-GPC.

Based on these pathway changes, gene expression patterns of enzymes in the pathways were queried against the global human gene array data (Affymetrix) for the 48 h treatment of selenite vs. control. It should be noted that the large number (>2,000) of statistically significant changes in expression events in response to selenite made it impractical to perform de novo association of gene pathways. Figure 24 displayed selenite-induced change in

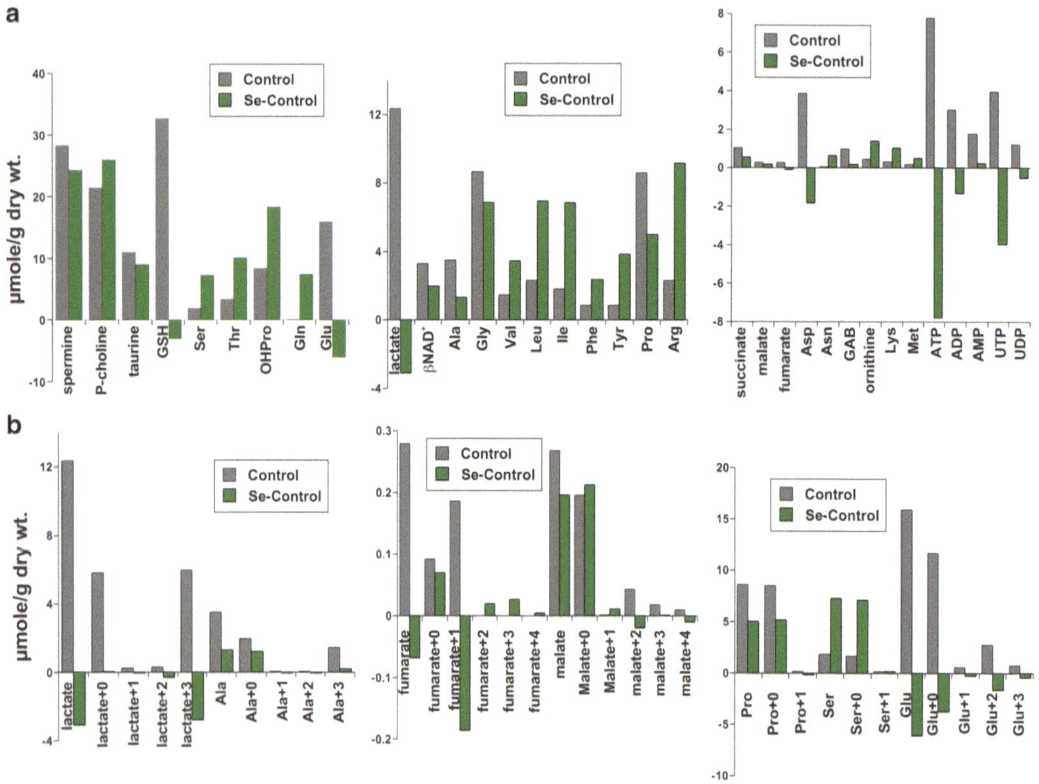

Fig. 23. ^{1}H NMR, GC-MS, and HPLC quantification of changes in metabolite and ^{13}C isotopomer profiles in A549 cell extracts in response to selenite treatment (from ref. (15) with permission). P-choline, taurine, and GSH were quantified by ^{1}H NMR, nucleotides by HPLC, and the rest by GC-MS. The ^{1}H NMR quantification used lactate as an internal standard (108) The *gray* and *solid bars* represent metabolite concentration from control and selenite-treated minus control treatments, respectively. Total metabolite concentrations are shown in (**a**) while the ^{13}C-mass isotopomer distribution for selected metabolite is shown in (**b**) along with the total concentration. Metabolite + 0, +1, +2, +3, +4 are ^{12}C, singly, doubly, triply, and quadruply ^{13}C-labeled mass isotopomers, respectively.

mRNA expression (calculated as base 2 signal log ratio or SLR of selenite-treated vs. control) in the context of glycolysis, PPP, Krebs cycle, glutaminolysis, fatty acid synthesis, phospholipid metabolism, and GSH synthesis. Also shown in blue text are the measured changes in metabolite and ^{13}C-isotopomer profiles.

The following gene expression events in response to selenite were found to be consistent with the metabolomic data. Decreased transcription of five glycolytic genes (particularly 6-phosphofructo-2-kinase [PFK2] which modulates the glycolytic PFK-1 activity) was related to reduced synthesis of lactate or decrease in glycolytic flux. Likewise, reduced gene expression of mitochondrial pyruvate dehydrogenase (PDH), α-KG DH, isocitrate dehydrogenase (Isocitrate DH), and malate dehydrogenase (MDH) may underlie the attenuated Krebs cycle activity, which together with the reduced glycolytic flux led to the reduced synthesis of citrate, malate,

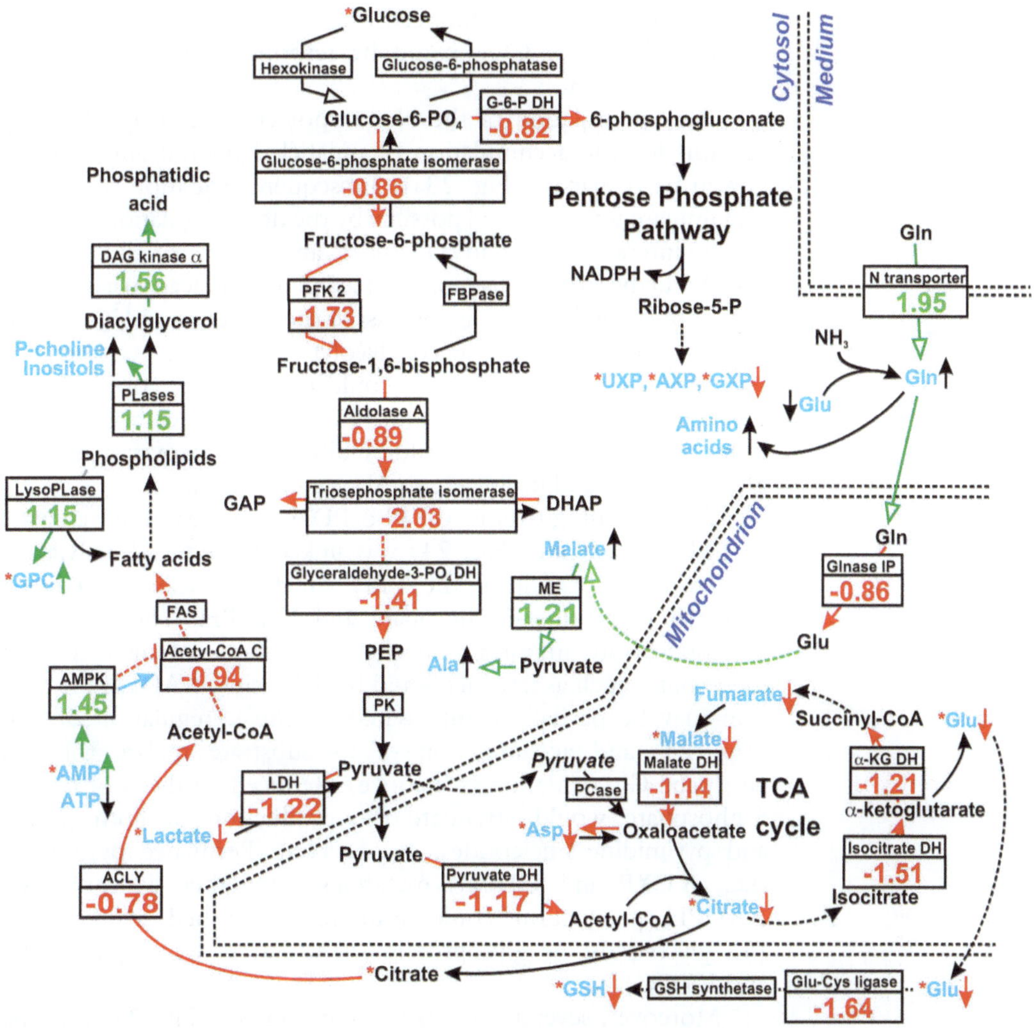

Fig. 24. Metabolomics-edited transcriptomic analysis for selenite-induced perturbations of glycolysis, pentose phosphate pathway, Krebs cycle, glutaminolysis, PL metabolism, and GSH synthesis in A549 cells. The signal log ratio of Se-treated vs. control mRNA expression in A549 cells is listed below each protein into which the mRNA was translated. Negative and positive values indicate a decrease and increase in expression, respectively. *Red arrows* indicate downregulation of genes, inhibition of protein activity, or depletion of ^{13}C-labeled metabolites (denoted by *). *Green arrows* indicate upregulation of genes, activation of protein activity, or accumulation of ^{13}C-labeled metabolites. *Black arrows* trace reactions, transport processes, and changes in concentration of unlabeled metabolites. The *open green arrows* delineate glutaminolysis of unlabeled Gln taken up from the medium and subsequent oxidation to generate unlabeled malate, which can be converted to Ala via ME. As such, unlabeled malate or ^{13}C-malate (*malate) (Fig. 23b) represented respectively the carbon flow via glutaminolysis or glycolysis-Krebs cycle sequence to the malate hub. *Dashed arrows* indicate multiple or postulated reaction steps. *Acetyl-CoA C* acetyl-CoA carboxylase; *AMPK* 5′-AMP-activated protein kinase; *DAG* diacylglycerol; *PLases* phospholipases; *LysoPlase* lysophospholipase; *P-choline* phosphorylcholine; *GPC* glycerophosphorylcholine; *G-6-P DH* glucose-6-phosphate dehydrogenase; *PFK2* phosphofructokinase 2; *FPBase* fructose bisphosphatase; *GAP* glyceraldehyde-3-phosphate; *DHAP* dihydroxyacetone phosphate; *PEP* phosphoenolpyruvate; *PK* pyruvate kinase; *LDH* lactate dehydrogenase; *Pyruvate DH* pyruvate dehydrogenase; *PCase* pyruvate carboxylase; *ACLY* ATP-citrate lyase; *α-KG DH* α-ketoglutarate dehydrogenase; *Malate DH* malate dehydrogenase; *OAA* oxaloacetate; *ME* malic enzyme; *Glnase IP* glutaminase interacting protein; *N transporter* neutral amino acid transporter; *Glu-Cys ligase* glutamyl-cysteinyl ligase (adapted from ref. (15)).

and Glu from glucose. Reduced availability of Glu coupled with downregulation of GCL could be responsible for the reduced synthesis of GSH.

The upregulation of the N transporter (102) (Fig. 24) may account for the accumulation of unlabeled neutral amino acids, Gln in particular (cf. Fig. 23a). Subsequent oxidation of Gln via glutaminase was enhanced possibly by the downregulation of glutaminase interacting protein (Glnase IP, an inhibitor of glutaminase) (103). Further metabolism of oxidized Gln could lead to accumulation of unlabeled malate, as contrast to the depletion of ^{13}C-labeled malate resulting from reduced glycolytic and Krebs cycle activity. Increased ME gene expression could enhance the conversion of unlabeled malate to Ala. Without the integrated metabolomic and transcriptomic analysis, it would be difficult to uncover stimulated glutaminolysis and its linkage to Ala accumulation.

The downregulation of G-6-PDH (the gateway enzyme to PPP) by selenite (Fig. 24) was linked to reduced activity of the oxidative branch of the PPP, which can lead to reduced synthesis of ribulose-5-phosphate and NADPH. The latter two metabolites are important in the biosynthesis of many central metabolites such as fatty acids and nucleic acids. NADPH production may be partially compensated by the upregulation of ME (Fig. 24) and accumulation of its substrate malate through enhanced Gln oxidation (see above). Reduced synthesis of ribose-5-phosphate would attenuate the production of both purine and pyrimidine nucleotides, as observed. Perturbed pyrimidine (i.e., 5′UXP and UDPG) metabolism together with reduced NADPH production could lead to diminished synthesis of PL, glycolipids, or glycoproteins, (the latter two require UTP and UDPG).

Moreover, several gene expression events in Fig. 24 could be linked to perturbations of lipid metabolism by selenite, i.e., the upregulation of AMPK, PLases, lyophospholipase (LysoPlase), and diacylglycerol (DAG) kinase α (DAGKα) as well as downregulation of ACC. Enhanced AMPK expression coupled with increased AMP/ATP ratio (a result of mitochondrial dysfunction) can potentiate AMPK activity in phosphorylating ACC (37), which is the entry and key regulatory enzyme of fatty acid synthesis (104). ACC phosphorylation inactivates its activity, which together with decreased gene expression was relatable to the attenuated synthesis of fatty acids (see also the first example above). The upregulation of PLases and LysoPlases (105) could enhance PL degradation, leading to the accumulation of P-choline, inositols, and ^{13}C-labeled glycerophosphorylcholine (GPC). Enhanced expression of PLases could also increase DAG production, thereby activating protein kinase C (PKC). On the other hand, the upregulation of DAGKα could terminate DAG-induced PKC activation via the production of phosphatidic acid (106). Phosphatidic acid could directly activate mTOR (cf. Fig. 2), thereby partially counteracting AMPK-mediated inhibition of mTOR. As illustrated in Fig. 2, inhibition of mTOR would have a profound impact on protein biosynthesis, which could contribute to the observed buildup of many protein amino acids (cf. Fig. 23). Again, without coupling transcriptomic with metabolomic profiles, it would be difficult to postulate and resolve such complex regulations of lipid and protein metabolism.

Finally, it should be noted that the selenite-associated metabolic dysregulations in A549 cells were linked to the observed phenotypic changes, i.e., growth inhibition, reduced mitochondrial redox potential and cytoskeleton disintegration (cf. Figs. 15 and 16). This is consistent with the lack of SeM effect on comparable phenotypic attributes and metabolic networks perturbed by selenite.

4. Conclusions

In conclusion, the above two examples illustrate how ^{13}C-tracers and ^{13}C-isotopomer profiling can be utilized and are necessary to map metabolic networks. They also demonstrate how such network information is integrated with transcriptomic data (i.e., META) to link drug or toxicant-induced changes in metabolic functions to regulatory pathways, as well as to phenotypic attributes. The approach enables systematic generation of highly specific working hypotheses and facilitates subsequent hypothesis validation for complex drug or toxicant action(s). It is generally applicable to any biological system including human body, as we have recently demonstrated (107).

Acknowledgments

This work was supported in part by the National Cancer Institute grant # 1 R01 CA101199-01, NIH Grant Number RR018733 from the National Center for Research Resources, National Science Foundation EPSCoR grant # EPS-0447479, Kentucky Challenge for Excellence, and the Brown Foundation. We thank Dr. Laura Bandura and Ms. Vennila Arumugum for A549 cell culturing, sample processing, and extraction.

Glossary

META	Metabolomics-edited transcriptomics analysis
Systems biology	Holistic and integrated analysis of biological processes as a system, not as individual parts

References

1. Griffiths JR, Stubbs M. Opportunities for studying cancer by metabolomics: preliminary observations on tumors deficient in hypoxia-inducible factor 1. Adv Enzyme Regul. 2003;43:67–76.
2. Watkins SM, et al. Lipid metabolome-wide effects of the PPARgamma agonist rosiglitazone. J Lipid Res. 2002;43(11):1809–17.
3. Hirai MY, et al. Integration of transcriptomics and metabolomics for understanding of global responses to nutritional stresses in Arabidopsis thaliana. Proc Natl Acad Sci U S A. 2004;101(27):10205–10.
4. Boros LG. Metabolic targeted therapy of cancer: current tracer technologies and future drug design strategies in the old metabolic network. Metabolomics. 2005;1(1):11–5.
5. Suzuki KT. Metabolomics of selenium: Se metabolites based on speciation studies. J Health Sci. 2005;51(2):107–14
6. Lafaye A, et al. Combined proteome and metabolite-profiling analyses reveal surprising insights into yeast sulfur metabolism. J Biol Chem. 2005;280(26):24723–30.
7. Smith MT, et al. Use of "Omic" technologies to study humans exposed to benzene. Chem Biol Interact. 2005;153:123–7.
8. Heijne WHM, et al. Profiles of metabolites and gene expression in rats with chemically induced hepatic necrosis. Toxicol Pathol. 2005;33(4):425–33.
9. Tohge T, et al. Functional genomics by integrated analysis of metabolome and transcriptome of Arabidopsis plants over-expressing an MYB transcription factor. Plant J. 2005;42(2):218–35.
10. Verhoeckx KCM, et al. Characterization of anti-inflammatory compounds using transcriptomics, proteomics, and metabolomics in combination with multivariate data analysis. Int Immunopharmacol. 2004;4(12):1499–5
11. Lenz EM, et al. Qualitative high field 1 H-NMR spectroscopy for the characterization of endogenous metabolites in earthworms with biochemical biomarker potential. Metabolomics. 2005;1(2):123–36.
12. Troy H, et al. Metabolic profiling of hypoxia-inducible factor-1β-deficient and wild type Hepa-1 cells: effects of hypoxia measured by 1H magnetic resonance spectroscopy. Metabolomics. 2005;1:1–11.
13. Whitehead T, Monzavi-Karbassi B, Kieber-Emmons T. 1H-NMR metabolomics analysis of sera differentiates between mammary tumor-bearing mice and healthy controls. Metabolomics. 2005;1:1–10.
14. Lutz NW. From metabolic to metabolomic NMR spectroscopy of apoptotic cells. Metabolomics. 2005;1:1–18.
15. Fan T, et al. Metabolomics-edited transcriptomics analysis of Se anticancer action in human lung cancer cells. Metabolomics J. 2005;1(4):325–39.
16. Rezzi S, et al. Application of 1H-NMR by metabolomics approach to exhaled breath condensate in childhood asthma. In: Abstracts of the 2nd scientific meeting of the metabolomics society, Boston, MA; 2006.
17. Yang L, et al. Metabolomic assays of the concentration and mass isotopomer distribution of gluconeogenic and citric acid cycle intermediates. Metabolomics. 2006;2(2):1573–3882.
18. Weljie AM, et al. Targeted profiling: quantitative analysis of H-1 NMR metabolomics data. Anal Chem. 2006;78(13):4430–42.
19. Fiehn O, et al. Metabolite profiling for plant functional genomics. Nat Biotechnol. 2000;18(11):1157–61.
20. Buchholz A, et al. Metabolomics: quantification of intracellular metabolite dynamics. Biomol Eng. 2002;19(1):5–15.
21. Baverel G, et al. Carbon 13 NMR spectroscopy: a powerful tool for studying renal metabolism. Biochimie. 2003;85(9):863–71.
22. Mesnard F, Ratcliffe RG. NMR analysis of plant nitrogen metabolism. Photosynth Res. 2005;83(2):163–80.
23. Robertson DG. Metabolomics in toxicology: a review. Toxicol Sci. 2005;85(2):809–22.

24. Whitehead TL, et al. H-1-NMR metabolomics analysis of zebrafish (Danio rerio) exposed to the environmentally-relevant EDC 17a-ethinylestradiol (EE2). In: Abstracts of papers of the American Chemical Society, Atlanta, GA; 2006. p. 231.
25. Lee WNP, Go VLW. Nutrient-gene interaction: tracer-based metabolomics. J Nutr. 2005;135(12):3027S–32.
26. Oresic M, et al. Serum metabolite patterns between birth and development of autoantibodies and overt type 1 diabetes: application of large-scale metabolomics to the Type 1 Diabetes Prediction and Prevention study (DIPP). Diabetologia. 2006;49:147.
27. Oresic M, Vidal-Puig A, Hanninen V. Metabolomic approaches to phenotype characterization and applications to complex diseases. Expert Rev Mol Diagn. 2006;6(4):575–85.
28. Chen HW, et al. Combining desorption electrospray ionization mass spectrometry and nuclear magnetic resonance for differential metabolomics without sample preparation. Rapid Commun Mass Spectrom. 2006;20 (10):1577–84.
29. Weeks ME, et al. A parallel proteomic and metabolomic analysis of the hydrogen peroxide- and Sty1p-dependent stress response in *Schizosaccharomyces pombe*. Proteomics. 2006;6(9):2772–96.
30. Zimmermann D, et al. Determination of volatile products of human colon cell line metabolism by GC/MS analysis. Metabolomics. 2007;3(1):13–7.
31. Miccheli A, et al. Metabolic profiling by C-13-NMR spectroscopy: 1,2-C-13(2) glucose reveals a heterogeneous metabolism in human leukemia T cells. Biochimie. 2006;88 (5):437–48.
32. Podrabsky JE, et al. Extreme anoxia tolerance in embryos of the annual killifish *Austrofundulus limnaeus*: insights from a metabolomics analysis. J Exp Biol. 2007;210 (Pt 13):2253–66.
33. Morvan D, Demidem A. Metabolomics by proton nuclear magnetic resonance spectroscopy of the response to chloroethylnitrosourea reveals drug efficacy and tumor adaptive metabolic pathways. Cancer Res. 2007;67(5):2150–9.
34. Ohta D, Shibata D, Kanaya S. Metabolic profiling using Fourier-transform ion-cyclotron-resonance mass spectrometry. Anal Bioanal Chem. 2007;389(5):1469–75.
35. Oikawa A, et al. Clarification of pathway-specific inhibition by Fourier transform ion cyclotron resonance/mass spectrometry-based metabolic phenotyping studies. Plant Physiol. 2006;142(2):398–413.
36. Lane AN, Fan TW-M. Quantification and identification of isotopomer distributions of metabolites in crude cell extracts using 1 H TOCSY. Metabolomics. 2007;3:79–86.
37. Lindsley JE, Rutter J. Nutrient sensing and metabolic decisions. Comp Biochem Physiol B Biochem Mol Biol. 2004;139(4):543–59.
38. Frederich M, Balschi JA. The relationship between AMP-activated protein kinase activity and AMP concentration in the isolated perfused rat heart. J Biol Chem. 2002;277 (3):1928–32.
39. Adams J, et al. Intrasteric control of AMPK via the gamma1 subunit AMP allosteric regulatory site. Protein Sci. 2004;13(1):155–65.
40. Hawley SA, et al. Complexes between the LKB1 tumor suppressor, STRAD alpha/beta and MO25 alpha/beta are upstream kinases in the AMP-activated protein kinase cascade. J Biol. 2003;2(4):28.
41. Zheng D, et al. Regulation of muscle GLUT-4 transcription by AMP-activated protein kinase. J Appl Physiol. 2001;91(3):1073–83.
42. Yamauchi T, et al. Adiponectin stimulates glucose utilization and fatty-acid oxidation by activating AMP-activated protein kinase. Nat Med. 2002;8(11):1288–95.
43. Jin Q, et al. Implication of AMP-activated protein kinase and Akt-regulated survivin in lung cancer chemopreventive activities of deguelin. Cancer Res. 2007;67(24):11630–9.
44. Carretero J, et al. Dysfunctional AMPK activity, signalling through mTOR and survival in response to energetic stress in LKB1-deficient lung cancer. Oncogene. 2007;26 (11):1616–25.
45. Zhong D, et al. LKB1 mutation in large cell carcinoma of the lung. Lung Cancer. 2006;53 (3):285–94.
46. Han S, Roman J. Rosiglitazone suppresses human lung carcinoma cell growth through PPARgamma-dependent and PPARgamma-independent signal pathways. Mol Cancer Ther. 2006;5(2):430–7.
47. Han S, Khuri FR, Roman J. Fibronectin stimulates non-small cell lung carcinoma cell growth through activation of Akt/mammalian target of rapamycin/S6 kinase and inactivation of LKB1/AMP-activated protein kinase signal pathways. Cancer Res. 2006;66 (1):315–23.
48. Mak BC, Yeung RS. The tuberous sclerosis complex genes in tumor development. Cancer Invest. 2004;22(4):588–603.

49. Ferré P, Azzout-Marniche D, Foufelle F. AMP-activated protein kinase and hepatic genes involved in glucose metabolism. Biochem Soc Trans. 2003;31(Pt 1):220–3.
50. Swinnen JV, et al. Androgens, lipogenesis and prostate cancer. J Steroid Biochem Mol Biol. 2004;92(4):273–9.
51. Uyeda K, Repa JJ. Carbohydrate response element binding protein, ChREBP, a transcription factor coupling hepatic glucose utilization and lipid synthesis. Cell Metab. 2006;4(2):107–10.
52. Swinnen JV, et al. Mimicry of a cellular low energy status blocks tumor cell anabolism and suppresses the malignant phenotype. Cancer Res. 2005;65(6):2441–8.
53. Ravnskjaer K, et al. Glucose-induced repression of PPAR{alpha} gene expression in pancreatic {beta}-cells involves PP2A activation and AMPK inactivation. J Mol Endocrinol. 2006;36(2):289–99.
54. Reid ME, et al. Selenium supplementation and lung cancer incidence: an update of the nutritional prevention of cancer trial. Cancer Epidemiol Biomarkers Prev. 2002;V11 (N11):1285–91.
55. Combs GFJ. Status of selenium in prostate cancer prevention. Br J Cancer. 2004;91:195–9.
56. Cohen V, Khuri FR. Chemoprevention of lung cancer. Curr Opin Pulm Med. 2004;10 (4):279–83.
57. Patrick L. Selenium biochemistry and cancer: a review of the literature. Altern Med Rev. 2004;9(3):239–58.
58. Rayman MP. The importance of selenium to human health. Lancet. 2000;356 (9225):233–41.
59. Reid ME, et al. A report of high-dose selenium supplementation: response and toxicities. J Trace Elem Med Biol. 2004;18(1):69–74.
60. Al-Taie OH, et al. Selenium supplementation enhances low selenium levels and stimulates glutathione peroxidase activity in peripheral blood and distal colon mucosa in past and present carriers of colon adenomas. Nutr Cancer. 2003;46(2):125–30.
61. Ganther HE. Selenium metabolism, selenoproteins and mechanisms of cancer prevention: complexities with thioredoxin reductase. Carcinogenesis (Oxford). 1999;20(9):1657–66.
62. Arner ESJ, Holmgren A. Physiological functions of thioredoxin and thioredoxin reductase. Eur J Biochem. 2000;267(20):6102–9.
63. Frenkel GD, Gong YH. Effect of selenite on tumor cell invasiveness. Cancer Lett. 1994;78 (1–3):195–9.
64. Kryukov GV, et al. Characterization of mammalian selenoproteomes. Science. 2003;300 (5624):1439–43.
65. Stadtman TC. Selenocysteine. Annu Rev Biochem. 1996;65:83–100.
66. Clark LC, et al. Decreased incidence of prostate cancer with selenium supplementation: results of a double-blind cancer prevention trial. Br J Urol. 1998;81(5):730–4.
67. Ip C, et al. In vitro and in vivo studies of methylseleninic acid: evidence that a monomethylated selenium metabolite is critical for cancer chemoprevention. Cancer Res. 2000;60(11):2882–6.
68. Tanaka T, et al. Suppressing effects of dietary supplementation of the organoselenium 1,4-phenylenebis(methylene)selenocyanate and the Citrus antioxidant auraptene on lung metastasis of melanoma cells in mice. Cancer Res. 2000;60(14):3713–6.
69. Yan L, et al. Dietary supplementation of selenomethionine reduces metastasis of melanoma cells in mice. Anticancer Res. 1999;19 (2A):1337–42.
70. Yan L, et al. Effect of dietary supplementation of selenite on pulmonary metastasis of melanoma cells in mice. Nutr Cancer. 1997;28 (2):165–9.
71. Yoon SO, Kim MM, Chung AS. Inhibitory effect of selenite on invasion of HT1080 tumor cells. J Biol Chem. 2001;276 (23):20085–92.
72. Ip C, et al. Chemical speciation influences comparative activity of selenium-enriched garlic and yeast in mammary cancer prevention. J Agric Food Chem. 2000;48(6):2062–70.
73. Li L, et al. Characteristics of selenazolidine prodrugs of selenocysteine: toxicity, selenium levels, and glutathione peroxidase induction in A/J mice. Life Sci. 2004;75(4):447–59.
74. Rudolf E, et al. Combined effect of sodium selenite and campthotecin on cervical carcinoma cells. Neoplasma (Bratislava). 2004;51 (2):127–35.
75. Hu H, et al. Methylseleninic acid potentiates apoptosis induced by chemotherapeutic drugs in androgen-independent prostate cancer cells. Clin Cancer Res. 2005;11(6):2379–88.
76. Vadgama JV, et al. Effect of selenium in combination with Adriamycin or Taxol on several different cancer cells. Anticancer Res. 2000;20(3A):1391–4
77. Juliger S, et al. Chemosensitization of B-cell lymphomas by methylseleninic acid involves nuclear factor-kappaB inhibition and the rapid generation of other selenium species. Cancer Res. 2007;67(22):10984–92.

78. Li S, et al. Doxorubicin and selenium cooperatively induce fas signaling in the absence of Fas/Fas ligand interaction. Anticancer Res. 2007;27(5A):3075–82.
79. Santos RA, Takahashi CS. Anticlastogenic and antigenotoxic effects of selenomethionine on doxorubicin-induced damage in vitro in human lymphocytes. Food Chem Toxicol. 2008;46(2):671–7.
80. Li S, et al. Selenium sensitizes MCF-7 breast cancer cells to doxorubicin-induced apoptosis through modulation of phospho-Akt and its downstream substrates. Mol Cancer Ther. 2007;6(3):1031–8.
81. Zhang J, et al. Attenuating the toxicity of cisplatin by using selenosulfate with reduced risk of selenium toxicity as compared with selenite. Toxicol Appl Pharmacol. 2008;226(3):521–9.
82. Medina D, et al. Se-methylselenocysteine: a new compound for chemoprevention of breast cancer. Nutr Cancer. 2001;40(1):12–7.
83. Ma X, et al. Regulation of interferon and retinoic acid-induced cell death activation through thioredoxin reductase. J Biol Chem. 2001;276(27):24843–54.
84. Sinha R, et al. Methylseleninic acid, a potent growth inhibitor of synchronized mouse mammary epithelial tumor cells in vitro. Biochem Pharmacol. 2001;61(3):311–7.
85. Zhu Z, et al. Mechanisms of cell cycle arrest by methylseleninic acid. Cancer Res. 2002;62(1):156–64.
86. Tapiero H, Townsend DM, Tew KD. The antioxidant role of selenium and seleno-compounds. Biomed Pharmacother. 2003;57(3–4):134–44.
87. Stewart MS, et al. Selenium compounds have disparate abilities to impose oxidative stress and induce apoptosis. Free Radic Biol Med. 1999;26(1–2):42–8.
88. Shilo S, et al. Selenite sensitizes mitochondrial permeability transition pore opening in vitro and in vivo: a possible mechanism for chemo-protection. Biochem J. 2003;370(1):283–90.
89. Zheng Y, Zhong L, Shen X. Effect of selenium-supplement on the calcium signaling in human endothelial cells. J Cell Physiol. 2005;205(1):97–106.
90. Swede H, et al. Cell cycle arrest biomarkers in human lung cancer cells after treatment with selenium in culture. Cancer Epidemiol Biomarkers Prev. 2003;12(11):1248–52.
91. Becker K, et al. Thioredoxin reductase as a pathophysiological factor and drug target. Eur J Biochem. 2000;267(20):6118–25.
92. Huang LE, et al. Activation of hypoxia-inducible transcription factor depends primarily upon redox-sensitive stabilization of its alpha subunit. J Biol Chem. 1996;271(50):32253–9.
93. Hayashi T, Ueno Y, Okamoto T. Oxidoreductive regulation of nuclear factor kappa B: involvement of a cellular reducing catalyst thioredoxin. J Biol Chem. 1993;268(15):11380–8.
94. Schenk H, et al. Distinct effects of thioredoxin and antioxidants on the activation of transcription factors NF-{kappa}B and AP-1. Proc Natl Acad Sci. 1994;91(5):1672–6.
95. Arredondo J, et al. A receptor-mediated mechanism of nicotine toxicity in oral keratinocytes. Lab Invest. 2001;81(12):1653–68.
96. Merrill GF, Dowell P, Pearson GD. The human p53 negative regulatory domain mediates inhibition of reporter gene transactivation in yeast lacking thioredoxin reductase. Cancer Res. 1999;59(13):3175–9.
97. Kaeck M, et al. Differential induction of growth arrest inducible genes by selenium compounds. Biochem Pharmacol. 1997;53(7):921–6.
98. Chae HZ, Kang SW, Rhee SG. Isoforms of mammalian peroxiredoxin that reduce peroxides in presence of thioredoxin. In: Packer L, (ed.) Methods in Enzymology: Oxidants and antioxidants, part B, Academic: San Diego; 1999. p. 219–26.
99. Saitoh M, et al. Mammalian thioredoxin is a direct inhibitor of apoptosis signal-regulating kinase (ASK) 1. EMBO J. 1998;17(9):2596–606.
100. Fan TWM, Higashi RM, Lane AN. Integrating metabolomics and transcriptomics for probing Se anticancer mechanisms. Drug Metab Rev. 2006;38(4):707–32.
101. Fan T, et al. Metabolomics-edited transcriptomics analysis of Se anticancer action in human lung cancer cells. Metabolomics J. 2006;1(4):325–39.
102. Vasta V, et al. Glutamine transport and enzymatic-activities involved in glutaminolysis in human platelets. Biochim Biophys Acta. 1995;1243(1):43–8.
103. Aledo JC, et al. Identification of two human glutaminase loci and tissue-specific expression of the two related genes. Mamm Genome. 2000;11(12):1107–10.
104. Carling D, Zammit VA, Hardie DG. A common bicyclic protein-kinase cascade inactivates the regulatory enzymes of fatty-acid and cholesterol-biosynthesis. FEBS Lett. 1987;223(2):217–22.
105. Farber SA, Slack BE, Blusztajn JK. Acceleration of phosphatidylcholine synthesis and breakdown by inhibitors of mitochondrial

function in neuronal cells: a model of the membrane defect of Alzheimer's disease. FASEB J. 2000;14(14):2198–206.

106. Sanjuan MA, et al. Role of diacylglycerol kinase alpha in the attenuation of receptor signaling. J Cell Biol. 2001;153(1):207–20.

107. Fan TW-M, et al. Altered regulation of metabolic pathways in human lung cancer discerned by ^{13}C stable isotope-resolved metabolomics (SIRM). Mol Cancer 2009; 8:41–60.

108. Fan TWM, et al. Determination of metabolites by proton nmr and gc analysis for organic osmolytes in crude tissue extracts. Anal Biochem. 1993;214(1):260–71.

INDEX

Teresa Whei-Mei Fan et al. (eds.), *The Handbook of Metabolomics*, Methods in Pharmacology and Toxicology, DOI 10.1007/978-1-61779-618-0, © Springer Science+Business Media New York 2012

T

U

MIX
Papier aus verantwortungsvollen Quellen
Paper from responsible sources
FSC® C105338

If you have any concerns about our products,
you can contact us on
ProductSafety@springernature.com

In case Publisher is established outside the EU,
the EU authorized representative is:
Springer Nature Customer Service Center GmbH
Europaplatz 3, 69115 Heidelberg, Germany

Printed by Libri Plureos GmbH
in Hamburg, Germany